Ovulation Induction Simplified

Ovulation Induction Simplified

Editors

Sunita Tandulwadkar
MD (Obs & Gyne) FICS (Gyne-Endoscopy) FICOG
Gynecological Endoscopist and ART & IVF Specialist
Chief and Medical Director
IVF and Endoscopy Centre, Ruby Hall Clinic, Pune
Dr DY Patil IVF and Endoscopy Centre, Pune
Director, Solo Clinic IVF—Center for Excellence in Infertility
Founder and Medical Advisor
Solo Stem Cells—Stem Cell Research and Application Center
Pune, Maharashtra, India

Ameet S Patki
MD DNB FCPS FICOG FRCOG (UK)
Medical Director
Department of Reproductive Endocrinology and Infertility
IKAN Fertility Associates LLP
Mumbai, Maharashtra, India
President, ISAR (2024–2026)

Seema Pandey
MBBS MD (Obs & Gyne)
Infertility Specialist
Gynecologist, Reproductive Endocrinologist (Infertility)
Seema Hospitals and Eva Fertility Clinic and IVF Center
Azamgarh, Uttar Pradesh, India

Forewords
Sir Sabaratnam Arulkumaran
Clare Boothroyd

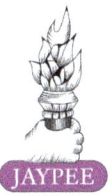

JAYPEE BROTHERS MEDICAL PUBLISHERS
The Health Sciences Publisher
New Delhi | London

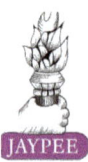

Jaypee Brothers Medical Publishers (P) Ltd

Headquarters
Jaypee Brothers Medical Publishers (P) Ltd
EMCA House, 23/23-B
Ansari Road, Daryaganj
New Delhi 110 002, India
Landline: +91-11-23272143, +91-11-23272703
+91-11-23282021, +91-11-23245672
Email: jaypee@jaypeebrothers.com

Corporate Office
Jaypee Brothers Medical Publishers (P) Ltd
4838/24, Ansari Road, Daryaganj
New Delhi 110 002, India
Phone: +91-11-43574357
Fax: +91-11-43574314
Email: jaypee@jaypeebrothers.com

Overseas Office
JP Medical Ltd.
83, Victoria Street, London
SW1H 0HW (UK)
Phone: +44 20 3170 8910
Email: info@jpmedpub.com

EU GPSR Authorised Representative
Logos Europe, 9 rue Nicolas Poussin
17000, La Rochelle, France
Phone: +33 (0) 6 67 93 73 78
E-mail: Contact@logoseurope.eu

Website: www.jaypeebrothers.com
Website: www.jaypeedigital.com

© 2025, Jaypee Brothers Medical Publishers

The views and opinions expressed in this book are solely those of the original contributor(s)/author(s) and do not necessarily represent those of editor(s) or publisher of the book.

All rights reserved. No part of this publication may be reproduced, stored or transmitted in any form or by any means, electronic, mechanical, photocopying, recording or otherwise, without the prior permission in writing of the publishers.

All brand names and product names used in this book are trade names, service marks, trademarks or registered trademarks of their respective owners. The publisher is not associated with any product or vendor mentioned in this book.

Medical knowledge and practice change constantly. This book is designed to provide accurate, authoritative information about the subject matter in question. However, readers are advised to check the most current information available on procedures included and check information from the manufacturer of each product to be administered, to verify the recommended dose, formula, method and duration of administration, adverse effects and contraindications. It is the responsibility of the practitioner to take all appropriate safety precautions. Neither the publisher nor the author(s)/editor(s) assume any liability for any injury and/or damage to persons or property arising from or related to use of material in this book.

This book is sold on the understanding that the publisher is not engaged in providing professional medical services. If such advice or services are required, the services of a competent medical professional should be sought.

Every effort has been made where necessary to contact holders of copyright to obtain permission to reproduce copyright material. If any have been inadvertently overlooked, the publisher will be pleased to make the necessary arrangements at the first opportunity.

Inquiries for bulk sales may be solicited at: jaypee@jaypeebrothers.com

Ovulation Induction Simplified

First Edition: **2025**

ISBN: 978-93-5465-941-6

Dedicated to
*All the passionate
learners of reproductive medicine*

Contributors

Aleyamma TK MD DNB Fellow
(Reproductive Medicine)
Senior Professor
Department of Reproductive Medicine
and Surgery
Christian Medical College Hospital
Vellore, Tamil Nadu, India

Ameet S Patki
MD DNB FCPS FICOG FRCOG (UK)
Medical Director
Department of Reproductive
Endocrinology and Infertility
IKAN Fertility Associates LLP
Mumbai, Maharashtra, India
President, ISAR (2024–2026)

Anil Gudi MD FRCOG
Director
Department of Fertility
Fertility Plus
Greater London, UK

Anu Chawla
MRCOG MD DNB FICOG FRM FMAS
Director
Department of Reproductive Medicine
London Fertility Clinic
London, UK

Anupama Ravi Futela MBBS MD
Appropriate Authority
Uttarakhand ART and Surrogacy Board
Senior Consultant and Medical
Superintendent
Department of Reproductive Medicine
Futela Hospital
Rudrapur, Uttarakhand, India

Arnav Hrishikesh Pai
MBBS MS (Obs & Gyne)
Department of Obstetrics and
Gynecology
Budget Fertility Center
Prabhadevi, Maharashtra, India

Ashadeep Chandrareddy MD
Senior Consultant
Department of Reproductive
Endocrinology, Infertility
and Laparoscopic Surgery
Asha Health Care
Bengaluru, Karnataka, India

Ashita Punjabi Hakhoo
MBBS MD (Obs & Gyne) FNB Reproductive
Medicine
Attending Consultant
Department of Obstetrics and
Gynecology
Sarvodaya Hospital
Faridabad, Haryana, India

Bhavana Mittal
MBBS DGO DNB FNB MNAMS FICOG
Senior Consultant
Department of IVF
Shivam IVF & Infertility Centre
New Delhi, India

Biswanath Ghosh Dastidar
MS (Obs & Gyne) MSc in Clinical Embryology
Obstetrician and Gynecologist
Assistant Professor
Department of Obstetrics and
Gynecology
IPGMER and SSKM Hospital
Director, GD Institute for Fertility
Research
Kolkata, West Bengal, India

Contributors

Bushra Khan MBBS MS (Obs & Gyne) FRM
IVF Consultant and Gynecologist
Department of IVF and Endoscopy
Dr DY Patil Medical College
Pune, Maharashtra, India

Chaitanya Nagori MD DGO
Director
Department of Reproductive Medicine
Dr Nagori's Institute for
Infertility and IVF
Ahmedabad, Gujarat, India

Chandana Bhat
Consultant
Department of Reproductive Medicine
Vishvas Fertility and Gynaecology
Centre, Marathahalli
Bengaluru, Karnataka, India

Einat Shalom-Paz MD
Professor of Reproductive
Endocrinology and Infertility
IVF Unit Director
Department of Obstetrics and
Gynecology
Hillel Yaffe
Hadera, Israel

Elpiniki Chronopoulou MBBS MRCOG
Consultant
Reproductive Medicine
CRGH London, UK

Gautam Khastgir MD FRCS FRCOG
Medical Director
Department of Reproductive Medicine
and Surgery
Bengal Infertility and Reproductive
Therapy Hospital Pvt Ltd
Kolkata, West Bengal, India

Hazel Mehlawat Final Year BSc
Student
Population Health Sciences
University College London
UCL- London, UK

Hrishikesh D Pai
MD FRCOG (UK-HON) FCPS FICOG MSc (USA)
Founder and Medical Director
Bloom IVF Group and Lilavati Hospital
IVF Centre, Mumbai
Professor
Department of Reproductive Medicine
DY Patil University
Navi Mumbai, Maharashtra, India
President, FOGSI (2022–2023)

Jaideep Malhotra
MBBS MD FICOG FICS FIUMB FICMCH FMAS
FRCPI FRCOG FIMS FICRM
Managing Director
Department of Infertility
ART Rainbow IVF
Agra, Uttar Pradesh, India

Jayapriya Jayakumaran MD
Obstetrician and Gynecologist
Department of Obstetrics and
Gynecology
HCA Florida Osceola Hospital
Florida, USA

Kalyani Shrimali
DNB (Obs & Gyne) MRM DRM (Germany)
Senior Fertility Consultant
Department of Infertility and
Reproductive Medicine
Nova IVF Fertility Clinic
Indore, Madhya Pradesh, India

Kamal Ojha MBBS MD FRCOG
Gynecologist
Consultant Gynecologists and
Honorary Senior Lecturer
Department of Obstetrics and
Gynecology
St George's University Hospital
London, UK

Kedar Ganla
MD (Obs & Gyne) MBBS MD DGO DFP FCPS
Consultant
Department of Reproductive Medicine
Ankoor Fertility Clinic
Mumbai, Maharashtra, India

Contributors

Khyati R Pandya
MBBS DGO Fellowships in Laparoscopy and IVF
Obstetrician and Gynecologist
Associate
Fertility Associates, Mumbai
Mumbai, Maharashtra, India

Laurel Stadtmauer MD PhD
Director of Third Party Reproduction
Reproductive Endocrinology
and Infertility
The IVF Center
Winter Park Florida
Professor
Department of Obstetrics and
Gynecology
University of Central Florida
Orlando, Florida, USA

M Lipika
MS (Obs & Gyn) Fellowship in Reproductive Medicine and Clinical Embryology
Chief Consultant
Arogyam Clinics
Consultant (IVF, Sexual Medicine & PCOS)
Odigyn Fertility Care
Cuttack, Odisha, India

Madhuri Patil MD DGO DFP FCPS FICOG
Clinical Director
Reproductive Endocrinology ART and
Endoscopy
Dr Patil's Fertility and Endoscopy Clinic
Bengaluru, Karnataka, India

Manisha Nandi
Diploma in Reproductive Medicine MS FRM DRME (Germany)
Consultant Gynecologist
Reproductive Endocrinologist
Reproductive Medicine
Indira IVF
Mumbai, Maharashtra, India

Meenakshi Choudhary
MBBS MD PhD FRCOG
Consultant in Reproductive Medicine
Newcastle Fertility Centre at Life
Newcastle upon Tyne Hospitals
NHS Foundation Trust
Newcastle upon Tyne
England, UK

Megha Gupta
MBBS DNB FRM FMAS FCG PGDMLS MICMCH
Consultant
Department of Reproductive Medicine
Vanshati Infertility and IVF Center
Lucknow, Uttar Pradesh, India

Mohan Shashikant Kamath
MS DNB FRCOG (ad eundem) MSc (UK) Fellow (Reproductive Medicine)
Professor and Head
Department of Reproductive Medicine
and Surgery
Christian Medical College Hospital
Vellore, Tamil Nadu, India

Mrinmayi Dharmadhikari
MS MRCOG DNB (Obs & Gyne)
Consultant
Department of Obstetrics &
Gynecology and Reproductive
Medicine
Silver Lining IVF and Endoscopy Centre
Pune, Maharashtra, India

N Sanjeeva Reddy MD DGO
Professor
Reproductive Medicine and Surgery
Sri Ramachandra Medical College and
Research Institute
Chennai, Tamil Nadu, India

Nandita Palshetkar
MD FCPS FICOG FRCOG (UK)
Professor Emeritus
Department of Obstetrics and
Gynecology
DY Patil School of Medicine
Navi Mumbai, Maharashtra, India
Infertility Specialist, Lilavati Hospital IVF
Center, Mumbai
Scientific Director and Co-Founder,
Bloom IVF and BAUFICI Genetics
President, Indian Society for Assisted
Reproduction (2022–2024)
President, Association of Maharashtra
Obstetric and Gynaecological Societies
(2020–2022)
Past President, FOGSI, IAGE, MOGS
and MSR

Contributors

Neharika Malhotra
MBBS MD (Gold Medalist) DRM (Germany) DMIS FICMCH FMAS FICOG ICOG Fellowship in Reproductive Medicine, DGC
Managing Director
Department of Obstetrics and Gynecology
Malhotra Nursing and Maternity Home
Agra, Uttar Pradesh, India

Padma Rekha Jirge
MRCOG (UK) FICOG MBA (Health Care Management) PG DMLE (Med Law & Ethics)
Scientific Director
Department of Reproductive Medicine
Shreyas Hospital and Sushrut Assisted Conception Clinic
Shreyas Hospital & Sushrut Assisted Conception Clinic
Kolhapur, Maharashtra, India

Priya Bhave MBBS MD DNB MRCOG
Consultant
Department of Reproductive Medicine
Bansal Hospital
Bhopal, Madhya Pradesh, India

Priyanka Harshavardhan Vora
MBBS DGO DFP FCPS BIMIE Masters in Reproductive Medicine (UK), Diploma in ART (Germany), MICOG, FCCS-Obs
Consultant
Department of Reproductive Medicine
Ankoor Fertility Clinic
Mumbai, Maharashtra, India

Rachana Sameer Deshpande
MS (Obs & Gyne) FICOG (Reproductive Medicine)
Director Infinity Fertility Centre
Department of Obstetrics and Gynecology
Reproductive Medicine Infinity Medisurge Centre
Infinity Prime Speciality Hospital
Thane West, Maharashtra, India

Radha Vembu MBBS DGO DNB PhD
Professor and Head
Department of Reproductive Medicine and Surgery
Sri Ramachandra Medical College and Research Institute
Chennai, Tamil Nadu, India

Rana Choudhary
MBBS DNB DGO DFP FCPS Masters in Reproductive Medicine (UK), Diploma in ART (Germany), FCPS, FICOG FICMCH
Consultant
Department of Reproductive Medicine
Ankoor Fertility Clinic
Mumbai, Maharashtra, India

Rashmika Gandhi
MBBS MS (Obs & Gyne) DNB Fellowship in Reproductive Medicine, Fellowship in Gyne Endoscopy IVF and Laparoscopy
Consultant
Department of IVF and Endoscopy, Obstetrics & Gynecology
Sukhmani Hospital
New Delhi, India

Rekha Pillai MBBS PhD MRCOG
Consultant in Reproductive Medicine
Newcastle Fertility Centre at Life
Newcastle upon Tyne Hospitals
NHS Foundation Trust
Newcastle upon Tyne
London, UK

Rishma Dhillon Pai
MD FRCOG DNB FCPS FICOG
Consultant Gynecologist and Infertility Specialist
Department of Obstetrics and Gynecology, IVF
Lilavati, Jaslok, and Hinduja Hospital
Mumbai, Maharashtra, India

Rohan Palshetkar
MS FRM BDRME ADRME
Professor and Head of Unit, Bloom IVF
Department of Reproductive Medicine
DY Patil School of Medicine and Bloom IVF
Mumbai, Maharashtra, India

Sapna Ahuja
MBBS DGO DNB (Obs and Gyne) DFFP MRCOG (Gold Medal) FRCOG
Consultant Reproductive Medicine
Deputy Medical Director
ARGC IVF Clinic, London
Department of Reproductive Medicine
Assisted Reproduction and Gynaecology Centre (ARGC)
London, Kent, UK

Contributors

Seema Pandey MBBS MD FICOG FISR
Director Eva & Vanshati Fertility UP
HOD Reproductive Medicine
Vivekanand Poly Clinic
Lucknow, Uttar Pradesh, India

Sheetal Sawankar
MBBS DNB MNAMS FICOG Diploma in
Reproductive Medicine (UK)
Masters in Reproductive Medicine (Germany)
Fellowship in Reproductive Medicine (India)
Fellowship in Reproductive Medicine
(BudMunder, Germany)
Certificate Course in Clinical Embryology & IVF
Laboratory Process (UK)
Founder and Director
Department of IVF
Avisa IVF and Fertility Center
Mumbai, Maharashtra, India

Shreya Gowni
MS (Obs & Gyne) DRME MRM
Consultant and Medical Director
Department of Infertility and
Reproductive Medicine
Matrika Fertility Centre
Warangal, Telangana, India

Sini Venugopal
MBBS MD (Obs & Gyne) FMAS DMAS FICMCH
Senior Fertility Consultant
Department of Fertility and IVF Unit
Genix Fertility Care
Bhubaneswar, Odisha, India

Sonal Karia
MBBS (University of Mumbai) MD (Obstetrics
and Gynecology—University of Mumbai)
FRANZCOG (Royal Australian and New Zealand
College of Obstetricians and Gynecologists)
CREI (Royal Australian and New Zealand
College of Obstetricians and Gynecologists)
Consultant (Reproductive
Endocrinology and Infertility)—
Genea—World Leading Fertility
Consultant (Obstetrics and
Gynecology)—McArthur Health
Service, NSW, Australia
Department of Obstetrics and
Gynecology & Reproductive
Endocrinology and Infertility
Genea—World Leading Fertility
Liverpool, NSW, Australia

Sonal Panchal MD PhD
Ultrasound Consultant
Dr Nagori's Institute for Infertility and IVF
Ahmedabad, Gujarat, India

Sujata Kar MD DNB (Obs & Gyne)
Managing Director
Department of Obstetrics and
Gynecology
Kar Clinic & Hospital (KCHPL)
Bhubaneswar, Odisha, India

Sunita Tandulwadkar
MD (Obs & Gyne) FICS (Gyne-Endoscopy)
FICOG
Gynecological Endoscopist and ART &
IVF Specialist
Chief and Medical Director
IVF and Endoscopy Centre
Ruby Hall Clinic, Pune
Dr DY Patil IVF and
Endoscopy Centre, Pune
Director, Solo Clinic IVF—Center for
Excellence in Infertility
Founder and Medical Advisor
Solo Stem Cells—Stem Cell Research
and Application Center
Pune, Maharashtra, India

Treasa Joseph
MS MRCOG Fellow (Reproductive Medicine)
Associate Professor
Department of Reproductive Medicine
and Surgery
Christian Medical College Hospital
Vellore, Tamil Nadu, India

Unnati Mamtora
MBBS DGO DNB Fellowship in Reproductive
Medicine and Endoscopy, Diploma in
Reproductive
IVF Consultant
Obstetrician, Gynecology and Infertility
Specialist
Medicine and Embryology (Kiel
University, Germany)
IVF Department
Lilavati Hospital
Mumbai, Maharashtra, India

Utpala Sen MD
Consultant
Department of Reproductive Medicine and Surgery
Bengal Infertility and Reproductive Therapy Hospital Pvt Ltd
Kolkata, West Bengal, India

Vidhu Modgil
MBBS MD (Obs & Gyne) FICOG
Director and Consultant
Suman Hospital and New Infertility & Research

Xuaochong Liu MD
Reproductive Endocrinologist
Kindbody Washington DC
Maryland, USA

Yuval Atzmon MD
Doctor
Reproductive Endocrinology and Infertility
Senior Physician
Department of Obstetrics and Gynecology
Hillel Yaffe
Hadera, Israel

Foreword

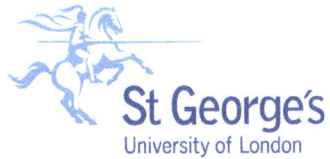

Medicine, Biomedical Sciences
Health and Social Care Science
Cranmer Terrace
London SW17 0RE
e.mail;sarulkum@sgul.ac.uk

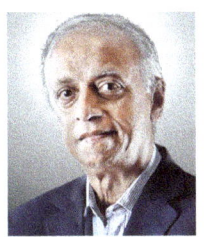

It is with great pleasure that I write the foreword for this highly educational and practical book *"Ovulation Induction Simplified",* authored by a galaxy of well-renowned academic clinicians and edited by stalwarts in the field of reproductive medicine Professors Sunita Tandulwadkar, Ameet S Patki, and Seema Pandey. The book is a distillation of clinical experience and advanced knowledge in the field of reproductive endocrinology. Ovulation induction appears to be a simple clinical practice, but the care and attention that need to be given to result in a pregnancy become more apparent once we read this book and understand the implications of such practice.

The book justifiably starts with endocrinology of stimulated and nonstimulated cycles in the follicular phase followed by the mystery in the luteal phase. One of the concerns in subfertility is that of ovarian reserve in elderly women. Knowledge of how to determine this before ovarian stimulation is amply explained in the chapters dealing with biomarkers of ovarian reserve and the use of other modalities such as the ultrasound. Color mapping of follicle in controlled ovarian stimulation and the evaluation of the endometrium are discussed in detail. The role of selective estrogen receptor modulators such as clomiphene citrate and tamoxifen and the use of aromatic inhibitors and finally the use of gonadotropins are described. The tricks of the trade of triggering at the right time with the right dose of human chorionic gonadotropin and the new issues of dual trigger are discussed. The issues related to downregulation with gonadotropin hormone analogs and antagonists and the pretreatment in in vitro fertilization (IVF) are explained. Optimal protocol in assisted reproduction is important, and this is described in the chapters on intrauterine insemination and as protocols for nonresponders, hyper-responders, and poor responders.

The debate about adjuvant therapy in assisted reproduction with insulin sensitizers like metformin and luteal phase support are useful to understand to maximize clinical benefits. These important issues are discussed in relation to in utero insemination cycles and in assisted reproduction cycles including with fresh and frozen embryo transfer. One should not forget the complications of hyperstimulation which can be prior to or during oocyte retrieval. Knowledge on the management of ovarian hyperstimulation syndrome that can cause severe morbidity and occasional mortality is provided. Consideration is given to issues which crop up from time to time such as mild and minimal stimulation, dual stimulation, low-cost IVF, and issues of occasional concern like immunotherapy. The final chapter deals with fertility toolbox which is a useful way of approaching subfertility management.

The book is organized in sections for easy navigation. The chapters are well written with plenty of figures and tables to make the readers understand the concepts well. Each chapter ends with several key points that are of practical value. I would highly recommend this book to be used by trainees and most certainly by embryologists and clinicians practicing reproductive medicine.

Sir Sabaratnam Arulkumaran
PhD DSc FRCS FRCOG
Professor Emeritus of Obstetrics & Gynaecology
Past President of FIGO, BMA, and RCOG
28.08.2024.

Foreword

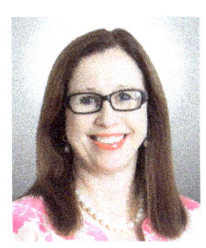

I am delighted to introduce this comprehensive work on all aspects of ovarian stimulation, both physiological and in the context of all types of medically-assisted reproduction. *Ovulation Induction Simplified* is intended for early career specialists and subspecialists in fertility and will without doubt become a useful resource for many healthcare workers in fertility practice, within the Indian subcontinent and beyond.

Most cases requiring ovulation induction have polycystic ovarian syndrome (PCOS), and India not only is now the most populous nation in the world, but also has a high prevalence of PCOS. It is therefore timely that expertise should come from and is most needed in India. In addition, the total fertility rate (TFR) of India has been falling for some time and this year reached the critical value of 2.1, which is deemed replacement rate for a population if other factors such as longevity and immigration remain stable. What the future TFR for India will be is uncertain, but if nearby and neighboring countries are any example, it will be an ongoing fall. The place of ovulation induction and assisted reproduction in mitigating that decline in TFR is uncertain.

This book, with its large number of authors with great expertise, brings together basic physiology and current-day practice in ovulation induction for coitus, intrauterine insemination, and assisted reproductive technologies. Without doubt, it will contribute enormously to the expertise of doctors and nurses working in fertility care. Many of the authors are my friends and colleagues with whom I have connected via the Asia Pacific Initiative on Reproduction (ASPIRE), and it is an honor to commend their work.

Clare Boothroyd
MBBS (Hons) MMedSci MBA (Exec)
FRACP FRANZCOG CREI GAICD
President, ASPIRE

Preface

In recent years, significant advancements have been made in assisted reproductive technology (ART), particularly in the comprehensive understanding of the fundamental endocrinology of a stimulated cycle. It has become apparent that the optimal dosage and duration of stimulation are pivotal factors underlying the success of any stimulated cycle. Beyond the mere quantification of eggs and the selection of pharmaceuticals, the overall milieu during the follicular and luteal phases has been found to play a crucial role.

Considering these insights, Dr Sunita Tandulwadkar, Chairperson of MSAR, and Dr Ameet S Patki, Secretary of MSAR, conceived the idea of producing the book *"Ovulation Induction Simplified."* This publication is intended to benefit practicing ART consultants, gynecologists on a global scale, and aspiring postgraduate students seeking clarity on the basic endocrinology of ovulation induction.

Amidst the challenges imposed by the COVID-19 pandemic, this book has emerged as a guiding light, inspiring the pursuit of meaningful endeavors. Moreover, it provided a platform for a series of virtual meetings through which contributions from leading experts in the field of reproductive medicine were solicited to imbue readers with a heightened interest in reproductive endocrinology.

We express our deep gratitude to both national and international luminaries whose generous allocation of time from their demanding schedules facilitated this collaborative effort. We also extend our appreciation to M/s Jaypee Brothers Medical Publishers, New Delhi, India, our esteemed publisher, for their steadfast support and invaluable technical guidance.

The distinguished editorial team, comprising Dr Sunita Tandulwadkar, President of the Maharashtra Chapter of ISAR, an esteemed ART Consultant and Academician, and Dr Ameet S Patki, Secretary of MISAR, well regarded for his scholarly contributions within the ART community, warrant special acknowledgments. Notably, the significant contributions and collaborative efforts of Dr Seema Pandey, an accomplished ART specialist and academician, were pivotal in the research, coordination, and realization of this publication.

Sunita Tandulwadkar
Ameet S Patki
Seema Pandey

Acknowledgments

Writing a book is tedious but a group effort. *Ovulation Induction Simplified* is going to be a big help to all the postgraduate students, fellows of reproductive medicine, and general practitioners in revisiting the basic concept of ovulation induction and controlled ovarian stimulation.

As coeditors of this book, we would like to thank all our esteemed authors who contributed their best in the book. M/s Jaypee Brothers Medical Publishers, New Delhi, India and their team as well as our friends and family deserve our thanks for their wonderful contributions.

Last but not least, we would like to thank our readers who keep liking our books and encourage us to give our best.

Contents

SECTION 1: Endocrinology of Nonstimulated and Stimulated Cycles

1. Endocrinology of Stimulated and
   Nonstimulated Cycle: Follicular Phase 3
   Jaideep Malhotra, Kalyani Shrimali, Neharika Malhotra

2. Luteal Phase Mystery of Nonstimulated and Stimulated Cycles 13
   Sonal Karia

SECTION 2: Ovarian Reserve Markers

3. Biomarkers of Ovarian Reserve: Appraisal of
   Prediction and Results 25
   Seema Pandey

4. Markers of Ovarian Reserve 38
   Elpiniki Chronopoulou, Anil Gudi

SECTION 3: Flow Matters

5. Color Mapping of Follicle in Controlled
   Ovarian Hyperstimulation 49
   Sonal Panchal, Chaitanya Nagori

6. Evaluation and Monitoring of Endometrium in
   Controlled Ovarian Hyperstimulation 67
   Sonal Panchal, M Lipika

SECTION 4: Ovulation Induction/Ovarian Stimulation—Armamentarium of Ovulogens

7. Selective Estrogen Receptor Modulators:
   Clomiphene Citrate and Tamoxifen 87
   Sujata Kar, Megha Gupta

8. Aromatase Inhibitors 100
   Rekha Pillai, Hazel Mehlawat, Meenakshi Choudhary

9. Gonadotropins: Follicle-stimulating Hormone,
   Luteinizing Hormone, and Human Menopausal Gonadotropin 113
   Rishma Dhillon Pai, Unnati Mamtora, Arnav Hrishikesh Pai

SECTION 5: Trigger it Right

10. Human Chorionic Gonadotropin: Not a Panacea Anymore 127
    Anupama Ravi Futela, Ashadeep Chandrareddy

11. Analog Trigger: Are We Missing the Target? 147
    Yuval Atzmon, Einat Shalom-Paz

12. Dual Trigger: It Works! 159
    Rachana Sameer Deshpande, Padma Rekha Jirge

SECTION 6: Downregulate it Right

13. Gonadotropin-releasing Hormone Analogs:
    Agonist and Antagonist 173
    Madhuri Patil

14. Pretreatment in In Vitro Fertilization Cycles: Does it Work? 194
    Aleyamma TK, Treasa Joseph, Mohan Shashikant Kamath

SECTION 7: Determinants of an Optimal Protocol

15. Determinants of an Optimal Protocol 211
    Seema Pandey, Shreya Gowni, Vidhu Modgil

SECTION 8: Ovarian Stimulation Protocols for IUI Cycle

16. Ovarian Stimulation Protocols in Intrauterine Insemination 231
    Sunita Tandulwadkar, Bushra Khan, Rashmika Gandhi

17. Ovarian Stimulation Protocols for Normoresponders 245
    Laurel Stadtmauer, Xuaochong Liu, Jayapriya Jayakumaran

18. Ovarian Stimulation Protocols for Hyper-responders 257
    Seema Pandey, Sini Venugopal

19. Ovarian Stimulation Protocols for Poor Responders 275
    Gautam Khastgir, Utpala Sen

20. Stimulation Protocols for Fertility Preservation 288
    Kamal Ojha, Biswanath Ghosh Dastidar

SECTION 9: Adjuvants: Do they Work?

21. Adjuvants in Assisted Reproductive Technology 301
    Nandita Palshetkar, Rohan Palshetkar

22. Insulin Sensitizers: Metformin and Inositols 310
    N Sanjeeva Reddy, Radha Vembu

SECTION 10: Luteal Phase Support

23. Luteal Phase Support in Intrauterine Insemination Cycles 329
    Bhavana Mittal, Chandana Bhat

24. Luteal Phase Support in Assisted Reproductive
    Technology Cycles: Fresh and Frozen Embryo Transfer 339
    Anu Chawla, Manisha Nandi

SECTION 11: Complications of Ovarian Stimulation

25. Complications Encountered during Oocyte Retrieval 345
    Ameet S Patki, Khyati R Pandya

26. Ovarian Hyperstimulation Syndrome: Prevention and Cure 352
    Kedar Ganla, Rana Choudhary, Priyanka Harshavardhan Vora

SECTION 12: Mixed Bag

27. Mild and Minimal Stimulation 369
    Bushra Khan, Sunita Tandulwadkar

28. Dual Stimulation 379
    Hrishikesh D Pai, Sheetal Sawankar

29. Low-cost In Vitro Fertilization 390
    Priya Bhave, Ashita Punjabi Hakhoo

30. Immunotherapy in Assisted Reproduction Treatment 398
    Sapna Ahuja

31. Fertility Toolbox 415
    Mrinmayi Dharmadhikari, Ameet S Patki

Index 435

Section 1

Endocrinology of Nonstimulated and Stimulated Cycles

- Endocrinology of Stimulated and Nonstimulated Cycle: Follicular Phase
  Jaideep Malhotra, Kalyani Shrimali, Neharika Malhotra
- Luteal Phase Mystery of Nonstimulated and Stimulated Cycles
  Sonal Karia

Chapter 1

Endocrinology of Stimulated and Nonstimulated Cycle: Follicular Phase

Jaideep Malhotra, Kalyani Shrimali, Neharika Malhotra

■ INTRODUCTION

The reproductive organs of the female are responsible for the procreation. The ovaries are paired pelvic organs with two functions. Firstly, they secrete the cyclic hormones and secondly, they are the source for reproduction by secreting or releasing oocytes.

We all know that ovary contains a finite number of follicles and when their number is reduced to few thousand, the ovary ceases its cyclic activity. For a pregnancy to be established naturally, it requires regular ovarian activity and the fecundity reduces with age and reaches low levels as age advances and ovarian reserve decreases.

Assisted reproductive technology (ART) has undergone significant evolution in the treatment of infertility in couples. In this process, clinical scenarios are meticulously assessed and addressed. Controlled ovarian stimulation (COS) is utilized to simultaneously induce the development of an ample number of follicles in women who are otherwise cycling regularly.

■ ORGANOGENESIS

The primitive gonad develops and forms the gonadal ridge at 5 weeks of gestation. The flat granulosa cells surround the primary oocyte which is called as primordial follicle. These primordial follicles numbers and the speed with which they enter the growth phase determine a woman's reproductive period.

Numerous autocrine and paracrine effects of growth factors are observed, emanating from the oocyte itself, as well as the granulosa and theca cells. Certain factors possess the ability to impede entry into the growth phase, such as anti-Müllerian hormone (AMH), forkhead box L2 (FOXL2), and the tumor suppressor tuberous sclerosis complexes I. These factors exert regulatory influences on the process.[1-3]

The oocyte surrounded by the granulosa cells is called secondary oocyte. The preantral follicle is the ones who has the initial expression of follicle-stimulating hormone (FSH) receptors. This is independent of gonadotropin but local factors (BMP, activin, etc.) influence it **(Fig. 1)**.[1-3]

Along with this follicular growth, the neighboring stroma gets converted into theca cells. Theca cells are the source for androgen production, which is the precursor for estradiol synthesis, it also brings blood supply to the oocyte.

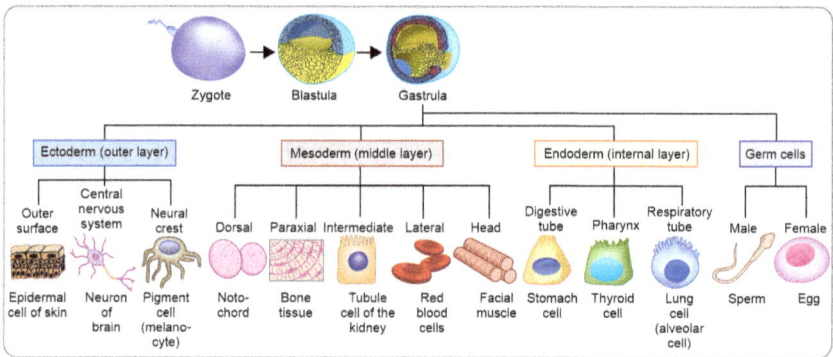

Fig. 1: Germ layers.

As the primordial follicles enter the growth phase, others undergo atresia. By birth, the number of follicles is reduced to 1–2 million and by puberty 400,000–500,000, due to atresia.[4]

■ MALFUNCTION IN OVARIAN DEVELOPMENT

Gonadal dysgenesis results when the germ cells fail to migrate into primitive gonad which is responsible for gonadal development. This leads to regressions of primitive gonad and hence gonadal dysgenesis.

Turners syndrome (X0) that is absence of one of the X chromosomes is the most common form of gonadal dysgenesis which affects the normal development of primary and secondary sexual characteristics.

There are several inhibitory factors that prevent the follicles from entering the growth phase. Certain genetic mutation can lead to malfunctioning and leads to rapid deterioration of follicle pool (e.g., FOXL2) and leads to premature ovarian failure (POF).[5]

Gonadotoxic effects of chemotherapy and radiotherapy destroy the follicle pool and thus shorten the reproductive lifespan of ovaries. Once follicles are lost, they cannot be regenerated or replaced, underscoring the necessity for donation programs involving donor oocytes.[6]

■ FOLLICULOGENESIS

Follicle growth or recruitment starts from puberty and goes up to menopause till the follicle pool is depleted. It takes almost 85 days from follicle activation until it ovulates. The majority of these 85 days of oocyte growth are gonadotropin independent and mostly controlled by autocrine and paracrine effects on growth factors **(Fig. 2)**.[1-4]

■ NEUROENDOCRINE CONTROL

The last 2–3 weeks of follicle growth is influenced majorly by FSH and luteinizing hormone (LH) from antral stage. These hormones are peptide

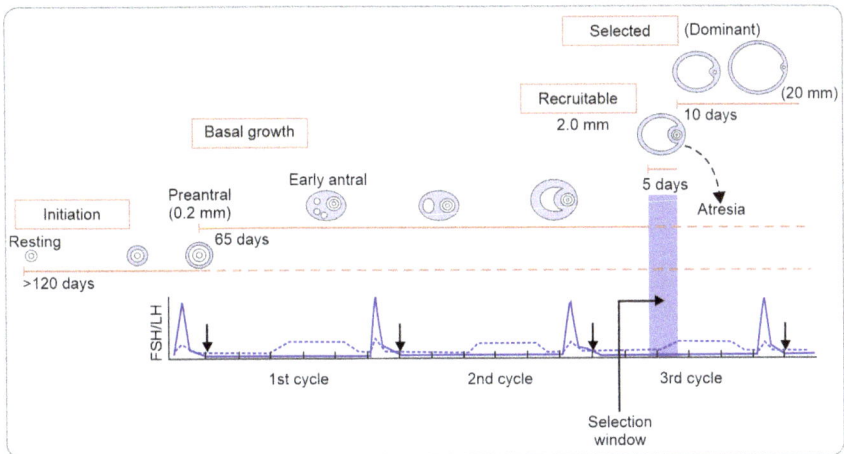

Fig. 2: Diagram of folliculogenesis, starting from preantral (late secondary). (FSH: follicle-stimulating hormone; LH: luteinizing hormone)
Courtesy: NCBI https://www.ncbi.nlm.nih.gov

based and are released by anterior aspect of pituitary gland under influence of hypothalamic gonadotropin-releasing hormone (GnRH) pulses.

Gonadotropin-releasing hormone is a decapeptide which is synthesized and released by the hypothalamus. Its release into the portal vessels from which it is supplied to pituitary is pulsatile (every 60–90 minutes in follicular phase and 120–240 minutes in luteal phase). As soon as it reaches the anterior lobe of pituitary gland, it attaches to the surface receptors and releases the stored FSH and LH.

Mechanism

There are two mechanisms/feedbacks by which the follicle growth and ovulation are controlled **(Fig. 3)**.

Negative Feedback

The primary action of FSH is on the granulosa cells, where it stimulates granulosa cell proliferation, increases aromatase activity, and increases granulosa cell FSH receptors and theca cell LH receptor expression.

Luteinizing hormone acts on the theca cells which leads to androgen production. These androgens are responsible for the estradiol synthesis with the help of aromatase enzyme. Estradiol is released into the bloodstream and upon reaching hypothalamus induces negative feedback leading to decreased production of FSH and LH.[7]

Positive Feedback

The dominant follicle will secrete estradiol and as it reaches a sufficiently high level and if its levels are maintained, it will lead to positive feedback and ultimately leads ovulation and release of the oocyte midcycle.

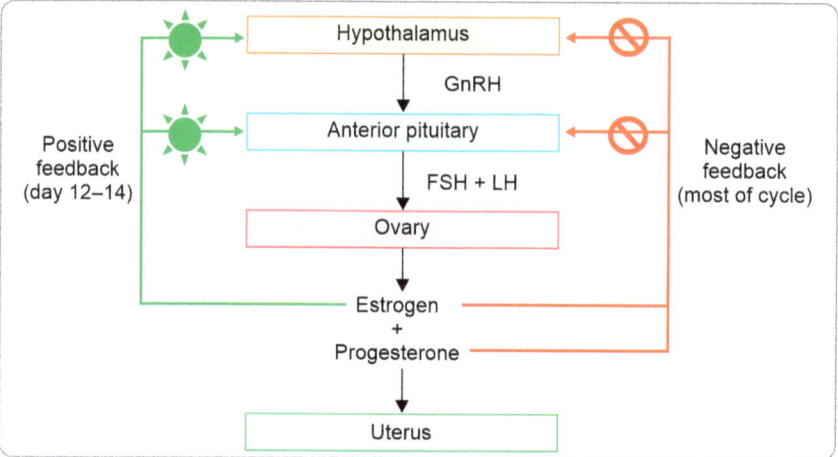

Fig. 3: This diagram shows how hormones control the menstrual cycle with negative and positive feedback. (FSH: follicle-stimulating hormone; GnRH: gonadotropin-releasing hormone; LH: luteinizing hormone)
Courtesy: Guerin L. Biology Advanced Concepts Ch17. The Menstrual Cycle Advanced

DISRUPTION OF NEUROENDOCRINE CONTROL OF FOLLICULOGENESIS AND ITS EFFECTS

- *Kallmann's syndrome:* GnRH neurons not reaching the hypothalamus during the organogenesis
- GnRH neurons destroyed during surgery of tumor, or compression of tumor, hemorrhage

The above would lead to minimal release of FSH and LH, insufficient enough to maintain the follicular growth.

Hypothalamus stalk destroyed too can lead to above scenario even though the hypothalamus is intact as it disrupts the portal circulation.

The treatment for these situations would be either to administer GnRH (when pituitary circulation is intact) to stimulate pituitary release of FSH and LH or the other would be to use gonadotropins like FSH and LH to induce folliculogenesis. To make a note is that only FSH will be insufficient to induce folliculogenesis in such cases as estradiol synthesis will be minimal due to lack of androgens as there is no LH release.[8] Therefore, in cases of hypogonadotropic hypogonadism, both FSH and LH are required for successful stimulation.[9]

PITUITARY AND OVARIAN HORMONAL CONTROL OF FOLLICULOGENESIS

The negative feedback diminishes as the corpus luteum starts to regress leading to decrease in estradiol, progesterone, and inhibin A levels. Hence, the hypothalamus and pituitary are released from their suppression and lead to production of intercycle increase of FSH which is responsible for the follicles entering the final stage of folliculogenesis.

Activins and inhibins are secretory products of growing follicles.

Inhibins are of two types which is inhibin A—alpha A and beta A chains. It is the main product of corpus luteum.

Inhibin B—alpha B and beta B chains. It is the main product of smaller follicles.

As the follicle increases in size, it increases the production of inhibin B. It also exerts negative effect on pituitary FSH release. It also has other roles like augmenting theca cells for androgen production.[1,3,4] There are many other growth factors that affect the FSH and LH sensitivity and fine tune the growth of follicles.

As the estradiol and inhibin levels increase, it leads to decreased pituitary FSH output and hence only those follicles survive that have the highest FSH receptor expression. These follicles will also express LH receptors on their theca cells and from midfollicular phase, on granulosa cells as well. The follicles respond to the falling FSH, they also have the capability now to grow and synthesize the steroid hormones in response to LH as well.[4]

As the follicle keeps growing, it starts secreting inhibin instead of activin. Again, inhibin has a negative influence on FSH release. Along with inhibin, follistatin also is a negative regulator of FSH release. The net effect of these hormonal changes leads to decrease in FSH levels, and this shortage leads to atresia. Only those follicles which have adequate FSH receptors and subsequently LH receptors will maintain their growth and activity even when the influence of gonadotropins is decreased and then one of these follicles will become dominant follicle.[1,2,4,10,11]

CLINICAL APPLICATIONS DURING CONTROLLED OVARIAN STIMULATION

Controlled ovarian stimulation is intrinsic to the assisted reproduction process because it increases the number of oocytes undergoing development. Of the initially recruited follicles, only few are competent for fertilization and to form viable embryos.

In controlled ovarian stimulation (COS), multiple follicles are induced to grow simultaneously to attain numerous mature, healthy oocytes.

The stimulation protocols are designed in such a way to override the selection of single dominant follicle and grow multiple follicles.

ROLE OF GnRH ANALOGS AND ANTAGONIST IN STIMULATED CYCLES

In the part of this COS, the biggest worry is the premature luteinization caused by multiple follicular growth. Hence, a hypogonadotropic state is induced on purpose with the aim to prevent premature luteinization. The two methods exist to prevent this premature luteinization or to prevent the spontaneous LH release from the pituitary.

The GnRH agonists are synthetic analogs of GnRH which are naturally occurring hormones made by substituting the amino acids at position 6 and 10. The purpose of this modification is to extend the half-life when bound to the receptor. The outcome is the desensitization and downregulation of the pituitary after initial flare effect. The protocol is called as long protocol for COS.[12]

The other protocol is known as the antagonist protocol which is widely used now. Here, the antagonists are also produced with similar modifications and act by competitive inhibition of the natural GnRH and do not cause receptor downregulation. This inhibition can be overcome with bolus of GnRH. The effect is immediate and there is no flare effect.[12]

ROLE OF GONADOTROPINS IN FOLLICULOGENESIS AND OVULATION

As discussed already that the initial growth of primordial follicle to preantral follicle is independent of gonadotropins. The two cell, two-gonadotropin concept, for the subsequent follicular growth requires both FSH and LH.[13]

Follicle-stimulating hormone is responsible for the growth and development of follicles as well as for estradiol production. During the follicular phase, serum estradiol levels rise in parallel to the growth of follicle size as well as to the increasing number of granulosa cells. FSH receptors exist exclusively on the granulosa cell membranes. Increasing FSH levels during the late luteal phase lead to an increase in the number of FSH receptors and ultimately to an increase in estradiol secretion by granulosa cells.

Luteinizing hormone receptors are located on the theca cells and LH is responsible for the production of androgens. LH principally stimulates androstenedione production, and to a lesser degree testosterone production in theca cells. Androstenedione is then transported to the granulosa cells where it is aromatized to estrone and finally converted to estradiol by 17-β-hydroxysteroid dehydrogenase type I by the aromatase enzyme. This is known as the two-cell, two-gonadotropin hypothesis of regulation of estrogen synthesis in the human ovary.

Also, it induces LH receptors which allow ovulation and development of corpus luteum in response to LH surge. Hence, both are needed for normal follicular maturation.

This is also known as the two cells–two gonadotropins theory as depicted in **Figure 4**.

All forms of FSH, including hMG, uFSH, HP-FSH, and rFSH, have successfully been used to achieve pregnancies.

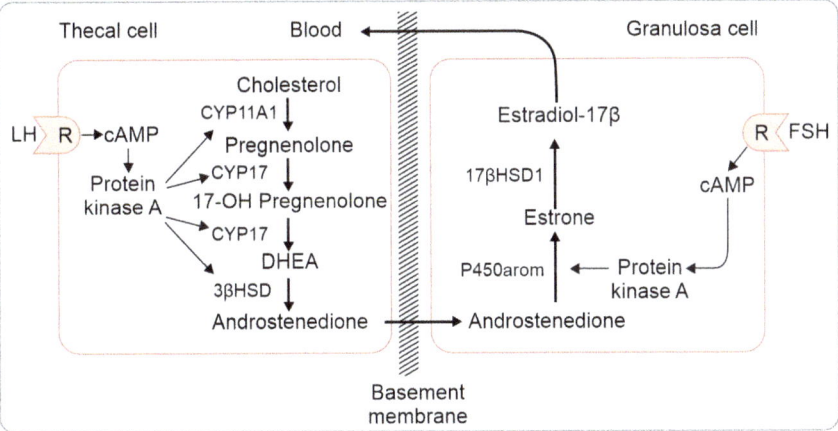

Fig. 4: Two-cell, two-gonadotropin hypothesis of regulation of estrogen synthesis in the human ovary.[14] (DHEA: dehydroepiandrosterone; FSH: follicle-stimulating hormone; LH: luteinizing hormone)

■ ROLE OF LH DURING COS

There are no consensus currently on which patients will benefit from LH supplementation while undergoing COS. A negative impact of deeply suppressed as well as elevated LH levels has been described (threshold effect, ceiling effect).[15]

The addition of antagonist or agonist to the COS regimen alters the LH levels leading to decrease in the LH production sometimes very low levels. LH levels are needed for androgen production and thus estradiol levels. FSH alone is capable of follicular growth, but estradiol production will remain low.[12,13] Hence, in patients with hypogonadotropic hypogonadism, the stimulation will need both FSH and LH. While in patients with normal hypogonadotropic axis is normal, may be able to produce some levels of LH even when GnRH analogs are used and this small amount of LH will lead to multiple follicular development.

In older patients (>35 years), poor responders, those with slow response to stimulation, and those with LH < 0.5 IU/L, addition of LH may be helpful.[16,17]

In the newer classification of POSEIDON (Patient-oriented Strategies Encompassing Individualized Oocyte Number), group 3 and 4 patients are the poor ovarian response (POR) patients according to Bologna criteria. These groups benefit by adding the LH in the stimulation protocol.

A retrospective analysis of 999 poor prognosis patients (defined as AFC < 11 and AMH < 1.1 ng/mL) in the long downregulation protocol and comparing a rLH + rFSH regimen to hMG showed that rLH + rFSH was superior to hMG regarding the clinical pregnancy rate per started cycle (12.5 vs. 8.1%, $p < 0.02$).[18]

■ ROLE OF TRIGGERING IN FINAL OOCYTE MATURATION

The folliculogenesis in a natural cycle results in a single dominant follicle that will be fertilized and produce a healthy pregnancy. The oocyte or egg is arrested at the prophase of the first meiotic division during the follicular phase. This needs the final maturation by converting into meiotic phase 2. The ovulation is controlled by pituitary, firing a biochemical trigger (LH and FSH surges) when all is set. After 18 hours of surge the resumption of meiosis, while 28–36 hours into surge, metaphase II oocytes can be harvested.[19]

Human chorionic gonadotropin is routinely used to trigger ovulation in COS cycles. It is a glycoprotein which contains 30% carbohydrate and consists of alpha and beta units. The beta subunit is conferring the specific activity to the hormone. The human chorionic gonadotropin (hCG) and LH have a similar homology in the beta subunit. This similarity enables hCG to serve as an effective ligand for the LH receptor in the follicular unit, hence its use for the trigger.

The FSH/LH surge ends in 48 hours but the hCG-mediated LH activity spans for almost 8 days. This LH levels overstimulate the corpus lutea, leading to high serum estradiol levels, which decreases internal LH secretion.[20] Due to the decrease in the internal LH level, luteal defects occur and hence the luteal support is needed in the COS cycles in order to maintain receptive endometrium.

Newly introduced GnRH agonist (triptorelin 0.2 mg SC or Buserelin 0.5 SC or 1 mg leuprolide acetate) induces the release of LH from pituitary gland and is used nowadays to prevent ovarian hyperstimulation syndrome (OHSS). The agonist trigger causes LH surge for 24 hours compared to 48 hours in natural cycle. Also, it has more luteolytic effect resulting in luteal phase defects due to decrease LH levels and no hCG support to support the corpora lutea for the progesterone secretion. This has led to decrease in pregnancy rates in agonist trigger.[21] In contrast to hCG whose luteotrophic activity for 7–10 days agonist trigger has shorter. The LH has the circulatory half-life of approximately 60 minutes which prevents OHSS.

■ CONCLUSION

The menstrual cycle is regulated and controlled by various hormones. In the advanced technologies, modifications of various hormones have been possible to alter the endocrine milieu to our benefit of COS. The use of gonadotropins and GnRH analogs influences the buildup of follicles as well as endometrium. The stimulation protocols helpful in COS have been developed by the understanding of the normal phases of menstrual cycles. However, current stimulation protocols are not optimal for patient groups. In near future, adoption of individual COS and implementation of personalized protocols would be seen.

KEY POINTS

- *Hormonal regulation:* In the follicular phase of the menstrual cycle, follicle-stimulating hormone from the pituitary gland stimulates the growth and development of ovarian follicles.
- *Estrogen production:* As follicles mature, they produce increasing levels of estrogen. Estrogen is responsible for thickening the endometrial lining in preparation for potential implantation of a fertilized egg.
- *Luteinizing hormone surge:* In a natural, nonstimulated cycle, a surge in luteinizing hormone triggers ovulation, releasing a mature egg from the dominant follicle.
- *Controlled ovarian stimulation:* In stimulated cycles for assisted reproductive technology procedures, exogenous gonadotropins are administered to promote the development of multiple follicles simultaneously.
- *Monitoring:* Close monitoring of hormone levels and follicular growth is crucial during stimulated cycles to prevent complications such as ovarian hyperstimulation syndrome and to optimize the timing of egg retrieval.
- *Endometrial preparation:* While COS primarily focuses on follicular development, attention must also be paid to the endometrium to ensure its receptivity for embryo implantation.
- *Timing of trigger:* In both stimulated and nonstimulated cycles, the LH surge or a trigger shot of human chorionic gonadotropin is essential for final follicular maturation and ovulation.
- *Role of inhibitory factors:* Factors like anti-Müllerian hormone and inhibin regulate follicular recruitment and growth, contributing to the fine-tuning of the follicular phase.

Understanding the endocrinology of both stimulated and nonstimulated cycles during the follicular phase is crucial for successful fertility treatments and reproductive outcomes.

REFERENCES

1. Okem O, Urman B. Understanding follicle growth in vivo. Hum Reprod. 2010;25:2944-54.
2. Sirotkin AV. Cytokines: signaling molecules controlling Ovarian functions. Int J Biochem Cell Biol. 2011;43:857-61.
3. Hiller SG. Paracrine support of ovarian stimulation. Mol Hum Reprod. 2009;15:843-50.
4. Gougeon A. regulation of follicular ovarian development in primates: facts and hypothesis. Endocr Rev. 1996;17:121-55.
5. De Baere E, Copelli S, Caburet S, Laissue P, Beysen D, Christin-Maitre S, et al. Premature Ovarian failure and forkhead transcription factor FOXL2:blepharophimosis-ptosis epicanthus inversus syndrome and ovarian dysfunction. Pediatr Endocrinol Rev. 2005;2(4):653-60.

6. Damewood MD, Growchow LB. Prospects for fertility after chemotherapy or radiation for neoplastic disease. Fertil Steril. 1986;45:443-59.
7. Moenter SM, Defezio RA, Straume M, Nunemaker CS. Steroid regulation of GnRH neurons. Ann N Y acd Sci. 2003;1007:143-52.
8. Burgues S. Spanish collaborative group of female hypogonadotropic hypogonadism. The effectiveness and safety of recombinant LH to support follicular development induced by recombinant hum FSH in WHO group I anovulation; evidence for a multicentric study in Spain. Hum Reprod. 2001;16:2525-32.
9. Shoham Z, Balen A, Patel A, Jacobs HS. Results of ovulation induction using human menopausal gonadotropin or purified follicle stimulating hormone in hypogonadotropic hypogonadism patients. Fertil Steril. 1991;56(6):1048-53.
10. Gregory SJ, Kaiser UB. Regulation of gonadotropins by inhibin and activin. Semin Reprod Med. 2004;22:253-67.
11. Hillier SG, Yong EL, Illingworth PJ, Baird DT, Schwall RH, Mason AJ. Effect of recombinant inhibin on androgen synthesis in cultured human thecal cells. Moll Cell Endocrinol. 1991;75:R1-6.
12. Chillik C, Acosta A. The role of LHRH agonists and antagonists. Reprod Biomed Online. 2001;2(2):120-8.
13. Kobayashi M, Nakano R, Ooshima A. Immunohistochemical localization of pituitary gonadotropins and gonadal steroids confirms the "two cell, two gonadotropins" hypothesis of steroidogenesis in the human ovary. J Endocrinol. 1990;126:483-8.
14. Carr BR. Diseases of the ovary and Reproductive Tract. In: Wilson JD, Foster DW, Kronenberg HM, Larsen PR (Eds). Williams Textbook of Endocrinology, 9th edition. Philadelphia: WB Saunders; 1998. pp.751-817.
15. Shoham Z. The clinical therapeutic window of luteinizing hormone in controlled ovarian stimulation. Fertiil Steril. 2002;77:1170-7.
16. Humaidan P, Bungum M, Bungim L, Yding Anderson C. Effect of recombinant LH supplementation in women undergoing assisted reproduction with GnRH agonist down-regulation and stimulation with recombinant FSH: an opening study. Reprod Biomed Online. 2004;8:635-43.
17. Lisi F, Rinaldi L, Fishel S, Caserta D, Lisi R, Campbell A. Evaluation of two doses of recombinant LH supplementation in an unselected group of women undergoing follicular stimulation for an in vitro fertilization. Fertil Steril. 2005;83:309-15.
18. Mignini Renzini M, Brigante C, Coticchio G, Dal Canto M, Caliari I, Comi R, et al. Retrospective analysis of treatments with recombinant FSH and recombinant LH versus human menopausal gonadotropin in women with reduced ovarian reserve. J Assist Reprod Genet. 2017;34(12):1645-51.
19. Siebel MM, Smith DM, Levesque L, Barten M, Taymor ML. The temporal relationship between the luteinizing hormone surge and human oocyte maturation. Am J Obstet Gynecol. 1982;142(5):568-72.
20. Fauser BC, Devroey P. Reproductive biology and IVF: ovarian stimulation and luteal phase consequences. Trends Endocrinol Metab. 2003;14(5):236-42.
21. Humaidan P, Papanikolaou EG, Kyrou D, Alsbjerg B, Polyzos NP, Devroey P, et al. The luteal phase after GnRH agonist triggering of ovulation: present and future perspectives. Reprod Biomed Online. 2012;24:134-41.

Chapter 2

Luteal Phase Mystery of Nonstimulated and Stimulated Cycles

Sonal Karia

■ INTRODUCTION

The ovary, one of the most dynamic organs in the human body, undergoes a sequence of cyclical changes relevant to menstruation and reproduction in human beings. The events during a normal menstrual cycle result from an interplay of stimulatory and inhibitory events controlled by hormonal, autocrine, and paracrine factors.

The menstrual cycle in human beings is largely divided into two main phases:
1. *Follicular phase:* Phase of recruitment of a cohort of follicles in the ovary followed by sequence of changes leading to progressive growth and development of usually one follicle from primordial to preantral, antral, and preovulatory stages. This phase begins with the onset of menstruation and continues until just prior to the preovulatory surge of luteinizing hormone (LH).
2. *Luteal phase* which comprises two main events:
   a. *Ovulation:* A sequence of changes, primarily controlled by a rise in LH, resulting in a preovulatory LH surge and release of a mature fertilizable oocyte from the ovarian follicle.
   b. *Postovulatory phase:* Begins with the formation of a corpus luteum (CL) and ends either in a pregnancy or luteolysis, which culminates, with the initiation of the next menstrual cycle

The usual menstrual cycle lasts from 28 to 35 days, with the luteal phase remaining relatively constant in duration in most women (approximately 12-14 days). In this chapter, we will focus on the physiological and pathological changes during the luteal phase of the cycle.

■ PHYSIOLOGY OF LUTEAL PHASE

To understand the physiology of the luteal phase, a basic understanding of the role of LH hormone in the ovarian cycle is essential. LH hormone plays a key role in resumption of oocyte meiosis, luteinization of granulosa cells, and production of progesterone. It also plays an important role in the expansion of the cumulus and prostaglandin production, which are essential for follicular rupture, and oocyte release.[1,2]

Luteinizing Hormone

- LH is a glycoprotein dimer composed of two glycosylated noncovalently linked subunits:
  - Alpha subunit (92 amino acids, long arm of chromosome 6)
  - Beta subunit (121 amino acids, long arm of chromosome 19)
- The beta subunit is unique and determines LH immunologic and biologic activity.
- Half-life of LH is 20 minutes.
- LH receptor, and mutations of the LH receptor can lead to inactivity or overactivation of LH.

LH receptor:
- LH and human chorionic gonadotropin (hCG) bind to and activate a common receptor, the LH/choriogonadotropin receptor (LHCGR), also known as the LH or lutropin receptor (LHR).[3,4]
- Comprised of 675 amino acids, it is a G-protein-coupled receptor—a member of the rhodopsin subfamily of glycoprotein hormone receptors
- Like all G-protein coupled receptors, LHCGR is anchored within the cell membrane by seven transmembrane domains.
- Unlike some of the other transmembrane receptors, leucine-rich repeats and multiple sites for glycosylation characterize the large extracellular domain of LHCGR.
- The gene for LHR is located on chromosome 2p21, in the same general region as the FSH receptor.[5]

LH effect at the molecular level: The sequences of events resulting in LH effect are as follows:
- LH/hCG binds to LHCGR.
- Conformational change in LHCGR leading to activation of stimulatory G protein (Gs)
- Activation of adenylate cyclase leading to increase in intracellular cAMP
- Cyclic adenosine monophosphate/protein kinase A (cAMP/PKA) pathway is a significant effector of downstream events that lead to ovulation and steroid biosynthesis.
- LHCGR stimulation also activates the phospholipase C/inositol phosphate (PLC/IP) signaling pathway.[6]
- Phospholipase C (PLC)-based signaling only occurs during the preovulatory LH surge and during pregnancy.

CHAPTER 2: Luteal Phase Mystery of Nonstimulated and Stimulated Cycles

- Other signaling molecules—extracellular signal-regulated protein kinases 1 and 2 (ERK1/2)—contribute to regulation of oocyte and follicle maturation.[7]

LUTEAL PHASE ENDOCRINE CHANGES

Following ovulation, the follicle is reorganized into a unique structure called corpus luteum (CL). The CL plays a central role in the regulation of the estrous cycle and in the maintenance of pregnancy. Effectively, the CL functions as a transient endocrine gland largely through the production of progesterone.

Formation and Role of Corpus Luteum

Even before the release of the ovum, the follicular granulosa cells start increasing in size and accumulate a yellow pigment called lutein. This transformation of the follicular cells to luteal cells takes place within hours.[8] Angiogenesis is an important feature of CL formation. It is mediated by the effect of angiogenic factors like vascular endothelial growth factor (VEGF) and angiopoietins.[9,10] These factors are produced in the luteinized granulosa cells. The process leads to formation of a dense capillary network responsible for supplying nutrients, hormones, and lipoprotein-bound cholesterol to the luteal cells, which is a necessary substrate for production of progesterone, the main ovarian hormone in the luteal phase.[11]

At least two distinct luteal cell types have been identified, i.e., large luteal cells and small luteal cells. The large luteal cells are formed from granulosa cells and are responsible for production of a variety of peptides including oxytocin, relaxin, inhibin, gonadotropin-releasing hormone (GnRH), growth factors, and prostaglandins. Compared to the small luteal cells, they are more active in steroidogenesis, with higher progesterone production and greater aromatase activity for conversion of androgens to estrogens. Regulation of steroidogenesis in the CL is determined in part by LH secretory pattern and LH receptors as well as variations in the levels of the enzymes regulating steroid hormone production, such as 3-β-hydroxysteroid dehydrogenase (3β-HSD), CYP17, CYP19, or side chain cleavage enzyme **(Fig. 1)**.[12]

Progesterone production:[13] The key steps resulting in progesterone production include:
- Import of LDL bound cholesterol esters into the cell
- Increase in cAMP and protein kinase A (PKA) resulting from LH action via binding to LH receptors.
- *PKA causes:*
  - Increased internalization of the cholesterol-LDL molecule
  - Activation of cholesterol esterase
  - Increased cholesterol uptake by mitochondria
  - Probable role in regulating conversion of pregnenolone to progesterone in smooth endoplasmic reticulum.

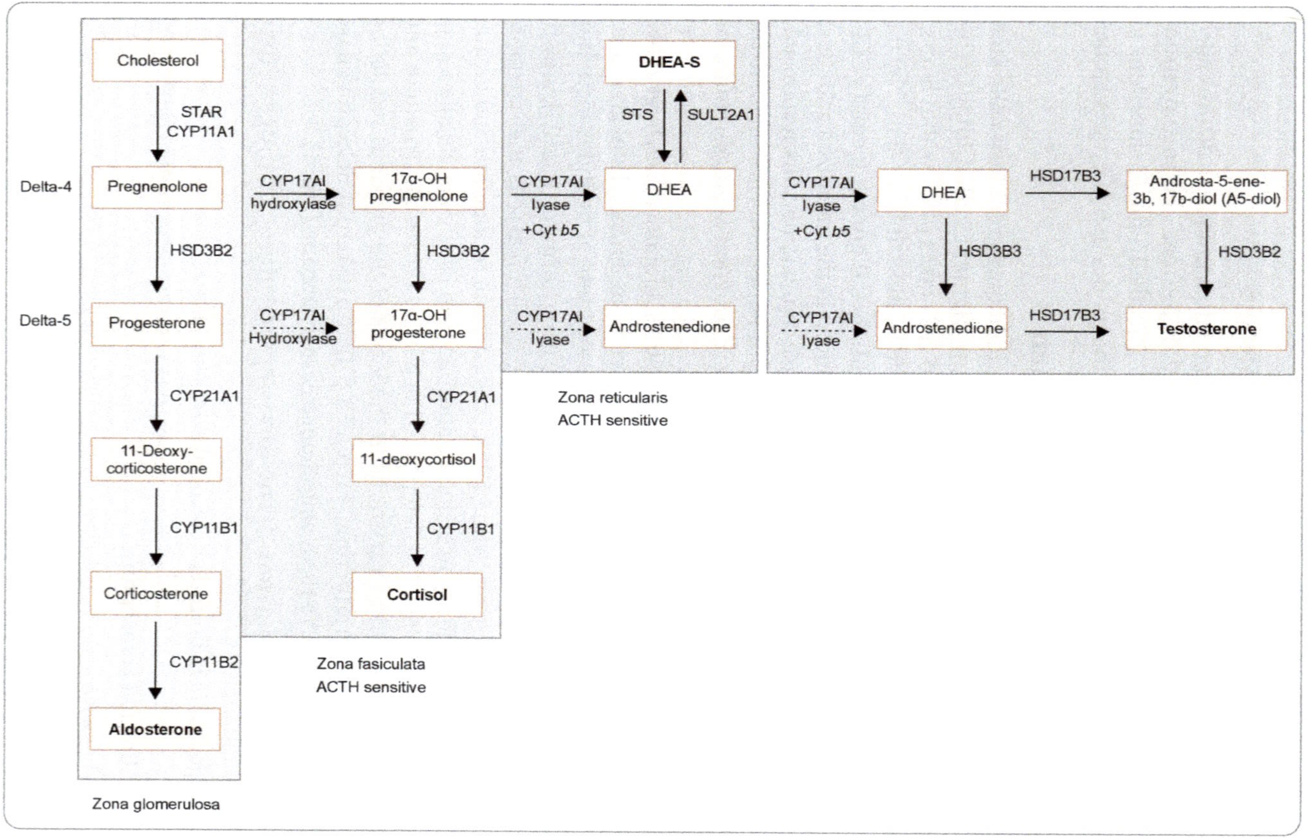

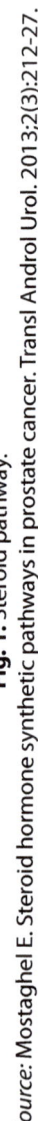

Fig. 1: Steroid pathway.

Source: Mostaghel E. Steroid hormone synthetic pathways in prostate cancer. Transl Androl Urol. 2013;2(3):212-27.

CHAPTER 2: Luteal Phase Mystery of Nonstimulated and Stimulated Cycles

ROLE OF PROGESTERONE

Progesterone exerts its effect primarily through nuclear progesterone receptor (PR-A and PR-B).[14] A third isoform of nPR, PR-C, is abundantly found in myometrial tissue. The PR-C isoform may play an important role in initiation of labor.[15] The effects of progesterone are summarized here.

Reproductive system:
- Endometrium—converts an estrogen primed proliferative endometrium into a secretory one, which is receptive to the blastocyst
- Cervical mucous thickening—prevention of bacterial and sperm entry
- Reduction in myometrial contractility and local vasodilatation by inducing N_2O in the decidua
- Lactation inhibition
- Role in onset of labor

Immune system:[16]
- Modifies the activity of the T cell population—suppression of T helper cells 1 (pro-inflammatory) and favors the T helper cell 2 (anti-inflammatory) type cytokine secretions, inhibits the cytotoxicity of T cells and increases the differentiation of Th0 cells as T regs.
- Inhibitory effect exerted by progesterone on the activities of natural killer (NK cells)
- Alteration of dendritic cells and upregulation of immunomodulatory proteins secreted by mesenchymal stem cells

Central nervous system:[17]
Neuroprotective and neuromodulatory effect through promotion of myelination via conversion to allopregnanolone.

Progesterone—role in implantation and trophoblast invasion:[18]
- Inhibition of the proliferative effect of estrogen on uterine epithelial cells
- Facilitates stromal cell proliferation, decidual growth and the expression of adhesion molecules, which play a key role in implantation.
- It acts as a negative regulator of trophoblast invasiveness by controlling matrix metalloproteinase activity, and also modulates trophoblast migration via diverse pathways.
- Suppression of deleterious maternal immune responses.

Other effects:
- Increase in core body temperature
- Smooth muscle relaxation and reduction of muscular spasm
- Endometrial protection, prevention of endometrial hyperplasia and cancer by regulating the effect of estrogen on the endometrium—an effect that is used as a therapeutic option for endometrial protection in women at high risk of endometrial pathology resulting from unopposed estrogen exposure such as in polycystic ovary syndrome (PCOS).

- Progesterone increases insulin basal levels and promotes insulin release after carbohydrate intake[13]

■ LUTEOLYSIS

In a nonconception cycle, the CL undergoes a process of regression, known as luteolysis. There is a loss of functional integrity, which leads to decrease in progesterone production as well as loss of structural integrity, which is associated with different forms of cell death. Reduction in the production of progesterone, which is a hallmark feature of luteolysis, is initiated with a decline in expression of the *StAR* gene and protein. Several molecules, including prostaglandin F_2-α (PGF_2-α), TNF-α, IL-1β, endothelin, monocyte chemoattractant (MCP-1) as well as estrogens, and reactive oxygen species have been implicated in the luteolytic process.[12]

■ CORPUS LUTEUM RESCUE IN CONCEPTION CYCLES

There is reasonable evidence for the role of trophoblastic production of hCG in prevention of the regression of the CL in fertile cycles. The levels of LH and estradiol are significantly higher in conception cycles approximately 4 days after the peak midcycle LH levels. These changes are suggestive of alterations in signaling in the hypothalamic-pituitary-ovarian axis. There is a progressive rise in serum hCG which is first detected around the time of implantation and rises until the first 12 weeks of pregnancy. There is a significant increase in the volume of the CL as well as a positive correlation between CL volume, relaxin, and hCG serum concentrations.[12]

■ LUTEAL PHASE DEFECT

In spite of the first reports being published as early as 1949,[19] there is no consensus on the scientific definition of luteal phase defect/deficiency (LPD). Attempts have been made to define this entity based on endometrial biopsies to check for a lag in endometrial maturation. However, this concept has not been validated due to the fact that there is evidence for higher prevalence of abnormal endometrial maturation in fertile women compared to subfertile women.[20] LPD is sometimes clinically manifested by a shortened luteal phase lasting less than 9 days, from the day of ovulation to menstrual bleeding. It is also suspected when spotting begins many days before menstruation without an identifiable organic cause. LPD has been implicated as a cause of irregular menstrual bleeding, infertility, and recurrent pregnancy loss.[21] The proposed mechanisms causing LPD include impaired function of the CL resulting in insufficient progesterone and estradiol secretion or an inability of the endometrium to mount a proper response to appropriate estradiol and progesterone exposure.[22,23] Measurement of serum progesterone levels for diagnosis of LPD seems inadequate due to pulsatile release of progesterone from the CL with as high as eightfold variation in levels in a 90-minute period in the mid-luteal phase of the cycle.[24] The American Society of Reproductive Medicine does not consider LPD as an independent subfertility factor at present.

LUTEAL PHASE IN ART CYCLES

The luteal phase is known to be defective in fresh assisted reproductive technology (ART) cycles. The following mechanisms have been proposed for this occurrence:
- Removal of large quantities of granulosa cells during oocyte retrieval (not supported in natural cycles)
- Prolonged pituitary recovery following GnRH agonist co-treatment leading to lack of support of the CL
- HCG trigger could potentially cause a LPD via a short-loop feedback mechanism (not supported in natural cycles)
- GnRH antagonist cycles—rapid recovery of the pituitary but initiation of premature luteolysis leads to significant reduction in the luteal phase length
- Supraphysiologic levels of steroids secreted by a high number of corpora lutea during the early luteal phase, which directly inhibits LH release via negative feedback actions at the level of the hypothalamic–pituitary axis—this seems to be the main and most accepted mechanism for LPD in ART cycles.[25]

Given the above proposed and plausible mechanisms, luteal phase support with hCG/progesterone is recommended for all stimulated cycles as well most frozen ART cycle. This will be dealt with in detail in subsequent chapters.

KEY POINTS

- LH plays a key role in inducing resumption of oocyte meiotic maturation and completion of reduction division in the oocyte with release of first polar body.
- Progesterone plays a significant role in reproduction apart from secretory transformation of the endometrium in the luteal phase.
- Supraphysiological levels of steroids secreted by high number of CL in early luteal phase seem to be the main contributor to deficient luteal phase in stimulated ART cycles.
- LPDs are associated with but not considered a definite cause of subfertility due to lack of consensus in definition and diagnosis.
- Luteal phase support with hCG/progesterone plays a key role in ART pregnancies.

REFERENCES

1. Richards JS, Russell DL, Robker RL, Dajee M, Alliston TN. Molecular mechanisms of ovulation and luteinization. Mol Cell Endocrinol. 1998;145(1-2):47-54.
2. Richards JS. Hormonal control of gene expression in the ovary. Endocr Rev. 1994;15(6):725.
3. Ascoli M, Fanelli F, Segaloff D. The lutropin/choriogonadotropin receptor, a 2002 perspective. Endocr Rev. 2002;23(2):141-74.
4. Puett D, Angelova K, Rocha da Costa M, Warrenfeltz S, Fanelli F. The luteinizing hormone receptor: Insights into structure-function relationships and hormone-receptor-mediated changes in gene expression in ovarian cancer cell. Mol Cell Endocrinol. 2010;329(1-2):47-55.
5. Rousseau-Merck MF, Atger M, Loosfelt H, Milgrom E, Berger R. The chromosomal localization of the human follicle-stimulating hormone receptor gene (FSHR) on 2p21-p16 is similar to that of the luteinizing hormone receptor gene. Genomics. 1993;15(1):222-4.
6. Gilchrist R, Ryu K, Ji I, Ji T. The luteinizing hormone/chorionic gonadotropin receptor has distinct transmembrane conductors for cAMP and inositol phosphate signals. J Biol Chem. 1996;271(32):19283-7.
7. Fan H, Sun Q. Involvement of mitogen-activated protein kinase cascade during oocyte maturation and fertilization in mammals. Biol Reprod. 2004;70(3): 535-47.
8. Richards JS, Russell DL, Ochsner S, Espey LL. Ovulation: new dimensions and new regulators of the inflammatory-like response. Annu Rev Physiol. 2002;64:69-92.
9. Ferrara N, Chen H, Davis-Smyth T, Gerber H, Nguyen T, Peers D, et al. Vascular endothelial growth factor is essential for corpus luteum angiogenesis. Nat Med. 1998;4:336-40.
10. LeCouter J, Lin R, Ferrara N. Endocrine gland-derived VEGF and the emerging hypothesis of organ-specific regulation of angiogenesis. Nat Med. 2002;8:913-7.
11. Reynolds L, Grazul-Bilska A, Redmer D. Angiogenesis in the corpus luteum. Endocrine. 2000;12:1-9.
12. Devoto L, Fuentes A, Kohen P, Céspedes P, Palomino A, Pommer R, et al. The human corpus luteum: life cycle and function in natural cycles. Fertil Steril. 2009;92:1067-79.
13. Taraborelli S. Physiology, production and action of progesterone. Acta Obstet Gynecol Scand. 2015;94 Suppl 161:8-16.
14. Gellersen B, Fernandes M, Brosens J. Non-genomic progesterone actions in female reproduction. Hum Reprod Update. 2009;15(1):119-38.
15. Condon JC, Hardy DB, Kovaric K, Mendelson CR. Up-regulation of the progesterone receptor C isoform in laboring myometrium by activation of nuclear factor B may contribute to the onset of labor through inhibition of PR function. Mol Endocrinol. 2006;20:764-75.
16. Shah N, Lai P, Imami N, Johnson M. Progesterone related immune modulation of pregnancy and labour. Front Endocrinol. 2019;10:198.
17. Wang JM. Regeneration in a degenerating brain: potential of allopregnanolone as a neuroregenerative agent. Curr Alzheimer Res. 2007;4(5):510-7.
18. Halasz M, Szekeres-Bartho J. The role of progesterone in implantation and trophoblast invasion. J Reprod Immunol. 2013;97(1):43-50.

19. Jones GS. Some newer aspects of the management of infertility. JAMA. 1949;141(16):1123-9.
20. Coutifaris C, Myers ER, Guzick DS, Diamond MP, Carson SA, Legro RS, et al. Histological dating of timed endometrial biopsy tissue is not related to fertility status. Fertil Steril. 2004;82(5):1264.
21. Schliep KC, Mumford SL, Hammoud AO, Stanford JB, Kissell KA, Sjaarda LA, et al. Luteal phase deficiency in regularly menstruating women: prevalence and overlap in identification based on clinical and biochemical diagnostic criteria. J Clin Endocrinol Metab. 2014;99(6):E1007-14.
22. Boutzios G, Karalaki M, Zapanti E. Common pathophysiological mechanisms involved in luteal phase deficiency and polycystic ovary syndrome. Impact on fertility. Endocrine. 2013;43(2):314-7.
23. Usadi RS, Groll JM, Lessey BA, Lininger RA, Zaino RJ, Fritz MA, et al. Endometrial development and function in experimentally induced luteal phase deficiency. J Clin Endocrinol Metab. 2008;93(10):4058-6.
24. Mesen T, Young S. Progesterone and the Luteal Phase. A Requisite to Reproduction. Obstet Gynecol Clin North Am. 2015;42(1):135-51.
25. Fatemi H. Simplifying luteal phase support in stimulated assisted reproduction cycles. Fertil Steril. 2018;110(6):1035-6.

Section

2

Ovarian Reserve Markers

❏ **Biomarkers of Ovarian Reserve: Appraisal of Prediction and Results**
   Seema Pandey
❏ **Markers of Ovarian Reserve**
   Elpiniki Chronopoulou, Anil Gudi

Chapter 3

Biomarkers of Ovarian Reserve: Appraisal of Prediction and Results

Seema Pandey

■ INTRODUCTION

Partly due to present social trends, financial requirements, and personal goals and deadlines, many women delay having children until later ages, such as after having entered their 30s and mid-30s. While the choice remains entirely personal, it can sometimes lead to distress resulting from subfertility. Subfertility or difficulty conceiving at later ages can result from decreased quantity and quality of oocytes. Since the number of primary follicles that are present in each female ovary is predetermined at birth, only a few of these ever mature into oocytes. With advancing age, the number of remaining follicles in the ovaries decreases and this may cause difficulty in conception. Diminishing ovarian reserve is typically seen in women in the mid- to late-30s but may also occur earlier in cases such as premature ovarian failure. In women struggling to conceive, the estimation of ovarian reserve can be a good predictor of the probability of conception and the response to fertility treatments such as ovarian induction and in vitro fertilization (IVF), etc.[1]

Assessment of ovarian reserve is necessary for employing targeted assisted reproductive technology (ART) to optimize the chances of successful conception. This also prevents falsely classifying and treating a patient for having diminished ovarian reserve (DOR) when the actual cause of their subfertility may be something else.

Ovarian reserve defines the number of primordial follicles in both the ovaries and their quality at a particular age and time. It is impacted by factors such as age, genetics, and environmental influences. Ovarian reserve testing has been extensively studied in the last 20 years. Measurement of this parameter can provide clinicians and patients with valuable information about the present fertility status and potential for success in an assisted fertility program. However, there is no consensus on which tests should be used to assess ovarian reserve. Ovarian reserve is a complex concept that has 2 distinct windows of interpretation. It can be divided into the biological concept of ovarian reserve, or that which we can measure in a laboratory or with an ultrasound machine, and the clinical concept of ovarian reserve, which we can measure with outcome data. The biological concept of ovarian reserve is based on the accepted concept that the number of oocytes within a woman's ovary declines over time. This natural decline is influenced by a number of different factors including age, genetics, and environmental factors. Unlike sperm generation in the male, the follicular pool in women is unidirectional, and the rate of decrease progresses fast as a woman ages. There is no accepted method to predict this decline over time in an individual woman, it can vary in women of same age too. Biological markers indicating ovarian reserve are touted as prospective measures of a woman's chances of conception and live birth despite a lack of standardized and reproducible evidence of their efficacy. The article intends to review the ovarian reserve biomarkers, their implications, and how to best serve patients with aberrant results during their assisted fertility journey.

Ovarian reserve is the quality and quantity of eggs that are viable inside a patient's ovaries. This quantity starts as an inflexible number from birth and gradually declines as women age. It can be measured by testing for ovarian reserve biomarkers in the blood supported by medical imaging. The markers for ovarian reserve in **Flowchart 1** can be classified as follows:

1. *Biological:* Chronological age of the patient can be taken as an indicator of the ovarian reserve. Since the primordial follicle pool diminishes with age, advancing age indicates a lesser ovarian count in general. The ovarian follicle pool begins to decrease in the 20s and drastic decreases are observed in the late 30s. This decline, however, varies greatly among women. The nonuniformity of observed decline makes it an unreliable tool, especially if used alone. The schematic illustration of the quantitative and qualitative decline of the ovarian follicle pool in **Figure 1** (Jirge, 2011) is assumed to dictate the onset of the important reproductive events.

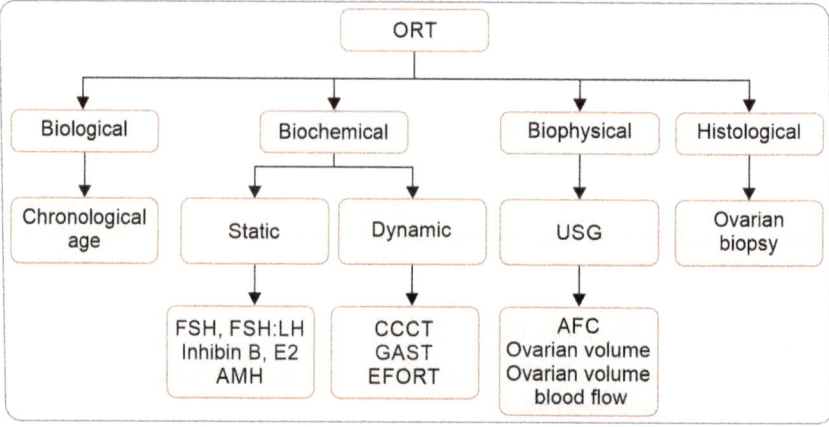

Flowchart 1: Types of ovarian reserve tests.

(AMH: anti-Müllerian hormone; CCCT: clomiphene citrate challenge test; EFORT: exogenous follicle-stimulating hormone response test; FSH: follicle-stimulating hormone; LH: luteinizing hormone; ORT: ovarian reserve test; USG: ultrasonography)
Source: Jirge PR. Ovarian reserve tests. J Hum Reprod Sci. 2011;4(3):108-13.[2]

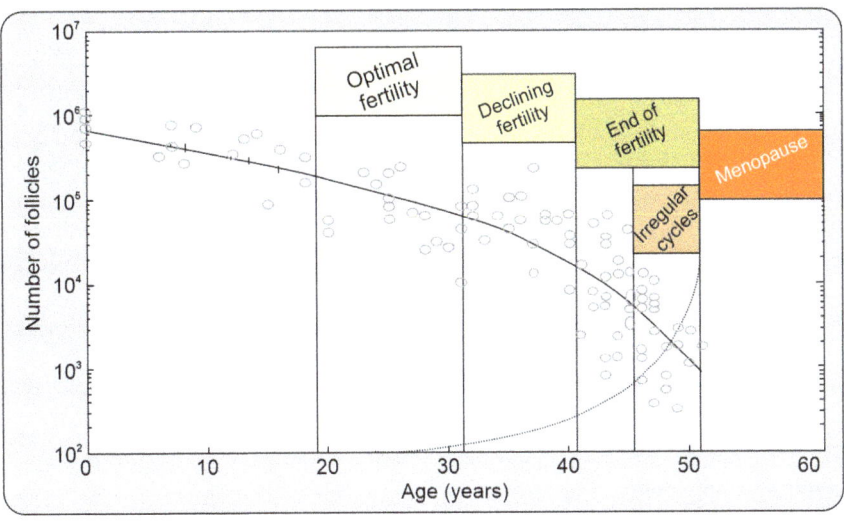

Fig. 1: Schematic illustration of the quantitative and qualitative decline of the ovarian follicle pool.
Source: Jirge PR. Ovarian reserve tests. J Hum Reprod Sci. 2011;4(3):108-13.[2]

2. *Biochemical:* These are further subdivided as:
   - *Static:* A static biochemical ovarian reserve test is a fertility test that measures certain hormone levels in a woman's blood in order to indirectly determine her remaining eggs (oocytes). As a result of these tests, a woman's ovarian reserve is assessed at the time of testing, without stimulating the ovaries. The model of anti-Müllerian hormone (AMH) actions in the ovary in **Figure 2** depicts AMH, produced by the granulosa cells of small growing follicles, inhibits initial follicle recruitment and follicle-stimulating hormone (FSH)-dependent growth and selection of preantral and small antral follicles. In addition, AMH remains highly expressed in cumulus cells of mature follicles. The inset shows in more detail the inhibitory effect of AMH on FSH-induced CYP19a1 expression leading to reduced estradiol (E2) levels, and the inhibitory effect of E2 itself on AMH expression.
   - *Follicle-stimulating hormone:* Serum FSH levels are measured in the beginning of the follicular phase (day 2-4). The values vary both intra- and intercycle and are also affected by the influence of exogenous gonadotropins. FSH levels should be interpreted using serum estradiol levels.[4] With present assessment modalities, serum FSH levels that are >10 IU/L (10-20 IU/L) are highly specific (80-100%), but not very sensitive (10-30%) for prediction of poor response to follicular stimulation. However, levels that are >18 IU/L have a 100% specificity for predicting failure to give birth to a live baby.[5]

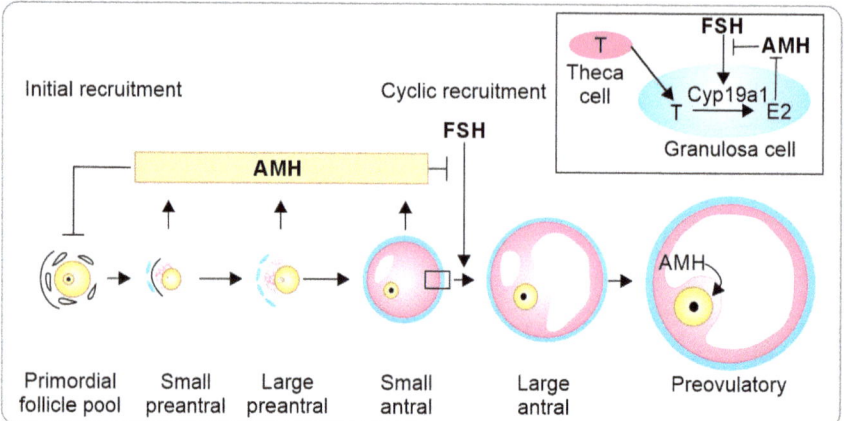

Fig. 2: Model of AMH actions in the ovary. (AMH: anti-Müllerian hormone; FSH: follicle-stimulating hormone)
Source: Dumont A, Robin G, Catteau-Jonard S, Dewailly D. Role of anti-Müllerian hormone in pathophysiology, diagnosis and treatment of polycystic ovary syndrome: a review. Reprod Biol Endocrinol. 2015;13:137. Figure modified from van Houten et al. (2010)[3]

- *Estradiol:* When measured by itself, E2 has limited value as a predictor of ovarian reserve. It is usually measured on days 2–4 and used in concordance with FSH. An increased level of E2 (>60–80 pg/mL) with normal basal FSH levels indicates a higher probability of poor response to stimulation, thereby decreasing the chances of pregnancy.[6]
- *Inhibin B:* This is also measured during days 2–4 of the early follicular phase. The cut-off value for inhibin B is 40–45 pg/mL. Because of large variations in intra- and intercycle levels as well as the lack of a uniform method for commercial assay, it is difficult to interpret and should not be routinely used.[7]
- *Clomiphene citrate challenge test (CCCT):* This requires serial measurement of FSH on days 3 and 10. Cut off value is >10 IU/L on any day. Abnormal values indicate diminished ovarian reserve.
- *Dynamic:* These include GAST and EFFORT which are not only costly and difficult to interpret, but their predictive value is no better than that of FSH, AMH, and antral follicle count (AFC).

3. *Biophysical:* The biophysical parameters used for the measurement of ovarian reserve include:
    - *AFC:* The antral follicle count is measured in the beginning of the follicular phase. The number of remaining primordial follicles in both ovaries is estimated after visualization using a transvaginal probe. The results may vary due to interobserver variation. An AFC of 3–4 is highly specific (73–100%) and not very sensitive (9–73%) for the prediction of poor response.[8]

- *Ovarian volume:* This is calculated by taking ovarian measurements in three different planes and applying the formula $D1 \times D2 \times D3 \times 0.52$. 3 mL is taken as the cut-off value.[9] This test is not very valuable for the prediction of poor stimulatory response.[10]
- *Ovarian blood flow:* The increase in blood flow on Doppler studies due to ovarian stimulation is not considered to have any additional value to AFC and is, therefore, not recommended.[11]

4. *Histology:*
   - *Ovarian biopsy:* It is an invasive procedure and presents an additional risk of formation of intrabdominal adhesions and other surgical complications. It is of limited value in guiding the treatment of subfertility and is mainly used for research purposes only.[12]

ANTI-MÜLLERIAN HORMONE

This hormone is a member of the transforming growth factor-β (TGF-β) family of secretory proteins. It is secreted by the preantral and small antral follicles. It is a preferred tool for the prediction of stimulatory response because it remains largely unaffected by the variations in the menstrual cycle. Therefore, its serum value can be taken throughout the cycle. Additionally, it remains uninfluenced by exogenous gonadotropins and intake of OCPs, etc.

Low levels of AMH are specific for poor ovarian reserve. They do not, however, predict the chances of conception. Therefore, this tool is not useful for screening purposes in populations that are at low risk for DOR. When compared to FSH, AMH shows better predictability of live births in women of different age groups undergoing treatment for subfertility and infertility.[13]

A study was conducted to correlate the predictive accuracy of serum AMH levels in relation to conception and live pregnancy outcomes. The cut-off value for serum AMH levels indicating poor response to stimulation was taken as 1.05 ng/mL, this had a sensitivity of 74% and a specificity of 87%. Hyper-response cut-off value was considered to be 3.55 ng/mL (94% sensitive and 81% specific). The study group under consideration was stratified according to the serum AMH levels (low: <1.05 ng/mL, moderate: 1.05–3.55 ng/mL, and high: >3.55 ng/mL). These stratified groups did not show any statistical variability in the rate of formation of mature oocyte (71.6% vs. 76.5% vs. 74.8%) or rates of fertilization (76.9% vs. 76.6% vs. 73.8%). They did, however, show significant variability in the rates of clinical pregnancy (21.7% vs. 24.1% vs. 40.8%, $p = 0.017$) **(Table 1)**.[14]

HOW TO PREDICT RESPONSE TO ART?

Women with impaired ovarian reserve, or who have demonstrated a history of poor response to standard exogenous gonadotropin stimulation treatments, may necessitate additional testing to comprehensively address

TABLE 1: Summary of the value of ovarian reserve screening tests.

Test	Cut point	Poor response to ovarian stimulation		Nonpregnancy		Reliability	Advantages	Limitations
		Sensitivity	Specificity	Sensitivity	Specificity			
FSH (international units/L)	10–20	10–80	83–100	7–58	43–100	Limited	Widespread use	• Reliability • Low sensitivity
AMH (ng/mL)	0.2–0.7	40–97	78–92	–	–	Good	Reliability	• Limit of detectability • Two commercial assays • Does not predict nonpregnancy
AFC (n)	3–10	9–73	73–100	8–33	64–100	Good	• Reliability • Widespread use	Low sensitivity
Inhibin B (pg/mL)	40–45	40–80	64–90	–	–	Limited	–	• Reliability • Does not predict nonpregnancy
CCCT, day 10 FSH (international units/L)	10–22	35–98	68–98	23–61	67–100	Limited	Higher sensitivity than basal FSH	• Reliability • Limited additional value to basal FSH • Requires drug administration

(AFC: antral follicle count; AMH: anti-Müllerian hormone; CCCT: clomiphene citrate challenge test; FSH: follicle-stimulating hormone)

Sources:
1. Practice Committee of the American Society for Reproductive Medicine. Testing and interpreting measures of ovarian reserve: a committee opinion. Fertil Steril. 2012;98:1407-15.
2. Amato P. Ovarian Reserve Testing. Clinical Reproductive Medicine and Surgery: A Practical Guide, 4th edition. Switzerland: C Springer Nature Switzerland AG; 2022.[18]

the underlying causation and make informed fertility decisions. The benefits of a comprehensive ovarian reserve testing approach are to reduce incurring additional costs or iatrogenic effects during their reproductive treatments. Three comprehensive testing paths have emerged to address these challenges:
1. Poseidon
2. Ovarian response prediction index (ORPI)
3. Bologna

Bologna Criteria

Bologna criteria were developed by the European Society of Human Reproduction and Embryology (ESHRE) 20 years ago to add clarity to who may or may not benefit from additional fertility intervention.[15]

Primarily concerned with oocyte quality without distinguishing quantity, the Bologna criteria are of limited scope and deficient real-world value for predicting and managing infertility.[16] A key limitation of the Bologna criteria for demonstrating any affinity toward the prediction of suboptimal fertility results among those with poor ovarian response to gonadotropin stimulation is the prerequisite of meeting two or more of the following three criteria to qualify as a predictably poor responder to stimulation:
1. Maternal age of 40 years or more, or the presence of any other risk factor
2. A history of poor response to ovarian stimulation (cycles cancelled or oocytes 3 or less in number)
3. Decreased serum value of biomarkers of ovarian reserve (AFC of <5-7 follicles or serum AMH of <0.5-1.1 ng/mL).

The Bologna criteria are not currently employed during the evaluation for treatment with ARTs because of the standardized exclusions and limited reciprocity of predictability based on the outcomes.

The better present-day application, the Bologna criteria need to take into consideration the current range for AMH (from 0.7 to 1.3 ng/mL). The values for AFC should, however, remain the same **(Figs. 3 to 6)**.[17]

Ovarian reserve testing before the first IVF cycle would allow the practitioner to classify patients as expected to have a poor, normal, or increased response to stimulation. **Table 2** shows the correlation of various markers and their sensitivity to predict a response.

Ovarian Response Prediction Index

Ovarian response prediction index subscribes to an indexed score based on the AMH results, FSH values, and age for prediction of the ovarian stimulation response. The ORPI index predicts the likeliness of pregnancy at different points in time during the ovarian stimulation process based on observations of how eggs are developing. The index is calculated using the following six variables:
1. Antral follicular count
2. FSH levels

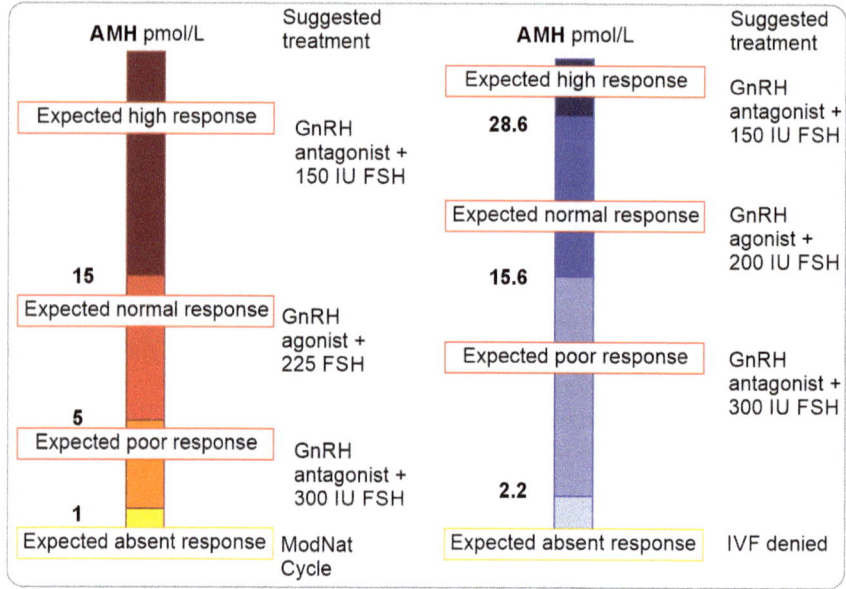

Fig. 3: Strategic modeling of COS on the basis of OR markers.[16] (AMH: anti-Müllerian hormone; COS: controlled ovarian stimulation; FSH: follicle-stimulating hormone; GnRH: gonadotropin-releasing hormone; IVF: in vitro fertilization)

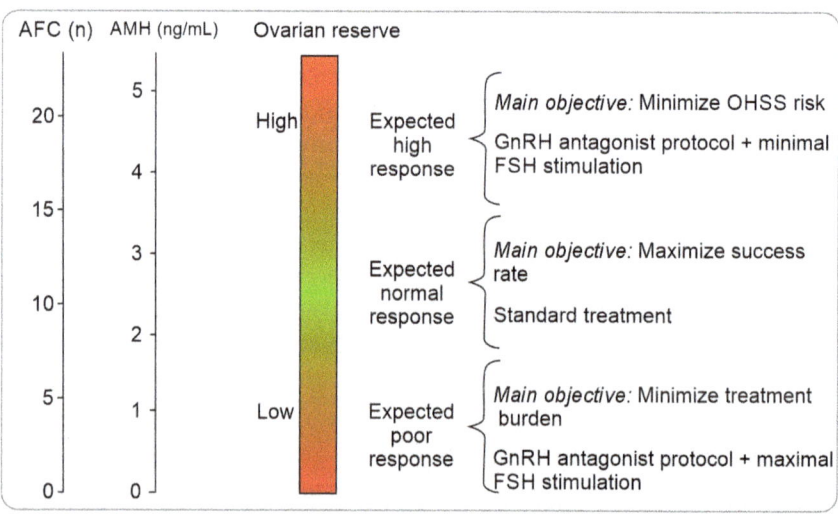

Fig. 4: Prediction of ovarian response—AMH and AFC (AMH: anti-Müllerian hormone; FSH: follicle-stimulating hormone; GnRH: gonadotropin-releasing hormone; OHSS: ovarian hyperstimulation syndrome)

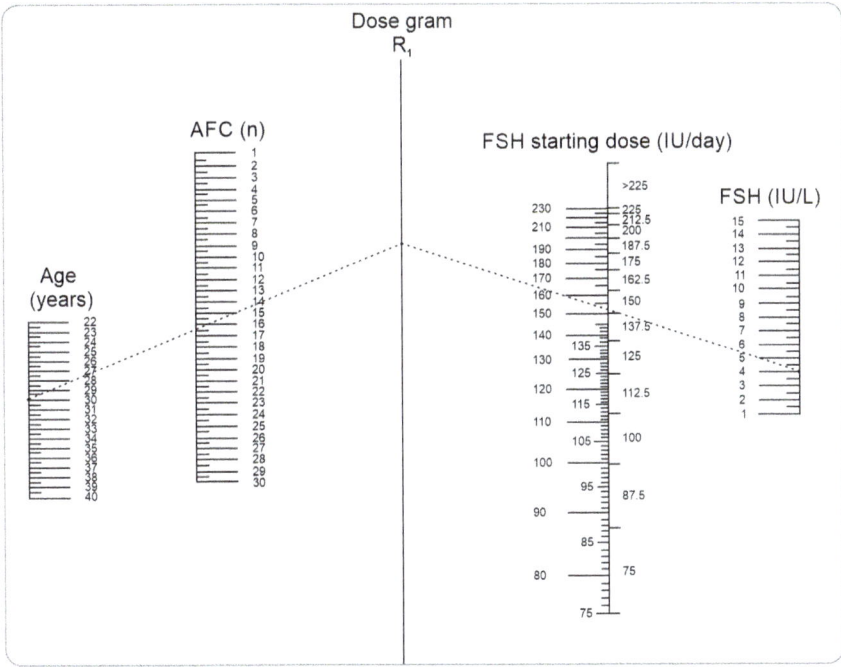

Fig. 5: Nomogram for calculation of the FSH starting dose based on age, AFC, and day 3 serum FSH.[16] (AFC: antral follicle count; FSH: follicle-stimulating hormone)
Source: La Marca A, Sunkara SK. Individualization of controlled ovarian stimulation in IVF using ovarian reserve markers: from theory to practice. Hum Reprod Update. 2014;20(1):124-40.

3. Day 3 estradiol level
4. Luteal phase progesterone level
5. Age in years at menopause (natural or surgical)
6. Number of prior pregnancies.

This method of predicting the ovarian response to stimulation is calculated by multiplication of the serum AMH (ng/mL) level by the number of observed antral follicles (2-9 mm) on the transvaginal scan, and then by dividing the result by the patient's age (in years).

$$ORPI = AMH (ng) \times AFC (2\text{-}9 MM)/Age (years)$$

It considers three variables and offers a good prediction of the response to ovarian stimulation and the possibility of collecting greater than four MII oocytes. If analyzed correctly, ORPI can help in eliminating ovarian hyperresponse by standardization of FSH doses so that hyperstimulation does not occur **(Fig. 6)**.

Clinicians may identify women who are at high risk of not responding well to ovarian stimulation treatments with the ORPI index to make fully informed and highly personalized choices.

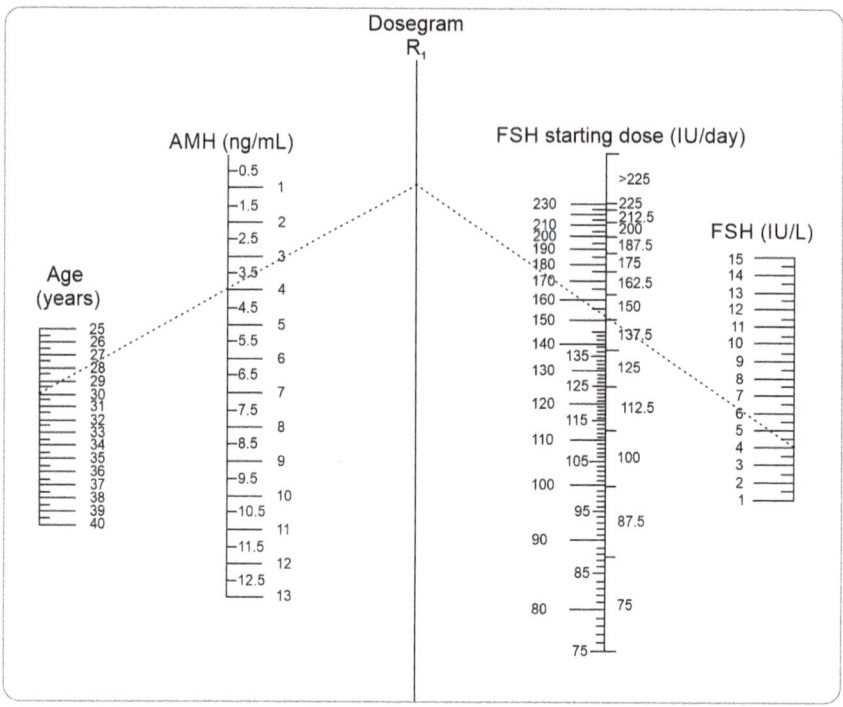

Fig. 6: Nomogram for calculation of the FSH starting dose based on age, AMH, and day 3 serum FSH. (AMH: anti-Müllerian hormone; FSH: follicle-stimulating hormone)

TABLE 2: Characteristics of good ovarian reserve marker and prediction of ovarian response.

Characteristics for a good marker	Age	AMH	FSH	AFC
Prediction of poor response	+	+++	++	+++
Prediction of hyper-response	+	+++	–	++
Low intercycle variability	+++	++	–	++
Low intracycle variability	+++	++	–	++
Applicable to all patients	+++	+++	+	+
Cheapness	+++	–	–	–

(AFC: antral follicle count; AMH: anti-Müllerian hormone; FSH: follicle-stimulating hormone)

POSEIDON Criteria for "Low Prognosis" Patients Undergoing ART

The POSEIDON (Patient-Oriented Strategies Encompassing Individualized Oocyte Number) concept primarily attempts to stratify women with decreased chances of a good response to ART and individualization of target therapeutic approaches in each group, with the number of oocytes required

CHAPTER 3: Biomarkers of Ovarian Reserve: Appraisal of Prediction...

POSEIDON group 1	POSEIDON group 2
Young patients <35 years with adequate ovarian reserve parameters (AFC ≥5; AMH ≥1.2 ng/mL) and with an unexpected poor or suboptimal ovarian response: • *Subgroup 1a:* <4 oocytes* • *Subgroup 1b:* 4–9 oocytes retrieved* *After standard ovarian stimulation	Older patients ≥35 years with adequate ovarian reserve parameters (AFC ≥5; AMH ≥1.2 ng/mL) and with an unexpected poor or suboptimal ovarian response: • *Subgroup 2a:* <4 oocytes* • *Subgroup 2b:* 4–9 oocytes retrieved* *After standard ovarian stimulation
POSEIDON group 3	POSEIDON group 4
Young patients (<35 years) with poor ovarian reserve prestimulation parameters (AFC <5; AMH <1.2 ng/mL)	Older patients (≥35 years) with poor ovarian reserve prestimulation parameters (AFC <5; AMH <1.2 ng/mL)

Fig. 7: Four groups of "low prognosis patients" in assisted reproductive technology according to the POSEIDON's stratification based on oocyte quantity and quality. (AFC: antral follicle count; AMH: anti-Müllerian hormone)
Source: Adapted with permission from Elsevier: Poseidon Group (Patient-Oriented Strategies Encompassing IndividualizeD Oocyte Number), Alviggi C, Andersen CY, Buehler K, Conforti A, De Placido G, et al. A new more detailed stratification of low responders to ovarian stimulation: from a poor ovarian response to a low prognosis concept. Fertil Steril. 2016;105(6):1452-3.

to have at least one euploid embryo for transfer in each patient as the targeted end point **(Fig. 7)**.

■ CONCLUSION

One of the most common indications for performing an ovarian reserve test is to evaluate the health of a woman's ovaries before undergoing fertility-preserving surgery. Predicting ovarian response in advance of starting interventional assisted fertility shares benefits between the patient and the fertilization specialists. Developing a standardized set of rules for personalized testing could enhance the safety and affinity of modalities of ovarian stimulation by providing guidance for the selection of fertility procedures consistent with the needs of each individualized patient presentation.

The clinical evidence for any of the currently available ovarian reserve markers is insufficient to recommend their use as a single criterion for determination of response to ART. FSH is the most commonly used screening test for poor ovarian reserve. However, studies have shown that AFC and AMH show less variability during the cycle and, therefore, are promising predictors of ovarian reserve.

■ KEY POINTS

- Ovarian reserve testing is the mainstay of any fertility treatment program.
- Till date there is not a single test which can predict the quantitative as well as qualitative reserve.

- Multiple criteria were adopted to measure the response but none of these criteria could be used single handedly for all the age or groups.
- They both give good quantitative prediction, however AFC has inter and intraobserver variation while AMH has laboratory to lab variations.
- Ovarian response prediction is good tool to predict ovarian reserve which gives an indirect evidence of the quality and direct of quality.

■ REFERENCES

1. Coccia ME, Rizzello F. Ovarian reserve. Ann N Y Acad Sci. 2008;1127:27-30.
2. Jirge PR. Ovarian reserve tests. J Hum Reprod Sci. 2011;4(3):108-13.
3. Dumont A, Robin G, Catteau-Jonard S, Dewailly D. Role of anti-Müllerian hormone in pathophysiology, diagnosis and treatment of polycystic ovary syndrome: a review. Reprod Biol Endocrinol. 2015;13:137.
4. Broekmans FJ, Kwee J, Hendriks DJ, Mol BW, Lambalk CB. A systematic review of tests predicting ovarian reserve and IVF outcome. Hum Reprod Update. 2006;12(6):685-718.
5. Scott RT, Elkind-Hirsch KE, Styne-Gross A, Miller KA, Frattarelli JL. The predictive value for in vitro fertility delivery rates is greatly impacted by the method used to select the threshold between normal and elevated basal follicle-stimulating hormone. Fertil Steril. 2008;89(4):868-78.
6. Bancsi LF, Broekmans FJ, Eijkemans MJ, de Jong FH, Habbema JD, te Velde ER. Predictors of poor ovarian response in in vitro fertilization: a prospective study comparing basal markers of ovarian reserve. Fertil Steril. 2002;77(2):328-36.
7. Muttukrishna S, Suharjono H, McGarrigle H, Sathanandan M. Inhibin B and anti-Mullerian hormone: markers of ovarian response in IVF/ICSI patients? BJOG. 2004;111(11):1248-53.
8. Frattarelli JL, Levi AJ, Miller BT, Segars JH. A prospective assessment of the predictive value of basal antral follicles in in vitro fertilization cycles. Fertil Steril. 2003;80(2):350-5.
9. Gibreel A, Maheshwari A, Bhattacharya S, Johnson NP. (2009). Ultrasound tests of ovarian reserve: a systematic review of accuracy in predicting fertility outcomes. [online] Available from https://www.ncbi.nlm.nih.gov/books/NBK76802/. [Last accessed May, 2024]
10. Hendriks DJ, Kwee J, Mol BW, te Velde ER, Broekmans FJ. Ultrasonography as a tool for the prediction of outcome in IVF patients: a comparative meta-analysis of ovarian volume and antral follicle count. Fertil Steril. 2007;87(4):764-75.
11. Practice Committee of the American Society for Reproductive Medicine. (2015). Testing and interpreting measures of ovarian reserve: a committee opinion. [online] Available from https://www.fertstert.org/article/S0015-0282(14)02518-7/pdf. [Last accessed May, 2024]
12. Wang S, Zhang Y, Mensah V, Huber WJ, Huang YT, Alvero R. Discordant anti-müllerian hormone (AMH) and follicle stimulating hormone (FSH) among women undergoing in vitro fertilization (IVF): which one is the better predictor for live birth? J Ovarian Res. 2018;11(1):60.
13. Choi MH, Yoo JH, Kim HO, Cha SH, Park CW, Yang KM, et al. Serum anti-Müllerian hormone levels as a predictor of the ovarian response and IVF outcomes. Clin Exp Reprod Med. 2011;38(3):153-8.

14. Ferraretti AP, La Marca A, Fauser BC, Tarlatzis B, Nargund G, Gianaroli L. ESHRE consensus on the definition of "poor response" to ovarian stimulation for in vitro fertilization: the Bologna criteria. Hum Reprod. 2011;26(7):1616-24.
15. Ferraretti AP, Gianaroli L. The Bologna criteria for the definition of poor ovarian responders: is there a need for revision? Hum Reprod. 2014;29(9):1842-5.
16. La Marca A, Sunkara SK. Individualization of controlled ovarian stimulation in IVF using ovarian reserve markers: from theory to practice. Hum Reprod Update. 2014;20(1):124-40.
17. Oliveira JB, Franco JG Jr. The ovarian response prediction index (ORPI) as a clinical internal quality control to prevent ovarian hyperstimulation syndrome. JBRA Assist Reprod. 2016;20(3):91-2.
18. Amato P. Ovarian Reserve Testing. In: Falcone T, Hurd WW (Eds). Clinical Reproductive Medicine and Surgery: A Practical Guide, 4th edition. Cham: Springer; 2022.

Chapter 4

Markers of Ovarian Reserve

Elpiniki Chronopoulou, Anil Gudi

◾ INTRODUCTION

Ovarian reserve has many measures and many meanings. For clinicians, it is a way to plan treatment and measure anticipated risks and success rates. For scientists, it is a fascinating look into the complex matter of ovarian function, folliculogenesis, and follicular atresia. For women, it is the million-dollar question of what their individual reproductive potential is; how much time they have to create a family. The research around ovarian reserve markers and significance is myriad and yet it remains a subject poorly understood and largely misinterpreted.[1]

The birth of Louise Brown was the beginning of a success story for the world of assisted reproductive technology (ART). Despite the significant advances in this field and the intense research into ovarian function, ovarian reserve still remains the black box of human reproduction. We know this is determined by multiple factors—modifiable (environmental and lifestyle factors) and nonmodifiable (age, genetics, ethnicity, and disease). We also know age-related fertility decline is rapid and irreversible. Women who use the contraceptive pill for years without having monthly ovulations, women who undergo multiple cycles of superovulation, and women who have multiple pregnancies, as well as nulliparous women will all, unavoidably, go into menopause at a similar age on average. Woman's age remains the best predictor of chances of conception both for natural conception and for in vitro fertilization (IVF). However, the number of eggs at a certain age can vary significantly. A woman with a high ovarian reserve at the age of 30 years may have 100 times more follicles in total than a woman of similar age with poor ovarian reserve.[1] Women want to know a personalized estimate of their reproductive lifespan in order to make informed decisions. 70% of women who attended a Fertility Assessment and Counselling clinic in Denmark wanted to know how long they could safely postpone childbearing. Ovarian reserve testing can help as approach this question.[2]

Ovarian reserve describes the functional capability of the ovary in terms of number of remaining oocytes. This differs from oocyte quality which relates to the potential of a fertilized oocyte to result to live birth as highlighted by the Practice Committee of the American Society for Reproductive Medicine (2020), but evidence suggests that there is interplay between the two concepts.[1,3] There is currently no consensus on how to diagnose and how to define reduced ovarian reserve. Definitions are conflicted with no widely accepted age specific cutoffs.[4,5] Many efforts have been made to identify the best marker of ovarian reserve and most of these studies have been conducted in the ART setting. Such a marker should be characterized by good predictive value, specificity, replicability, consistency, and affordability and measurements should be standardized, noninvasive, and with no intracycle and intercycle variation.[6] The marker should be able to detect fertility decline early in order to offer a window to act on the results if needed.

The most widely known marker is anti-Müllerian hormone (AMH) which has been studied in numerous publications.[1,5,7] Other markers which have been proposed historically is follicle-stimulating hormone (FSH), clomiphene citrate challenge test, gonadotropin-releasing hormone (GnRH) agonist stimulation test, and inhibin B. The challenge tests have been largely abandoned for logistical and practical reasons. Several direct to consumer fertility tests are currently advertised online and promise to provide accurate fertility predictions by measuring AMH, FSH, and inhibin B. These markers provide very limited information out of context (age, genetic predisposition, medical and surgical history, concurrent gynecological conditions, etc.) and should be interpreted with caution. Besides, significant intralaboratory variations for biomarker assays have been reported in the literature and are documented in the everyday clinical practice even though automated assays are being introduced. Variations in blood collection process and handling and storing samples can also affect results.[2] Cost of these blood tests and waiting time for the result remains a concern and commercialization is unavoidable. Seen in isolation, these results could provide false reassurance or intense anxiety, leading to rushed decisions or unnecessary fertility treatments. These markers are helpful in the ART setting to predict response, plan protocols, and assess risks of hyperstimulation. However, it should be noted that AMH has limited value in predicting chances of natural conception. It is a measure of follicular quantity rather than quality. Two meta-analyses have shown AMH to be a poor predictor of live birth following ART.[3,7] Even though the norm has been that AMH does not fluctuate within the menstrual cycle, there is evidence of significantly lower AMH levels in the luteal phase compared to early follicular.[8]

Gynecological ultrasound (US) has been proposed as another means to assess ovarian reserve which has the potential to bypass the issues surrounding serum markers.

ULTRASOUND AS A TOOL FOR OVARIAN RESERVE ESTIMATE

In contrast to indirect markers, US examination can offer a more direct estimate of the number of recruitable follicles and of the appearance and volume of ovary. Transvaginal US (TVUS) is minimally invasive and relatively inexpensive.[4] Simultaneously, it offers a thorough assessment of coexisting gynecological conditions such as endometriosis, ovarian cysts, fibroids, and uterine abnormalities which could also affect fertility outcomes. The main limitation is intraobserver variation. Patient characteristics such as obesity could also potentially affect the TVUS views, compromising precision. Experienced operators, standardized training of operators, and appropriate machine settings remain of paramount importance.[1,5]

ANTRAL FOLLICLE COUNT

High-resolution TVUS scanning is used to count small antral follicles 2-10 mm in mean diameter on two-dimensional (2D) plane in both ovaries.[1,2,6] New evidence has highlighted that the day of the cycle may not actually be important, challenging the old concept which was based on measurements performed during the early follicular phase of the menstrual cycle (traditionally, days 2-4).[1,2,3,9] The technological advancements in the field of ultrasonography have rendered visualization of small follicles possible.[2,8] Primordial follicles cannot be seen by US since they are too small (<0.05 mm in diameter). Antral follicle count (AFC) should be performed using a TVUS probe with frequency ≥7 MHz. The operator should be able to adjust the machine settings in order to achieve the best contrast between follicular fluid and ovarian stroma and should choose the best method for counting ovarian follicles based on availability of resources and on their own preference and skill as described in a 2017 practical guide on the principles of counting antral follicles by US. Follicles <2 mm should be included in the count with caution to avoid measuring artifacts/blood vessels/other small anechoic structures. Standardization of US settings, techniques, and methods used are of paramount importance to facilitate the scientific dialogue as significant differences in AFC estimates have been observed within the same unit and between different centers.[1,5] Measurement-enabled three-dimensional (3D) methods are being rapidly introduced in the everyday clinical practice and have their own limitations.

Antral follicle count represents the antral (fluid-filled) follicles that can be visualized on US at the specific time point in the cycle, which could defer among days of the cycle and in between cycles. AMH, on the other hand, gives an insight into the pool (primordial follicles that start maturation) or the "functional ovarian reserve." Follicular development into large antral and preovulatory follicles is characterized by reduced AMH expression and increased FSH dependence and thus, the US image may not correlate with AMH value. AFC depicts numbers and not FSH sensitivity and it has been reported that half the follicles (or more) seen on US could be atretic. The size of follicles also matters and should be documented as follicular size offers an insight into ovarian resistance to stimulation. Small antral follicles may prove more difficult to stimulate as they are less responsive to FSH.

Low AFC has been shown to be associated with infertility in all age groups. AFC has been considered a reflection of ovarian aging and has also been associated with the risk of fetal aneuploidy. AFC can help predict response during ovarian stimulation with good accuracy in terms of number of oocytes retrieved, chances of cycle cancellation, and risk of hyperresponse.[1,6] The literature debate comparing AMH and AFC for this purpose has yielded conflicted results. However, AFC does not seem to have consistent results on predicting embryo quality and live birth rate and further research is needed in this field.[2,3]

■ OVARIAN VOLUME

While traditionally, the AFC has been the main focus of interest during TVUS to assess ovarian reserve and function, the appearance of the ovary, in terms of volume and stroma, also offers significant information. These markers are often overlooked in clinical practice as their assessment has largely been subjective and difficult to quantify.

The ovarian volume acts as repository for nongrowing follicles and there is a strong positive correlation between ovarian volume and follicular pool for the 25-51 years' age group. Therefore, as an indirect marker of the ovarian follicle pool and ovarian volume has been shown to correlate with response to ovarian stimulation. Low ovarian volume in linked with higher chances of cycle cancellation (when either ovary measures <3 cm^3). Reduction in single dimensions (particularly width) also seems to be indicative of fertility decline and poor response in the ART setting. The association of ovarian volume with success of ovulation induction in polycystic ovary syndrome (PCOS) population has also been examined and remains controversial. As expected, the ovarian volume correlates with values of AMH, androgens, and LH/FSH ratio.

There is some sparse evidence that with advanced age comes a reduction in ovarian volume as estimated by 2D and 3D US, but these results were not consistent. The age-related reduction of ovarian volume is well documented postmenopause but not necessarily during the premenopausal years. Several authors documented that menopausal status determines ovarian volume more than age. In an attempt to create a model for assessment of ovarian volume throughout life, Kelsey et al. (2013) showed that 69% of variation of ovarian volume is due to age alone.[4] The authors found that the peak volume reached at the age of 20 years is 7.7 mL on average and declines to about 2.8 mL at menopause. This model could help determine age-specific ovarian volume limits moving away from subjective measurements and aiming to create standardized ranges. Ovarian volume is not routinely used in isolation as marker of ovarian reserve in the general population but has a role in the prediction of response to superovulation and more research is needed into its use for the assessment of ovarian reserve in conjunction with other markers.

■ OVARIAN STROMA

The cortex is the outer lining of the ovary and has a key role in defining fertility in women as it harbors the ovarian reserve. The ovarian stroma represents the supporting tissue of the ovary, the components that are not ovarian follicles. It contains multiple different cell types including immune cells and stem cells and ovarian extracellular matrix. Some studies have used the term "theca interstitial stroma." The Hilar cells produce and secrete androgen in response to luteinizing hormone (LH). The theca therefore could give an idea of the ovarian androgen. The stroma is dynamic and subjected to cyclical changes in response to ovulation, corpus luteum formation, etc. Changes are also noted during the reproductive lifespan. The support provided by the ovarian stroma is essential for follicular maintenance and folliculogenesis and further research is needed to detect the correlation between stroma and ovarian volume with clinical outcomes. The ovarian stroma has gained lots of attention recently not only as marker of ovarian reserve but also for its role in ovarian function and carcinogenesis. Ovarian stromal blood flow indices were not found predictive of ovarian response in a prospective study by Ng et al. (2005) in contrast to previous studies.[10] However, Younis et al. (2007) in a prospective study showed that undetectable basal stroma blood flow in at least one ovary is suggestive of low ovarian reserve for women undergoing IVF.[11] Blood vessel density in deep cortical stroma has been shown to decrease with age, while superficial cortical stroma vascularization increases as it is inversely correlated with the density of small follicles.

The example of PCOS shows the significance of ovarian volume and stroma. PCOS is characterized by significantly increased ovarian volume, stromal volume, and stromal peak blood flow velocity as compared to controls. The ratio of ovarian stromal area to total ovarian area by US has been proposed as part of the Rotterdam PCOS definition. Studies trying to correlate ovarian stromal area with hormone profile in PCOS yielded conflicting results. This is important to investigate further as increased stroma volume associated with increased ovarian androgen could provide an indication of resistance to stimulation. Ovarian angiogenesis dysfunction has also been proposed as a mechanism of stroma alterations in PCOS. Ovaries from women with PCOS were characterized by a twofold increase in blood vessel density in both superficial and deep cortical stroma compared to controls.

■ RECENT ADVANCES

Recent studies have provided new insights into ovarian reserve markers and their implications:

- *Endometriosis and ovarian reserve:* Endometriosis has been shown to negatively impact ovarian reserve through various mechanisms, including inflammation and oxidative stress. The presence of autoimmunity in endometriosis patients further exacerbates the decline in ovarian reserve.[3,7,9]
- *Nutritional status:* Nutritional status, including body mass index (BMI) and waist-to-hip ratio, has been found to influence ovarian reserve. Higher BMI is associated with a decrease in ovarian reserve, particularly in women with polycystic ovary syndrome (PCOS).[1,6]
- *Vitamin D:* Vitamin D has been linked to ovarian reserve markers and reproductive health. Supplementation of vitamin D has shown promising results in improving ovarian reserve metrics and reducing depressive symptoms in women with normal or diminished ovarian reserve.[1-3]
- *Progestin-primed ovarian stimulation (PPOS):* PPOS has been found to be more effective than clomiphene citrate or letrozole plus gonadotropin in improving clinical pregnancy rates, optimal embryo rates, and cumulative pregnancy rates in women with diminished ovarian reserve undergoing IVF/ICSI treatment.[5]
- *Long non-coding RNAs (lncRNAs):* lncRNAs have been identified as key regulators in the pathogenesis of diminished ovarian reserve (DOR). They influence follicular development, atresia, and hormone synthesis, making them potential prognostic markers and treatment targets for DOR.[3,5]
- *Immune checkpoint inhibitors (ICIs):* ICIs, used in cancer treatment, have been shown to decrease ovarian follicular reserve and impair oocyte maturation in mouse models. This raises concerns about their impact on fertility in young women undergoing such treatments.[1,7]

■ CONCLUSION

At the moment, there is no ideal test of ovarian reserve. Combination of different markers and individualization of decisions remains the current practice. However, there are no easily applicable standardized models for this combined approach. The combination of AMH, inhibin B, and 3D assessment of AFC and ovarian volume showed no better results compared to the results of each test performed individually. Conventional ovarian reserve markers do not necessarily correlate with follicle output rate (FORT) and follicle to oocyte index (FOI). Discordant findings among ovarian reserve markers are often challenging to interpret.

Many traditional dogmas adopted arbitrarily several decades ago have now been challenged. The use of TVUS as a tool to explore ovarian reserve is gaining more and more space in the field of ART and goes beyond the day 2–4 count of antral follicles. Careful assessment of the size of follicles, of ovarian volume and stroma, vascularization, and ovarian pathology are required for a complete assessment of ovarian function. Quantity versus quality is also important. There is some evidence that decreased ovarian reserve as defined by AFC and AMH is significantly associated with unexplained cases of recurrent pregnancy loss, implying an association with impaired embryo quality.[8] Further research is warranted to explore the observed associations.

The ultimate question is if ovarian reserve markers should be widely used outside the scope of fertility treatment for general population screening and this needs careful consideration. The current consensus is that none of the existing markers should be used to predict inability to conceive naturally. Precise quantification of the ovarian reserve would undoubtedly be a scientific breakthrough.

■ KEY POINTS

- There is no ideal test for ovarian reserve till date.
- The most commonly used ovarian reserve are AMH and AFC, and both are equally good.
- Ovarian reserve testing provides only quantitative assessment but not the qualitative one.

■ REFERENCES

1. Tal R, Seifer DB. Ovarian reserve testing: a user's guide. Am J Obstet Gynecol. 2017;217(2):129-40.
2. Practice Committee of the American Society for Reproductive Medicine. Testing and interpreting measures of ovarian reserve: a committee opinion. Fertil Steril. 2020;114(6):1151-7.
3. La Marca A, Sunkara SK. Individualization of controlled ovarian stimulation in IVF using ovarian reserve markers: from theory to practice. Hum Reprod Update. 2014;20(1):124-40.
4. Dewailly D, Andersen CY, Balen A, Broekmans F, Dilaver N, Fanchin R, et al. The physiology and clinical utility of anti-Mullerian hormone in women. Hum Reprod Update. 2014;20(3):370-85.
5. Fleming R, Seifer DB, Frattarelli JL, Ruman J. Assessing ovarian response: antral follicle count versus anti-Müllerian hormone. Reprod Biomed Online. 2015;31(4):486-96.
6. Iliodromiti S, Anderson RA, Nelson SM. Technical and performance characteristics of anti-Müllerian hormone and antral follicle count as biomarkers of ovarian response. Hum Reprod Update. 2015;21(6):698-710.

7. Broekmans FJ, Kwee J, Hendriks DJ, Mol BW, Lambalk CB. A systematic review of tests predicting ovarian reserve and IVF outcome. Hum Reprod Update. 2006;12(6):685-718.
8. Broer SL, Mol BW, Hendriks D, Broekmans FJ. The role of antimullerian hormone in prediction of outcome after IVF: comparison with the antral follicle count. Fertil Steril. 2009;91(3):705-14.
9. Gleicher N, Weghofer A, Barad DH. Defining ovarian reserve to better understand ovarian aging. Reprod Biol Endocrinol. 2011;9:23.
10. Ng EHY, Tang OS, Chan CCW, Ho PC. Ovarian stromal blood flow in the prediction of ovarian response during in vitro fertilization treatment. Human Reproduction. 2005;20(11):3147-51.
11. Younis JS, Jadaon J, Izhaki I, Haddad S, Radin O, Bar-Ami S, et al. Undetectable basal ovarian stromal blood flow in infertile women is related to low ovarian reserve. Fertil Steril. 2007;88(2):351-6.

Section 3

Flow Matters

- Color Mapping of Follicle in Controlled Ovarian Hyperstimulation
  Sonal Panchal, Chaitanya Nagori
- Evaluation and Monitoring of Endometrium in Controlled Ovarian Hyperstimulation
  Sonal Panchal, M Lipika

Chapter 5

Color Mapping of Follicle in Controlled Ovarian Hyperstimulation

Sonal Panchal, Chaitanya Nagori

■ INTRODUCTION

Ovary is a receptor organ for follicle-stimulating hormone (FSH) and luteinizing hormone (LH) and produces steroids, estrogen and progesterone, anti-Müllerian hormone, inhibin A, etc. These hormonal changes represent various stages of follicular development and are responsible for endometrial changes occurring during the cycle. The hormonal changes are closely related to morphological and vascular changes in the ovary and the endometrium. We shall discuss the follicular changes in this chapter. Doppler has an important role to play as vascular changes more closely correlate with and represent the hormonal changes.

■ TECHNIQUE OF ULTRASOUND AND DOPPLER STUDY FOR FOLLICLE

1. Follow the transverse section of the uterus to locate ovary, along the adnexal soft tissue.
2. Rotate the probe to find out the long plane of the ovary and then the probe is spanned across this plane to find out the longest section.
3. This image is stored as one frame on a dual screen.
4. Then probe is rotated 90° with no other movements of the probe to get a true transverse section of the ovary.
5. Measure the largest longitudinal diameter.
6. Anteroposterior (AP) diameter is the longest diameter perpendicular to long diameter on long section **(Fig. 1)**.
7. Transverse diameter is side to side diameter on transverse section.
8. Ovarian volume is calculated by the formula (x × y × z × 0.523).
9. Antral follicles are counted by eyeballing, when spanning across the ovary in any one plane, without rotation of the probe.
10. After B mode assessment, the color is switched on to assess the stromal vessels.
11. The color box should be large enough to include the entire ovary only.

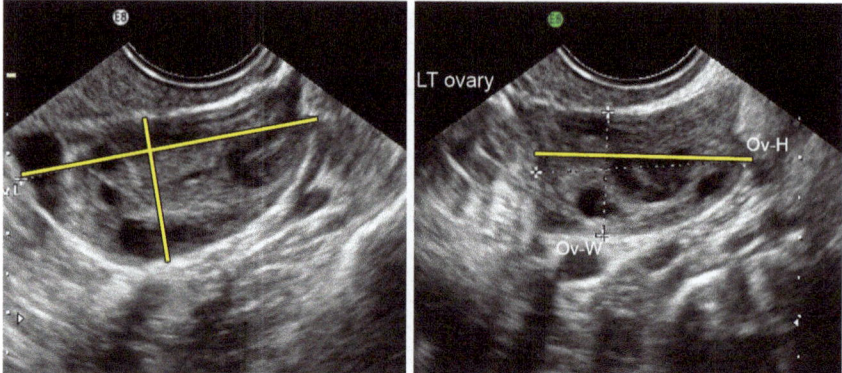

Fig. 1: Measurement of three orthogonal diameters of ovary on B mode ultrasound. (LT: left)

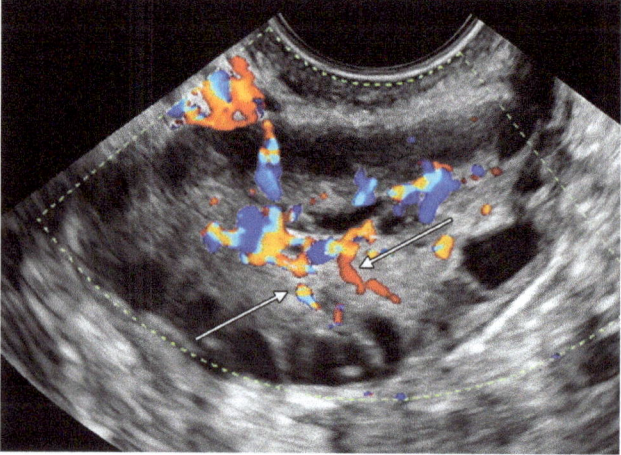

Fig. 2: Color Doppler image of the ovary showing stromal vessels.

12. The vessels that are in the middle of the stroma and not close to the follicles and not also in direct continuation with the ovarian artery, entering in the ovary, are stromal vessels **(Fig. 2)**.
13. For color Doppler assessment, pulse repetition frequency (PRF) is set at 0.3–0.4, optimum gains and wall filter are set at the lowest for both color and the power Doppler. Sample volume for spectral Doppler is usually 2 mm for follicular, corpus luteal, and endometrial scans. Angle correction is essential for these scans.
    - For pulse Doppler, PRF is set at 1.3 but may be lowered if required and the wall filters are set at 30 Hz as stromal flows at baseline scan are low velocity flows.
14. For the preovulatory scan perifollicular blood vessels, vessels that overlap the follicular margin are to be considered as perifollicular and blood flow in these vessels is also assessed by spectral Doppler **(Fig. 3)**.

CHAPTER 5: Color Mapping of Follicle in Controlled Ovarian Hyperstimulation

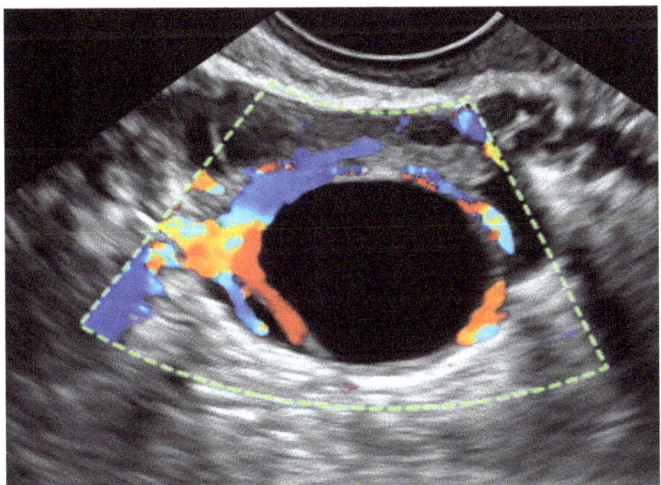

Fig. 3: Color Doppler image of the follicle showing perifollicular vessels.

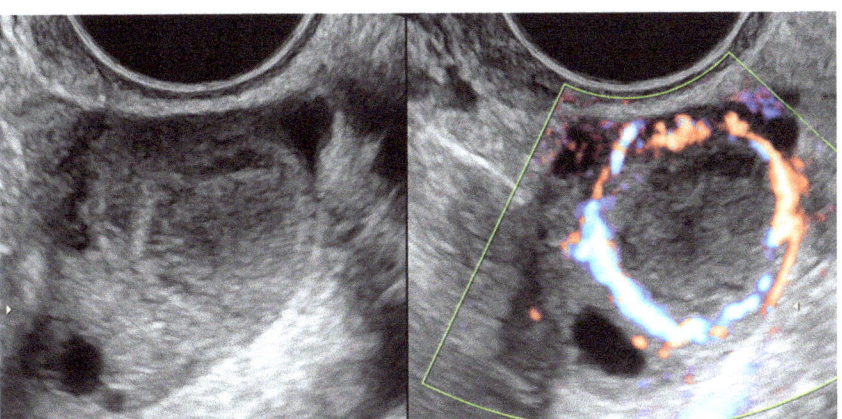

Fig. 4: B mode and high-definition (HD) flow image of the corpus luteum and its peripheral blood flow.

15. Pick up the brightest vessels for spectral Doppler assessment. Take at least three measurements and select the combination of lowest resistance index (RI) and highest peak systolic velocity (PSV) for decision-making.
16. Corpus luteal flow is similarly assessed, especially in the midluteal phase **(Fig. 4)**.

Vascular studies may be more precisely quantified by three-dimensional (3D) power Doppler indices. Vascularity index (VI) indicates the abundance of the flow in the entire ovary, flow index (FI) indicates the average intensity of the flow in the calculated volume, and vascularity FI (VFI) indicates the perfusion in the volume calculated by VOCAL software **(Fig. 5)**.

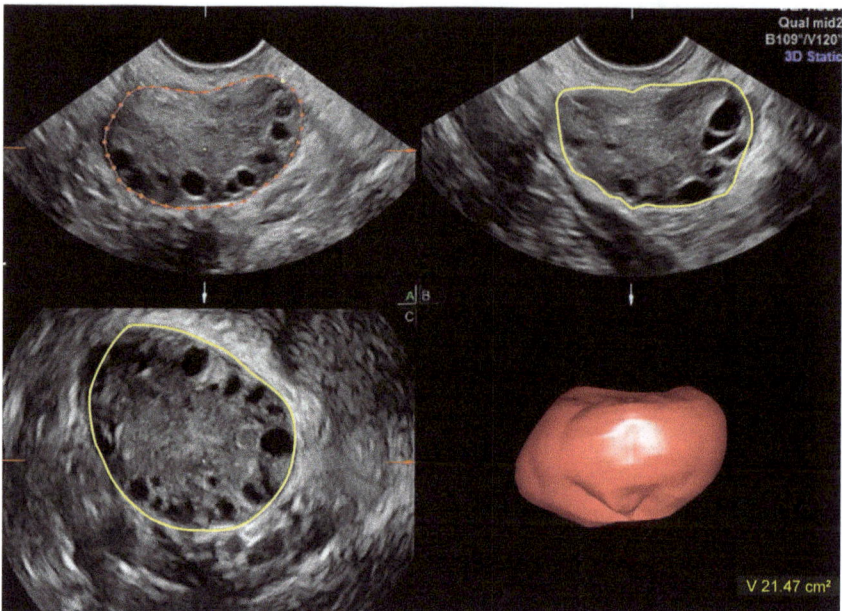

Fig. 5: Three-dimensional (3D) ultrasound acquired volume of the ovary—process by VOCAL showing calculated ovarian volume.

VOCAL calculates volume of any structure by rotating it 180°. A rotating step of 6–30° angle can be selected. A circumference is drawn around the structure of interest at every rotation step and at the end of 180°, total volume is calculated by the scanner computer. On this calculated ovarian volume with power Doppler, applying volume histogram gives values of 3D power Doppler indices, VI, FI, and VFI. VI is an index for abundance of flow in the selected volume, FI is an index for average intensity of flow in a selected volume, and VFI is a perfusion index **(Fig. 6)**.

FOLLICULAR TRACKING IN CONTROLLED OVARIAN HYPERSTIMULATION

Controlled ovarian hyperstimulation (COH) is used for all available assisted reproductive technologies (ART). The purpose is to grow more than one follicle that will increase the chance of pregnancy per cycle. It is claimed that it improves the follicle quality too. Gonadotropins are used for COH. Ultrasound (US) for Doppler plays an important role right from deciding the dose of gonadotropins in the early proliferative phase of the cycle to luteal phase. But for the ease of understanding, we shall divide this discussion into three parts:
1. Baseline scan and deciding the stimulation protocol
2. Preovulatory scan and decision on trigger
3. Luteal phase scan

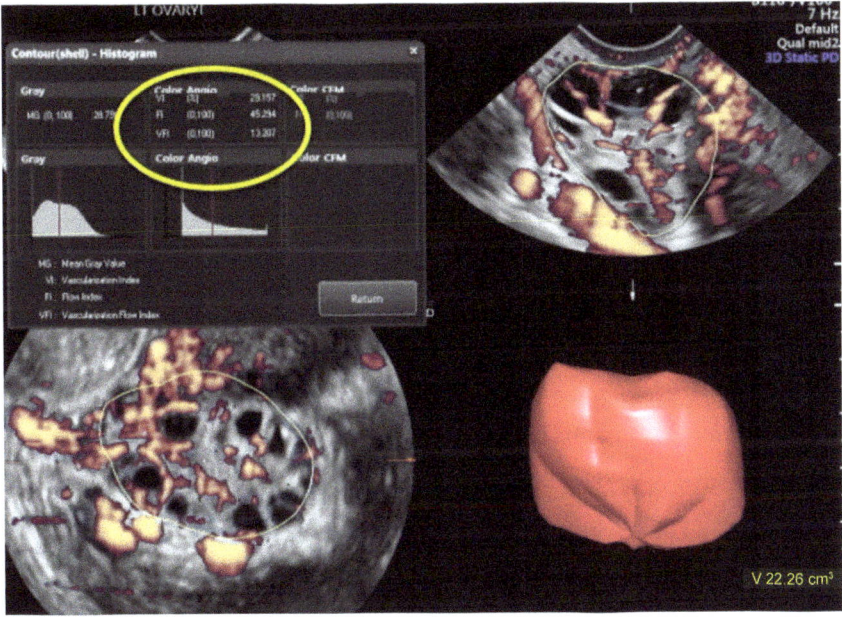

Fig. 6: 3D power Doppler acquired volume of the ovary, processed by VOCAL, followed by volume histogram software, showing VI, FI, and VFI values.

Baseline Scan and Deciding the Stimulation Protocol

This scan is done on day 2-3 of the menstrual cycle, when estrogen and progesterone levels are at baseline, ovaries are silent, and have no active follicle or corpus luteum (CL). Scan is always done transvaginally. This is done to assess ovarian reserve and response.

Reserve: Likely number of follicles that may develop or likely number of ova that may be retrieved—*antral follicle count (AFC) and ovarian volume.*

Response: Approximate doses that would be required to produce one or more mature follicle—*intraovarian flow.*

Therefore, this scan includes assessment of the ovarian size, AFC, and ovarian stromal flows—its RI and PSV. Secondary antral follicles (1-2 mm) are the first follicular structures that may be visualized on US **(Fig. 7)**.

The AFC and ovarian stromal flow parameters on the baseline scan were shown to be most predictive of the ovarian response after pituitary downregulation.[1] According to a study by Popovic-Todorovic et al.[2] also, total number of antral follicles and ovarian stromal blood flow were the two most significant predictors of ovarian response and ovarian volume was highly significant predictor of number of follicles and oocytes retrieved.

Measurement of ovarian stromal flow in early follicular phase is related to subsequent ovarian response in in vitro fertilization (IVF) treatment.

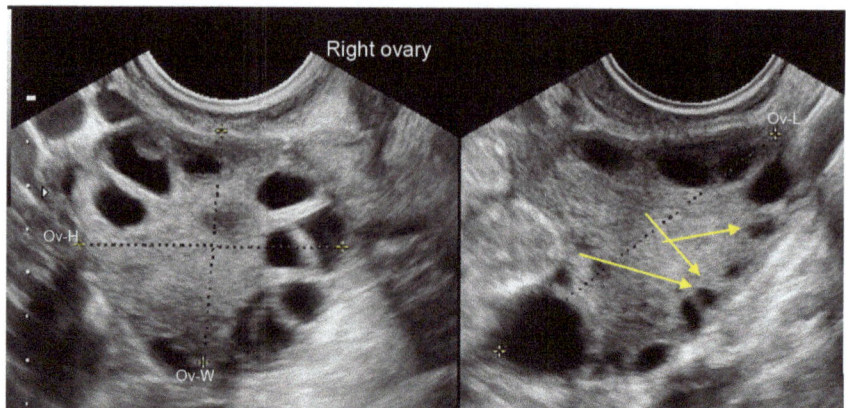

Fig. 7: B mode ultrasound of the ovary showing small secondary antral follicles.

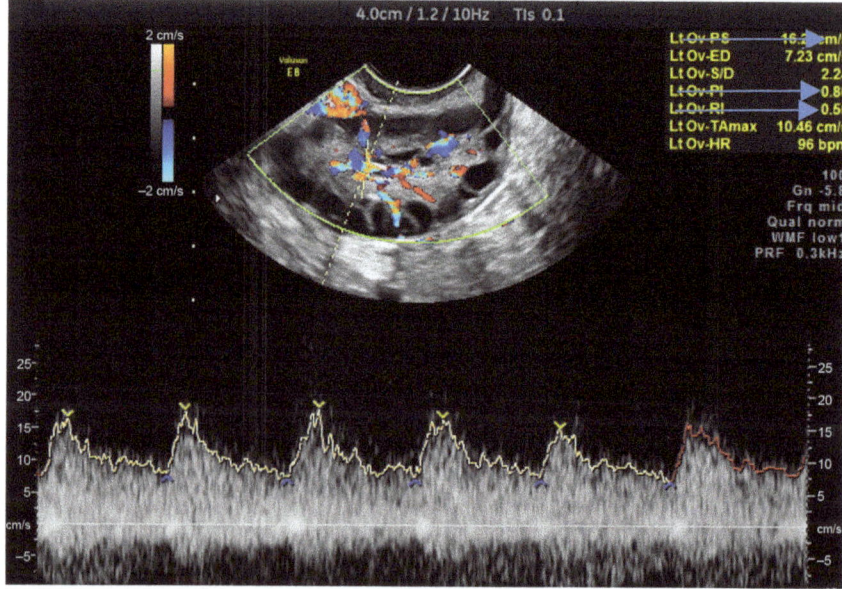

Fig. 8: Ovarian stromal flow as seen on color Doppler and pulsed wave Doppler and calculation of RI, PI, and PSV. (PI: pulsatility index; PSV: peak systolic velocity; RI: resistance index)

Those who had low stromal PSV in the early follicular phase were poor responders.[3] This can be measured by pulsed wave Doppler **(Fig. 8)**.

This means that Doppler can be used to decide the dose of gonadotropins to be used for ovulation induction. This is because if the flow to the ovarian stroma is more, more percentage of the drug loaded in the patient's system will flow into the ovary and so the total amount of gonadotropin required for ovulation induction is less, but if the ovarian stroma flow is less, then less percentage of total drug will be delivered in the ovary and so total dose required for stimulating that ovary will be more. Ovarian stromal flow is less

CHAPTER 5: Color Mapping of Follicle in Controlled Ovarian Hyperstimulation

in obese and in patients with advanced age; this explains why these patients require higher doses for stimulation[4] and there are several literature evidences for the same. Ovarian stromal PSV after pituitary suppression is predictive of ovarian responsiveness and outcome of IVF treatment.[5] Ovarian blood flow predicts ovarian responsiveness and hence provides a noninvasive and cost-effective prognostic factor of IVF outcome.[6] This low flow can be because of high resistance or low velocity. Based on all these facts and findings, it is understood that ovaries that have high resistance and low velocity flow require higher doses of gonadotropins for stimulation and vice versa.

Using age, body mass index (BMI), AFC, ovarian volume, stromal RI, and PSV as parameters to individualize the stimulation doses of gonadotropins, a scoring system has been devised. This method simplifies the dose calculation for individual patient and has proved to be an important guide for safe use of gonadotropins for ovulation induction in ART cycles[7,8] with zero severe ovarian hyperstimulation syndrome (OHSS) rates **(Tables 1 and 2)**.

The final dose calculation is based on factors given in **Tables 1 and 2**.[7,8]

Looking into the Literature to Justify these Parameters

Number of antral follicles, measuring 2–10 mm in diameter, correlates well with the female's age, ovarian reserve, and ovarian response to gonadotropin

TABLE 1: Baseline score calculation.

Score	1	2	3	4	5
Age	>40	35.1–40	30.1–35	25.1–30	<25
BMI	>30	30–28.1	28–25.1	25–22.1	<22
AFC	<5	5–10	10–15	15–20	>20
Ov volume	<3	3.1–5	5.1–7	7.1–10	>10
Stromal RI	>0.75	0.75–0.66	0.65–0.56	0.55–0.45	<0.45
Stromal PSV	<3	3.1–5	5.1–7	7.1–10	>10

(AFC: antral follicle count; BMI: body mass index; Ov volume: ovarian volume; PSV: peak systolic velocity; RI: resistance index)

TABLE 2: Dose calculation of rFSH for IUI and IVF cycles depending on the baseline score.

Score	IUI starting dose of rFSH	IVF starting dose of rFSH
≥25	25 IU	75 IU
21–24	37.5 IU	150 IU
16–20	75 IU	225 IU
11–15	112.5 IU	300 IU
6–10	150 IU	375 IU

(IUI: intrauterine insemination; IVF: in vitro fertilization; rFSH: recombinant follicle-stimulating hormone)

stimulation.[9] AFC <6 correlates well with reduced ovarian reserve **(Figs. 9A and B)** and poor response to ovarian stimulation with positive predictive value of 75%. Total AFC >21 could lead to the decision to adjust the gonadotropin dose in trying to prevent a hyperresponse leading to OHSS.[10] Ovarian volume of <3 cc indicates poor ovarian reserve **(Figs. 9A and B)**, whereas volume of >10 cc indicates polycystic ovary and risk of OHSS **(Fig. 5)**.

Measurement of ovarian stromal flow in early follicular phase is related to subsequent ovarian response in IVF treatment.[11] Ovarian stromal blood flow velocity after 2–3 weeks of pituitary suppression is a true representative of baseline ovarian blood flow and predictive of ovarian responsiveness and outcome of IVF treatment.[5] Ovarian stromal PSV was the most important single independent predictor of ovarian response in patients with normal basal serum FSH level. Therefore, Doppler of ovaries on baseline scan can be helpful to decide stimulation protocol.[3] It is known that follicles of <6 mm in diameter are less responsive to either endogenous or exogenous gonadotropins. If therefore all follicles are smaller than this, it would lead to higher total dose of gonadotropins consumption in a cycle. Age and BMI are the factors proved to alter ovarian response. After the stimulation is started, the scan is done on day 5 of stimulation, provided all the follicles on the day when stimulation is started are 10 mm or less. Once the follicle reaches 10 mm, it is a dominant follicle.

After Stimulation is Started

Once the stimulation is started, usually a follow-up scan is done after 5 days. If one of the follicles has reached dominance or the endometrium has started growing, it indicates the patient is responding to stimulation and the same dose is continued till follicle matures. But if the patient does not respond, the dose needs to be increased. A normal growth rate of a healthy dominant follicle is approximately 2 mm/day and reaches a size of 18–24 mm before ovulation.[12] The dominance of the follicle is proved by the blood vessels that

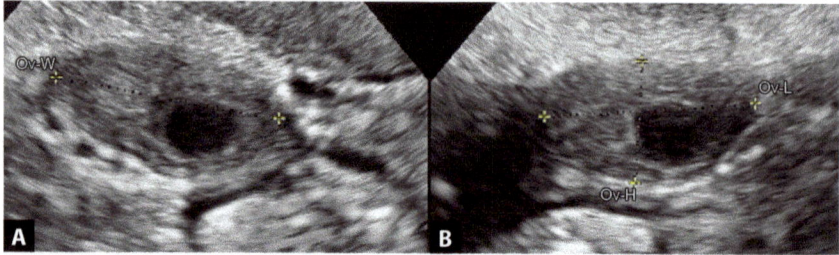

Figs. 9A and B: Small ovary with only one antral follicle—poor reserve ovary.

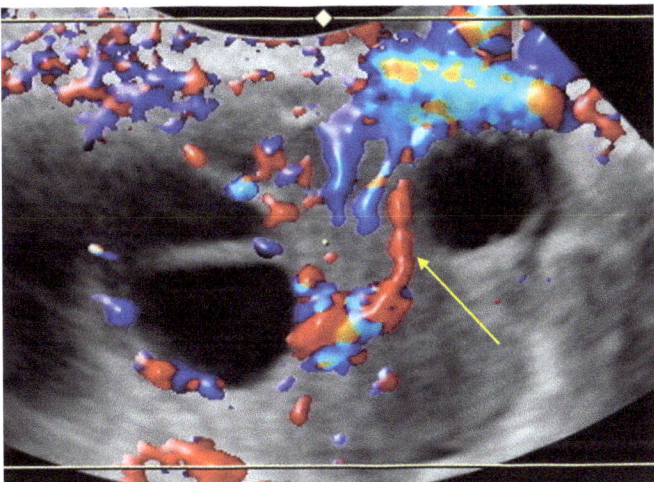

Fig. 10: Color Doppler image of the ovary showing the vessel heading toward the dominant follicle.

start growing toward the follicle **(Fig. 10)**. This starts as follicle size reaches 10 mm and as early as day 5–7 of the cycle.

Preovulatory Scan

Follicle

The *follicular size* can be measured as mean diameter or volume. The follicular diameter is measured as when the follicle is seen as a rounded structure on US image **(Fig. 11A)**. Mean diameter of the follicle is measured by first rotating the probe and finding out the longest follicular diameter on that same image AP diameter is measured as longest diameter perpendicular to this diameter. The probe is then rotated 90° and side to side longest diameter is transverse diameter **(Figs. 11B and C)**. Mean of these three orthogonal diameters is mean follicular diameter.

A follicular size of 17–18 mm is considered optimum for gonadotropin-stimulated cycle, whereas for clomiphene citrate-(CC)-stimulated cycles, minimum size of 18–20 mm is required.[13] A normal follicle—regular round shape and no echogenicity in the lumen and shows a thin hypoechoic rim surrounding the follicle **(Fig. 12)**. Though the size of the follicle has been considered a parameter for follicular maturity, this only assesses the anatomical maturity, not the follicular maturity, that would correlate with the ovum yield.

Doppler

Blood vessels start developing with the dominance of the follicle. This is in response to increase in granulosa cell mass and rise in estrogen.

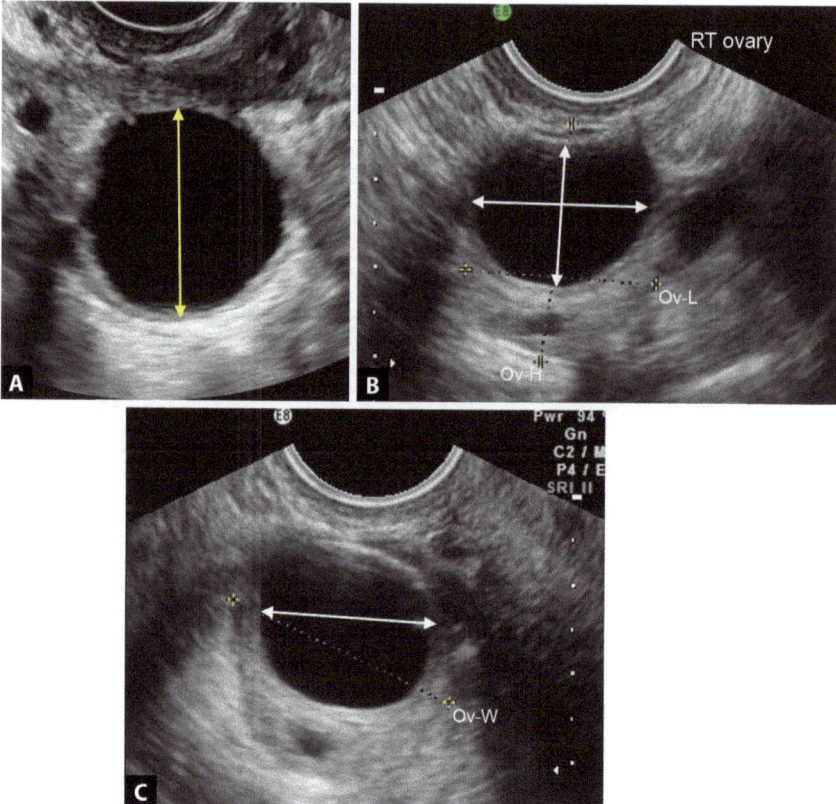

Figs. 11A to C: Measuring follicle size: (A) By single diameter when follicle is seen as almost round structure on screen, even on rotating the probe and (B and C) by three orthogonal diameters and mean of these is follicular mean diameter, when follicle does not appear round on screen. (RT: right)

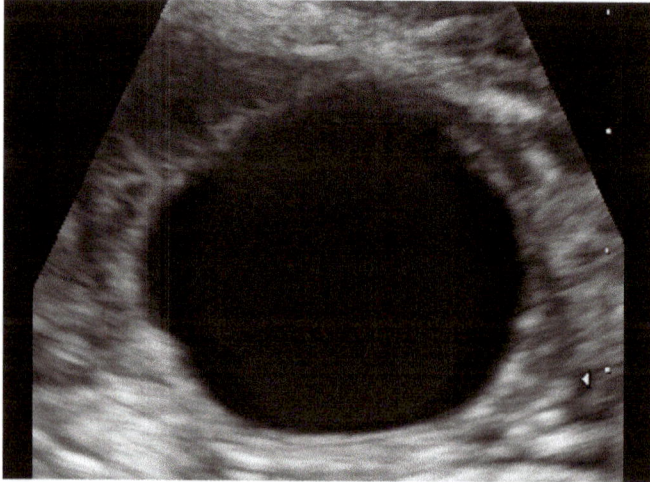

Fig. 12: B mode ultrasound image of a mature follicle.

About 2 days before ovulation, when estrogen peaks, the RI of these vessels starts falling.[14] The vessel that overlaps the follicular walls is perifollicular vessel. When functionally mature and capable of producing a fertilizable ovum, Doppler shows blood vessels covering two-thirds to three-fourths of the follicular circumference (**Fig. 13**). Chui et al. graded the follicular flow as grades 1–4 when in a single cross area slice, the flow covered <25%, 25–50%, 50–75%, and >75% of follicular circumference and related good ovum quality to grade 3–4 vascularity.[15] On pulse Doppler, these blood vessels show RI of 0.4–0.48[18] and PSV of >10 cm/s (**Fig. 14**). Fall in RI of the perifollicular vessels

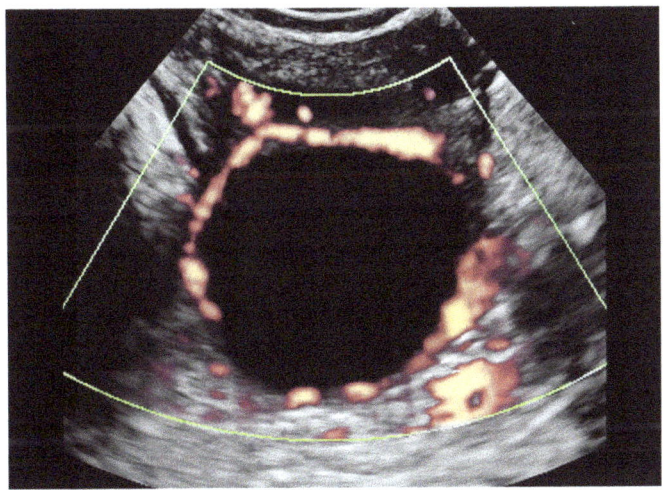

Fig. 13: Perifollicular vascularity seen on color Doppler.

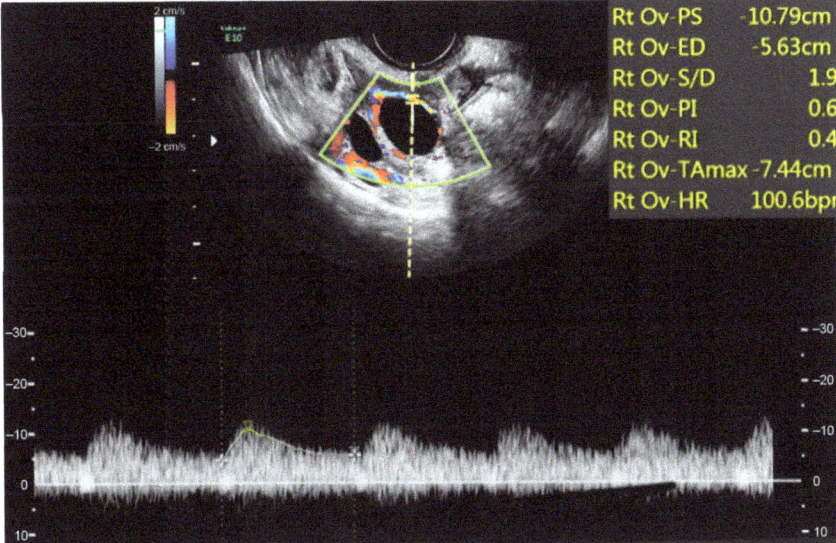

Fig. 14: Pulse Doppler image of the low-resistance perifollicular flow.

correlates with the estrogen peak at follicular maturity. This leads to positive feedback for LH release and negative feedback for FSH release. The rise in PSV to 10 cm/s can be correlated to the kick to LH.

Follicle flow correlates well with oocyte recovery rates and hence may be useful in determining the most appropriate time to administer trigger to optimize oocyte recovery rate. Our data of >1,000 intrauterine insemination (IUI) cycles has shown that when the perifollicular RI > 0.53 and PSV < 9 cm/s, 12 hours before human chorionic gonadotropin (hCG) injection, the conception rates were only 8.3% and 10%, respectively, as compared to 32.8% and 28.2%, respectively, and individually when perifollicular RI < 0.50 and PSV > 11 cm/s. We have therefore always preferred to wait with no extra medication when patient is on CC stimulation or continue with the same dose of gonadotropin till we get desired perifollicular RI and PSV, though sometimes the follicular size may reach up to 22 mm. Almost 90% of the times the desired RI and PSV are reached by the time follicular size is 22–24 mm maximum. Moreover, embryo produced by fertilization of the ovum obtained from follicle that had a perifollicular PSV of <10 cm/s is less likely to be grade I embryo and also have higher chance of chromosomal malformations.[16,17] Another study also documents that oocytes from severely hypoxic follicles are associated with high frequency of abnormalities of organization of chromosomes on metaphase spindle and may lead to segregation disorders and catastrophic mosaics in embryo[18] and follicles with more uniform perifollicular network contain oocytes capable to produce pregnancy[19] **(Fig. 15)**.

This can be best assessed by 3D power Doppler. We have found perifollicular VI between 6 and 20 and perifollicular FI > 35 as most optimum for best conception rates[20] **(Fig. 16)**. Although it is possible to assess the

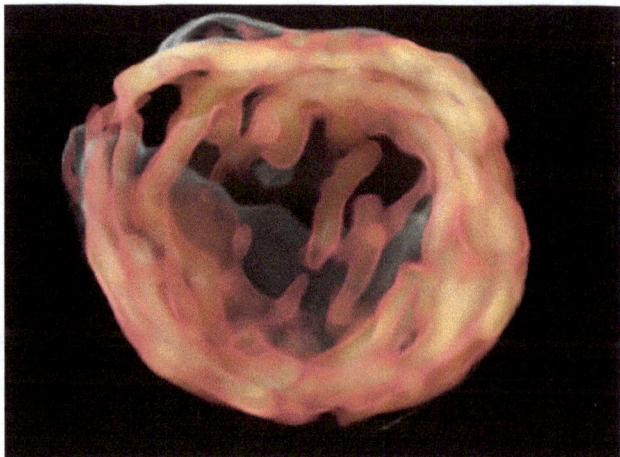

Fig. 15: Three-dimensional (3D) power Doppler image rendered in glass body mode showing uniformly distributed perifollicular flow.

CHAPTER 5: Color Mapping of Follicle in Controlled Ovarian Hyperstimulation

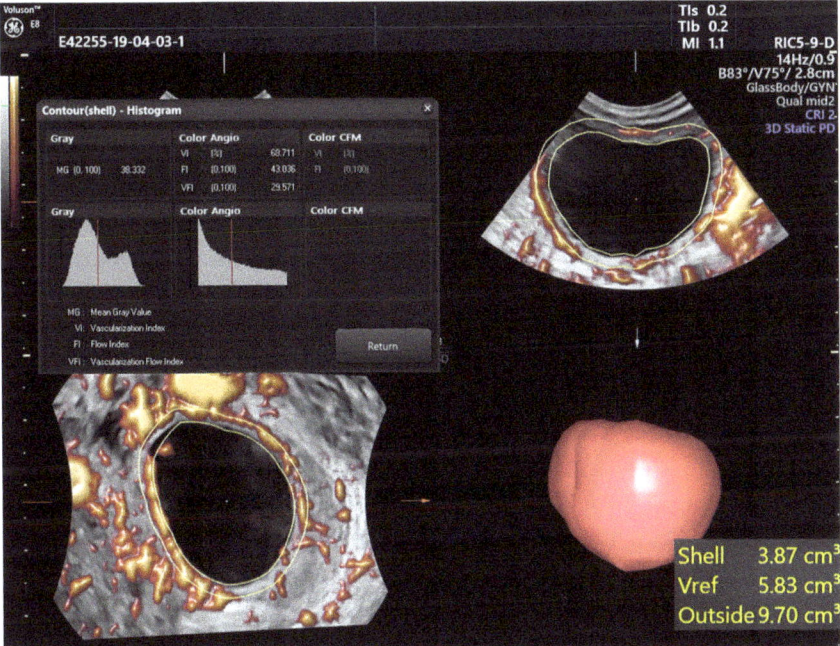

Fig. 16: 3D power Doppler ultrasound acquired image of the follicle, processed by VOCAL followed by volume histogram shows VI, FI, and VFI values of the follicle.

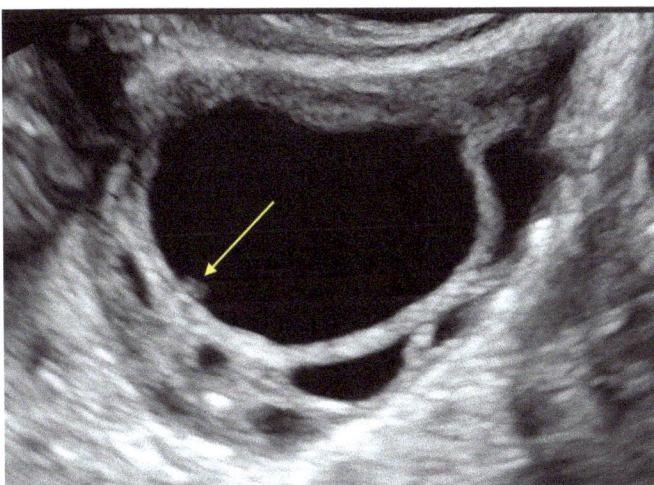

Fig. 17: B mode ultrasound image of the follicle showing cumulus.

follicular flow as expressed by the PSV and perifollicular color map,[21] it is the 3D power Doppler that gives the most precise information about the vascularization and follicular blood flow.[22]

In response to LH surge, resulting preovulatory changes in follicle are seen as appearance of a sonolucent halo surrounding the follicle and appearance of cumulus (a small solid projection from the follicle wall) 24–36 hours before ovulation **(Fig. 17)**.

Luteinizing hormone surge plays a major role in inducing influx of blood within follicles. At the LH surge, the perifollicular PSV is 10 cm/s. Vascular changes at the time of impending ovulation include increased vascularity of the inner wall of the follicle and a coincident surge in blood velocity just prior to eruption.[23] Under the effect of rising LH, the perifollicular PSV keeps on rising constantly.[23] The rise in PSV follows the rise in LH by approximately 12 hours. PSV increases 29 hours before the time of follicular rupture and continues for ≥72 hours after CL is formed.[24]

This derives that a rising PSV with steady low RI suggests that the follicle is progressing toward rupture. Instead, if PSV is steady or falling with rising RI, it suggests that the follicle may go into luteinized unruptured follicle (LUF). A marked increase in the PSV around the follicle, in the presence of a relatively constant PI, could be a sign of follicle maturity and impending ovulation.[18]

A study by Kupesic and Kurjak shows that when the ratio of follicular volume (FV) to blood FI (FV/FI) is between 0.4 and 0.6, the pregnancy rates are 39%; if >0.6, it is 52%; and when <0.4, it is only 21%.[1] The above data from different studies indicate that even when the follicle appeared mature according to the two-dimensional (2D) US and color and pulse Doppler parameters, the pregnancy rates were significantly better, when the follicle volume was between 3 and 7.5 cm^3, cumulus was present and the perifollicular VI and FI values were optimum as mentioned earlier. Although it is possible to assess the follicular flow as expressed by the PSV and perifollicular color map,[21] 3D power Doppler provides a more detailed quantitative information about the ovarian vascularization and perifollicular blood flow.[22]

Secretory Phase Assessment

This phase of the cycle is usually ignored, but its study can diagnose abnormalities like LUF and luteal phase defect (LPD) that can be prevented by proper follicle monitoring and timely trigger. The functional efficacy of the CL can be assessed by Doppler by assessing the pericorpus luteal vascularity. A clear correlation between RI of CL and plasma progesterone levels and CL RI (normal RI 0.35–0.50) can therefore be used as an adjunct to plasma progesterone assay as an index of luteal function[25] **(Fig. 18)**.

The receptor organ for progesterone also (such as estrogen) is endometrium and its vascular studies can be a reliable clue to adequate progesterone production. Soon after the surge starts, progesterone starts rising, the outer margin of the endometrium starts becoming fluffy and blurred. After a few hours of rupture, endometrial outer margin starts

CHAPTER 5: Color Mapping of Follicle in Controlled Ovarian Hyperstimulation

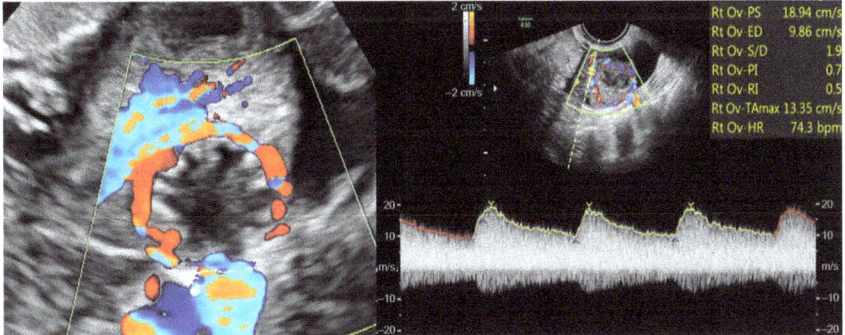

Fig. 18: Normal corpus luteal flow seen on color Doppler and pulse Doppler.

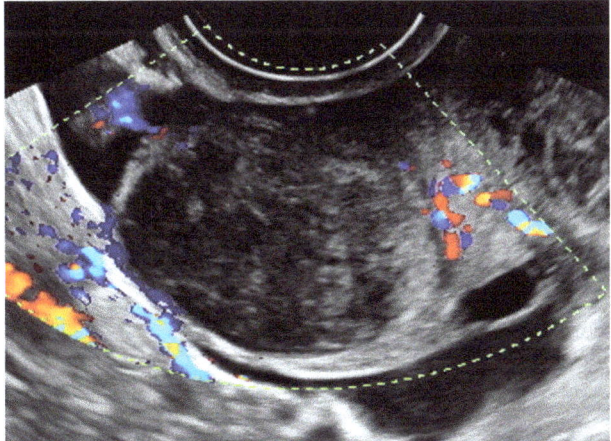

Fig. 19: Scanty pericorpus luteal flow seen on color Doppler image of the corpus luteum suggesting corpus luteum inadequacy.

becoming fluffy and later on hyperechoic. Hyperechogenicity progresses toward the central line of the endometrium to make the entire endometrium hyperechoic in the midluteal phase. With adequate progesterone levels in the midluteal phase, the spiral arteries show RI 0.48–0.52 (low resistance flow) and uterine artery shows PI of 2.0–2.5. The flow is assessed in the uterine artery of the dominant side (on the side of ovulation).

Inadequate progesterone production due to corpus luteal inadequacy is suggested by high resistance and scanty flow in corpus luteal vessels[25] **(Fig. 19)**, whereas high spiral artery resistance would suggest inadequate response of endometrium to progesterone. This is because of inadequate progesterone receptors in the endometrium or because of local endometrial cause, like endometrial injury or chronic endometritis.

In LPD, because of low progesterone levels, the resistance in the pericorpus luteal vessels is high. Because of low progesterone levels, there is inadequate relaxation of the muscularis of the uterine artery and therefore,

TABLE 3: Midluteal ultrasound parameters in normal luteal phase corpus luteal inadequacy, endometrial receptor inadequacy, and LUF.

	CL	Endometrium	Uterine artery
Normal luteal phase	RI < 0.5	RI < 0.5	PI < 2.5
CL inadequacy	RI > 0.6	RI > 0.6	PI > 3
Endometrial progesterone receptor inadequacy	RI < 0.5	RI > 0.6	PI > 3
LUF	RI 0.51–0.6	RI 0.51–0.6	PI 2.5–3.0

(CL: corpus luteum; LUF: luteinized unruptured follicle; PI: pulsatility index; RI: resistance index)

the uterine artery resistance is high along with higher resistance in its branches—the spiral vessels. But if it is because of inadequacy of progesterone receptors, corpus luteal flow is normal, but the spiral artery flow is high resistance.

Comparative values of corpus luteal RI and spiral artery RI in normal cycle and LPD[26] are shown in **Table 3**.

■ CONCLUSION

Ultrasound is an excellent tool for monitoring the follicles, understanding their behavior, and controlling their response to COH. Doppler is an excellent tool to understand hormonal changes. US with Doppler can be used as the only and a more relevant modality for cycle assessment in patients undergoing infertility treatment.

■ KEY POINTS

- Doppler on baseline scan is required to assess ovarian response and to correctly decide the dose of gonadotropins.
- Using the baseline scoring system is the safest way to decide ovulation induction protocol using gonadotropins.
- Doppler assessment of the follicle before ovulation trigger, can improve conception rate and reduce the incidence of chromosomal abnormalities in resulting embryo.
- Endometrial vascularity is more important than thickness and morphology for assessment of its receptivity and reduction in abortion rates.
- Luteal phase scan is important to diagnose luteal phase abnormalities and to guide towards the cause of the same.

■ REFERENCES

1. Kupesic S, Kurjak A. Predictors of IVF outcome by three-dimensional ultrasound. Hum Reprod. 2002;17(4):950-5.

2. Popovic-Todorovic B, Loft A, Lindhard A, Bangsboll S, Andersson AM, Anderson AN. A prospective study of predictive factors of ovarian response in 'standard' IVF/ICSI patients treated with recombinant FSH. A suggestion for recombinant FSH dosage normogram. Hum Reprod. 2003;18(4):781-7.
3. Zaidi J, Barber J, Kyei-Mensah A, Bekir J, Campbell S, Tan SL. Relationship of ovarian stromal blood flow at baseline ultrasound to subsequent follicular response in an in vitro fertilization program. Obstet Gynecol. 1996;88:779-84.
4. Lam PM, Johnson IR, Rainne-Fenning NJ. Three dimensional ultrasound features of the polycystic ovary and the effect of different phenotypic expressions on these parameters. Hum Reprod. 2007;22(12):3116-23.
5. Engmann L, Saldkevicius P, Agrawal R, Bekir JS, Campbell S, Tan S. Value of ovarian stromal blood flow velocity measurement after pituitary suppression in the prediction of ovarian responsiveness and outcome of in vitro fertilization treatment. Fertil Steril. 1999;71(1):22-9.
6. Arora A, Gainder S, Dhaliwal L, Suri V. Clinical significance of ovarian stromal blood flow in assessment of ovarian response in stimulated cycle for in vitro fertilization. Int J Reprod Contracept Obstet Gynecol. 2015;4(5):1380-3.
7. Panchal S, Nagori CB. Ultrasound based decision making on stimulation protocol for superovulated IUI cycles. IJIFM. 2016;7(1):7-13.
8. Panchal S, Nagori CB. Ultrasound based decision making on stimulation protocol in IVF. DSJUOG. 2016;10(3):330-7.
9. Scheffer GJ, Broekmans FJM, Looman CWN, Blankenstein M, Fauser BC, teJong FH, et al. The number of antral follicles in normal women with proven fertility is best reflection of reproductive age. Hum Reprod. 2003;18:700-6.
10. Kwee J, Elting ME, Schats R, McDonnell J, Lambalk CB. Ovarian volume and antral follicle count for the prediction of low and hyper responders with in vitro fertilization. Reprod Biol Endocrinol. 2007;5:9.
11. Lass A, Skull J, McVeigh E, Margara R, Winston RM. Measurement of ovarian volume by transvaginal sonography before ovulation induction with human menopausal gonadotrophin for in-vitro fertilization can predict poor response. Hum Reprod. 1992;12:294-7.
12. Hackeloer BJ, Fleming R, Robinson HP. Correlation of ultrasonic and endocrinological assessment of human follicular development. Am J Obstet Gynecol. 1979;135:122.
13. Luciano GN, Tarek AG. Ultrasonography and IVF. In: Rizk Botros RMB (Ed). Ultrasonography in Reproductive Medicine and Infertility. UK: Cambridge University Press; 2010. pp.193-201.
14. Jokubkeine L, Sladkevicius P, Rovas L, Valentine L. Assessment of changes in volume and vascularity of ovaries during the normal menstrual cycle using three dimensional power Doppler ultrasound. Hum Reprod. 2006;21(10):2661-8.
15. Chui KC, Pugh ND, Walker SM, Gregory L, Shaw RW. Follicular vascularity: the predictive value of transvaginal power Doppler ultrasonography in an in-vitro fertilization programme: a preliminary study. Hum Reprod. 1997;12(1):191-6.
16. Nargund G, Doyle PE, Bourne TH, Parsons JH, Cheng WC, Campbell S, et al. Ultrasound-deviced indices of follicular blood flow before HCG administration and prediction of oocyte recovery and preimplantation embryo quality. Hum Reprod. 1996;11:2512-7.

17. Nargund G, Bourne TH, Doyle PE, Parsons J, Cheng W, Campbell S, et al. Association between ultrasound indices of follicular blood flow, oocyte recovery and preimplantation embryo quality. Hum Reprod. 1996;11:109-13.
18. Van Blerkom, Antezak M, Schrader R. The developmental potential of human oocyte is related to the dissolved oxygen content of follicular fluid: association with vascular endothelial growth factor levels and perifollicular blood flow characteristics. Hum Reprod. 1997;12(5):1047-55.
19. Vlaisavljevic V, Reljic M, Gavric Lovrec V, Zazula D, Sergent N. Measurement of perifollicular blood flow of the dominant preovulatory follicle using three dimensional power doppler. Ultrasound Obstet Gynecol. 2003;22:520-6.
20. Panchal SY, Nagori CB. Can 3D PD be a better tool for assessing the pre HCG follicle and endometrium? A randomized study of 500 cases. Presented at 16th World Congress on Ultrasound in Obstetrics and Gynecology, 2006, London. J Ultrasound Obstet Gynecol. 2006;28(4):504.
21. Merce LT. Ultrasound markers of implantation. Ultrasound Rev Obstet Gynecol. 2002;2:110-23.
22. Merce LT, Barco MJ, Kupesic S, Kurjak A. 2D and 3D power Doppler ultrasound from ovulation to implantation. In: Kurjak A, Chervenak F (Eds). Textbook of Perinatal Medicine. London: Parthenon Publishing; 2005.
23. Bourne TH, Jurkovic D, Waterstone J, Campbell S, Collins WP. Intrafollicular blood flow during human ovulation. Ultrasound Obstet Gynecol. 1991;1:53-9.
24. Bourne TH, Athanasiou S, Bauer B. Ovulation and the periovulatory follicle. In: Bourne TH, Jauniaux E, Jurkovic D (Eds). Transvaginal Colour Doppler. Berlin: Springer-Verlag; 1995. pp. 119-30.
25. Glock JL, Brumsted JR. Colour flow pulsed Doppler ultrasound in diagnosing luteal phase defect. Fertil Steril. 1995;64:500-4.
26. Kupesić S, Kurjak A, Vujisić S, Petrović Z. Luteal phase defect: comparison between Doppler velocimetry, histological and hormonal markers. Ultrasound Obstet Gynecol. 1997;9(2):105-12.

Chapter 6

Evaluation and Monitoring of Endometrium in Controlled Ovarian Hyperstimulation

Sonal Panchal, M Lipika

■ INTRODUCTION

Endometrium is the mucous membrane that lines the inside of the uterus. It has a cell-rich connective tissue that surrounds the endometrial glands. It is composed of two layers: (1) the superficial functional layer and (2) the deeper basal layer. In each menstrual cycle, the superficial functional layer of the endometrium is shed and regenerates from the underlying basal layer. Its thickness, morphology, and vascularity change throughout the menstrual cycle in women of reproductive age.

■ EVALUATION OF ENDOMETRIUM

Systematic evaluation of the endometrium can be done based on IETA (International Endometrial Tumor Analysis group) consensus statement that has been published by a panel of experts (IETA consensus group).[1]

The evaluation of the endometrium and uterine cavity can be done both by transabdominal sonography (TAS) and transvaginal sonography (TVS). The TVS route is considered ideal for evaluating the endometrium. However, TAS may help, particularly in the presence of fibroids, an enlarged uterus or a mid-positioned (axially placed) uterus. Transrectal ultrasound scan should be considered if TVS is not possible due to any condition like vaginismus. It is best to do both a TAS and a TVS scan, because very often they complement each other.

The uterus is scanned (on 2D) in the sagittal plane from one cornu to the other and in the transverse plane from the cervix to the fundus. 3D US is useful for visualization of the coronal section of the uterus and EMJ (endomyometrial junction). Once the overview is done on ultrasound, the magnification should be increased focusing on the area of interest, i.e., the endometrium.

Evaluation of endometrial morphology is best done when endometrium is perpendicular to the sound beam. In a mid-positioned uterus, because sound beam is parallel to the endometrial long axis, endometrium appears hyperechoic and lesions are difficult to demonstrate. In such cases, one can place the probe in the anterior or posterior fornix and push on the cervix to retrovert or antevert the uterus further, to try and make the endometrium more perpendicular to the beam. TAS in such cases may provide better idea about endometrial morphology. If visualization is suboptimal, then that must be mentioned in the report. Saline or gel instillation (sonohysterogram) may help in better evaluation of the endometrium in cases where assessment is difficult or in those with an intracavitary pathology.

■ MEASUREMENT METHOD

Uterocervical length is measured from the fundal serosa to external os, measured as a continuous trace and physiological uterocervical length or endometrial trace is measured from fundal end of the endometrium to the external os **(Fig. 1)**.

The endometrium is measured in midsagittal plane, perpendicular to the endometrial midline, where the endometrium is thickest, from outer margin of anterior hyperechoic line to outer margin of posterior hyperechoic line **(Fig. 2)**. When there is fluid in the endometrial cavity, individual measurement of both endometrial lips is taken and are added. When the endometrium cannot be visualized clearly, as is sometimes the case with a mid-positioned uterus, it should be reported as "nonmeasurable".

Intracavitary pathology like polyp is included in the total endometrial thickness. Myoma should not be included in the measurement of endometrial thickness. Lesions like polyps or myomas are measured as three longest orthogonal diameters. Intracavitary fluid should be measured as largest measurement in the sagittal plane.

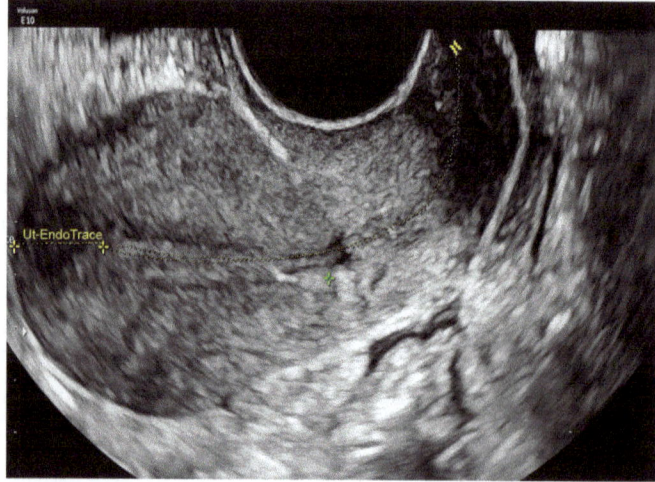

Fig. 1: B-mode ultrasound image of midsagittal section of the uterus, showing measurement of anatomical and physiological uterocervical length.

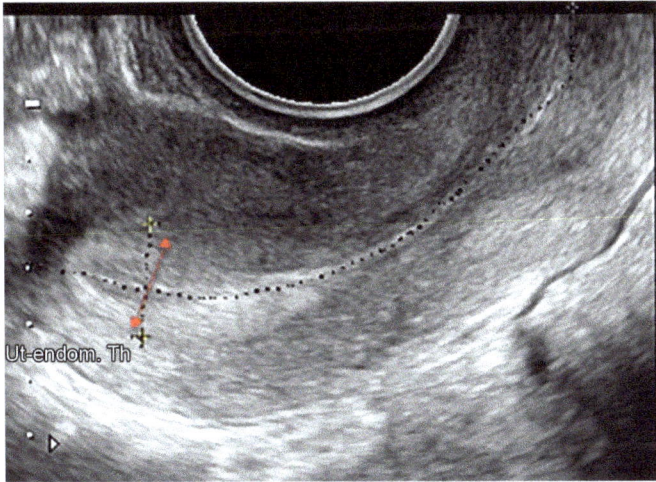

Fig. 2: B-mode ultrasound image if midsagittal section of uterus, with red arrowed line showing measurement of endometrial thickness.

■ QUALITATIVE ASSESSMENT OF THE ENDOMETRIUM

This includes the assessment of the endometrial echogenicity, the endometrial midline, and the EMJ:

- The echogenicity of the endometrium is compared with that of the myometrium. It could be hyperechoic, isoechoic, or hypoechoic.
- The endometrial echogenicity is considered uniform, if the endometrium is multilayered or homogeneous with symmetrical anterior and posterior walls. The echogenicity is termed nonuniform, if the endometrium appears heterogeneous. In case of nonuniform endometrium, it is to be mentioned it is due to hyperechoic/cystic shadows.
- The endometrial midline is the interface between the opposing surfaces of the two endometrial walls. It is defined as "linear" if it is straight and hyperechogenic; "nonlinear" if it is waved, "irregular", interrupted, or "not defined" in the absence of any distinct midline echoes.
- Endomyometrial junction is described as regular, irregular, interrupted, or not defined.
- When an intracavitary lesion is present, a bright line is generally seen at the interface between the lesion and the endometrial walls, particularly if the lesion is smooth walled. If any lesion is seen within the cavity, its morphology should be described, i.e., its margins, echogenicity, and vascularity.
- IETA also includes saline infusion sonohysterogram (SIS) findings. On SIS, the lesion is defined as "extended" if the endometrial abnormality involves 25% or more of the endometrial surface, and as localized if <25% of the endometrial surface is involved.

- Localized lesions are defined as "pedunculated", if the maximum transverse diameter is more than the diameter of its base, and "sessile" if their maximum transverse diameter is less than the diameter of its base.
- On SIS, the endometrial outline is defined as "smooth" if it appears regular, as having endometrial folds if there are multiple thickened "undulating" areas with a regular profile; as "polypoid" if there are deep indentations; or as "irregular" if the surface is cauliflower-like or sharply toothed (spiky).

ULTRASOUND DIAGNOSIS OF COMMON ENDOMETRIAL PATHOLOGIES

Endometrial Polyp

Endometrial polyp is growth arising from the endometrial lining of the uterus and may present as intermenstrual spotting and infertility/subfertility or may be asymptomatic.

Ultrasound Features of Endometrial Polyps (Figs. 3A to D)

A polyp typically appears as well-circumscribed hyperechoic homogenous lesion within the endometrial cavity, better seen in a proliferative endometrium. The presence of this hyperechoic line often helps in delineating a polyp on 2D. Heterogenicity of the polyp may indicate adenomyomatous polyp or atypia. Blood clots may sometimes mimic polyp but it does not have vascularity. Large or multiple polyps can mimic endometrial hyperplasia on 2D ultrasound.

On Doppler, a "single feeder vessel"/"pedicle artery sign" is seen in the polyp[2] **(Fig. 3B)**.

This vessel may show branching within the polyp. For gynecological scans, pulse repetition frequency (PRF) for color and power Doppler is set

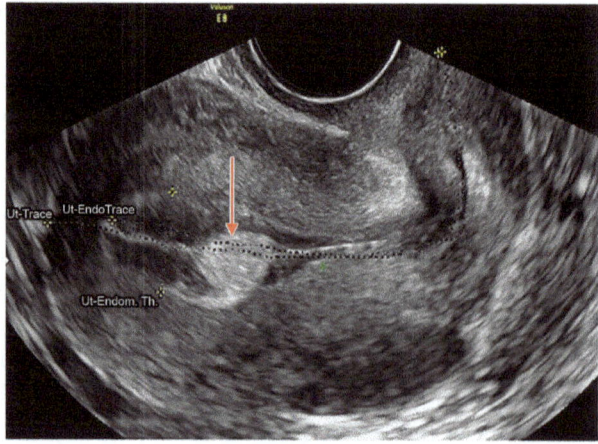

Fig. 3A

CHAPTER 6: Evaluation and Monitoring of Endometrium in...

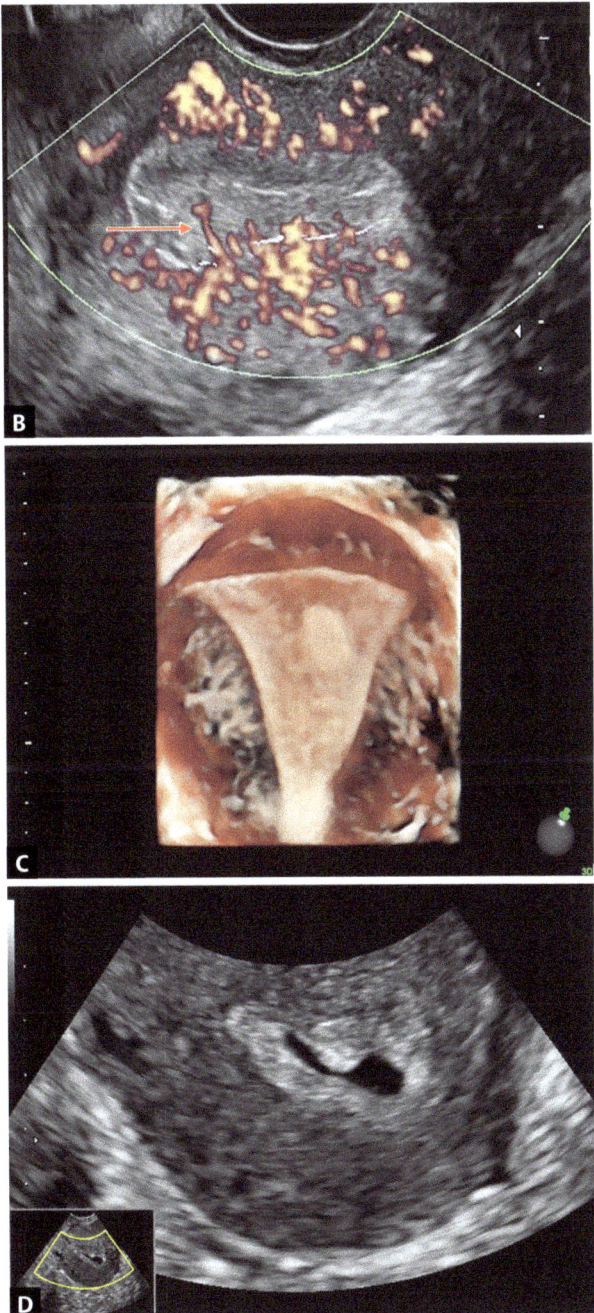

Figs. 3B to D

Figs. 3A to D: (A) B-mode ultrasound image of midsagittal section of uterus showing polyp (arrow); (B) Power Doppler image of endometrium showing single feeding vessel in polyp (arrow); (C) 3D ultrasound of the uterus with polyp; (D) Polyp on 2D ultrasound with saline infusion sonohysterography.

between 0.3 and 0.6. Polyps are often visualized well on 3D rendered coronal images of the uterine cavity **(Fig. 3C)**. Polyps could be multiple, each with its individual feeder vessel. Polyps are well demonstrated on SIS and especially with 3D ultrasound **(Fig. 3D)**.

Asherman's Syndrome or Intrauterine Adhesions

Intrauterine adhesions or endometrial scarring is usually post-traumatic or postsurgical, or as a result of chronic infection.

Depending on the extent of scarring, patients with Asherman's syndrome have scanty or absent periods. Some patients may complain of cyclical pain due to obstruction to the outflow of menstrual blood (from the functional endometrium not affected by scarring).

Ultrasound Features of Asherman's Syndrome or Intrauterine Adhesions

Persistently thin endometrium with at times hypoechoic breaks in endometrial continuity and sometimes hyperechoic strands may indicate intrauterine adhesions. Small fluid-filled locules may be seen in the endometrial shadow **(Fig. 4A)**. Subendometrial fibrosis may present as subendometrial hyperechoic flecks. 3D evaluation of the endometrial cavity is useful in assessing the extent of scarring. On sonohysterography, the synechiae appear as avascular echogenic bands bridging the uterine cavity **(Fig. 4B)**. In some cases, there may be restricted distention of endometrial cavity, if the scarring is significant. Hysteroscopy is not only useful in diagnosis and hysteroscopic adhesiolysis.

Endometritis

Acute endometritis presents as thick endometrium in early proliferative phase with increased vascularity and irregular junctional zone.

Chronic endometritis presents as persistently thin endometrium with no or scanty vascularity in endometrium and subendometrium. Intracavitary fluid may be seen with or without echogenicities **(Fig. 5A)**, which may be minimal. It is usually turbid (blood and/or pus). This fluid may show some hyperechoic debris within. Hyperechoic foci may be seen along the EMJ, in endometrium or in myometrium **(Fig. 5B)**. In infection with anaerobic organisms, there may be air within the endometrial cavity which is seen as bright scattered echoes with dirty acoustic shadowing. There may be associated ultrasound signs of pelvic inflammatory disease (PID) like free fluid in pelvis, hydrosalpinx, etc.

Adenomyosis

It may be a cause of persistently thin endometrium or bad endometrial receptivity. On ultrasound, it presents with irregular, obliterated or in

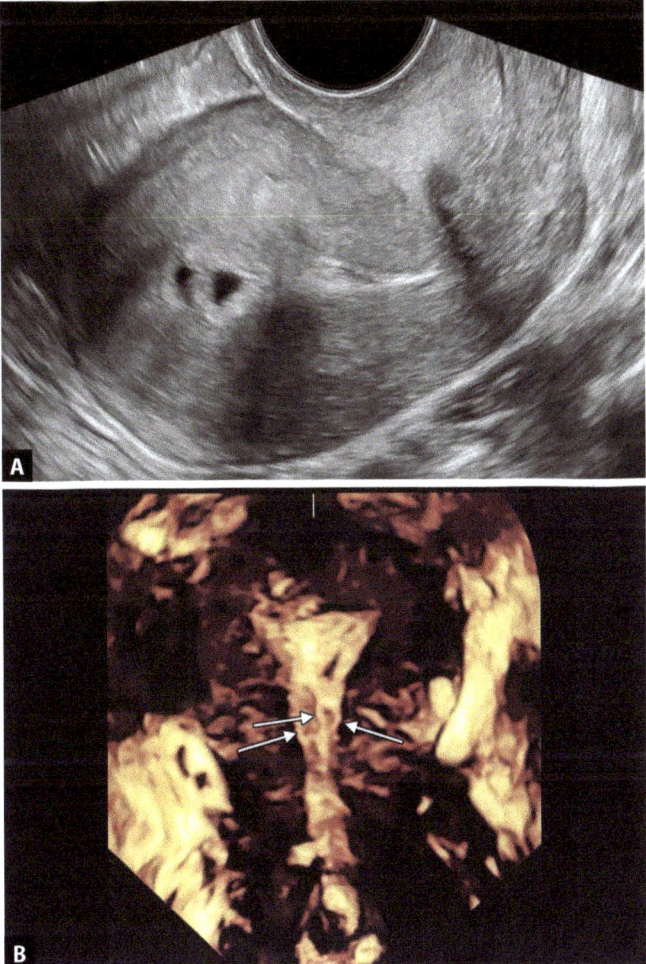

Figs. 4A and B: (A) 2D image of endometrium with tiny loculi, suggestive of synechiae; (B) 3D ultrasound of the endometrium showing synechiae (arrows).

accessible junctional zone with heterogeneous myometrium. This is due to hyperechoic dots, lines, islands, and anechoic myometrial cysts. There are alternate hyper- and hypoechoic vertical shadows (fan shadows). Moreover, there may also be reverse curvature of the fundal endometrium beyond the midbody of the uterus. On Doppler, it shows translesional vascularity, no peripheral vascularity.[3]

ENDOMETRIAL EVALUATION FOR RECEPTIVITY

Endometrium is a receptor organ to the reproductive steroids—estrogen and progesterone. Receptivity of endometrium to embryo is affected by the delicate equilibrium of these steroids. The changes in these hormones reflect as morphological and vascular changes in the endometrium.

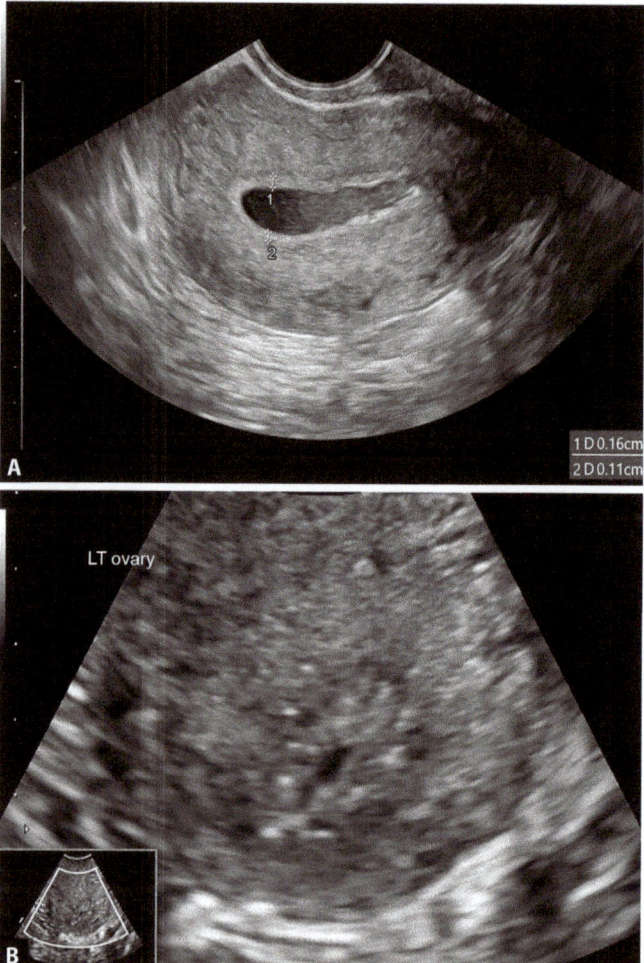

Figs. 5A and B: (A) B-mode ultrasound image of the uterus showing fluid with echogenicities in the endometrium; (B) B-mode ultrasound image of the uterus showing tiny hyperechogenicities in the junctional zone due to chronic endometritis.

These can be studied by ultrasound and Doppler in natural and stimulated cycles. Monitoring of continuous changes occurring in the uterus and endometrium are as important as monitoring of the follicle.

At the start of the menstrual cycle when the whole endometrium has shed off, the endometrium appears thin and linear. Endometrial thickness is <5 mm in early follicular phase and slightly more echogenic than the myometrium areas. Fresh blood appears hyperechoic. Doppler is of help to differentiate between the two. Blood never shows any blood vessels inside. Endometrium starts becoming triple line around 6th day of the cycle, soon after follicular dominance. It grows at a rate of 1–2 mm/day in mid-follicular phase. Endometrial thickness can be correlated with the rise in estradiol.[4] Though relationship of endometrial thickness to histological dating is controversial.

Endometrial peristalsis that initiates in the junctional zone is highest in the periovulatory period and is in cervicofundal direction, and in 30-40% of spontaneous cycles, its rate is 3-4/min.[5] At 24-36 hours before ovulation, cervix shows mucous as anechoic strip in the cervical canal. At times, minimal endometrial fluid is also seen as a result of estrogen rise. Endometrial and subendometrial vascular flow increases to its maximum 3 days prior to ovulation and then decreases until fifth postovulatory day (due to probably vasodilatation of subepithelial capillary plexus leading to stromal edema) and then again increases for the rest of the luteal phase.[6] Blood flow in the uterine vascular bed can be correlated to the estrogen/progesterone ratio.[7] At start of the luteinizing hormone (LH) surge, the spiral vessels that supply the endometrium show resistance index (RI) of <0.6. Its thickness decreases by 0.5 mm on the day of LH surge. With the advancing LH surge, the outer hyperechoic line of the endometrium starts getting fluffy, before ovulation.

During the secretory phase, the endometrium starts becoming echogenic from the periphery and proceeds toward the central line and is described as *"endometrial ring sign"*,[8] and increases by 2 mm during first half of luteal phase.[9] At about midluteal phase, the whole endometrium appears thickened and hyperechoic. The endometrial blood flow resistance remains low till the midluteal phase.

At the time of LH surge, the uterine artery resistance also falls to pulsatility index (PI) < 3.2. The RI of the uterine artery flow is 0.88 ± 0.04 till day 13 of the 28-day menstrual cycle.[10] It is due to postovulatory drop in serum estradiol concentration that leads to increased resistance in uterine artery, 3 days after LH peak with highest resistance on day 16.[11,12] The uterine artery resistance then falls. Low resistance in the uterine artery is maintained till the midluteal phase. In conception cycles, this resistance remains low or keeps on falling further whereas in nonconception cycles, the resistance of the uterine artery increases beyond the midluteal phase, with decreasing progesterone levels.

Though in anovulatory cycles, this fall is not seen and there is persistent rise in the uterine artery RI.[8] Blood flow to the endometrium, which is by spiral arteries, follows a similar pattern as the uterine arteries but shows a lower resistance and lower velocity than the uterine arteries.[13]

■ BASELINE SCAN

Monitoring of the uterus and endometrium also starts in early proliferative phase, days 2-3 of the cycle along with the baseline scan of the ovaries. Doppler of the uterine artery is an important part of this assessment. Uterine artery RI > 0.79 indicates that high doses of stimulation will be required for endometrial maturation.[14] On day 2, ovaries are silent, estrogen and progesterone levels are very low, and therefore no endometrial vascularity is expected normally. If endometrium is thick or flow is present, it is either high basal estrogen or high progesterone or inflammation of the endometrium leading to increased vascularity. High estrogen may be seen in polycystic ovarian syndrome patients or in patients with early recruitment of the follicle which can be confirmed by scanning the ovaries. High progesterone may be due to residual active corpus luteum that can be confirmed by ovarian scan showing corpus luteum with low-resistance blood flow. In both cases, endometrial-myometrial junction is intact but the endometrium shows vascularity.

B-MODE FEATURES OF ENDOMETRIUM WITH GOOD RECEPTIVITY

Endometrial growth does not significantly differ in stimulated and nonstimulated cycles. However, in clomiphene citrate (CC)-stimulated cycle, the endometrial thickness may increase only during late proliferative phase, because of release of estrogen receptors. But in gonadotropin-stimulated cycles, the endometrial thickness is greater than in spontaneous cycles.[15] Growth rate of endometrial thickness in stimulated cycles:

- *Days 7–9 of stimulation:* 1.9 mm
- *Days 9–11:* 0.9 mm
- *Day 11 till human chorionic gonadotropin (hCG):* 0.6 mm
- *hCG to embryo transfer (ET):* 0.5 mm

On TVS, an endometrial thickness of 6 mm is considered minimum that is required on the day of trigger for a successful outcome, although 8 mm is generally considered optimum.[16] Even when pregnancy occurs with endometrial thickness of 6–8 mm on the day of trigger, the rates of preclinical miscarriage (biochemical pregnancy) and clinical miscarriage were 21.9% and 15.6%, respectively, as compared to 0% and 12.9%, respectively, when endometrial thickness was >8 mm.[17] Endometrial thickness has more negative predictive value for implantation.[18] In healthy endometrium, the endometrial-myometrial interface is always seen as a clear hypoechoic halo surrounding the whole endometrium. Breach or irregularity of endometrial-myometrial junction may also be an indication of unhealthy endometrium and therefore poor receptivity.

Morphology of the endometrium is as important as thickness of the endometrium. Morphologically, the endometrium is grade A, when it is a triple line endometrium with echogenicities in the intervening area, not more echogenic than the anterior myometrium **(Fig. 6A)**. The echogenicity is attributed to the development of multiple vessels penetrating in the endometrium producing multiple tissue interfaces, stromal edema, or secretions in endometrial glands[19] and due to glycogen storage in the endometrial columnar epithelium. The endometrium is graded as grade B when it is multilayered with severely hypoechoic **(Fig. 6B)** or almost anechoic intervening area. Grade C endometrium is homogeneous isoechoic (isoechoic to myometrium) endometrium[20] **(Fig. 6C)**. All these morphologies indicate estrogen dominated endometrium.

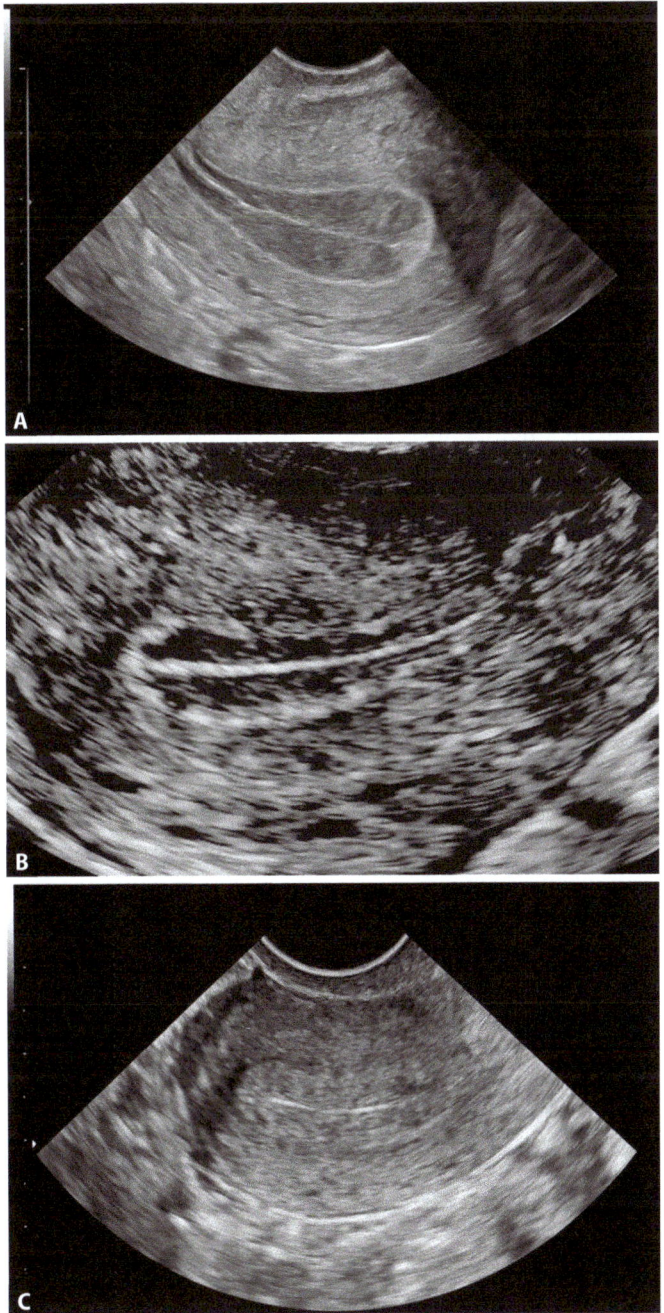

Figs. 6A to C: (A) Grade A endometrium on 2D US; (B) Grade B endometrium on 2D US; (C) Grade C endometrium on 2D US.

■ DOPPLER FEATURES OF RECEPTIVE ENDOMETRIUM

For Doppler evaluation of the endometrium, the color/power Doppler box should include the entire length of endometrium with minimal surrounding myometrium. Magnification is important and the Doppler setting (PRF 0.3, consistently, wall filter low, gains consistent) should be optimized to ensure maximal sensitivity for blood flow.

There are several reports by different groups[21] that agree on the fact that implantation rates can be more correlated to the vascularity of the endometrium rather than the thickness and morphology of the endometrium. Segmental uterine artery perfusion demonstrates significant correlation with hormonal and histological markers of uterine receptivity, reaching the highest sensitivity for subendometrial blood flow.[22] The endometrial neoangiogenesis differs in natural and stimulated cycles. In stimulated cycles, there may be 35% decrease in endometrial and subendometrial vascularity.[23]

On Color Doppler, the endometrium which has vascularity in zones 3 and 4 or in subendometrial and endometrial layers has been reported to have a high degree of endometrial receptivity. The zones of vascularity are defined according to Applebaum as:[24]

- *Zone 1*, when the vascularity on power Doppler is seen only at endometrial-myometrial junction
- *Zone 2*, when vessels penetrate through the hyperechogenic endometrial edge
- *Zone 3*, when vessels reach intervening hypoechogenic zone **(Fig. 7A)**
- *Zone 4*, when vessels reach the endometrial cavity (the central endometrial line) **(Fig. 7B)**

The pregnancy rates related to the zones of vascular penetration during in vitro fertilization (IVF) were 26.7% for zone 1, 36.4% for zone 2, and 37.9% for zone 3.[25] Another comparative study has also shown similar results with pregnancy rates for zones 1, 2, 3, and 4 of 5.2%, 28.7%, 52%, and 74%, respectively.[25]

Zaidi et al. have shown that absent subendometrial and intraendometrial vascularization on the day of trigger appears to be a useful predictor of failure of implantation in IVF, irrespective of morphological appearance.[19] Endometrial and subendometrial vascularization may serve as a prognostic marker for ongoing pregnancy, unlike any other markers of endometrial receptivity.

The vessels that reach the endometrium covering ≥ 5 mm^2 area of the endometrium are reported to be a good prognostic factor.[26] Those women with an intraendometrial power Doppler area (EPDA) <5 mm^2 achieved a significantly lower pregnancy rate (23.5% vs. 47.5%, $p = 0.021$) and implantation rate (8.1% vs. 20.2%, $p = 0.003$) than those with an EPDA >5 mm^2.[27]

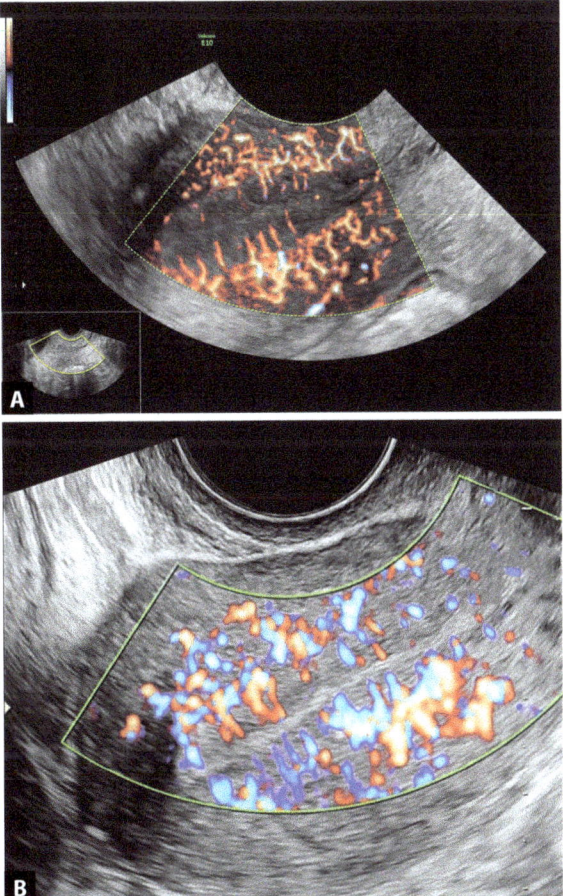

Figs. 7A and B: (A) Power Doppler image of the endometrium in midsagittal plane, showing zone 3 vascularity; (B) HD flow Doppler image of the endometrium in midsagittal plane, showing zone 4 vascularity.

The pulse Doppler of these arteries indicating RI between 0.49 and 0.59 and PI between 1.1 and 2.3 has also been reported to be a good prognostic factor.[28]

UTERINE ARTERY DOPPLER

Pulse Doppler analysis of the uterine artery waveform is also reported to be predictive of endometrial receptivity with its PI <3.2 being desirable.

Several authors have shown that the optimum uterine receptivity was obtained when average PI of the uterine artery was between 2 and 3 on the day of transfer or on the day of trigger.[29,30] Coulam et al. and Cacciatore et al. have also reported that no pregnancy was achieved after ET when uterine artery PI was above 3.3 in an IVF program.[31,32]

In our data of >1,000 IUI cycles, when color Doppler studies were done 12 hours before trigger injection, no conceptions were documented when uterine artery PI >3.5.[33,34] The hypothesis is that the high-resistance blood flow in the uterine artery may lead to higher resistance flow in endometrial vessels and inadequate endometrial estrogen priming and oxygenation and causes low implantation rates.

Doppler study for uterine receptivity should be done on the day of trigger on the dominant side, as LH surge induces significant increase in the resistance of uterine artery for 48 hours which can affect its evaluation on the day of follicular aspiration/rupture.[14,35]

3D AND 3D PD FEATURES OF GOOD ENDOMETRIAL RECEPTIVITY

The correlation of IVF outcome with 3D US volume of the endometrium has been reported to be better than with endometrial thickness.[34] It has been reported that pregnancy and implantation rates were significantly lower when endometrial volume was 1-2 mL[28,36] (**Fig. 8**). In IVF population, no pregnancy was observed in the group with endometrial volume of <2 cc on the day of ovulation trigger.[34,37] The pregnancy rates were 16.7%, 47%, and 62%, respectively, when the endometrial volume was 2-3, 3-5, and 5-7 cm³, respectively.

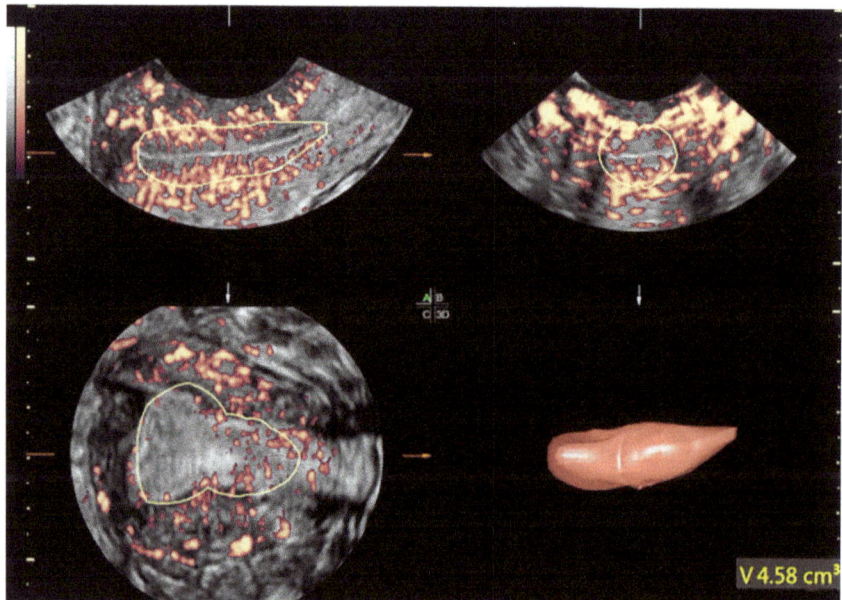

Fig. 8: 3D ultrasound power Doppler image of the endometrium with VOCAL calculated endometrium volume.

While there is no consensus regarding the role of 3D power Doppler indices in predicting endometrial receptivity, a study by Kupesic et al.[28] reported a subendometrial ad FI (flow index) of <11 on the day of ET as a cutoff level for predicting poor implantation. FI is a 3D power Doppler vascular index that speaks about average intensity of the flow in the defined volume. No pregnancies occurred when FI was <11 and the conception group showed FI of 13.2 ± 22. As there are conflicting reports, the routine application of 3D power Doppler indices for predicting endometrial receptivity in women undergoing assisted reproduction treatment currently is limited.

3D/4D ultrasound allows visualization of coronal plane of uterus and has been recommended by some researchers to identify the point of maximum implantation potential (MIP) within the endometrium.[38] ETs at the MIP were reported to be associated with good implantation and pregnancy rates. The MIP point is an intersection of two lines that are drawn parallel to both cornua on a mid-coronal section of uterus. This was hypothesized as the MIP point, as this point of endometrium is in the trajectory line when the embryo falls into the uterus during the process of natural conception and is thought to be the thickest and having the greatest blood flow.[39]

CONCLUSION

Endometrial monitoring with Doppler may be a tool that may unveil some of the mysteries of implantation failure. Volume assessment for endometrium may add a new dimension to this understanding as with 3D power Doppler it gives idea about the global vascularity of endometrium. Though larger studies and standardization of ultrasound parameters and settings are required to establish more precise values for follicular and endometrial VI, FI, and VFI, the results are fairly promising.

KEY POINTS

- Endometrial scanning if done with color Doppler flow gives an extra insight about the implantation potential and future pregnancies continuation. Though we need good and large RCTs.
- An applebaum uterine scoring system are good way of predicting the good ART outcome.
- A good 3D 4D ultrasound is good enough to assist the uterine cavity and excludes the need of routine hysteroscopy.

REFERENCES

1. Leone FP, Timmerman D, Bourne T, Valentin L, Epstein E, Goldstein SR, et al. Terms, definitions and measurements to describe the sonographic features of the endometrium and intrauterine lesions: a consensus opinion from the

International Endometrial Tumor Analysis (IETA) Group. Ultrasound Obstet Gynecol. 2010;35:103-12.
2. Richman TS, Viscomi GN, Cherney AD, Polan A. Fallopian tubal patency assessment by ultrasound following fluid injection. Radiology. 1984;152:507-10.
3. Van den Bosch T, Dueholm M, Leone FPG, Valentin L, Rasmussen CK, Votino A, et al. Terms, definitions and measurements to describe sonographic features of myometrium and uterine masses: a consensus opinion from the Morphological Uterus Sonographic Assessment (MUSA) group. UOG. 2015;46(5): 284-98.
4. Bakos O, Lundkvist O, Bergh T. Transvaginal sonographic evaluation of endometrial growth and texture in spontaneous ovulatory cycles—a descriptive study. Hum Reprod. 1993;8:799-806.
5. Ijland MM, Evers JLH, Dunselman GAJ, van Katwijk C, Lo CR, Hoogland HJ. Endometrial wavelike movements during menstrual cycle. Fertil Steril. 1996;65:746-9.
6. Rainne-Fenning NJ, Campbell BK, Kendall NR, Clewes JS, Johnson IR. Quantifying the changes in endometrial vascularity throughout the normal menstrual cycle with three-dimensional power Doppler angiography. Hum Reprod. 2004:19:330-8.
7. Killam AP, Rosenfeld C, Battaglia FC, Makowski EL, Meschia G. Effect of oestrogens on the uterine blood flow in oophorectomized ewes. Am J Obstet Gynecol. 1973:115;1045-50.
8. Bald R, Hackeloer BJ. Ultrasound imaging of different endometrial forms. In: Otto R, Jan FX (Eds). Ultrasound diagnostics 1982. Stuttgart: Thieme; 1983. p. 187.
9. Randall JM, Fisk MM, McTavish A, Templeton AA. Transvaginal ultrasonic assessment of endometrial growth in spontaneous and hyperstimulated menstrual cycles. Br J Obstet Gynecol. 1989;96:954-9.
10. Kurjak A, Kupesic-Urek S, Schulman H, Zalud I. Transvaginal colour Doppler in the assessment of ovarian and uterine blood flow in infertile women. Fertil Steril.1991:56:870.
11. Goswamy RK, Steptoe PC. Doppler ultrasound studies of the uterine artery in spontaneous ovarian cycles. Hum Reprod. 1988;3:721-5.
12. Sholtes MCW, Wladimiroff JW, van Rijen HJM, Hop WCI. Uterine and ovarian flow velocity wave forms in the normal menstrual cycle: a transvaginal study. Fertil Steril. 1989;52:981-5.
13. Andreotti RF, Thompson GH, Janowitz W. Endovaginal and transabdominal sonography of ovarian follicle. J Ultrasound Med. 1989;8:555.
14. Bassil S. Magritte IP. Roth J, Nisolle M, Donnez J, Gordts S. Uterine vascularity during stimulation and its correlation with implantation in in-vitro fertilization. Hum Reprod. 1995;10:1497-501.
15. Yagel S, Ben-Chetrit A, Anteby E, Zacut D, Hochner-Celnikier D, Ron M. The effect of ethinyl estradiol on endometrial thickness and uterine volume during ovulation induction by clomiphene citrate. Fertil Steril. 1992;57:33-6.
16. Dickey RP, Olar TT, Taylor SN, Curole DN, Harrigill K. Relationship of biochemical pregnancy to preovulatory endometrial thickness and pattern in patients undergoing ovulation induction. Hum Reprod. 1993;8:327-30.
17. Boue J, Boue A, Lazar P. Retrospective and prospective epidemiological studies of 1500 karyotyped spontaneous human abortions. Tetralogy. 1975;12:11-26.

18. Weissman A, Gotlieb L, Casper RF. The detrimental effect of increased endometrial thickness on implantation and pregnancy rates and outcome in an in vitro fertilization program. Fertil Steril. 1999:71:147-9.
19. Fleischer AC, Kepple DM. Benign conditions of the uterus, cervix, and endometrium. In: Nyberg DA, Hill LM, Bohm-Velez, Mendelson EB (Eds). Transvaginal ultrasound. St. Louis: Mosby Year Book; 1992. pp. 21-43.
20. Smith B, Porter R, Ahuja K, Craft I. Ultrasonic assessment of endometrial changes in stimulated cycles in an in vitro fertilization and embryo transfer program. J In Vitro Fert Embryo Transf. 1984;1:233-8.
21. Zaidi J, Campbell S, Pittrof R, Tan SL. Endometrial thickness, morphology, vascular penetration and velocimetry in predicting implantation in an in vitro fertilization program. Ultrasound Obstet Gynecol. 1995;6:191-8.
22. Kupesic S, Kurjak A. Prediction of IVF outcome by three-dimensional ultrasound. Hum Reprod. 2002;17:950-5.
23. Ng EH, Chan CC, Tang OS, Yeung WS, Ho PC. Comparison of endometrial and subendometrial blood flow measured by three-dimensional power Doppler ultrasound between stimulated and natural cycles in the same patients. Hum Reprod. 2004;19:2385-90.
24. Applebaum M. The 'steel' or 'teflon' endometrium-ultrasound visualization of endometrial vascularity in IVF patients and outcome. Presented at the third World Congress of Ultrasound in Obstetrics and Gynaecology. Ultrasound Obstet Gynecol. 1993;3(Suppl 2):10.
25. Merce IT, Barco MJ, Bau S, Troyano JM. Prediction of ovarian response and IVF/ICSI outcome by three-dimensional ultrasonography and power Doppler angiography. Eur J Obstet Gynecol Reprod Biol. 2007;132:93-100.
26. Yang JH, Wu MY, Chen CD, Jiang MC, Ho HN, Yang YS. Association of endometrial blood flow as determined by a modified colour Doppler technique with subsequent outcome of in vitro fertilization. Hum Reprod. 1999;14:1606-10.
27. Merce LT, Barco MJ, Bau S, Troyano JM. Are endometrial parameters by three-dimensional ultrasound and power Doppler angiography related to in vitro fertilization/embryo transfer outcome? Fertil Steril. 2008;89(1):111-7.
28. Kupesic S, Bekavac I, Bjelos D, Kurjak A. Assessment of endometrial receptivity by transvaginal colour Doppler and three-dimensional power Doppler ultrasonography in patients undergoing in vitro fertilization procedures. J Ultrasound Med. 2001;20:125-34.
29. Steer CV, Campbell S, Tan SL, Crayford T, Mills C, Mason BA, et al. The use of transvaginal colour flow imaging after in vitro fertilization to identify optimum uterine conditions before embryo transfer. Fertil Steril. 1992:57:372-6.
30. Zaidi J, Pittrof R, Shaker A, Kyei-Mensah A, Campbell S, Tan SL. Assessment of uterine artery blood flow on the day of human chorionic gonadotrophin administration by transvaginal colour Doppler ultrasound in an in vitro fertilization program. Fertil Steril. 1996;65:377-81.
31. Coulam CB, Stern JJ, Soenksen DM, Britten S, Bustillo M. Comparison of pulsatility indexes on the day of oocyte retrieval and embryo transfer. Hum Reprod. 1995:10:82-4.
32. Cacciatore B, Simberg N, Fusaro P, Titinen A. Transvaginal Doppler study of uterine artery blood flow in in vitro fertilization embryo transfer cycles. Fertil Steril. 1996,66:130-4.

33. Salle B, Bied-Damon V, benchalb M, Desperes S. Gaucherand P, Rudigoz RC. Preliminary report of an ultrasonography and colour Doppler uterine score to predict uterine receptivity in an IVF programme. Hum Reprod. 1998:13(6):1669-73.
34. Panchal SY, Nagori CB. Can 3D PD be a better tool for assessing the pre-HCG follicle and endometrium? A randomized study of 500 cases. Presented at 16th World Congress on Ultrasound in Obstetrics and Gynecology, 2006, London. J Ultrasound Obstet Gynecol. 2006:28:504.
35. Wittmack FM, Kreger DO, Blasco L, Tureck RW, Mastroianni L Jr, Lessey BA. Effect of follicular size on oocyte retrieval, fertilization, cleavage and embryo quality in in vitro fertilization cycles: a 6 year data collection. Fertil Steril. 1994:62:1205-10.
36. Raga F, Bonilla-Musoles F, Casan EM, Klein O, Bonilla F. Assessment of endometrial volume by three-dimensional ultrasound prior to embryo transfer: clues to endometrial receptivity. Hum Reprod. 1999;14:2851-4.
37. Panchal SY, Nagori CB. Role of 3D and 3D power Doppler to assess endometrial receptivity. IJIFM. 2010:1:19-24.
38. Gergely RZ, DeUgrate CM, Danzer H, Surrey M, Hill D, DeCherney AH. Three-dimensional/four dimensional ultrasound guided embryo transfer using the maximal implantation potential point. Fertil Steril. 2005;84:500-3.
39. Tang Y, Fisendahi C. An Update on Experimental Therapeutic Strategies for Thin Endometrium. Endocrines. 2023;4(4):672-84.

Section 4

Ovulation Induction/Ovarian Stimulation—Armamentarium of Ovulogens

- **Selective Estrogen Receptor Modulators: Clomiphene Citrate and Tamoxifen**
  Sujata Kar, Megha Gupta
- **Aromatase Inhibitors**
  Rekha Pillai, Hazel Mehlawat, Meenakshi Choudhary
- **Gonadotropins: Follicle-stimulating Hormone, Luteinizing Hormone, and Human Menopausal Gonadotropin**
  Rishma Dhillon Pai, Unnati Mamtora, Arnav Hrishikesh Pai

Chapter 7

Selective Estrogen Receptor Modulators: Clomiphene Citrate and Tamoxifen

Sujata Kar, Megha Gupta

HISTORY OF SELECTIVE ESTROGEN RECEPTOR MODULATORS

"These are my Clomid babies"—It was a blessing to hear from people about Mr Palopoli's accomplishments, when the drug clomiphene citrate (CC) was born and, therefore, so were many children. Frank Palopoli, a chemist, and his team of researchers invented Clomid in 1965. His efforts have put clomiphene on the World Health Organization's list of essential medicines. Oral contraception, ovulation induction, and treatment of specific estrogen-dependent tumor types were anticipated clinical applications.

Merrell had his initial conversations with clinical investigators during the April 1960 sessions of the American Society for the Study of Sterility (ASSS), which is now known as the American Society of Reproductive Medicine (ASRM), in Cincinnati, Ohio. In 1960, clinical research got underway.

The first human clinical test findings for clomiphene, then known as MRL-41, were published in the Journal of the American Medical Association (JAMA) in October 1961 by Greenblatt et al. The authors concluded, "Although the mechanism of action of this compound is not clear at the present time, it is heartening to find a drug which holds much promise of inducing ovulatory type menses with considerable regularity in anovulatory women."

On February 1, 1967, the US Food and Drug Administration (FDA) approved the sale and marketing of CC (Clomid) for the "treatment of ovulatory dysfunction in women desiring pregnancy".

One pharmaceutical product whose present use is the outcome of the combined and sequential research efforts of industry, government, university, and private practice physicians is CC. It has been 40 years since the chemical synthesis was initially created, and 36 years since the initial clinical studies were conducted.

The noble goal of chemoprevention has been attained in the fight against breast cancer. However, in the 1930s, therapeutic expertise was lacking; therefore, it was unable to progress in humans. More than 20 years would pass until the first antiestrogens were documented, in the late 1950s. When the first nonsteroidal antiestrogen, MER25, was discovered in 1958, the nonsteroidal antiestrogens had little clinical effect for the first 10 years. The early chemicals were investigated in the laboratory as antifertility drugs, but clomiphene worked the opposite way in people, and subfertile women were effectively induced to ovulate. This medical advancement paved the way for later discoveries in molecular pharmacology and pharmaceuticals during the second half of the 20th century. Since clomiphene was used to induce ovulation in healthy women, its endocrine system was extensively studied. However, toxicological concerns hindered the development of additional drugs for potential uses in women's health, such as the prevention and treatment of breast cancer. Next came tamoxifen, also known as ICI 46474. The treatment of metastatic breast cancer in postmenopausal women and the inducement of ovulation in infertile women proved safe and efficient based on preliminary clinical research, which consequently prolonged the lives of millions of women worldwide.

A cluster of translational studies focused on the uterus, breast (mammary gland), and bone together created the data base for further confirmatory studies and the clinical trials by the pharmaceutical industry that resulted in the reinvention of the failed breast cancer drug keoxifene to become raloxifene the first clinically available selective estrogen receptor modulator (SERM) to prevent both osteoporosis and breast cancer **(Fig. 1)**.

WHAT ARE SELECTIVE ESTROGEN RECEPTOR MODULATORS?

About 40 years ago, the first descriptions of hormone receptors—more especially, estrogen receptors—were given. There are two receptors for estrogens: (1) estrogen receptor β (ERβ) and (2) estrogen receptor alpha (ERα). The two receptors have distinct gene codes, and various organs express them differently in their tissues. ERβ is found in several tissues including bone, endothelium, lungs, urogenital tract, ovaries, central nervous system, and prostate. ERα is mostly expressed in reproductive tissues (uterus, breast, and ovaries), also in liver and central nervous system. There have been around seventy SERMs class compounds reported so far. Tetraphenylethylene, benzothiophenes, tetrahedron-acetylenes, indoles, and benzopyrans are the five chemical groups. These nonhormonal substances can all activate the endoplasmic reticulum (ER), lower the rate of bone turnover, and, as an antiresorptive, demonstrably increase bone density.

CLASSIFICATION OF SELECTIVE ESTROGEN RECEPTOR MODULATORS

Classification of SERMs is described in **Table 1**.

USES OF SELECTIVE ESTROGEN RECEPTOR MODULATORS

Uses of SERMs are given in **Table 2**.

CHAPTER 7: Selective Estrogen Receptor Modulators: Clomiphene...

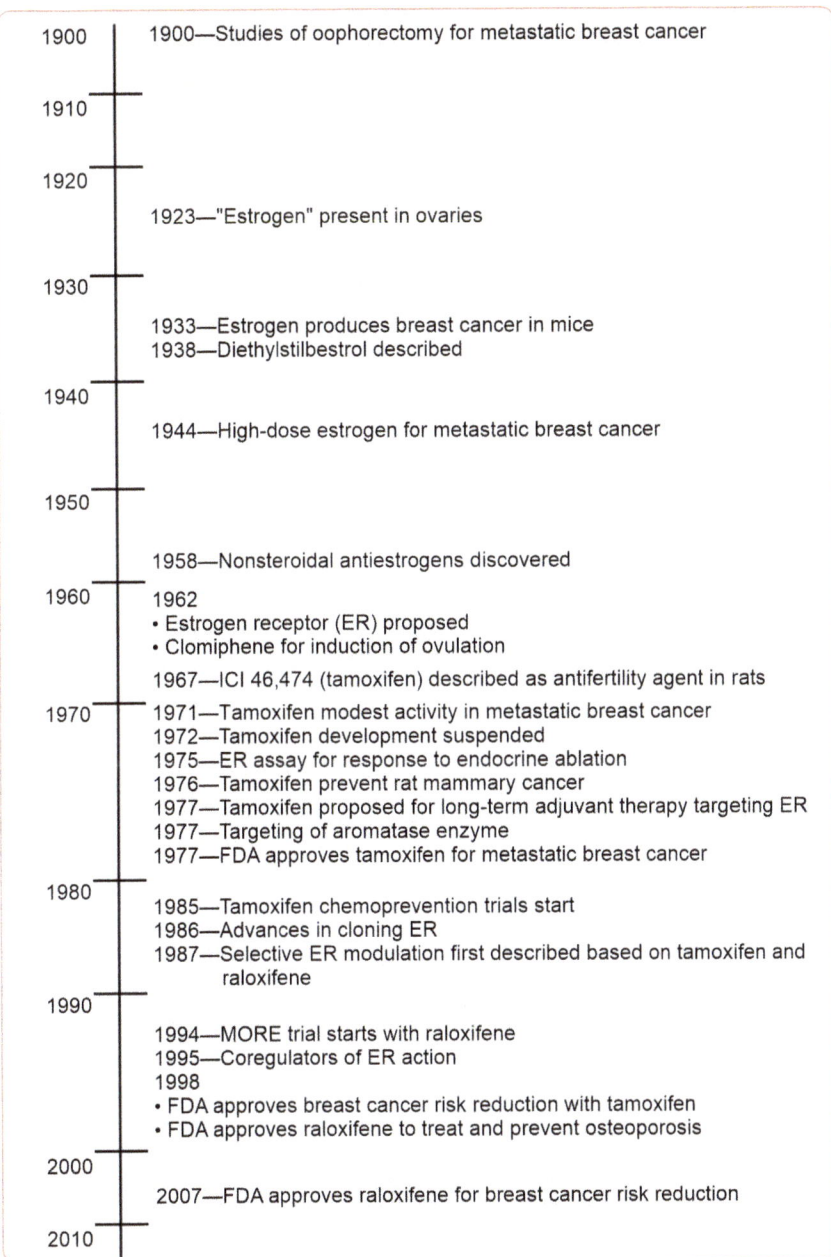

Fig. 1: Evolution of selective estrogen receptor modulators (SERMs).

Clomiphene Citrate

Clomiphene citrate has been the most widely used in treatment for fertility enhancement for the past 40 years. Clomiphene was a revolutionary advancement in reproductive medicine and quickly became popular for

TABLE 1: Classification of SERMs.

Pharmacological group	Generic drug
Triphenylethylene derivatives	Clomiphene, tamoxifen, toremifene, ospemifene (1271a), droloxifene, idoxifene, TAT-59, and GW5638
Other nonsteroidal compounds	EM-800, EM-652, raloxifene, arzoxifene, LY353381 (SERM3), LY 357489
Naphthalenes	Lasofoxifene (CP 336, 156)
Benzopyrans	Ormeloxifene, levormeloxifene, EM-800 (SCH 57050)
Findoles	Pipendoxifenes (ERA-923), Bazedoxifenes (TSE-424, WAY-140424)
Steroidal compounds	IC1182, 780 (Fulvestrant)

(SERMs: selective estrogen receptor modulators)

TABLE 2: Uses of SERMs.

Triphenylethylene derivatives	Antitumor activity and antiestrogenic
Nonsteroidal compounds	Prevention and treatment of osteoporosis
Naphthalenes	Prevention of osteoporosis and vaginal atrophy
Benzopyrans	Nonsteroidal oral contraceptive
Findoles	Antitumor activity
Steroidal compounds	Antitumor activity

(SERMs: selective estrogen receptor modulators)

induction of ovulation because of its ease of administration and minimal side effects.

Chemically speaking, CC is a derivative of nonsteroidal triphenylethylene and, like other similar compounds (e.g., tamoxifen), it can act as an estrogen agonist or antagonist, depending on the degree of endogenous estrogen that is present **(Fig. 2)**. Only very low endogenous estrogen levels cause the features of an estrogen agonist to become apparent. If not, CC just has antiestrogen properties.

Pharmacokinetics of Clomiphene Citrate

Clomiphene is excreted in stool after being cleared by the liver; 85% of a dose taken is normally gone after 6 days, while remnants may linger in the blood for much longer. As it is now prescribed, CC is a racemic combination of two separate stereoisomers with distinctive characteristics, zuclomiphene and enclomiphene. The research that is now available suggests that the more potent isomer, enclomiphene, is mainly responsible for CC's ability to induce ovulation. After being administered, enclomiphene levels rise quickly and quickly drop to undetectable quantities.

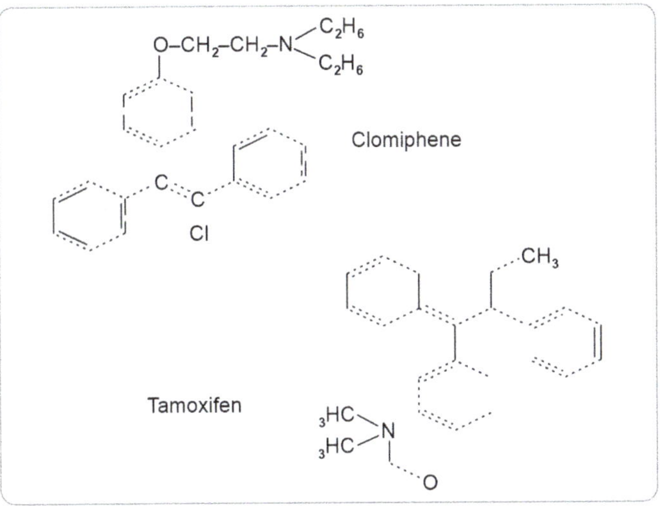

Fig. 2: Chemical structure of SERMs. (SERMs: selective estrogen receptor modulators)

Mechanism of Action

Clomiphene: It works by altering feedback mechanisms in the hypothalamic and pituitary ovarian axis by occupying estrogen receptors.[1] Because of their structural resemblance to estrogen, clomiphene and endogenous estrogen can compete for nuclear estrogen receptors at various reproductive system locations. But unlike estrogen, clomiphene attaches to nuclear estrogen receptors and stays there for a long period, interfering with the recycling of the receptor and lowering receptor concentrations.

Because estrogen receptor depletion obscures the interpretation of circulating estrogen levels at the hypothalamus level, circulating estrogen levels are misinterpreted as being lower than they actually are. Decreased negative feedback from estrogen stimulates natural counterregulatory processes that change the pattern of gonadotropin-releasing hormone (GnRH) production and enhance the release of gonadotropin from the pituitary, which in turn promotes the growth of ovarian follicles.

Clomiphene may potentially enhance gonadotrophs' sensitivity to GnRH activation at the pituitary level. Clomiphene elevates GnRH pulse frequency in ovulatory women. Clomiphene only increases pulse amplitude in anovulatory women with polycystic ovarian syndrome (PCOS). Serum levels of follicle-stimulating hormone (FSH) and luteinizing hormone (LH) increase while on clomiphene medication and then quickly return to baseline levels following the standard 5-day course of treatment. All things considered, the main way that clomiphene acts is by promoting the hypothalamus pituitary-ovarian feedback axis.

Indications:
- Clomiphene citrate is the drug of choice for ovulation induction in anovulatory subfertile women with normal thyroid function, normal serum prolactin levels, and normal endogenous estrogen production or a normal menstrual response to a progestin challenge (WHO Group II) with—normal tubal function and normal semen analysis.
- *Luteal phase deficiency:* Progesterone levels are typically higher after CC treatment than in spontaneous cycles, reflecting improved preovulatory follicle and corpus luteum development.
- *Unexplained infertility:* CC may be justified, particularly in young couples with short duration of infertility and in those unwilling or unable to pursue more aggressive therapies involving greater costs, risks, and logical demands.
- *Hypothalamic/pituitary dysfunction:* In PCOS, CC is the first line of treatment for ovulation induction.
- *Intrauterine insemination (IUI)/in vitro fertilization (IVF):* CC is now being used as an important drug for mild stimulation IVF.
- *Endometriosis:* CC is the choice of drug for ovulation induction in young women with stage 1 or 2 endometriosis.

Patient Selection Criteria for Clomiphene Treatment
- Patients with following conditions are not suitable for clomifene citrate.
- Hypersensitivity to clomiphene citrate or components of the formulation
- Pregnancy
- Breastfeeding
- History of hepatic impairment
- Hepatic disease
- Abnormal uterine bleeding
- Uncontrolled adrenal dysfunction
- Non-PCOS-related ovarian cyst
- Organic intracranial lesions
- Uncontrolled thyroid disease
- Pituitary tumor
- Risk of hypertriglyceridemia
- Endometrial cancer

Adverse Effects
Treatment with clomiphene is typically well tolerated.

The following minor side effects are rather common:
- Transient hot flushes, which happen in 10–20% of cases.
- Swings in mood are also somewhat common.
- Headache, breast discomfort, pelvic pressure or pain, and nausea are some milder and less frequent adverse effects.

- Although reports of persistent "afterimages" (palinopsia) and light sensitivity (photophobia) make visual disturbances (blurred or double vision, scotomata, and light sensitivity) uncommon (1-2%) and reversible, they are nonetheless unsettling, and treatment should be stopped when such symptoms appear.
- Antiestrogenic action on the cervix and endometrial

Risks and Complications

Clomiphene treatment has risks, but serious complications are rare.
- *Multiple pregnancy:* The risks for multiple pregnancy is approximately 8% (10-20%) due to multifollicular development
- *Birth defects:* There is no proof that taking clomiphene raises the chance of any one type of aberration or birth abnormalities in general. Furthermore, there is no proof that giving birth to a child while on clomiphene therapy raises the child's risk of learning disabilities or developmental delays.
- *Miscarriage:* Some research has reported that the rate of spontaneous miscarriage in pregnancies treated with clomiphene may be higher than in pregnancies conceived naturally, although other studies have found no difference in miscarriage rates.
- *Ovarian hyperstimulation syndrome (OHSS):* Mild OHSS (moderate ovarian enlargement) is relatively common, severe OHSS (massive ovarian enlargement, progressive weight gain, severe abdominal pain, nausea and vomiting, hypovolemia, ascites, and oliguria) rarely occurs.
- *Ovarian cancer:* Patients with concerns should be counseled that no causal relationship between ovulation inducing drugs and ovarian cancer has yet been established and no change in prescribing practices is warranted.[2] In any case, prolonged treatment with CC is generally futile and should, therefore, be avoided **(Table 3)**.

TABLE 3: Indications and contraindications of clomiphene.

Good response	*In patients with:* • Anovulation (e.g., PCOS) • Adequate endogenous estrogen production
Poor response	• FSH ≥ 40 mIU/mL • Low estrogen levels (failure to respond to progesterone challenge)
Contraindications	• Pregnancy • Uncontrolled thyroid/adrenal dysfunction • Organic intracranial lesion • Liver disease/history of liver dysfunction • Abnormal uterine bleeding • Ovarian cysts/enlargement (not PCOS)

(FSH: follicle-stimulating hormone; PCOS: polycystic ovarian syndrome)

COMPARISON BETWEEN SELECTIVE ESTROGEN RECEPTOR MODULATORS FOR OVULATION INDUCTION

Clomiphene versus Tamoxifen

Tamoxifen and CC both work equally well to induce ovulation. Despite the paucity of information on pregnancy outcomes and rates, there does not seem to be a discernible difference between the two medications.[3]

Ovulation Rate and Pregnancy Rate

A recent prospective randomized controlled trial compared the efficacy of tamoxifen with that of CC for ovulation induction in anovulatory women. The overall rates of ovulation and pregnancy were similar in both groups.[4]

Other studies have suggested that tamoxifen may be superior to CC in that it does not appear to have an adverse effect on the endometrium.

Future research could clarify the clinical circumstances in which one medication might be more effective than the other. Tamoxifen has been shown to be successful in the treatment of anovulation, even in patients in whom CC treatment has failed, but it has yet to be tested for superovulation.

Live Birth Rate and Miscarriage Rate

There are no appreciable differences in live birth rate and miscarriage rate after treatment with tamoxifen or clomiphene for subfertile couple with anovulation.

Clomiphene and Raloxifene

No statistically significant difference in ovulation was observed between raloxifene and CC in patients with PCOS with ovulatory dysfunction.[5]

TREATMENT PROTOCOLS

Clomiphene Citrate

Standard Therapy

Starting on the 3rd to 5th day following the start of spontaneous or progestin-induced menses, CC is taken orally. Regardless of whether therapy starts on cycle day 2, 3, 4, or 5, ovulation rates, conception rates, and pregnancy outcomes are identical in anovulatory women. Even though the amount needed to induce ovulation correlates with body weight, it is impossible to determine with any degree of accuracy what a given woman will require. As a result, using CC to induce ovulation is similar to doing an empirical incremental titration to determine the lowest dose that works best for each individual **(Fig. 3)**.

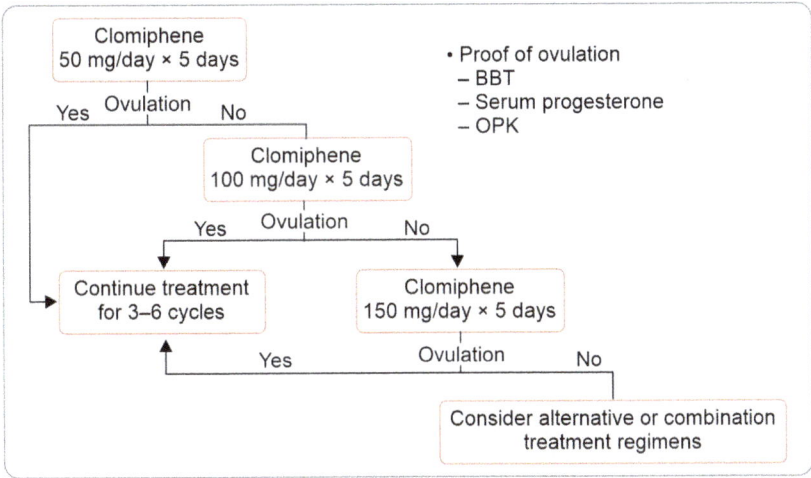

Fig. 3: Dosage schedule of clomiphene citrate. (BBT: basal body temperature; OPK: ovulation predictor kit)

Extended Course Clomiphene Treatment

Longer courses of CC treatment may be helpful for certain CC-resistant anovulatory women who, even at greater dosage levels, do not respond to a typical 5-day treatment schedule. When shorter courses of medication are unsuccessful, an 8-day high-dose treatment regimen (e.g., 200–250 mg/day) may be helpful.

Stair Step Protocol

It is believed that Hurst et al.'s 2009[6] innovative clomiphene stair step procedure may shorten the time it takes for ovulation in people with PCOS.

On the 2nd day following spontaneous or progestogen-induced withdrawal bleeding, 50 mg of clomiphene was administered for 5 days. Days 11–14 are spent doing TVS. A week following the initial TVS on day 21, USG is performed again, and 100 mg of clomiphene is started right away for 5 days if there is no response (no follicle larger than 10 mm). If there is no improvement, 150 mg of clomiphene is started again right away and given for 5 days. One week following the second U/S (on day 28), a USG is done. TVS follicular monitoring confirmed ovulation for the stair-step cycles. A mature follicle is thought to be 18–24 mm in size.

Traditional Protocol

A conventional strategy can be applied to PCOS patients, starting the clomiphene drug on day 2 following spontaneous or progestin-induced withdrawal bleeding. For the first 5 days in a row, the starting dose was 50 mg/day. The patient received 10 mg of medroxyprogesterone acetate (MPA) for 10 days if there was no response. In the following cycle, CC dosages were raised by 50 mg per day, for a total of three treatment cycles. From days 11 to 14 of every cycle, TVS monitored the growth of follicles. The endpoint was the first ovulation, and the follow-up period was three treatment cycles (up to 150 mg). Using TVS monitoring of follicle growth, ovulation was evaluated. A mature follicle is thought to be 18–24 mm in size.

The CC is also used in mild IVF cycle where it can be used alone or in combination with gonadotropins.

Mild Stimulation IVF

A fixed low-dose FSH or human menopausal gonadotropin (hMG) (up to 150 IU/day) is administered in a GnRH antagonist cotreatment cycle. The treatment cycle is monitored by TVS or by serum estradiol measurements. Antiestrogens like CC were used for ovarian stimulation in IVF either alone or in combination with exogenous gonadotropins (with or without GnRH antagonist cotreatment) **(Fig. 4)**. Luteal phase support is given either in the form of human chorionic gonadotropin (hCG) or progesterone.[7]

Kato Protocol

Briefly CC (50-100 mg/day) was administrated orally with an extended regimen from cycle day 3 until the day before inducing final oocyte maturation. hMG or recombinant FSH was added in the form of injections (50-150 IU/every other day) or nasal spray in order to obtain 1-4 mature follicles. Monitoring involving ultrasound scan and hormonal profile

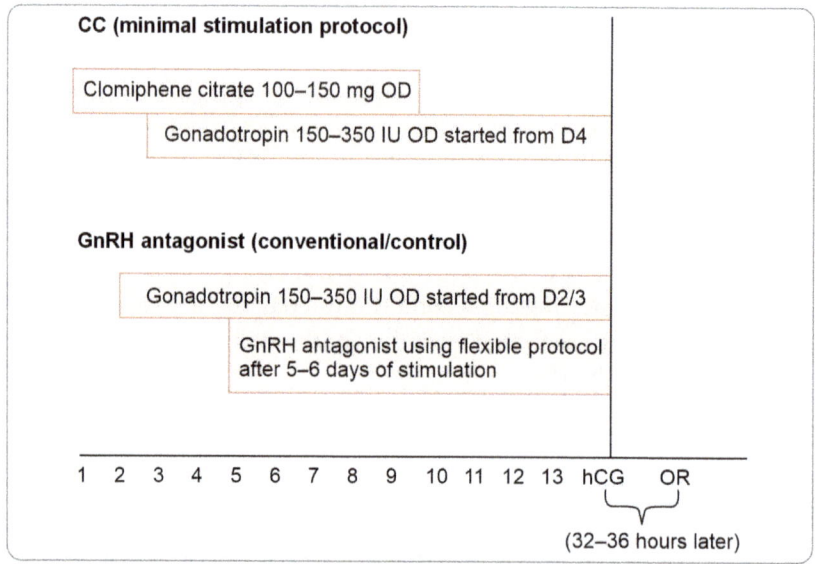

Fig. 4: Minimal stimulation protocol (CC). (CC: clomiphene citrate; GnRH: gonadotropin-releasing hormone; hCG: human chorionic gonadotropin)

(E2, LH, and progesterone) was usually started on day 8 and continued every other day until triggering day. Ovulation triggering was performed with a GnRH agonist, buserelin, 600 µg, administered in a nasal spray form.[8] Cycle was clomiphene based as it efficiently blocks the premature LH surge by its extended regimen until the day of trigger.[9] Oocyte retrieval was usually performed 30-34 hours after triggering.

Shanghai Protocol

Stage 1: Starting on cycle day 3, letrozole 2.5 mg/day and CC 25 mg/day are administered as cotreatments. Before the trigger day, CC is taken constantly and letrozole is only administered for 4 days. On cycle day 6, patients began receiving injections of 150 IU of hMG every other day. Beginning on cycle day 10, follicular monitoring is done every 2-4 days using a TVS to count the number of follicles forming and measure the levels of progesterone, estradiol, LH, and FSH in the serum. Triptorelin 100 g is used to initiate the last stage of oocyte maturation when one or two dominant follicles reach 18 mm in diameter. Ibuprofen 0.6 g is then administered on the triggering day and the following day to avoid potential follicle rupture prior to oocyte retrieval. Oocyte retrieval under TVS guidance took place 32-36 hours after the GnRH agonist was administered. Every follicle smaller than 10 mm was not removed and was instead sent to the luteal phase's second step of stimulation.

Stage 2: After oocyte retrieval, TVS is performed to decide whether to proceed with the second ovarian stimulation. The existence of two or more antral follicles with a diameter of 2-8 mm is required for extended stimulation. On the day of or the day following oocyte retrieval, 225 IU hMG and 2.5 mg of letrozole are given daily. The number of growing follicles and the serum concentrations of FSH, LH, estradiol, and progesterone are recorded during the first round of second stage follicular monitoring, which is carried out 5-7 days later and then every 2-4 days. The administration of letrozole is discontinued upon the dominant follicles' sizes of 12 mm. In cases where postovulation follicle size is less than 14 mm in diameter and stimulation is required for many more days, daily administration of 10 mg of MPA is added starting on stimulation day 12. In order to reduce the possibility of infection from the treatment, menstruation is delayed and oocyte retrieval is avoided during menstruation. The last stage of oocyte maturation is again triggered by injection with 100 g of triptorelin when three dominant follicles had diameters of 18 mm or one mature dominant follicle had diameters more than 20 mm. Ibuprofen 0.6 g is once again given on the day that oocyte maturation is triggered and the day that followed. TVS-guided oocyte retrieval is carried out 36-38 hours following the administration of GnRH agonist.[10] **Figure 5** shows the double stimulation protocol for the luteal and follicular phases.

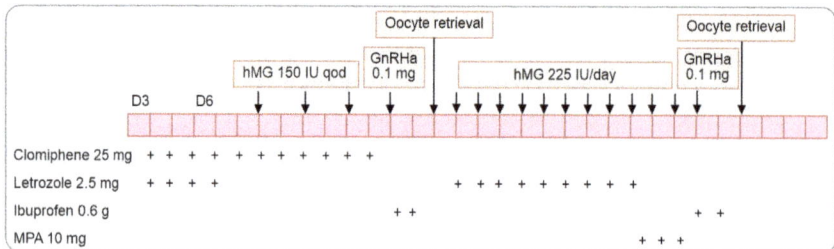

Fig. 5: Shanghai protocol. (GnRHa: gonadotropin-releasing hormone agonist; hMG: human menopausal gonadotropin; MPA: medroxyprogesterone acetate)

Tamoxifen

Tamoxifen can also reduce the estrogen receptivity. The mechanism of tamoxifen in improving folliculogenesis may involve direct action on the ovary without intervention of the hypothalamic-pituitary-adrenal axis.

It is administered orally, starting on the 2nd to 6th day after the onset of spontaneous or progestin-induced menses. It can be used in the dose of 20–80 mg. Transvaginal ultrasound was used for follicular monitoring from day 10 and on every alternate day till the day of ovulation or till the 20th day of the cycle.

Raloxifene

Raloxifene is an oral SERM that induces ovulation in a manner similar to CC.

■ CONCLUSION

Selective estrogen receptor modulators are medications that can both mimic and block estrogen's effects in different tissues. They do this by interacting with estrogen receptors in different cells. SERMs are often used to treat estrogen-related conditions, such as infertility. Most widely used SERM in infertility is CC.

It is a racemic mixture of two stereochemical isomers—zuclomiphene (cis) and enclomiphene (trans) in the ratio of 38% and 62%, respectively. CC is administered orally from early follicular phase of the menstrual cycle in a dose of 50–150 mg daily for 5 days. CC is widely used in anovulatory infertility (PCOS), unexplained infertility, luteal phase defect, and stages 1 and 2 endometriosis. CC is a well-tolerated drug. As such there is no causal relationship between ovulation inducing agent and ovarian cancer. There are various treatment protocols, one promising and recently used protocol is stair step protocol used in anovulatory infertility (PCOS). Various other SERMs have been used for ovulation induction like tamoxifen and raloxifene. No statistically significant difference in ovulation was observed between raloxifene versus CC and tamoxifen versus clomiphene in patients with PCOS with ovulatory dysfunction. CC is also used in mild IVF stimulation protocol. As extended dose of CC efficiently prevents premature LH surge, this action is utilized in ovarian stimulation (e.g., KATO protocol).

■ KEY POINTS

- Selective estrogen receptor modulators are a versatile group of molecules, useful in various scenarios of reproduction.
- Clomiphene citrate has a wide variety of usage in different scenarios starting from anovulation to minimal stimulation and not to mention double stimulation like Shanghai protocol.
- Where clomiphene is not working, other molecules like tamoxifen can be used especially where thickness of the endometrium is a concern.

■ REFERENCES

1. Imani B, Eijkemans MJ, te Velde ER, Habbema JD, Fauser BC. A nomogram to predict the probability of live birth after clomiphene citrate induction of ovulation in normogonadotropic oligoamenorrheic infertility. Fertil Steril. 2002;77:91-7.
2. Impicciatore GG, Tiboni GM. Ovulation inducing agents and cancer risk: review of literature. Curr Drug Saf. 2011;6(4):250-8.
3. Steiner AZ, Terplan M, Paulson RJ. Comparison of tamoxifen and clomiphene citrate for ovulation induction: a meta-analysis. Hum Reprod. 2005;20(6):1511-5.
4. Kar S. Clomiphene citrate or letrozole as first line of ovulation induction drug in infertile PCOS women: a Prospective randomized trial. J Human Reprod Sci. 2012;5(3):262-5.
5. de Paula Guedes Neto E, Savaris RF, von Eye Corleta H, de Moraes GS, do Amaral Cristovam R, Lessey BA. Prospective, randomized comparison between raloxifene and clomiphene citrate for ovulation induction in polycystic ovary syndrome. Fertil Steril. 2011;96(3):769-73.
6. Hurst BS, Hickman JM, Matthews ML, Usadi RS, Marshburn PB. Novel clomiphene "stair-step" protocol reduces time to ovulation in women with polycystic ovarian syndrome. Am J Obstet Gynecol. 2009;200:510.e1-4.
7. Baart EB, Martini E, Eijkemans MJ, Van Opstal D, Beckers NG, Verhoeff A, et al. Milder ovarian stimulation for in vitro fertilization reduces aneuploidy in the human preimplantation embryo: a randomized controlled trial. Hum Reprod. 2007;22(4):980-8.
8. Teramoto S, Kato O. Minimal ovarian stimulation with clomiphene citrate: a large-scale retrospective study. Reprod Biomed Online. 2007;15:134-48.
9. Kawachiya S, Segawa T, Kato K, Takehara Y, Teramoto S, Kato O. The effectiveness of clomiphene citrate in suppressing the LH surge in the minimal stimulation protocol. Fertil Steril. 2006;86(412):751.
10. Kuang Y, Chen Q, Hong Q, Lyu Q, Ai A, Fu Y, et al. Double stimulations during the follicular and luteal phases of poor responders in IVF/ICSI programmes (Shanghai protocol). Reprod Biomed Online. 2014;29:684-91.

Chapter 8

Aromatase Inhibitors

Rekha Pillai, Hazel Mehlawat, Meenakshi Choudhary

■ INTRODUCTION

Ovulatory dysfunction is one of the main causes of female infertility and accounts for about 32% of the cause of female infertility.[1] For over five decades, clomiphene citrate has been the mainstay of management of anovulation and oligo-ovulation followed by more expensive and complicated gonadotropins in clomiphene-resistant patients. Recently, the international evidence-based guideline for the assessment and management of polycystic ovarian syndrome (PCOS) published in 2018 suggested letrozole as the first-line drug for ovulation induction in women with PCOS.[2] Letrozole is a third-line aromatase inhibitor which prevents the conversion of testosterone to estrogen, thereby stopping the negative feedback of estrogen in the hypothalamus.[3] This chapter explores the role of aromatase inhibitors in ovulation induction and details the mechanism of action, pharmacology, and various other indications for its use in reproductive medicine and gynecology.

■ HISTORY

Aminoglutethimide was the first aromatase inhibitor to be licensed in 1981.[4] This was followed by the synthesis of the second-generation aromatase inhibitor fadrozole and third-generation aromatase inhibitor letrozole in 1996.[3] Following extensive research demonstrating its beneficial effects, letrozole was widely used for the treatment of advanced breast cancer.[4] Anastrozole is another third-generation aromatase inhibitor which is currently in wide use. Its use has been extended to the management of various conditions in pediatrics and gynecology, including managing anovulation.[4]

■ MECHANISM OF ACTION

The enzyme aromatase catalyzes the conversion of androstenedione and testosterone to estrone and estradiol, respectively. Inhibition of the enzyme will block estrogen production from all sources and stop the estrogen-mediated negative feedback on the hypothalamic–pituitary axis without depletion of the estrogen receptors. This will increase the gonadotropin secretion and stimulate follicular growth. On the other hand, clomiphene acts by blocking and depleting the estrogen receptors.[5]

The decrease in estrogen production increases the secretion of activins which is produced from a wide variety of tissues, including the pituitary gland. These activins will also stimulate follicle-stimulating hormone (FSH) synthesis by acting on the gonadotropins. Aromatase inhibitors have relatively shorter half-life compared to clomiphene citrate and hence get eliminated from the body rapidly[5] (**Fig. 1**).

Since aromatase inhibitors will not deplete the estrogen receptors as in clomiphene citrate, the normal central feedback mechanism by estrogen remains intact. This negative feedback results in suppression of FSH and atresia of smaller follicles, facilitating the growth of a single dominant follicle and thus mono-ovulation. This is particularly useful as it reduces the incidence of ovarian hyperstimulation syndrome (OHSS) and multiple pregnancies.[5]

Another hypothesis is as the conversion of androgen substrate to estrogen is blocked, this causes accumulation of the intraovarian androgens. Intraovarian androgens are found to increase the sensitivity of the FSH to the follicles, causing maturation of the follicles. Aromatase inhibitors cause upregulation of the estrogen receptors in the endometrium due to the lack of estrogen in the circulation. This can cause rapid growth of the endometrium

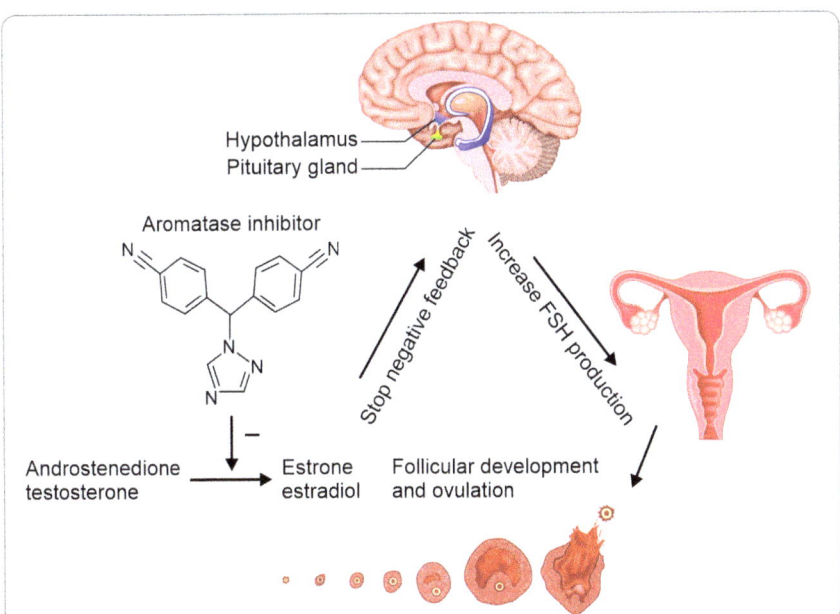

Fig. 1: Mechanism of action of aromatase inhibitor in ovulation pathway. (FSH: follicle-stimulating hormone)
Source: Illustrated by Mehlawat H using Inkscape software.

once the estrogen levels are restored. As a result, normal endometrial development occurs by the time of follicular maturation.[5]

AROMATASE INHIBITORS CLASSIFICATION

Based on the chemical structure, there are two different classes of aromatase inhibitors—type 1 steroidal inhibitors and type 2 nonsteroidal inhibitors **(Table 1)**.

Aminoglutethimide was a nonselective aromatase inhibitor and hence, it blocked multiple adrenal steroid production requiring cortisol replacement. This led to the development of selective aromatase inhibitors. Selective type 1 inhibitors or steroidal inhibitors are formestane and exemestane. Currently, only exemestane is in clinical use as formestane needed to be administered as painful intramuscular injections. Type 2 inhibitors or nonsteroidal inhibitors include fadrozole, rogletimide, vorozole, anastrozole, and letrozole. Currently, only anastrozole and letrozole are in clinical use.[6] Among these, letrozole is mainly used for ovulation induction in women with anovulatory subfertility.[7]

INDICATIONS IN GYNECOLOGY

There are currently three main indications in gynecology.

Ovulation Induction in Polycystic Ovary Syndrome

Aromatase inhibitor licensed in 1997 to treat advanced breast cancer was soon found to be useful to treat an array of conditions. Over the years, clomiphene citrate has been used to induce ovulation in oligo/anovulation in women. Though clomiphene citrate is 75% successful in inducing ovulation, the efficacy has been tampered by less fulfilling pregnancy rates of 10%. This was primarily thought to be due to the antiestrogenic effect of clomiphene citrate on the endometrium and the cervical mucus. The introduction of aromatase inhibitor brought out the possibility of increasing the effect of endogenous FSH without the antiestrogenic effect on the endometrium. Currently, letrozole is considered as the first-line pharmacological measure

TABLE 1: Classification of aromatase inhibitors.

Generation	Type 1	Type 2
Nonselective inhibitor		Aminoglutethimide
Selective inhibitor (not in clinical use)	Formestane	• Fadrozole • Rogletimide • Vorozole
Selective inhibitor (in clinical use)	Exemestane	• Anastrozole • Letrozole

to treat anovulatory subfertility in women with PCOS to improve ovulation, clinical pregnancy rate (CPR), and live birth rate (LBR).[8] LBR percentage increases by 40–60% with letrozole compared to clomiphene. Multiple pregnancy rate and occurrence of hot flushes are less likely with letrozole compared to clomiphene.[2] Currently, treatment with letrozole is off license as the drug company has not applied for a license for its use in fertility.

Fertility Preservation in Estrogen-dependent Cancers

Fertility preservation in breast cancer is challenging as most of these cancers are estrogen sensitive. Ovarian stimulation generates supraphysiological estrogen levels which can theoretically cause proliferation of the malignant cells. Administering an aromatase inhibitor or selective estrogen receptor modulators during ovarian stimulation help to reduce potential harm due to elevated estrogen levels. The European Society of Human Reproduction and Endocrinology (ESHRE) guideline on COS recommends the coadministration of antiestrogens such as letrozole or tamoxifen for fertility preservation in women with estrogen-sensitive disease. However, the quality of evidence is still low due to the observational nature of the studies, low sample size, and short duration of patient follow-up.[9]

Management of Endometriosis-associated Pain in Rectovaginal Endometriosis

Aromatase inhibitors are found to be beneficial for the management of pain associated with rectovaginal endometriosis which is refractory to medical and surgical management. It is found to be particularly useful when used in combination with oral contraceptive pills, progestogens, or gonadotropin-releasing hormone (GnRH) analogs.[10]

■ SIDE EFFECTS

The commonly reported side effects are alopecia, arthralgia, depression, dizziness, diarrhea, headache, hot flushes, hypertension, myalgia, edema, skin reaction, vaginal bleeding, vomiting, weight change, hyperhidrosis, and hypercholesterolemia.[11]

The uncommon side effects are anxiety, arthritis, breast pain, carpal tunnel syndrome, cataract, cerebrovascular insufficiency, cough, drowsiness, dry mouth, dyspnea, embolism, eye irritation, fever, insomnia, irritability, ischemic heart disease, leukopenia, memory loss, palpitation, stomatitis, altered taste, increased urinary frequency, blurred vision, and vulvovaginal disorder.[11]

However, for ovulation induction, the duration of use is only short and hence, it is unlikely to experience any serious long-term side effects.

SAFETY PROFILE

Manufacturers recommend avoiding use in pregnancy as concerns have been raised on potential teratogenic effects in an isolated peer-reviewed abstract.[12] However, subsequently published case reviews[13-16] and multicenter randomized controlled trials (RCTs)[17,18] failed to demonstrate an increased risk of congenital anomalies and they reported a rate of 5% for both letrozole and clomiphene. The expected incidence of congenital anomaly rate in this population was 5–8%. Manufacturers also advise to avoid breastfeeding and to exercise caution in severe hepatic and renal impairment.[11]

DOSE AND ADMINISTRATION PROTOCOL

There were only two studies that investigated the administration protocol of letrozole. One study compared 10-day course versus 5-day course of letrozole[19] and another study compared 3–5 day course versus 5–9 day course of letrozole.[20] For comparison of dosage, there was only one study that investigated between 2.5 and 5 mg/day versus 7.5 mg/day of letrozole[21] and the evidence was insufficient to comment on the best dose or the administration protocol for letrozole. However, studies have used a dose ranging from 2.5 to 7.5 mg/day for 5 days, starting from day 3 of the cycle. A retrospective study of 4,251 cycles looked into the ideal starting dose for letrozole and the study has found that a dose of 5 mg/day yields higher pregnancy rate than 7.5 mg/day, with lesser multiple pregnancy and miscarriage rates.[22]

The widely used dose of anastrozole is 1 mg/day for 5 days, starting on day 3 of menstruation. Tredway et al. in 2011 conducted a phase II, prospective, randomized, double-blind, multicenter, dose-finding, noninferiority study and they compared among 1, 5, and 10 mg/day dose of anastrozole with 50 mg/day of clomiphene citrate. The ovulation rates for 1, 5, and 10 mg/day were 30.4%, 36.8%, and 35.9%, respectively, compared with 64.9% for clomiphene citrate at 50 mg/day. The authors concluded that the ovulation rate of anastrozole was less effective than clomiphene citrate at 50 mg/day.[23]

COMPARISON OF AROMATASE INHIBITORS WITH OTHER OVULATION INDUCTION METHODS IN WOMEN WITH POLYCYSTIC OVARY SYNDROME

Aromatase Inhibitor versus Placebo

The Cochrane review conducted in women with anovulatory PCOS had two RCTs that compared letrozole versus placebo. Of these, only one trial reported on the LBR and there was insufficient evidence to suggest a difference in LBR. Two studies investigated CPR and showed that pregnancy rate was higher in the letrozole group compared to placebo [odds ratio (OR) 2.88; 95% confidence interval (CI) 1.08–7.66]. There was insufficient data to compare the OHSS rate and multiple pregnancy rate.[24]

Aromatase Inhibitor versus Clomiphene Citrate

Eight studies compared letrozole (2.5 mg to 7.5 mg/day) to clomiphene citrate (50 mg to 150 mg/day) in the Cochrane review for women with PCOS and reported an increased LBR in the letrozole group (OR 1.79; 95% CI 1.42-2.25). Only one study compared letrozole with clomiphene citrate and metformin and it showed no difference in the LBR between two groups (OR 1.05; 95% CI 0.60-1.81). Meta-analysis of the studies comparing aromatase inhibitor and metformin to clomiphene citrate and metformin, aromatase inhibitor and FSH to clomiphene citrate and FSH, and aromatase inhibitor versus clomiphene citrate and estradiol did not show any difference in the LBR.[24]

A comparison of CPR in women with PCOS showed a higher CPR in the letrozole group compared to clomiphene citrate with or without adjuvants (OR 1.56; 95% CI 1.37-1.78). The review showed similar frequency of OHSS (RD 0.00; 95% CI −0.01 to 0.00) and no difference in the multiple pregnancy rate between letrozole and clomiphene citrate (OR 0.73; 95% CI 0.43-1.24). The results were slightly in favor for clomiphene citrate for miscarriage (OR 1.39; 95% CI 1.07-1.81). However, when both groups were compared per pregnancy, no difference in the miscarriage rate was seen between the two groups (OR 0.94; 95% CI 0.70-1.26).[24]

Aromatase Inhibitor versus Clomiphene Citrate for Intrauterine Insemination

There was insufficient evidence of a difference in the OHSS risk, multiple pregnancy risk, and miscarriage risk between the two groups. The analysis showed CPR in favor of the letrozole group (OR 1.71; 95% CI 1.30-2.25).

Aromatase Inhibitor versus Gonadotropin

Hasan et al. compared letrozole 2.5 mg twice daily and 75 IU of FSH starting from day 3 of menstruation in 140 women.[25] The study did not show sufficient evidence to demonstrate a difference between the two groups on CPR, multiple pregnancy rate, and miscarriage rate. The study did not report on LBR or OHSS.[24]

Aromatase Inhibitor versus Ovarian Drilling

The Cochrane review showed low-quality evidence of no difference in LBR between two groups (OR 1.38; 95% CI 0.95-2.02). Comparison of CPR showed low-quality evidence of no difference between the letrozole with or without metformin to laparoscopic ovarian drilling (OR 1.28; 95% CI 0.94-1.74). The review showed insufficient evidence to show a difference between the two groups for OHSS (RD 0.00; 95% CI −0.01 to 0.01) and moderate-quality evidence of no difference between two groups for miscarriage rate (OR 0.81;

95% CI 0.38–1.70). For multiple pregnancy rate, the review demonstrated low-quality evidence of no difference between the two groups (OR 3.00; 95% CI 0.12–74.90)[24,26] **(Table 2)**.

Letrozole versus Anastrozole

Two studies compared letrozole to anastrozole. Letrozole 2.5 mg/day and anastrozole 1 mg/day was used starting from day 3 of the cycle. Both studies did not report LBR and there was insufficient evidence to report a difference in CPR, miscarriage rate, multiple pregnancy rate, and OHSS rate.[24,27,28]

EVIDENCE OF USE OF AROMATASE INHIBITORS IN VARIOUS CLINICAL CATEGORIES

Polycystic Ovary Syndrome

The current international guideline for the assessment and management of PCOS recommended letrozole as the first-line pharmacological agent to treat anovulatory subfertility to improve ovulation, pregnancy, and LBR.[2] This recommendation is based on the Cochrane review by Franik et al., which concluded that letrozole compared to clomiphene appears to improve LBR and CPR in anovulatory subfertility due to PCOS. There is high-quality evidence of no difference in OHSS rates, miscarriage rates, and multiple pregnancy rates between letrozole and clomiphene.[24]

TABLE 2: Showing whether there is evidence to favor aromatase inhibitor over the other method of ovulation induction in women with PCOS.

Comparison	LBR	CPR	OHSS	Multiple pregnancy	Miscarriage
Aromatase inhibitor vs. placebo	x	√	x	x	x
Aromatase inhibitor vs. clomiphene for sexual intercourse	√	√	x	x	x
Aromatase inhibitor vs. clomiphene for IUI	x	√	x	x	x
Aromatase inhibitor vs. gonadotropin	x	x	x	x	x
Aromatase inhibitor vs. ovarian drilling	x	x	x	x	x
Letrozole vs. anastrozole	x	x	x	x	x

(CPR: clinical pregnancy rate; IUI: intrauterine insemination; LBR: live birth rate; OHSS: ovarian hyperstimulation syndrome; PCOS: polycystic ovary syndrome)
√—Evidence in favor of aromatase inhibitor
x—No evidence of difference between aromatase inhibitor and the other method

Poor Responders in in-vitro Fertilization

Combining letrozole with gonadotropin has been suggested for ovarian stimulation, especially in poor responders.[29] Only three RCTs specifically investigated substituting letrozole for gonadotropin for ovarian stimulation, including 70, 20, and 50 women.[30-32] All three studies did not report any advantage in terms of improving CPR or ongoing pregnancy rate by adding letrozole. Hence, the ESHRE guideline on COS did not recommend letrozole as a substitute for gonadotropin for poor responders. They concluded that the number and size of the RCTs are small enough to make any concrete recommendations.[9]

High Responders in in-vitro Fertilization

There was only one retrospective study that investigated the role of letrozole in high responders and it did not report any difference in the CPR, OHSS rate, or the number of oocytes retrieved.[33] Hence, the ESHRE guideline on COS has reported that there is insufficient evidence for the use of letrozole alongside gonadotropins in high responders.[9]

Normal Responders

Two small RCTs investigated the addition of letrozole to FSH in GnRH antagonist protocol for ovarian stimulation.[31,34] There was no significant difference noted in the CPR or the number of oocytes retrieved in the letrozole added to the FSH group compared to FSH-alone group. One of the RCTs noted no OHSS in the letrozole group compared to seven OHSS in the control group. Based on this evidence, the ESHRE guidance on COS has concluded that addition of letrozole is not recommended for COS in predicted normal responders.[9]

Unexplained Infertility

A systematic review and meta-analysis compared letrozole with clomiphene citrate in women with unexplained infertility. The meta-analysis has demonstrated that in women with unexplained infertility, no difference in the clinical outcomes were observed between letrozole or clomiphene citrate.[35]

Frozen Embryo Transfer Cycles

A systematic review and meta-analysis published in 2020 compared the use of letrozole for endometrial preparation in the frozen embryo transfer (FET) cycles. They compared the use of letrozole for endometrial preparation compared with the natural cycle, artificial cycle, and artificial cycles with gonadotropin suppression for FET. No difference in the CPR or LBR was observed when letrozole was used compared with the natural cycle, artificial cycle, or cycles with gonadotropin suppression for FET.[36]

Fertility Preservation

A systematic review published in 2017 investigated the safety and efficacy of COS for fertility preservation in women with early breast cancer.[37] The systematic review had 12 prospective and retrospective studies that involved the administration of aromatase inhibitor protocol for fertility preservation. The review reported no evidence of a reduction in relapse-free survival period in women who had COS with letrozole compared with those who did not undergo fertility preservation procedures.[37] The recurrence rate reported in one of the largest studies included in the review was 5% (6/120) in the letrozole group compared to 5.5% (12/217) in those who did not undergo COS.[38] However, the review reported a lower peak estradiol concentration (337–829 pg/mL) in the letrozole group with no reduction in the oocyte retrieval rate.[37] and hence, the ESHRE guideline on COS recommended coadministering antiestrogens for fertility preservation in estrogen-sensitive breast cancer women. These results were supported by a subsequent review published in 2020.[39]

High Body Mass Index

It was proposed that aromatase inhibitor is beneficial for ovulation induction in high body mass index (BMI) women. The systematic review by Franik et al. compared letrozole with selective estrogen receptor modulator with or without adjuvants such as gonadotropins followed by timed intercourse and did a subgroup analysis based on the BMI of the women (less than a BMI of 25 kg/m^2 and more than a BMI of 25 kg/m^2). The subgroup analysis did not show a significant difference in the LBR or the OHSS rate between the two groups based on their mean BMI (p value 0.87).

Endometriosis

Aromatase inhibitors have been suggested to be potentially useful for the management of endometriosis-related pain. There are two systematic reviews published[40,41] on the benefit of aromatase inhibitors for management of endometriosis-related pain. All the included studies were on women with rectovaginal endometriosis who were refractory to previous medical and surgical management. Based on this evidence, the ESHRE guideline on management of endometriosis has suggested that aromatase inhibitors can be used in combination with the oral contraceptive pill, progestogens, or GnRH analogs in women with pain from rectovaginal endometriosis who are refractory to other medical or surgical management.[10] The guideline emphasizes that due to the side effects of the aromatase inhibitors, it should only be used if all other medical or surgical options are exhausted.

Fibroids

A Cochrane review was conducted in 2013 to investigate the effectiveness and safety of aromatase inhibitors in women with fibroid uterus.[42] The review identified only one trial[43] that compared aromatase inhibitors with GnRH analogs in managing women with fibroids and it reported on the side effects of the drugs and the reduction in fibroid volume. The aromatase inhibitors group saw a reduction in fibroid volume by 46% compared to 32% in the GnRH group which did not reach significance. The systematic review concluded that the evidence is not sufficient to support the use of aromatase inhibitors in women with fibroid uterus.

■ CONCLUSION

Aromatase inhibitors are a novel group of drugs which have established their role in reproductive medicine and have shown promising evidence to be used as the first-line agent for ovulation induction in women with PCOS. Due to its mechanism of action, it is beneficial for fertility preservation in a subgroup of women with estrogen-dependent tumors. However, its role in controlled ovarian stimulation lacks conclusive evidence.

■ KEY POINTS

- *Letrozole as a first-line treatment for ovulation induction in PCOS:* This chapter highlights Letrozole, a type of aromatase inhibitor, as the preferred medication for inducing ovulation in women with PCOS. Letrozole works by regulating the hypothalamus-pituitary-ovarian axis without affecting oestrogen receptors, unlike older medications like Clomiphene citrate.
- *Mechanism of action:* Aromatase inhibitors function by blocking the aromatase enzyme, which converts androgens into estrogens. This disrupts the negative feedback loop mediated by estrogen, stimulating the production of gonadotropins and promoting follicular growth.
- *Gynaecological applications beyond PCOS:* While the chapter focuses on PCOS, it also mentions other gynecological uses of aromatase inhibitors. These include:
  - *Fertility preservation in estrogen-sensitive cancers:* Letrozole can be used alongside ovarian stimulation to reduce estrogen levels and potentially minimize the risk of cancer recurrence.
  - *Management of endometriosis associated pain:* Aromatase inhibitors might offer relief for women with rectovaginal endometriosis who have not responded well to other treatments.
- *Safety and limitations:* The chapter acknowledges potential side effects of aromatase inhibitors and emphasizes the lack of conclusive evidence for their use in controlled ovarian stimulation (COS) procedures. It also highlights the need for further research in specific areas.

REFERENCES

1. Thonneau P, Marchand S, Tallec A, Ferial M, Ducot B, Lansac J, et al. Incidence and main causes of infertility in a resident population (1,850,000) of three French regions (1988-1989). Hum Reprod. 1991;6:811-6.
2. Teede HJ, Misso ML, Costello MF, Dokras A, Laven J, Moran L, et al. Recommendations from the international evidence-based guideline for the assessment and management of polycystic ovary syndrome. Hum Reprod. 2018;33:1602-18.
3. Lee VCY, Ledger W. Aromatase inhibitors for ovulation induction and ovarian stimulation. Clin Endocrinol (Oxf). 2011;74:537-46.
4. Santen R, Brodie H, Simpson E, Siiteri P, Brodie A. History of aromatase: saga of an important biological mediator and therapeutic target. Endocr Rev. 2009;30:343-75.
5. Casper RF, Mitwally MF. Aromatase inhibitors for ovulation induction. J Clin Endocrinol Metab. 2006;91:760-71.
6. Chumsri S. Clinical utilities of aromatase inhibitors in breast cancer. Int J Womens Health. 2015;7:493-9.
7. Usluogullari B, Duvan CZ, Usluogullari CA. Use of aromatase inhibitors in practice of gynecology. J Ovarian Res. 2015;8:1-7.
8. Gadalla MA, Norman RJ, Tay CT, Hiam DS, Melder A, Pundir J, et al. Medical and Surgical Treatment of Reproductive Outcomes in Polycystic Ovary Syndrome: An Overview of Systematic Reviews. Int J Fertil Steril. 2020;13:257-70.
9. Bosch E, Broer S, Griesinger G, Grynberg M, Humaidan P, Kolibianakis E, et al.; Ovarian Stimulation TEGGO. ESHRE guideline: ovarian stimulation for IVF/ICSI. Hum Reprod Open. 2020;2020:hoaa009.
10. Dunselman G, Vermeulen N, Becker C, Calhaz-Jorge C, D'Hooghe T, De Bie B, et al. ESHRE guideline: management of women with endometriosis. Hum Reprod. 2014;29:400-12.
11. Joint Formulary Committee. BNF 78. London: Pharmaceutical Press; 2020.
12. Biljan M, Hemmings R, Brassard N. The outcome of 150 babies following the treatment with letrozole or letrozole and gonadotropins. Fertil Steril. 2005;84:S95.
13. Forman R, Gill S, Moretti M, Tulandi T, Koren G, Casper R. Fetal safety of letrozole and clomiphene citrate for ovulation induction. J Obstet Gynaecol Can. 2007;29:668-71.
14. Sharma S, Ghosh S, Singh S, Chakravarty A, Ganesh A, Rajani S, et al. Congenital malformations among babies born following letrozole or clomiphene for infertility treatment. PloS One. 2014;9:e108219.
15. Tatsumi T, Jwa S, Kuwahara A, Irahara M, Kubota T, Saito H. No increased risk of major congenital anomalies or adverse pregnancy or neonatal outcomes following letrozole use in assisted reproductive technology. Hum Reprod. 2017;32:125-32.
16. Tulandi T, Martin J, Al-Fadhli R, Kabli N, Forman R, Hitkari J, et al. Congenital malformations among 911 newborns conceived after infertility treatment with letrozole or clomiphene citrate. Fertil Steril. 2006;85:1761-5.
17. Diamond MP, Legro RS, Coutifaris C, Alvero R, Robinson RD, Casson P, et al. Letrozole, gonadotropin, or clomiphene for unexplained infertility. N Engl J Med. 2015;373:1230-40.

18. Legro RS, Brzyski RG, Diamond MP, Coutifaris C, Schlaff WD, Casson P, et al. Letrozole versus clomiphene for infertility in the polycystic ovary syndrome. N Engl J Med. 2014;371:119-29.
19. Badawy A, Mosbah A, Tharwat A, Eid M. Extended letrozole therapy for ovulation induction in clomiphene-resistant women with polycystic ovary syndrome: a novel protocol. Fertil Steril. 2009;92:236-9.
20. Ghomian N, Khosravi A, Mousavifar N. A Randomized Clinical Trial on Comparing the cycle characteristics of two different initiation days of Letrozole Treatment in Clomiphene Citrate Resistant PCOS Patients in IUI Cycles. Int J Fertil Steril. 2015;9:17-26.
21. Ramezanzadeh F, Nasiri R, Yazdi MS, Baghrei M. A randomized trial of ovulation induction with two different doses of Letrozole in women with PCOS. Arch Gynecol Obstet. 2011;284:1029.
22. Rodriguez-Purata J, Lee JA, Whitehouse MC, Luna M, Mukherjee M, Pavilion K. What is the ideal starting dose for patients utilizing letrozole for ovulation induction (OI)? Analysis of 4251 cycles. Fertil Steril. 2015;104:e107-8.
23. Tredway D, Schertz JC, Bock D, Hemsey G, Diamond MP. Anastrozole vs. clomiphene citrate in infertile women with ovulatory dysfunction: a phase II, randomized, dose-finding study. Fertil Steril. 2011;95:1720-4.e8.
24. Franik S, Eltrop SM, Kremer JA, Kiesel L, Farquhar C. Aromatase inhibitors (letrozole) for subfertile women with polycystic ovary syndrome. Cochrane Database Syst Rev. 2018;5(5):CD010287.
25. Hassan A, Shehata N, Wahba A. Cost effectiveness of letrozole and purified urinary FSH in treating women with clomiphene citrate-resistant polycystic ovarian syndrome: a randomized controlled trial. Hum Fertil. 2017;20:37-42.
26. Yu Q, Hu S, Wang Y, Cheng G, Xia W, Zhu C. Letrozole versus laparoscopic ovarian drilling in clomiphene citrate-resistant women with polycystic ovary syndrome: a systematic review and meta-analysis of randomized controlled trials. Reprod Biol Endocrinol. 2019;17:1-7.
27. Al-Omari W, Sulaiman W, Al-Hadithi N. Comparison of two aromatase inhibitors in women with clomiphene-resistant polycystic ovary syndrome. Intl J Gynecol Obstet. 2004;85:289-91.
28. Badawy A, Mosbah A, Shady M. Anastrozole or letrozole for ovulation induction in clomiphene-resistant women with polycystic ovarian syndrome: a prospective randomized trial. Fertil Steril. 2008;89:1209-12.
29. Goswami S, Das T, Chattopadhyay R, Sawhney V, Kumar J, Chaudhury K, et al. A randomized single-blind controlled trial of letrozole as a low-cost IVF protocol in women with poor ovarian response: a preliminary report. Hum Reprod. 2004;19:2031-5.
30. Ebrahimi M, Akbari-Asbagh F, Ghalandar-Attar M. Letrozole + GnRH antagonist stimulation protocol in poor ovarian responders undergoing intracytoplasmic sperm injection cycles: An RCT. Int J Reprod Biomed. 2017;15:101-8.
31. Verpoest WM, Kolibianakis E, Papanikolaou E, Smitz J, Van Steirteghem A, Devroey P. Aromatase inhibitors in ovarian stimulation for IVF/ICSI: a pilot study. Reprod Biomed Online. 2006;13:166-72.
32. Yasa C, Bastu E, Dural O, Celik E, Ergun B. Evaluation of low-dose letrozole addition to ovulation induction in IVF. Clin Exp Obstet Gynecol. 2013;40:98-100.

33. Chen Y, Yang T, Hao C, Zhao J. A Retrospective Study of Letrozole Treatment Prior to Human Chorionic Gonadotropin in Women with Polycystic Ovary Syndrome Undergoing In Vitro Fertilization at Risk of Ovarian Hyperstimulation Syndrome. Med Sci Monit. 2018;24:4248-53.
34. Mukherjee S, Sharma S, Chakravarty BN. Letrozole in a low-cost in vitro fertilization protocol in intracytoplasmic sperm injection cycles for male factor infertility: A randomized controlled trial. J Hum Reprod Sci. 2012;5:170-4.
35. Eskew AM, Bedrick BS, Hardi A, Stoll CRT, Colditz GA, Tuuli MG, et al. Letrozole Compared With Clomiphene Citrate for Unexplained Infertility: A Systematic Review and Meta-analysis. Obstet Gynecol. 2019;133:437-44.
36. Chen D, Shen X, Fu Y, Ding C, Zhong Y, Zhou C. Pregnancy outcomes following letrozole use in frozen-thawed embryo transfer cycles: a systematic review and meta-analysis. Geburtshilfe Frauenheilkd. 2020;80:820.
37. Rodgers RJ, Reid GD, Koch J, Deans R, Ledger WL, Friedlander M, et al. The safety and efficacy of controlled ovarian hyperstimulation for fertility preservation in women with early breast cancer: a systematic review. Hum Reprod. 2017;32:1033-45.
38. Kim J, Turan V, Oktay K. Long-term safety of letrozole and gonadotropin stimulation for fertility preservation in women with breast cancer. J Clin Endocrinol Metab. 2016;101:1364-71.
39. Bonardi B, Massarotti C, Bruzzone M, Goldrat O, Mangili G, Anserini P, et al. Efficacy and safety of controlled ovarian stimulation with or without letrozole co-administration for fertility preservation: a systematic review and meta-analysis. Front Oncol. 2020;10:2008.
40. Ferrero S, Gillott DJ, Venturini PL, Remorgida V. Use of aromatase inhibitors to treat endometriosis-related pain symptoms: a systematic review. Reprod Biol Endocrinol. 2011;9:89.
41. Patwardhan S, Nawathe A, Yates D, Harrison G, Khan K. Systematic review of the effects of aromatase inhibitors on pain associated with endometriosis. BJOG. 2008;115:818-22.
42. Song H, Lu D, Navaratnam K, Shi G. Aromatase inhibitors for uterine fibroids. Cochrane Database Syst Rev. 2013;(10):CD009505.
43. Parsanezhad ME, Azmoon M, Alborzi S, Rajaeefard A, Zarei A, Kazerooni T, et al. A randomized, controlled clinical trial comparing the effects of aromatase inhibitor (letrozole) and gonadotropin-releasing hormone agonist (triptorelin) on uterine leiomyoma volume and hormonal status. Fertil Steril. 2010;93:192-8.

Chapter 9

Gonadotropins: Follicle-stimulating Hormone, Luteinizing Hormone, and Human Menopausal Gonadotropin

Rishma Dhillon Pai, Unnati Mamtora, Arnav Hrishikesh Pai

■ INTRODUCTION

Assisted reproductive technologies have been used since 1978 to help couples who have difficulty in conceiving. It first began with the birth of Louis Brown; however, that was through a natural cycle in vitro fertilization (IVF). The success rate of the natural cycle IVF was very low and hence, efforts were made to use drugs which produced a larger number of eggs which would help increase success rates. The first use of gonadotropins extracted from the human pituitary was reported in 1959. Initially gonadotropins were used in anovulatory women to induce ovulation and then its use was extended to ovulatory women as well in 1980s[1-3] and was followed by the use of gonadotropins for ovarian stimulation. Better pregnancy rates were reported by the use of clomiphene citrate and human menopausal gonadotropin (hMG) protocol which resulted in yield of higher number of eggs and embryos by the Monash Group.[4] However, these stimulation cycles were reportedly associated with 20–40% chances of premature luteinization and untimely ovulation. To combat this effect, a series of modifications of the gonadotropin-releasing hormone (GnRH) molecule were done which resulted in the development of the GnRH analogs with agonists and the antagonists. Gradually, the stimulation protocols were more simplified by the use of gonadotropins in the antagonist cycles to increase the beneficial effects and at the same time reduce the complications and risks.[5]

The development of gonadotropins has come a long way from the introduction of gonadotropins of urinary origin, then the highly purified forms, to recombinant gonadotropin preparations to more recently the long-acting preparations **(Table 1)**.

■ STRUCTURE OF GONADOTROPINS

The gonadotropin hormones belong to the glycoprotein hormone family. They consist of noncovalently bonded beta and alpha subunits. The alpha and beta subunits have the carbohydrate moieties attached. The alpha units are common to all the glycoprotein hormones and are composed of 92 amino acids. The beta subunit is unique and distinct; this confers the receptor

TABLE 1: History of development of gonadotropins.

Year	History of development
1927	Zondek and Aschheim demonstrated that blood and urine of pregnant women contain gonadotropin-like substance which was found to be hCG
1931	Commercial hCG was first available where hCG was prepared from the placental tissue culture
1940	Researchers were able to extract hCG from the urine
1949	Extraction of hMG from postmenopausal urine
1960	Urinary preparations of hCG and hMG introduced for commercial use
1980	Purified FSH only products became available
1993	Highly purified FSH-only products introduced
1995	rec-FSH became available
2000	rec-LH introduced
2001	rec-hCG was launched
2004	Introduction of the fill by mass rec-FSH—reducing the batch-to-batch variability
2010	Introduction of long-acting FSH preparation
2011	Pen projector devices for precise delivery of rec-FSH, rec-LH, and rec-hCG

(FSH: follicle-stimulating hormone; hCG: human chorionic gonadotropin; HMG: human menopausal gonadotropin; LH: luteinizing hormone; rec: recombinant)

activity of the glycoprotein molecule.[6] The attachment of the carbohydrate moiety provides the biological activity of the molecule by forming heterodimers. The bioactivities and half-lives of each glycoprotein differs depending on the extent of glycosylation of the molecules.[7] The glycosylation results in formation of sulfonated or sialic acid-linked molecules. The sulfonated isoforms clear faster from the circulation than the nonsulfonated ones. The sialic acid forms have more half-life.[8-10]

■ FOLLICLE-STIMULATING HORMONE

The follicle-stimulating hormone (FSH) stimulates the ovarian follicles and is involved in the selection of the dominant follicle for ovulation.

The beta subunit of the FSH is specific for FSH and is made of 111 amino acids **(Fig. 1)**. This beta subunit is encoded by the gene on chromosome number 11p13. All the glycoprotein hormones act on the receptor cells through the G-coupled receptors on the target cell surfaces. The FSH hormone acts through the FSH receptors (FSHR) present on the granulosa cells of the ovary by activation of the cyclic adenosine monophosphate (cAMP). The FSH stimulates the growth and proliferation of the follicles and cause P450 activation in turn, causing increase in the aromatase activity.

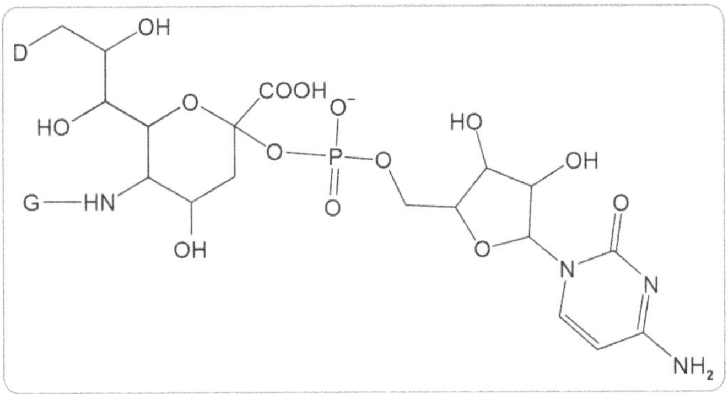

Fig. 1: Chemical structure of follicle-stimulating hormone (FSH).

The granulosa cells of the ovary produce inhibin and activin. They cause increase in the production of the FSHR by their autocrine activity, increasing the action of FSH.[11,12] There are two glycosylation sites on the alpha subunit and two glycosylation sites on the beta subunits. Thus, variable compositions are formed which create different isoforms. All of these hence have different plasma half-lives ranging from 3 to 4 hours and different bioactivities as well. Sialic residues are formed after glycosylation more often as compared to the sulfonated ones. This sialylation increases the metabolic stability of FSH by decreased glomerular filtration and decreased clearance by the liver sialoprotein receptors.[13,14]

■ LUTEINIZING HORMONE

The beta subunit of the luteinizing hormone (LH) contains 121 amino acids (**Fig. 2**). This confers its receptor specificity. The amino acids in the beta subunit of LH and human chorionic gonadotropin (hCG) are same, with hCG having additional 23 amino acids. The two hormones LH and hCG differ in their half-lives and biological activity due to the variation in the composition of the carbohydrate moieties. LH has shorter half-life of only 20–30 minutes.

■ HUMAN CHORIONIC GONADOTROPIN

The beta subunit of the hCG is similar to the LH, but additionally, it has a long carboxy terminal which contains additional 24 amino acids.

There are two sites for glycosylation in the hCG molecule compared to only two sites in the LH molecule. Due to this, it has a longer half-life of approximately 24 hours as compared to LH which is 30 minutes.

Due to the structural similarity between the hCG and the LH, hCG can be used to trigger the final stage of follicular maturation. Aspiration of follicles (egg retrieval procedure) are timed according to the timely hCG injections. The chemical structure of FSH, LH, and hCG is shown in **Figures 3A to C**.

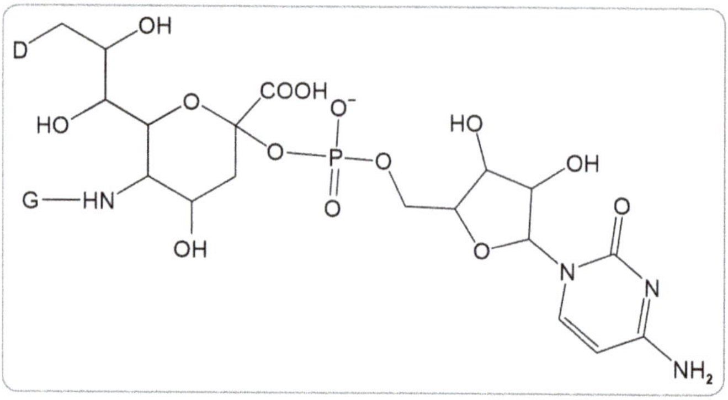

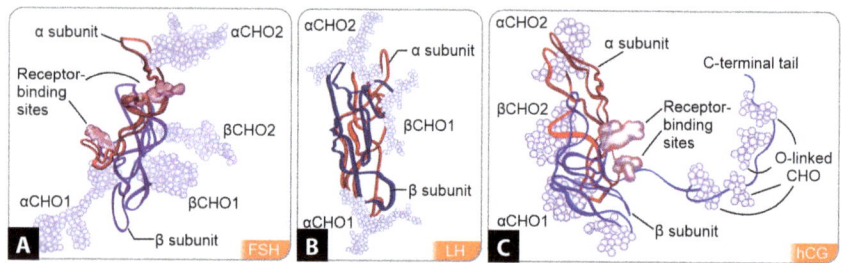

Fig. 2: Chemical structure of luteinizing hormone (LH).

Figs. 3A to C: Chemical structure of FSH, LH, and hCG. (FSH: follicle-stimulating hormone; hCG: human chorionic gonadotropin; LH: luteinizing hormone)

COMMERCIAL PREPARATIONS OF GONADOTROPINS

Human Menopausal Gonadotropin

Human menopausal gonadotropin is derived from postmenopausal urine. It contains FSH, LH, and hCG only in 5% purity.[3] The ratio of FSH and LH is 1:1 in hMG preparations.[15] hCG is responsible for the LH activity mostly and sometimes, it may be added from outside for attaining the desired amount.[2] They are available in both conventional and highly purified preparations.

Urinary Follicle-stimulating Hormone Preparations

Urinary preparations of FSH are made by removing the LH component. The process of preparation removed the LH component but still contained other urinary proteins.[16]

The LH component was initially removed by using polyclonal antibodies. There were further advances later and monoclonal antibodies were used in the preparation of highly purified forms. The availability of the highly purified preparation allowed subcutaneous delivery of the injections. This was convenient to the patients as it reduced the number of visits to the hospital as self-administration with the subcutaneously available injection was possible.[17,18]

Recombinant Follicle-stimulating Hormone

Recombinant technology has made it possible to make more reliable FSH preparations.

The nuclear deoxyribonucleic acid (DNA) of the host cell is incorporated by the genes that code for FSH (alpha and beta subunit) through a plasmid vector. The Chinese hamster ovary cell lines have now replaced the *Escherichia coli* (*E. coli*) that were initially used. They can be used to make large cell cultures and provide adequate production of biologically active gonadotropins.[2,19]

For clinical use, two types of recombinant (rec-) FSH preparations are used—the follitropin alpha and follitropin beta. The master cell bank for the follitropin alpha is made by using two vectors for each subunit in alpha and single vector used for beta follitropin.[19,20] The alpha and beta follitropin differ in their production, purifications, and glycosylation. The alpha unit is more acidic than the beta one. But the preparations have similar potency. rec-FSH preparations have half-lives of 2 hours and terminal half-lives of 7 hours.

Long-acting Recombinant Follicle-stimulating Hormone

Due to shorter half-lives of standard preparations, daily administration of the FSH injections is required. After the peak levels of FSH are reached in 12 hours, the levels begin to fall gradually. Steady levels of FSH are reached after 3–5 days of administration. Hence, dose adjustments are advised after 5 days. The serum levels of FSH have to be maintained above the threshold level for continuous growth of follicles.

This motivated the development of long-acting FSH. Using the gene transfer techniques and mutagenesis, the long-acting rec-FSH was developed.[21] hCG C-peptide terminal is combined with the rec-FSH to develop long-acting effects. Plasma half-life is of 65 hours.[21,22] First seven injections of the daily standard gonadotropin injections can be replaced by a single injection of corifollitropin alfa followed by daily injection of standard FSH preparation till the egg maturation is achieved.[23]

Gonadotropin Preparations with Luteinizing Hormone Activity

The current preparations with LH activity include:
- hMG (LH activity is mainly by the hCG component)
- rec-LH
- A combination of pure FSH and LH in fixed ratio of 2:1 manufactured through recombinant technology

Initially, only hMG preparations were available, but later rec-LH preparations were introduced, especially for women with gonadotropin deficiency.[24,25] rec-LH preparations can be self-administered by the subcutaneous route. The recombinant injections have advantages over the urinary preparations in terms of purity, specificity, and lower inter batch-to-batch variability.[26] Also, the serum LH activity is higher when the urinary preparations are used as the hCG component binds to the LHR with higher affinity. It takes 24–36 hours for it to be eliminated. Compared to this, the rec-LH has half-life of 10–12 hours as it is eliminated faster.[27-31]

Combination of recombinant human (rec-h) FSH and rec-h LH in the ratio of 2:1 was launched recently. It has an advantage of administering both the FSH and LH in a single injection, avoiding multiple pricks. Its efficacy and biological activity is similar to rec-FSH and rec-LH when administered alone.

Human Chorionic Gonadotropin

Human chorionic gonadotropin is administered in the ovulation induction and stimulation cycles to achieve the final step of ovulation instead of the natural LH surge. It has its structural similarities with the LH hormone, but it binds with more affinity to the LHR, with higher biological activity. Its half-life is more than the LH hormone. Cochrane meta-analyses have shown equal efficacy of both the urinary and recombinant preparations.[32] The recombinant injections can be given by subcutaneous route, allowing self-administration and is tolerated better.[33] This is advantageous over the urinary preparations which are given by the intramuscular route and hence need to be administered by a healthcare professional.

Gonadotropins are used in combination with the oral ovulogens or alone for the purpose of ovulation induction. Different protocols for controlled ovarian stimulation (COS) are followed depending upon the patient's profile, where the general aim of stimulation is to get adequate number of follicles without putting the women to risk of ovarian hyperstimulation.

■ USES OF GONADOTROPINS

- Ovulation induction in type 1 anovulatory women (hypogonadotropic hypogonadism)
- For induction of ovulation in women with type 2 anovulation, unexplained infertility, endometriosis, and recurrent pregnancy loss
- COS in intrauterine insemination (IUI) cycles, especially in patient not responding to letrozole/clomiphene
- COS for IVF/intracytoplasmic sperm injection (ICSI)
- Male infertility due to hypogonadotropic hypogonadism for induction of spermatogenesis and it can also be used in cases of severe oligoasthenoteratospermia.

The understanding of the concept of FSH window and LH threshold and LH ceiling is an important foundation to application of the knowledge for determination of the stimulation protocol to be used with individualized approach to every patient.

Various protocols and regimens are followed depending upon the age, the ovarian reserve, the body mass index (BMI) of the patient, previous history, and previous response to ovarian stimulation if any (discussed in detail in the subsequent chapters) **(Box 1)**.

DOSAGE OF GONADOTROPINS

- The dosage of gonadotropins mainly depends upon the indication of use.
- The dosage is much lower in IUI cycles. For ovulation induction (OI), 75 or 150 IU dosage is commonly used.
- For COS in IVF, dosage ranging from 150 to 300 IU is typically used, depending upon patient's age and ovarian reserve.

COMPARISON OF URINARY AND RECOMBINANT PREPARATIONS

The advantages of the recombinant preparations are:
- Preloaded pens available for subcutaneous use which can be self-administered with delivery of accurate dose ensured.
- Higher purity
- Specific activity
- Reduced batch-to-batch variability

The urinary preparations are cost-effective when compared to recombinant ones.

Studies have shown that the urinary hMG preparations and rec-FSH give similar results in terms of live birth rate, clinical pregnancy rate, and miscarriage rate.
- No statistically significant difference was found in the live birth rates and ovarian hyperstimulation syndrome (OHSS) rates when rec-FSH and hMG were compared.[34]

BOX 1: Practical guide to usage of the gonadotropins in IUI/IVF cycles.

- Patient comes on day 2/3/4 of periods
- Do TVS for the AFC, rule out ovarian cyst, residual follicle cyst, corpus luteum from previous cycle, establish thin endometrium (<5 mm)
- Do serum E2 levels, if needed
- Start gonadotropins (choice of Gn according to the protocol chosen)
- Dosage is decoded as per the age, AFC count, BMI, and previous cycle response history
- Injections can be started within first 5 days of commencement of menses
- Frequent monitoring with TVS and sometimes serum E2 levels to judge adequate response to stimulation

(AFC: antral follicle count; BMI: body mass index; E2: estradiol; Gn: gonadotropin; IUI: intrauterine insemination; IVF: in vitro fertilization; TVS: transvaginal ultrasound)

- It was studied that if the amount of total dosage of hormones required differs between rec-FSH and hMG to achieve a live birth, then the difference is statistically insignificant.[35]
- The live birth, clinical pregnancy rate, and miscarriage rate were found to be similar between urinary gonadotropins and rec-FSH in polycystic ovary syndrome (PCOS) women.[36,37]

■ FUTURE OF GONADOTROPINS[38]

Gonadotropins of both the natural and recombinant origins have been available since few decades, but there still remains a need for more reliable, less expensive, and easily administered preparations. Challenges exist in making oral preparations available for use. There exists a need for availability of preparations that require less injections that can reduce or minimize the complications of hyperstimulation and at the same time be equally efficacious.

Kisspeptin, for example, was used in ovulation induction effectively without risk of ovarian hyperstimulation.

Inactivating the mutation in the neurokinin B demonstrated normal FSH and low LH activity. Hence, neurokinin B antagonist oral preparations can effectively be used in patients of PCOS by reversing the high LH to FSH ratio. Hot flushes have been demonstrated to coincide with the LH pulses. The slowing of pulses by neurokinin B antagonists can help in reducing the hot flushes.

Impressive low molecular weight (LMW) oral, sustained release preparations of both FSHR and LHR agonists and antagonists are under development and may be available for commercial use after adequate human trials.

The LMW preparations have shown to demonstrate ability to restore the receptor function and inactivate the receptor mutation. This can offer broader usage in a spectrum of conditions arising from the receptor mutation along with application in reproductive medicine. Future roles and applications on extragonadal tissues are also emerging. However, the application and effect on the extragonadal tissues still remain to be fully explored.

■ CONCLUSION

We have come a long way since gonadotropin was first identified in currently available preparations. Medical practitioners can now individualize the treatment and provide better care due to the availability of recombinant preparations containing pure forms with accurate dosing. Available preparations can be injected subcutaneously and in pen forms for easy usage and more precise dose calculation. The newer advances in the preparations are still underway till orally active agonists and antagonists become available.

KEY POINTS

- Gonadotropins are used in combination with oral ovulogens or alone for ovulation induction. Different protocols for controlled ovarian stimulation (COS) are followed depending on the patient's profile where the general aim of stimulation is to get an adequate number of follicles without putting the women at risk of ovarian hyperstimulation.
- The understanding of the concept of the FSH window, LH threshold and LH ceiling is an important foundation to the application of the knowledge for the determination of the stimulation protocol to be used with an individualized approach to every patient.
- Various protocols and regimens are followed depending upon the age, the ovarian reserve the BMI of the patient the previous history, and previous response to ovarian stimulation if any.
- Advantages of the recombinant preparations:
  - Preloaded pens are available for subcutaneous use which can be self-administered with delivery of accurate dose ensured.
  - Higher purity
  - Specific activity
  - Reduced batch-to-batch variability
- The urinary preparations are cost-effective when compared to recombinant ones.
- Impressive low molecular weight (LMW) oral, sustained-release preparations of both FSHR and LHR agonists and antagonists are under development and may be available for commercial use after adequate human trials.

REFERENCES

1. Beall SA, DeCherney A. History and challenges surrounding ovarian stimulation in the treatment of infertility. Fertil Steril. 2012;97(4):785-801
2. Lunenfeld B. Historical perspectives in gonadotrophin therapy. Human Reprod Update. 2004;10(6):453-67.
3. Practice Committee of American Society for Reproductive Medicine, Birmingham, Alabama. Gonadotropin preparations: past, present, and future perspectives. Fertil Steril. 2008;90(5 Suppl):S13-20.
4. Trounson AO, Leeton JF, Wood EC, Webb J, Wood J. Pregnancies in humans by fertilization in vitro and embryo transfer in the controlled ovulatory cycle. Science. 1981;212:616.
5. Bosch E, Ezcurra D. Individualised controlled ovarian stimulation (iCOS): maximising success rates for assisted reproductive technology patients. Reprod Biol Endocrinol. 2011;21:82.
6. Vaitukaitis JL, Ross GT, Braunstein GD, Rayford PL. Gonadotropins and their subunits: basic and clinical studies. Recent Prog Horm Res. 1976;32:289-331.

7. Ulloa-Aguirre A, Espinoza R, Damian-Matsumura P, Chappel SC. Immunological and biological potencies of the different molecular species of gonadotrophins. Hum Reprod. 1988;3(4):491-501.
8. Wide L, Naessén T, Sundström-Poromaa I, Eriksson K. Sulfonation and sialylation of gonadotropins in women during the menstrual cycle, after menopause, and with polycystic ovarian syndrome and in men. J Clin Endocrinol Metab. 2007;92(11):4410-7.
9. Fiete D, Srivastava V, Hindsgaul O, Baenziger JU. A hepatic reticuloendothelial cell receptor specific for SO4-4GalNAc beta 1,4GlcNAc beta 1,2Man alpha that mediates rapid clearance of lutropin. Cell. 1991;67(6):1103-10.
10. Wide L, Eriksson K, Sluss PM, Hall JE. Serum half-life of pituitary gonadotropins is decreased by sulfonation and increased by sialylation in women. J Clin Endocrinol Metab. 2009;94(3):958-64.
11. Speroff L, Fritz MA. Regulation of the menstrual cycle. In: Speroff L, Fritz MA (Eds). The Clinical Gynecologic Endocrinology and Infertility, 7th edition. Philadelphia: Lippincott Williams & Wilkins; 2005. pp. 348-83.
12. Speroff L, Fritz MA (Eds). Hormone biosynthesis, metabolism, and mechanisms of action? The Clinical Gynecologic Endocrinology and Infertility, 7th edition. Philadelphia: Lippincott Williams & Wilkins; 2005. pp. 109-16.
13. Campbell RK. Molecular pharmacology of gonadotropins. Endocrine. 2005;26(3):291-6.
14. Morell AG, Gregoriadis G, Scheinberg IH, Hickman J, Ashwell G. The role of sialic acid in determining the survival of glycoproteins in the circulation. J Biol Chem. 1971;246(5):1461-7.
15. Esteves SC, Schertz JC, Verza S Jr, Schneider DT, Zabaglia SF. A comparison of menotropin, highly-purified menotropin and follitropin alfa in cycles of intracytoplasmic sperm injection. Reprod Biol Endocrinol. 2009;7:111.
16. Giudice E, Crisci C, Eshkol A, Papoian R. Composition of commercial gonadotrophin preparations extracted from human post-menopausal urine: characterization of non-gonadotrophin proteins. Hum Reprod. 1994;9(12):2291-9.
17. Alviggi C, Revelli A, Anserini P, Ranieri A, Fedele L, Strina I, et al. A prospective, randomised, controlled clinical study on the assessment of tolerability and of clinical efficacy of Merional (hMG-IBSA) administered subcutaneously versus Merional administered intramuscularly in women undergoing multifollicular ovarian stimulation in an ART programme (IVF). Reprod Biol Endocrinol. 2007;5:45.
18. Platteau P, Laurent E, Albano C, Osmanagaoglu K, Vernaeve V, Tournaye H, et al. An open, randomized single-centre study to compare the efficacy and convenience of follitropin beta administered by a pen device with follitropin alpha administered by a conventional syringe in women undergoing ovarian stimulation for IVF/ICSI. Hum Reprod. 2003;18(6):1200-4.
19. Howles CM. Genetic engineering of human FSH (Gonal-F). Hum Reprod Update. 1996;2(2):172-91.
20. Olijve W, de Boer W, Mulders JW, van Wezenbeek PM. Molecular biology and biochemistry of human recombinant follicle stimulating hormone (Puregon). Mol Hum Reprod. 1996;2(5):371-82.

21. Fauser BC, Mannaerts BM, Devroey P, Leader A, Boime I, Baird DT. Advances in recombinant DNA technology: corifollitropin alfa, a hybrid molecule with sustained follicle-stimulating activity and reduced injection frequency. Hum Reprod Update. 2009;15(3):309-21.
22. Fares FA, Suganuma N, Nishimori K, LaPolt PS, Hsueh AJ, Boime I. Design of a long-acting follitropin agonist by fusing the C-terminal sequence of the chorionic gonadotropin beta subunit to the follitropin beta subunit. Proc Natl Acad Sci USA. 1992;89(10):4304-8.
23. Balen AH, Mulders AG, Fauser BC, Schoot BC, Renier MA, Devroey P, et al. Pharmacodynamics of a single low dose of long-acting recombinant follicle-stimulating hormone (FSH-carboxy terminal peptide, corifollitropin alfa) in women with World Health Organization group II anovulatory infertility. J Clin Endocrinol Metab. 2004;89(12):6297-304.
24. Bosdou JK, Venetis CA, Kolibianakis EM, Toulis KA, Goulis DG, Zepiridis L, et al. The use of androgens or androgen-modulating agents in poor responders undergoing in vitro fertilization: a systematic review and meta-analysis. Hum Reprod Update. 2012;18(2):127-45.
25. Hill MJ, Levens ED, Levy G, Ryan ME, Csokmay JM, DeCherney AH, et al. The use of recombinant luteinizing hormone in patients undergoing assisted reproductive techniques with advanced reproductive age: a systematic review and meta-analysis. Fertil Steril. 2012;97(5):1108-14.e1.
26. Bassett RM, Driebergen R. Continued improvements in the quality and consistency of follitropin alfa, recombinant human FSH. Reprod Biomed Online. 2005;10(2):169-77.
27. le Cotonnec JY, Porchet HC, Beltrami V, Munafo A. Clinical pharmacology of recombinant human luteinizing hormone: Part I. Pharmacokinetics after intravenous administration to healthy female volunteers and comparison with urinary human luteinizing hormone. Fertil Steril. 1998;69(2):189-94.
28. Grøndahl ML, Borup R, Lee YB, Myrhøj V, Meinertz H, Sørensen S. Differences in gene expression of granulosa cells from women undergoing controlled ovarian hyperstimulation with either recombinant follicle-stimulating hormone or highly purified human menopausal gonadotropin. Fertil Steril. 2009;91(5):1820-30.
29. Menon KM, Munshi UM, Clouser CL, Nair AK. Regulation of luteinizing hormone/human chorionic gonadotropin receptor expression: a perspective. Biol Reprod. 2004;70(4):861-6.
30. Bosch E, Vidal C, Labarta E, Simon C, Remohi J, Pellicer A. Highly purified hMG versus recombinant FSH in ovarian hyperstimulation with GnRH antagonists—a randomized study. Hum Reprod. 2008;23(10):2346-51.
31. Venetis CA, Kolibianakis EM, Papanikolaou E, Bontis J, Devroey P, Tarlatzis BC. Is progesterone elevation on the day of human chorionic gonadotrophin administration associated with the probability of pregnancy in in vitro fertilization. A systematic review and meta-analysis. Hum Reprod Update. 2007;13(4):343-55.
32. Youssef MA, Al-Inany HG, Aboulghar M, Mansour R, Abou-Setta AM. Recombinant versus urinary human chorionic gonadotrophin for final oocyte maturation triggering in IVF and ICSI cycles. Cochrane Database Syst Rev. 2011;(4):CD003719.

33. Driscoll GL, Tyler JP, Hangan JT, Fisher PR, Birdsall MA, Knight DC. A prospective, randomized, controlled, double-blind, double-dummy comparison of recombinant and urinary HCG for inducing oocyte maturation and follicular luteinization in ovarian stimulation. Hum Reprod. 2000;15(6):1305-10.
34. Van Dorsselaer A, Carapito C, Delalande F, Schaeffer-Reiss C, Thierse D, Diemer H, et al. Detection of prion protein in urine-derived injectable fertility products by a targeted proteomic approach. PLoS One. 2011;6(3):e17815.
35. Van Wely M, Kwan I, Burt AL, Thomas J, Vail A, Van der Veen F, et al. Recombinant versus urinary gonadotrophin for ovarian stimulation in assisted reproductive technology cycles. Cochrane Database Syst Rev. 2011;(2):CD005354.
36. Bordewijk EM, Mol F, van der Veen F, Van Wely M. Required amount of rFSH, HP-hMG and HP-FSH to reach a live birth: a systematic review and meta-analysis. Hum Reprod Open. 2019;2019(3):hoz008.
37. Weiss NS, Kostova E, Nahuis M, Mol BWJ, van der Veen F, van Wely M. Gonadotrophins for ovulation induction in women with polycystic ovary syndrome. Cochrane Database Syst Rev. 2019;(1):CD010290.
38. Anderson RC, Newton CL, Anderson RA, Millar RP. Gonadotropins and their analogs: Current and Potential Clinical Applications. Endocr Rev. 2018;39(6):911-37.

Section 5

Trigger it Right

- **Human Chorionic Gonadotropin: Not a Panacea Anymore**
  Anupama Ravi Futela, Ashadeep Chandrareddy
- **Analog Trigger: Are We Missing the Target?**
  Yuval Atzmon, Einat Shalom-Paz
- **Dual Trigger: It Works!**
  Rachana Sameer Deshpande, Padma Rekha Jirge

Chapter 10

Human Chorionic Gonadotropin: Not a Panacea Anymore

Anupama Ravi Futela, Ashadeep Chandrareddy

■ INTRODUCTION

Trigger is the most crucial step that concludes ovarian stimulation and achieves final oocyte maturation and ovulation. Prior to maturation, oocytes are arrested in the diplotene of prophase stage of meiosis 1, also known as germinal vesicle. These oocytes must reach at least the early antral follicle stage to respond to follicle-stimulating hormone (FSH) and to be competent to resume meiosis. In late stages of follicular growth, luteinizing hormone (LH) receptors are induced by FSH. Therefore, only fully grown oocytes respond to LH surge in vivo to begin cytoplasmic and nuclear maturity. Nuclear maturation involves germinal vesicle breakdown, followed by resumption of meiosis, and finally, extrusion of the first polar body. Cytoplasmic maturity is more difficult to define but involves a number of factors preparing cytoplasm synchronously for fertilization and subsequent embryonic development.[1] Gonadotropins are used to induce ovulation in controlled ovarian stimulation (COS). After sufficient follicular growth, our goal shifts from prevention of a premature LH surge to induction of the LH surge and completion of oocyte maturation. Much like a Disney princess, an oocyte rests dormant for years in the glass casket of ovaries, waiting for the "true love's kiss" from her prince—the LH trigger **(Fig. 1)**.

Dr Robert G Edward, Nobel awardee for his work on human in vitro fertilization (IVF), studied the growth of mouse embryos at Edinburgh University in 1952. He had to identify female mice in estrus by taking tedious vaginal swabs, often at midnight. He discovered that pregnant mares' serum (PMS), which is rich in FSH and human chorionic gonadotropin (hCG), can be used to predictably induce estrus and ovulation. Incidentally, this is where he met his future wife, Ruth Fowler and they teamed up to test this approach of super ovulating adult mice. He gained considerable knowledge about control of estrus cycles, ovulation, and artificial insemination, which proved to be instrumental for his later clinical IVF work. He also discovered that gonadotropins could be used to mature oocytes, "in vitro" as well. In fact, they matured at the same rate as their counterparts "in vivo." He also learnt that the maturation timing for oocytes is species specific and he timed it at 37 hours in humans, later aspirating them at 36 hours.

We shall discuss the physiology of triggering and various proposed alterations later in the chapter after first getting to know about the various drugs used for triggers.

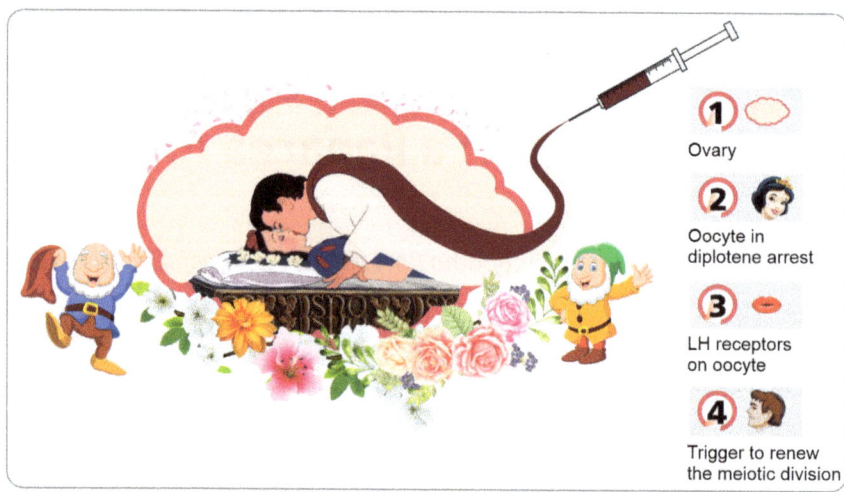

Fig. 1: Prince's kiss analogy illustrated: luteinizing hormone (LH) surge—the catalyst for ovulation in fairy tale form.
Courtesy: Dr Pragyat Futela, Dr Anupama Ravi Futela, and Mr Vinod Dudeja.

HUMAN CHORIONIC GONADOTROPIN: THE GOLD STANDARD

Human chorionic gonadotropin is the oldest known gonadotropin and has been a marvelous discovery. It is still the most commonly used trigger in varying forms. This prince has many feathers in its cap which makes it as wondrous. Both LH and hCG act on the same LH/hCG receptors (LHCG-R).[2] The key difference is that hCG has a significantly prolonged half-life due to sialic acid residues on its β-subunit. Also, hCG is best at supporting the luteal phase as it upregulates vascular endothelial growth factor (VEGF) expression in the corpus luteum. VEGF further improves angiogenesis and perfusion of Graafian follicles. On the other hand, VEGF is the key mediator of ovarian hyperstimulation syndrome (OHSS), which is a serious iatrogenic complication, exacerbated by hCG triggering and perpetuated by circulating hCG after implantation.

The hCG rescues corpus luteum like none other. It helps neoangiogenesis aiding in prevention of luteolysis (something contradictory of which happens after agonist trigger). hCG also causes relaxation of smooth muscles and myometrial vasodilatation—all leading to uterine quiescence to aid in implantation.[3] Also, one of the reason for better results of day 5 versus day 3 embryo transfer is hCG (due to better hCG expression from the embryo itself after its eight cell stage and h-hCG secretion in high local concentrations by blastocyst[4]) which helps in the embryo–endometrial crosstalk and trophoblastic invasion. Hence, hCG's role in improving implantation outcomes is unequivocal. The advantages as a trigger are manifold and **Table 1** enumerates a few.

TABLE 1: Biological functions of hCG and its implication in current perspective.[2-4]

hCG function	Implication
Rescues corpus luteum	Better progesterone production which takes over LH on day 8 postovulation
Surrogate LH surge	Causing resumption of meiosis in large- and medium-sized follicles, cumulus expansion, germinal vesicle (nuclear membrane) breakdown, granulosa cell luteinization, etc.
Trophoblastic invasion in decidua, gelatinase secretion, and NK cell activation	• Implantation regulation • The autocrine effect of hyperglycosylated hCG ensures this blastocyst cross talk with endometrium
Action on IGFBP-1 and stromal fibroblast function	• Improves endometrial receptivity and extends the implantation window (*high level of IGFBP-1 indicates closure of the window*)[4] • Inhibits apoptosis
Inhibition of myometrial contraction	Uterine quiescence aids in implantation
Differentiation of cytotrophoblast into multinucleated syncytiotrophoblast by fusion	Aids in implantation (reason of high hCG in normal pregnancy, even when placenta takes over the progesterone production is mainly that the fusion process has to continue for long)
Neoangiogenesis at follicle and myometrium	Ensures good blood supply to the follicles and uterus and also returns good progesterone supply back in circulation
VEGF secretion	Role for placental angiogenesis (but increases risk of OHSS too)
LH-like activity on LHCG-R[4]	Apart from stimulating follicle development, Low-dose hCG (60–200 u per day) alone can support development of large antral follicles who have acquired these receptors on granulosa cells
Collagenase production	Along with progesterone and prostaglandins this helps fracture the follicular vesicle wall and helps in oocyte extrusion
Inhibits macrophages and immunity regulation	Immune response from mother is repelled by the extremely negatively charged hCG molecules permitting survival of fetal allograft

(hCG: human chorionic gonadotropin; IGFBP-1: insulin-like growth factor-binding protein-1; LH: luteinizing hormone; LHCG-R: joint LH and hCG receptor; OHSS: ovarian hyperstimulation syndrome; NK: natural killer; VEGF: vascular endothelial growth factor)

When do we Trigger?

The triggering shots are often used with timed intercourse or assisted reproductive techniques (ART) procedures. During these procedures, trigger is timed according to several criteria for follicular maturity.[5,6]
- ≥2 follicles of at least 17–18 mm in diameter[5]
- Endometrial thickness in trilaminar pattern ≥8–9 mm is considered in intrauterine insemination (IUI) or natural transfer cycles.
- Serum estradiol (E2) ≥200 pg/mL/follicle or in COS cycles 70–140 pg/mL/oocyte on ≥11 mm follicles

The follicular size plays the main role in decision-making rather than hormone assessments and endometrial pattern (additional hormonal assays, that is, LH assessment was not found useful on trigger day).[6] The *United Kingdom (UK) Timing of hCG Group* has shown that addition of E2 levels/follicle seldom changed the trigger timings.[5] Prolongation of the stimulation offered no advantage in terms of oocyte or embryo quality.[7] However, prolongation of the follicular phase in patients does not affect oocyte or embryo quality but is associated with significantly lower ongoing pregnancy rates.[8] An artificial intelligence-based interpretable machine learning model for predicting the optimal day of trigger has been proposed recently in 2022 by Fanton et al. based on linear regression with follicle counts and E2 levels. Early triggers gave 2.3 fewer metaphase II oocytes (M2s), 1.8 fewer 2PNs, and 1.0 fewer blastocysts, whereas late triggers had on average 2.7 fewer M2s, 2.0 fewer 2PNs, and 0.7 fewer usable blastocysts compared with matched patients with on-time triggers.[9]

Human Chorionic Gonadotropin Dose as Trigger

Effective triggering dose of hCG has conventionally been 5,000[10] or 10,000 IU for ART. It is interesting to note that a dose of 1,000–1,200 IU is sufficient for oocyte maturation[11] and 3,300 IU for rupture of the follicle.[12] Since we do not require follicle rupture in IVF cycles, a dose of just 1,500–2,000 (27–30 IU/kg) prior to retrieval is sufficient when given along with GnRHa. A desirable blood hCG level is 50 mIU/mL[13,14] after 12 hours of injection and preferably should be <100 mIU/mL.[15] We do not need to give higher doses of hCG with a higher number of follicles.[12,16] In fact, owing to the risk of OHSS, it is advisable to give a lesser dose of hCG because the chances of OHSS do increase with a higher number of follicles as well as higher hCG doses.[15] It is also interesting to note that 12-hour levels of <10 mIU/mL were found to have high chances of empty follicle syndrome (EFS).[17] Lower doses of hCG, e.g., 300 IU of recombinant hCG (rec-hCG) can still induce nuclear maturation and granulosa cell luteinization, but they were not sufficient to ensure optimal cytoplasmic oocyte maturation for fertilization and corpora lutea function.[11]

Body mass index (BMI) also plays an important role while deciding the doses of hCG injection.[14]

CHAPTER 10: Human Chorionic Gonadotropin: Not a Panacea Anymore

- If BMI is ≤25 kg/m^2, then desired dose for oocyte maturation is 5,000 IU.
- If BMI is >25 kg/m^2, then >5,000 IU dose is advisable.
- If BMI is ≥30 kg/m^2, then a dose of ≥10,000 IU should be considered. Some clinicians practice triggering based on a sliding scale:[13]
  - 10,000 IU for E2 levels ≤ 1,500 pg/mL
  - 5,000 IU for E2 levels between 1,501 and 2,500 pg/mL
  - 4,000 IU for levels between 2,501 and 3,000 pg/mL
  - 3,300 IU for ≥3,001 pg/mL or else 1,500 IU hCG with 2 mg leuprolide (discussed in dual trigger later in this chapter)

There have been initial reservations about the efficacy of recombinant preparations of hCG, but recent evidence suggests equal efficacy compared to urinary hCG.[18,19] The comparison between the two is shared in **Table 2**. Recombinant preparations can be taken as an aristocratic *Maserati* which

TABLE 2: Urinary and recombinant varieties of hCG.[18,20-22]

	u-hCG	rec-hCG
Half-life	31–37 hours	28 hours
Reliability	Time tested and effective	• It has proven the same in last few years[18] • Some studies rate them superior[20,22]
Source	Production from uncontrolled urinary source makes the potency variable	Less batch-to-batch variability due to genetically engineered cell line production
Metabolism	Hepatic	Hepatic
Excretion	Urinary	Same
Route of administration	Intramuscular route-only restriction due to lack of purity[18]	Subcutaneous route making it user-friendly
Dose precision	Good	Excellent
Trigger doses are variable	5,000 IU is common. However, 500, 1,000, 1,500, 2,000 till 10,000 are used in different situations	250 μg = 6,500 IU Usually, 6,500–13,000 IU are used[20]
Safety	Well tolerated. Some itching, redness, pain, swelling, and bruising can occur[18]	Even better local tolerance
OHSS risk	Present	Same
Cost	Most pocket friendly	Costlier
Contaminants[21,22]	Uncommon (but 33 different nongonadotropin proteins have been identified)	Human prion peptides causing neurodegeneration are not identified

(OHSS: ovarian hyperstimulation syndrome; rec-hCG: recombinant human chorionic gonadotropin; u-hCG: urinary human chorionic gonadotropin)

albeit costly, provides a reliable surge and better local tolerance, can be given subcutaneously, and most of all is contamination free. The last advantage says it all, i.e., recombinant preparations are prion free and would be the author's personal choice.

Human Chorionic Gonadotropin: The Double-edged Sword

The very reason why hCG is so effective is the reason for it being the culprit for OHSS. hCG is no longer the sole primary trigger option due to two main reasons:

1. With the prototype shift in ART practices to improve safety and to achieve OHSS-free clinics, most laboratories are gradually adopting segmentation of IVF cycles, in which oocyte retrieval and embryo transfers are done in separate cycles, thanks to cryopreservation. Since fresh transfers are not done during segmentation, therefore hCG's main advantage of aiding in implantation is not required. Instead, we try to induce rapid luteolysis in a *freeze all* policy.
2. hCG acts as a surrogate on LHCG-R, whereas in natural cycles, the LH surge comes from the pituitary which in turn is ordered by GnRH. This GnRH order concomitantly surges the FSH as well. LH is primarily responsible for nuclear maturity of the oocyte, while FSH is required to promote cytoplasmic maturity as well as nuclear maturation, i.e., resumption of meiosis and cumulus expansion along with the function of inducing LH receptors formation in luteinizing granulosa cells, thus optimizing function of corpus luteum.[23] This is more physiological compared to hCG trigger and more close to natural surge pattern. Thus, a practical clinical answer has developed in the form of GnRH analogs.

AGONIST TRIGGERS: ANOTHER MILESTONE OF REPRODUCTIVE MEDICINE

Past century saw agonist downregulation as the most common protocol which mandated hCG as the only trigger option. Also in those days, since fresh cycle transfers were common, hCG was mandatory because it provided the much wanted aid on implantation. But the hanging sword of OHSS kept us looking for alternative options for triggering. hCG had ruled the ART kingdom for many decades of the last century like a *king*.[27] The younger princes, i.e., Agonist, LH, and kisspeptin (KISS-1), got the opportunity to enter the woods only in the last few decades **(Table 3)**.

Although the role of GnRH as plausible triggering agent was diagnosed as early as 1973,[28] it was only after the advent of GnRH antagonist and its ability to avoid premature luteinization that we realized how effective *agonist triggers* (GnRH analogs) can be. Owing to the FSH surge along with LH surge after agonist triggers, it enhances ooplasmic maturity and prevents

TABLE 3: Timeline of development of triggering options in the field of infertility.[24]

1927 hCG Identified	• Since inception, it was the sole gonadotropin researched and used for successful oocyte maturation • FSH and LH were identified in 1929 and animal pituitary gonadotropins were produced
1931 Commercial hCG available	• hMG extracted from postmenopausal urine (1950) • hMG found to produce ovarian stimulation in rats (1953)
1962 First reported ovarian stimulation	Superovulation strategies started. Clomiphene and gonadotropin use became common practice in the sixth decade of last century
1973	The WHO issues first guidance on diagnosis and management of infertile couples
1978 Birth of Louise Brown	• First live birth from IVF natural cycle • If luteal support was identified earlier, probably this would have happened a few years earlier
1981	• hMG for stimulation and hCG for trigger protocols were used for IVF • Hormone level assays and ultrasound imaging evolved
1983 Inception of human FET	First successful pregnancy after frozen thaw embryo transfer[25]
1984 GnRH agonists use started	Downregulation with agonists followed by triggering with hCG became the norm in those days. Risk of OHSS was high in that era
1995, 1996 Recombinant gonadotropin products	Respective follitropin alpha and beta marketing approval overcame the problem of finite donor supply and batch-to-batch variability
1999 Antagonists invented	Antagonist came into commercial use. Earlier hCG was the sole trigger option, but with antagonist protocols and its better acceptance, agonists' use started as trigger
2000 Rec-hCG approved	Better reliability
Agonist trigger[26] 1990 Early cases with agonist. Leuprolide acetate trigger reported	Leuprolide, buserelin, triptorelin, and nafarelin all are used and are now time tested. The time to OPU after injection has been the same as hCG (34–36 hours). However, their use was not universal due to poor pregnancy rates with fresh embryo transfers
2010 Cryopreservation	Vitrification programs evolved from slow freezing; its benefit gained worldwide acceptance. With segmentation of IVF cycles, agonist triggers matured as they gave better M2 yield

Contd...

Contd...

History	
2007 dual trigger[36]	Came into common use for they provided better luteal support and better clinical pregnancies. Dual trigger use continues till date even in freeze all cycles as M2 yield is better
2000 Rec-LH approved	High doses are required which makes it very expensive. This option is tried since the risk of OHSS is negligible. 5,000–30,000 IU SC dose is as effective as hCG
2003—*kisspeptin*	Still under research; it holds good promise for the future

(FET: frozen embryo transfer; FSH: follicle-stimulating hormone; GnRH: gonadotropin-releasing hormone; hCG: human chorionic gonadotropin; hMG: human menopausal gonadotropin; IVF: in vitro fertilization; LH: luteinizing hormone; M2: metaphase II oocyte; OHSS: ovarian hyperstimulation syndrome; OPU: oocyte pickup; rec: recombinant; SC: subcutaneous; WHO: World Health Organization)

asynchrony between nuclear and cytoplasmic maturation and thereby helps decondensation of sperm nucleus, oocyte activation, and fertilization. GnRHa have greater affinity to the GnRH receptors than GnRH antagonists do and can displace the antagonist to induce a more physiological LH and FSH surge, ensuring better M2 yield.[29] Also, agonists induce quick and reversible luteolysis and have decreased OHSS risk (*causes of luteolysis are downregulated pituitary due to analog usage and supraphysiological E2 causing further LH suppression*). However, due to this rapid luteolysis, despite the better M2 and better embryo quality, the advantage of agonist trigger ends when we talk about fresh transfers as it does not provide better pregnancy rates.[23,30] But for the donor population, additional benefits came in the form of decreased treatment burden on donors with lesser monitoring, lesser bloodwork, better luteolysis, shorter duration of luteal phase, reduced ovarian volume, diminished abdominal distension, and above all, less risk of OHSS. Thus, agonist triggers have worked wonders for simplifying egg donation programs both for donor and clinician.

The endogenous GnRH (a 10 amino acid peptide) has a half-life of 2–4 minutes only. However, the amino acid replacement at position 6 and 10 have given us analogs with longer half-life. Triptorelin ($t_{1/2}$—4 hours), leuprolide ($t_{1/2}$—1.5 hours), and buserelin ($t_{1/2}$—1.3 hours) are in common clinical use with no evidence of superiority over each other.[31] Endogenous pulsatile secretion causes a long-lasting surge of 48 hours, whereas the analog surges are short lived, usually for 24 hours.

Since fresh transfers were the flavor of the old season, a whole lot of work followed which elaborates on how to improve luteal phase support (LPS) to improve pregnancy rate after agonist triggers.[32] With good luteal support,

TABLE 4: Comparison between the two most common triggers.

hCG trigger	Analog/agonist trigger
Long duration of action on LHCG-R causing prolonged function of corpus luteum	Fast upsurge is followed by steep fall, causing shorter duration of action with resultant faster luteolysis
It is desirable when we want to rescue CL, i.e., in cases of fresh transfers	It is desirable when we want rapid luteolysis, e.g., in high responders, donors, and where FETs are planned
It improves implantation by virtue of help in trophoblastic invasion, myometrial relaxation and endometrial neoangiogenesis[3]	No extra help is provided for implantation
VEGF secretion plays role in higher chances of OHSS (4–17%)	There is no excess VEGF secretion, hence less chances of OHSS
• Chances of EFS are rare and usually due to human errors[33] • If EFS happens, then agonist triggers with antagonist protocol should offer more physiological options next time	EFS can occur in patients on long-term pills, very thin patients, and few missed hypogonadotropic hypogonadism patients, whose pituitary is inherently or iatrogenically suppressed[34]
Only option for agonist protocol and the WHO group 1 anovulatory patients	Useless for downregulated and hypogonadotropic hypogonadism patients

(CL: corpus luteum; EFS: empty follicle syndrome; FETs: frozen embryo transfers; hCG: human chorionic gonadotropin; LHCG-R: joint luteinizing hormone and hCG receptor; OHSS: ovarian hyperstimulation syndrome; VEGF: vascular endothelial growth factor; WHO: World Health Organization)

agonist-triggered cycles also started giving comparable clinical pregnancies (Table 4).

Best of Both Worlds: Dual Triggers

Further research utilized the best of the two (hCG and analogs) and *dual trigger* was devised. Dual trigger is the cotreatment of both GnRHa and low-dose hCG for triggering final oocyte maturation. This trigger has the advantage of both endogenous LH and FSH surges as well as surrogate LH in the form of hCG. This results in better oocyte and embryo quality [*as investigated in various messenger ribonucleic acid (mRNA) studies*].[35] Dual trigger ensures reduction of OHSS with acceptable fertilization, implantation, and clinical and ongoing pregnancy rates.

Agonists induce quick and reversible luteolysis and hence have decreased OHSS risk. hCG can revert this rapid luteolysis, aiding in implantation and therefore, a common clinical practice is to use both in combination and to ensure luteal support for better pregnancy outcomes even in fresh cycles. Since fresh transfers are uncommon, why go with dual and not just a singular agonist trigger? It is found that additional hCG does add impetus due to its angiogenic and cumulus mucinification function and also provides a much wanted backup action in case the agonist fails to act on pituitary. The chances of empty follicle are mainly due to human errors or rarely due to receptor insensitivity.[33] The most common reason for EFS in a donor has been found that they are on long-term pills and the pituitary is on long suppression. These borderline low LH and FSH patients, however above hypogonadotropic hypogonadism (hypo hypo) levels, would still run the risk of EFS with agonist trigger.[34] In such a situation, the sole agonist trigger *can* be a failure. It is a good practice to routinely check urinary/serum LH levels 12 hours post-trigger to avoid later disappointments in this group of patients who are on long-term pituitary suppression, for example, on oral contraceptive pills (OCPs). Also, routine dual trigger practice can save a clinic from such surprise empty follicles by adding hCG.

Dual trigger helps in oocyte maturation both by endogenous LH and FSH surge as well as surrogate LH in the form of hCG. Hence, it is an efficient alternative for improving the yield of oocytes in those with a low oocyte/follicle ratio. In such cases, GnRHa is an efficient alternative for egg maturation, while hCG provides sustained support for the luteal phase.

Different dosage combinations of GnRHa and hCG can enable individualizing the precise ovulation trigger. Statistically, dual triggers in normal responders significantly improves implantation, clinical pregnancy, and live birth rates in GnRH antagonist IVF cycles.[36] Shapiro et al. described a dual trigger protocol with hCG dose of ≤33 IU/kg body weight (ranging between 1,000 and 2,500 IU) achieving a pregnancy rate of 53.3%. A low-dose hCG (1,000–1,500 IU) is often used for hyperresponders and 1,500–2,000 IU for a normoresponder. Poor responders are usually triggered by 5,000–10,000 IU hCG along with agonist in dual triggers.

Benefits of dual trigger have been reported with all permutations of 1 mg, 2 mg, or 4 mg doses of GnRHa and 500, 1,000, 1,500, 2,000, 2,500, 5,000, and 10,000 IU doses of hCG. 2 mg leuprolide or 0.2 triptorelin along with 1,500 hCG is a very common practice adopted by many ART centers.

Dual trigger is ideal in all freeze cycles and also with patients giving poor follicle output ratio (FOR) in previous retrievals. In case of fresh transfers, hCG is added pre- or postretrieval along with dual/agonist triggers. Despite better stimulation outcomes, pregnancy outcomes were significantly worse in the group,[37] where dual trigger was done with low-dose hCG (500–1,500), with fresh transfer, as it did not provide adequate luteal support as compared to 10,000 hCG/250 Ovitrelle. Also, the reason being that multifolliculogenesis, higher levels of progesterone and drugs to prevent LH surge causes low LH levels in the early luteal phase as compared to natural cycle. Endogenous LH and endogenous or exogenous LH-like activity (hCG) plays a role not only in maintaining corpus luteum functions but also upregulation of growth factors and cytokines, for example, leukemia-inhibiting factor required for implantation.[38] The dual trigger also gives flexibility of taking a decision post- oocyte retrieval about possibility of fresh transfer or freeze all. Tailored LPS adds to this flexibility.[27,32] If the oocyte yield is less, risk of hyperstimulation is less, bloodwork also supports and we think of possible fresh embryo transfer, then we can add the rescue dose of hCG soon after the retrieval and repeat at transfer along with progesterone for luteal support. Studies suggest that women with >25 follicles, >11 mm in diameter, should be considered for freeze all strategy to eliminate OHSS risk.[32] GnRHa trigger combined with modified LPS is clinically more successful than hCG in reproductive outcomes on fresh IVF/intracytoplasmic sperm injection (ICSI) cycles and in OHSS prevention.

■ SURGE PHYSIOLOGY

Dramatic changes occur in the preovulatory follicles of most mammals between the time of gonadotropin surge and ovulation. Under the influence of LH, the granulosa cells separate from the basement membrane adjacent to the theca cells. The oocyte that has been arrested at diplotene of prophase 1 since the embryonic stage undergoes meiosis reactivation. This involves germinal vesicle (nuclear membrane) breakdown and first polar body extrusion.[1] Concomitant with these changes, the cumulus cells that surround the oocyte undergo expansion and mucification. The breakdown of the granulosa cells and cumulus expansion are vital parts of the ovulation process because they separate the oocyte cumulus complex (OCC) from the follicular wall and allow it to float freely in the follicular fluid, ready for extrusion at ovulation. The cumulus cells are typically expanded and luteinized and the corona radiata exhibits a sunburst pattern. A series of inflammatory responses initiate within the follicle to secure the structural changes required for follicular rupture and oocyte extrusion. Soon after the oocyte release, termination of this inflammation occurs and there is transformation of steroidogenic apparatus of theca and granulosa cells into lutein cells mainly focusing on progesterone secretion.[39]

The preovulatory natural gonadotropin surge lasts for about 2 days (49 ± 9 hours) and is composed of an ascending phase (14 hours), a plateau (14 hours), and slow descending phase (20 hours).[40] The LH level is usually 10-20 times the baseline LH (40-60 IU).[41] The restart of meiosis is identified at 18 hours after LH surge onset. For highest oocyte maturation, LH concentration should be retained over a threshold for 14-27 hours.[42-44] Usually, we expect the LH rise should be above 14 IU. Kummer et al. have proposed a value of >15 IU/L of LH and >3.5 ng/mL of progesterone after the trigger to predict successful surge.[45] Usually, these serum assessments are done 12 hours after trigger *(In unpublished data, the author has rarely found progesterone levels > 3.5 at 12 hours post-trigger, but LH levels did corroborate with the above. In a 35-patient series, we found LH levels to range from 13 to 93 with an average of 58 IU. The levels of <14 were in two patients only and both* had high BMI). However, we can find good oocytes at lower levels too since we might have missed the surge peak which can occur early with medications, especially agonist triggers where the peak occurs at 4 hours. Also, important to note is that studies have shown poor predictability of EFS by routine post-trigger evaluation. Moreover, single point LH estimation may not be useful as it is the duration of LH surge which better predicts oocyte maturation.[45] Surges of <14 hours duration yielded little effect, surges of 18–24 hours elicited oocyte maturation and initial luteinization of granulosa cells, and only surges of >36 hours had sustained luteal development and function.[11] Agonist surges which are short lived result in normal maturation of oocyte and ovulation, but shorter length of luteal phase mandates necessary LPS (*standard support*[23] *with progesterone is not as effective as modified support with additional 1,500 hCG*[46]). The shorter duration of LH surge causes insufficient luteinization of granulosa cells, hence impaired secretion and shorter life of these corpora lutea.[47]

Surge after hCG trigger lasts for a longer (120 hours) duration along with rapid and higher peak levels (130–300 IU).[39] The 12 hours level after natural cycle and hCG shows that five times average levels are seen (25 vs. 125 IU), pushing three times higher progesterone synthesis and exposing endometrium to high and early transformative concentrations of progesterone.[39] This too high, too soon, and too long progesterone might be possibly attenuating to implantation potential as it can advance the endometrium.[39]

Agonist triggers giving rise to LH surge have a fast ascending phase of 4 hours and a descending phase of 20 hours (total = 24 hours) **(Fig. 2)**.

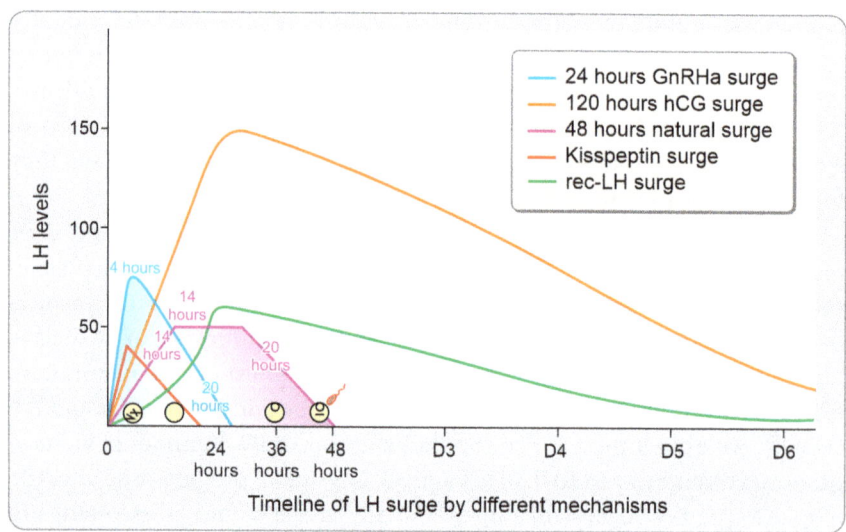

Fig. 2: Surge timeline by various triggers.[2,50] (GnRHa: gonadotropin-releasing hormone agonist; hCG: human chorionic gonadotropin; LH: luteinizing hormone; rec-LH: recombinant LH)

[*There is a statistically significant reduction in oocyte yield with serum LH concentration of <15 IU/L but not in maturity and fertilization rates.[48] The average post-trigger levels were 69.3 IU/L (10.5–133.3 IU/L[49]). However, the studies have concluded that measuring LH levels are not necessary and does not affect clinical outcomes.*] This shorter and thus inadequate surge can be a cause of empty follicle and immature oocyte retrieval due to short duration in some patients. To mimic the natural pattern, agonist needs to be used with hCG or a second dose of agonist is given after 12 hours to attain plateau and longer effect. These alterations are referred to as *double trigger*.

Double trigger is a combination of GnRHa and standard hCG, when used 40 and 34 hours prior to ovum pickup, respectively.[51] This trigger prolongs the time between ovulation trigger and ovum pickup, aiming to overcome granulosa cell dysfunction, facilitating cumulus cell expansion and meiotic maturation and thus results in retrieving more mature oocytes. *Double trigger has a role in patients with abnormal follicular maturation despite adequate stimulation.* In patients with <50% number of oocytes retrieved per number of dominant follicles on day of trigger, double trigger has led to significant increase in number of oocytes retrieved and number of high-quality embryos when compared to hCG alone. Double trigger has been offered in the treatment of immature oocyte syndrome, where <25% of the expected oocytes are retrieved or are with poor/low oocytes yield and EFS.

Some authors refer to a different schedule as a double trigger. Here, instead of giving two different types of triggers with a 6-hour gap, we give two doses of GnRHa with a 12-hour gap. This alteration has been suggested to make it mimic the physiological surge where we add a second agonist 12 hours later.[43,44] This will decrease the chances of empty follicles (EFS), especially in polycystic ovary (PCO) patients. The underlying mechanism proposed is that PCO women show neuroendocrine abnormalities [hypothalamic–pituitary–ovarian (HPO) axis dysfunction causing suboptimal response is more probable in them]; hence, abovementioned threshold levels are not sustained long enough. Another variant is suggested, to add a third dose after 24 hours of first injection. One confusion often arises as to if the repeated doses of agonists can cause poor flare owing to pituitary desensitization. But this has not been found true in antagonist-treated cycles as dynamics and endocrine profiles vary with antagonist *(It is interesting to observe that the hormone profiles consistent with pituitary suppression occur by 6 days of consistent microdose 40 µg bd agonist administration[52])*. Thus, the continued flare effect lasting for next 24 hours with the repeat dose of agonist 12 hours following the first dose results in better oocyte maturity.[43,44]

It is interesting to note that ovulation could be expected to occur early in ovulation induction cycles than in multifollicular cycles. It is also advisable to do ovum pick up a little early with hCG as compared to agonist triggers.[50]

However, the purpose of early retrieval is purely not to miss the OCC by in vivo extrusion. These should be kept in incubators for further maturation, timing of which can vary in different patients. GnRHa trigger has increased across ART practices, leading to promising case reports of successful use of GnRHa triggering in an in vivo-matured (IVM) cycle reflecting possible advantage of GnRHa in IVM cycles, especially those performed for fertility preservation.[53]

■ RECOMBINANT-LH: INFLATED BUBBLE DIFFUSED

Apart from hCG and agonist triggers, other two options are *recombinant LH (Rec-LH)* and Kisspeptins (KISS-1). Rec-LH is not routinely used as it is expensive and cumbersome in administration. The dose of 15,000–30,000 IU of rec-LH gave the highest safety to efficacy ratio.[54] Previous publications suggest using a conversion factor of 2.5, a dose of 12,500 IU rec-LH is as effective as 5,000 IU of hCG in humans.[41] Data on the rise of LH in the first 24 hours after injection are not clear; hence, timing of oocyte retrieval may not be optimal. The rise of LH is less certain and may peak higher or sooner. The serum LH at 24 hours following 5,000, 15,000, and 30,000 IU rec-LH was 20 IU/L, 60 IU/L, and 90 IU/L, respectively.[54]

Recombinant LH offers no additional advantage over hCG other than theoretical lesser OHSS risk. Therefore, it has not become a viable ovulation triggering option. Reduced clinical pregnancy rates and suboptimal decision of timing of oocyte retrieval in rec-LH group further restricts its use for ovulation triggering. A 2016 Cochrane analysis found that the quality of evidence regarding the rec-LH performance was very low[19] and after unpublished trials, the makers Serono decided not to register high-dose rec-LH into clinical use.[19] High cost of rec-LH is prohibiting and again it did not have the advantage of the dual FSH and LH natural surge, so probably this prince shall never fight the woods to reach Miss Snow White.

■ SUPREME BOSS: PLAUSIBLE PANACEA? KISSPEPTIN—YET TO BE EXPLORED

Kisspeptin is a hypothalamic neuropeptide that regulates HPO axis function.[55] Preovulatory rise in serum KISS-1 leads to its action on GnRH neurons in hypothalamus causing GnRH release which causes LH surge that triggers final oocyte maturation and ovulation. *KISS-1* which works at GnRH receptor level (as the central regulator of the neuroendocrine mechanisms) may offer a novel *natural* option. It appears to be a physiological answer available for triggering the surge. Recognized as the gatekeeper of the reproductive axis since 2003, it has proven to stimulate gonadotropin secretion in humans too.[56]

The GnRH neurons are devoid of estrogen receptor α (ERα), which are required to sense negative feedback. Since GnRH neurons do not express ERαs, the transmission of the ovulation trigger signal, forwarded from the gonads to the hypothalamic GnRH neurons, is likely mediated by a different, distinct neuronal population. So how does the negative feedback occur with high E2 levels? It is through these KISS-1 neurons at the brain's arcuate nucleus which have ERα receptors and which in turn governs GnRH release. Evidence obtained in recent studies indicate that KISS-1 neurons are the putative "missing link," mediating both negative and positive feedback of sex steroids.

The GnRH release has different responses and patterns depending on the sex and depending on various times of the cycle. In contrast to males where only tonic pulsatile secretion occurs, the females have two modes—pulsatile and surge modes which are dictated by oscillatory activity of KISS-1 neurons. Pulsatile mode occurs in follicular phase and depending on the pulse frequency, the preferential secretion is encoded—LH (on high frequency pattern) and FSH (on low frequency pattern). The cellular and molecular basis of such a dynamic and timely switch in patterns, which occurs only in adult females, had remained an enigma to a large extent until the discovery of the key roles of specific population of KISS-1 neurons in this phenomenon.

Can KISS-1's commercial production make this a viable option as a trigger or not—there is no immediate answer. Dosing of KISS-1 is in a single bolus of 1.6–12.8 nmol/kg or two boluses of 9.6 nmol/kg, 10 hour apart.[57] The second dose of KISS-1 provided an individualized LH response. It was found that the second dose of KISS-1 gave a good LH rise if the first dose gave poor response and minimal rise if the first dose gave robust LH rise.[58] KISS-1's role as trigger has an advantage of reduced OHSS risk. Whether rapid luteolysis story ensuing after analog repeats here with KISS-1 or not is to be seen and we need more studies on this drug. However, if made cost-effective, it might become the panacea, the successful prince Florian.

■ CONCLUSION

As evident, hCG the traditional prime trigger is not the only triggering option available in modern ART practice. Considering its risk of OHSS, the new prince, agonist has taken up this role in the new woods of antagonist protocol and freeze all cycles. **Table 5** gives the comparison of various trigger drugs. Author presumes that the future prince charming is the dual trigger. It looks like that the future books shall be recommending progesterone primed or antagonist protocol COS along with dual trigger and freeze all policy for majority patients in coming decade **(Table 5)**.

TABLE 5: Comparison between various trigger agents.[50]

Trigger for final oocyte maturation	Protocol	Dose and types	Action site	Peak concentration at	Risk of OHSS
hCG	• Agonist and antagonist both • Also, hypo hypo patients	u-hCG: 5,000–10,000 IU r-hCG: 250–500 µg	Ovaries—on LH receptors	20 hours	High
Analog or GnRHa	• Antagonist only • Not for hypo hypo	• Leuprolide: 0.5–4 mg • Decapeptyl: 0.2–0.4 mg • Buserelin: 0.5–4 mg	Pituitary—on GnRH receptors	4 hours	Less
Rec-LH	Both protocol	Rec-LH: 5,000–30,000 IU	Ovarian—LH	5 hours	Less
Kisspeptin	Antagonist only	Kisspeptin-54 a single bolus of 1.6–12.8 nmol/kg or two boluses of 9.6 nmol/kg 10 hour apart	Kisspeptin receptors on GnRH neurons in hypothalamus	4–6 hours	Least

(GnRH: gonadotropin-releasing hormone; GnRHa: GnRH agonist; hCG: human chorionic gonadotropin; hypo hypo: hypogonadotropic hypogonadism; LH: luteinizing hormone; OHSS: ovarian hyperstimulation syndrome; rec-LH: recombinant LH; r-hCG: recombinant hCG; u-hCG: urinary hCG)
Note: Dual and double triggers are combinations and variations in time schedule are discussed earlier.

■ KEY POINTS

- hCG is the oldest known gonadotropin used as trigger for timed oocyte retrieval in the prime era of long protocols.
- Agonist use as trigger was known for long but was primarily used as down regulating agent in those times.
- hCG remained the panacea till antagonist protocols became popular.
- Prototype shift in ART practices encouraging OHSS free clinics and segmentation of cycles have made agonist popular triggering choice.
- Luteal phase deficiency associated with agonist triggers gave poor pregnancy rates with fresh transfer due to early luteolysis. Hence volumes of luteal phase support studies have come up.
- Addition of low dose hCG with agonist was a great leveller using best of the two triggers.

CHAPTER 10: Human Chorionic Gonadotropin: Not a Panacea Anymore

- Dual trigger gives advantage of postponing the decision of fresh transfer vs freeze all after the oocyte retrieval and later. We can add more hCG later on for better luteal phase support if decision of same cycle transfer is taken.
- LH alone as a trigger is not reliable and is very costly.
- Kisspeptin is not in commercial production as yet and still under research.

REFERENCES

1. Speroff L, Fritz MA (Eds). Assisted reproductive technologies. Clinical Gynecologic Endocrinology and Infertility, 8th edition. India: Wolters Kluwer India Pvt. Ltd./Lippincott Williams & Wilkins South Asian edition; 2011. p. 1353.
2. Cole Laurence A. Biological functions of hCG and hCG-related molecules. Reprod Biol Endocrinol. 2010;8:102.
3. Keay SD, Vatish M, Karteris E, Hillhouse EW, Randeva HS. The role of hCG in reproductive medicine. BJOG. 2004;111:1218-28.
4. Filicori M, Fazleabas AT, Huhtaniemi I, Licht P, Rao ChV, Tesarik J, et al. Novel concepts of human chorionic gonadotropin; Reproductive system interactions and potential in the management of infertility. Fertil Steril. 2005;84(2):275-84.
5. Lass A; UK Timing of hCG Group. Monitoring of IVF-ET cycles by ultrasound and hormonal levels: a prospective, multicenter randomised study. Fertil Steril. 2003;80(1):80-5.
6. Loumaye E, Engrand P, Howles CM, O'Dea L. Assessment of the role of serum LH and Estradiol response to FSH on IVF treatment outcome. Fertil Steril. 1998;69(3):76S-85S.
7. Tan SL, Balen A, el Hussein E, Mills C, Campbell S, et al. A prospective randomised study of the optimum timing of hCG administration after pituitary desensitisation in IVF. Fertil Steril. 1992;57(6):1259-64.
8. Kolibianakis EM, Albano C, Camus M, Tournaye H, Van Steirteghem AC, Devroey P. Prolongation of the follicular phase in IVF results in a lower ongoing pregnancy rate in cycles stimulated with rec FSH and GnRH antagonists. Fertil Steril. 2004;82(1):102-7.
9. Fanton M, Nutting V, Solano F, Maeder-York P, Hariton E, Barash O, et al. An interpretable machine learning model for predicting the optimal day of trigger during ovarian stimulation. Fertil Steril. 2022;118(1):101-7.
10. Abdalla HI, Ah-Moye M, Brinsden P, Howe DL, Okonofua F, Craft I. The effect of the dose of hCG and the type of gonadotropin stimulation on oocyte recovery rates in an IVF program. Fertil Steril. 1987;48(6):958-63.
11. Zelinski-Wooten MB, Hutchison JS, Trinchard-Lugan I, Hess DL, Wolf DP, Stouffer RL. Initiation of periovulatory events in gonadotrophin stimulated macaques with varying doses of rec hCG. Hum Reprod. 1997;12:1877-85.
12. Schmidt DW, Maier DB, Nulsen JC, Benadiva CA. Reducing the dose of hCG in high responders does not affect the outcomes of IVF. Fertil Steril. 2004;82(4):841-6.
13. Gunnala V, Reichman D, Schattman G, Davis O, Rozenwaks Z. Analysis of Sliding scale hCG for reduction of ovarian hyperstimulation syndrome (OHSS) in 10,427 IVF-ICSI cycles. Fertil Steril. 2014;102(3):E118.

14. Irani M, Setton R, Gunnala V, Kligman I, Goldschlag DE, Rozenwaks Z. Dose of human chorionic gonadotropin to trigger final oocyte maturation. Fertil Steril. 2016;106(3):E262-3.
15. Shapiro BS, Daneshmand ST, Garner FC, Aguirre M, Ross R, Morris S. Effects of ovulatory serum concentration of hCG on the incidence of OHSS and success rates of IVF. Fertil Steril. 2005;84(1):93-8.
16. Kolibianakis EM, Papanikolaou EG, Tournaye H, Camus M, Van Steirteghem AC, Devroey P. Triggering final oocyte maturation using different doses of hCG: A randomised pilot study in patients with PCOS treated with GnRH antagonists and rec FSH. Fertil Steril. 2007;88(5):1382-8.
17. Ndukwe G, Thornton S, Fishel S, Dowell K, al-Hassan S, Hunter A. Predicting empty follicle syndrome. Fertil Steril. 1996;66:845-7.
18. Chang P, Kenley S, Burns T, Denton G, Currie K, DeVane G, et al. Recombinant human chorionic gonadotropin (rhCG) in assisted reproductive technology: Results of a clinical trial comparing two doses of rhCG (Ovidrel) to urinary hCG (Profasi) for induction of final follicular maturation in in vitro fertilization-embryo transfer. Fertil Steril. 2001;76(1):67-74.
19. Youssef MA, Abou-Setta AM, Lam WS. Recombinant vs urinary hCG for final oocyte maturation triggering in IVF and ICSI cycles. Cochrane Database Syst Rev. 2016;4(4)CD003719.
20. Zeke J, Kanyó K, Zeke H, Cseh A, Vásárhelyi B, Szilágyi A, et al. Pregnancy rates with recombinant versus urinary human chorionic gonadotropin in in vitro fertilization: An observational study. Sci World J. 2011;11:1781-87.
21. Dorsselaer AV, Carapito C, Delalande F, Schaeffer-Reiss C, Thierse D, Diemer H, et al. Detection of prion protein in urine derived injectable fertility products by a targeted proteomic approach. PLoS One. 2011;6(3):e17815.
22. Papanikolaou EG, Fatemi H, Camus M, Kyrou D, Polyzos NP, Humaidan P, et al. Higher birth rate after rec hCG triggering compared with urinary derived hCG in single blastocyst IVF antagonist cycles: a randomised controlled trial. Fertil Steril. 2010;94(7):2902-4.
23. Humaidan P, Bredkjaer H, Bungum L, Bungum M, Grøndahl ML, Westergaard L, et al. GnRH agonist (buserelin) or hCG for ovulation induction in GnRH antagonist IVF/ICSI cycles: a prospective randomised study. Hum Reprod. 2005;20(5):1213-20.
24. Lunenfeld B, Bilger W, Longobardi S, Alam V, D'Hooghe T, Sunkara SK. The Development of Gonadotropins for Clinical Use in the Treatment of Infertility. Front Endocrinol. 2019;10:429.
25. Trouson A, Mohr L. Human pregnancy following cryopreservation, thawing and transfer of an eight cell embryo. Nature. 1983;305:707-9.
26. Gogen Y, Balakier H, Powell W, Casper RF. Use of GnRH agonist to trigger follicular maturation for IVF. J Clin Endocrinol Metab. 1990;71(4):918-22.
27. Humaidan P, Polyzos NP. hCG vs GnRH agonist trigger in ART - "The king is dead, long live the king!" Fertil Steril. 2014;102(2):339-41.
28. Nakano R, Mizuno T, Kotsuji F, Katayama K, Wshio M, Tojo S. "Triggering" of ovulation after infusion of synthetic LH releasing factor. Acta Obstet Gynecol Scand. 1973;52:269-72.

29. Krishna D, Suvarna R, Sumi M, Snehal D, Arveen V, Anuja K, et al. hCG trigger vs GnRH agonist trigger in PCOS patients undergoing IVF cycles: frozen embryo transfer outcomes. JBRA Assist Reprod. 2021;25(1):48-58.
30. Shapiro BS, Andersen CY. Major drawbacks and additional benefits of agonist trigger - not OHSS related. Fertil Steril. 2015;103(4):874-8.
31. Castillo JC, Humaidan P, Bernabéu R. Pharmaceutical options for triggering of final oocyte maturation in ART. Biomed Res Int. 2014;2014:580171.
32. Humaidan P, Engmann L, Benadiva C. Luteal phase supplementation after GnRHa trigger in fresh embryo transfer: The American vs European approaches. Fertil Steril. 2015;103(4):879-85.
33. Stevenson TL, Lashen H. Empty follicle syndrome: the reality of a controversial syndrome, a systematic review. Fertil Steril. 2008;90(3):691-8.
34. Castillo JC, Garcia-Velasco J, Humaidan P. Empty follicle syndrome after GnRHa triggering vs hCG triggering in COS. J Assist Reprod Genet. 2012;29:249-53.
35. Haas J, Ophir L, Barzilay E, Machtinger R, Yung Y, Orvieto R, et al. Standard human chorionic gonadotropin vs double trigger for final oocyte maturation results in different granulosa cells gene expressions: a pilot study. Fertil Steril. 2016;106(3):653-9.
36. Shapiro BS, Daneshmand ST, Garner FC, Aguirre M, Thomas S. GnRHa combined with a reduced dose of hCG for final oocyte maturation in fresh autologous cycles of IVF. Fertil Steril. 2008;90(1):231-3.
37. Youssef MA, Van der Veen F, Al-Inany HG, Mochtar MH, Griesinger G, Nagi Mohesen M, et al. GnRH agonist vs hCG for oocyte triggering in antagonist assisted reproductive technology. Cochrane Database Syst Rev. 2014;10: CD008046.
38. Licht P, Russu V, Lehmeyer S, Wildt L. Molecular aspects of direct LH/hCG effects on human endometrium - lessons from intrauterine microdialysis in the human female in vivo. Reprod Biol. 2001;1:10-9.
39. Andersen CY, Kelsey T, Mamsen LS, Vuong LN. Shortcomings of an unphysiological triggering of oocyte maturation using hCG. Fertil Steril. 2020;114:200-8.
40. Hoff JD, Quigley ME, Yen SS. Hormonal dynamics at mid cycle: A reevaluation. J Clin Endocrinol Metab. 1983;57(4):792-6.
41. Drakakis P, Loutradis D, Beloukas A, Sypsa V, Anastasiadou V, Kalofolias G, et al. Early hCG addition to rFSH for ovarian stimulation in IVF provides better results and the cDNA copies of the hCG receptor may be indicator of successful stimulation. Reprod Biol Endocrinol. 2009;7:110.
42. Seibel MM, Smith DM, Levesque L, Borten M, Taymor ML. The temporal relationship between the luteinizing hormone surge and human oocyte maturation. Am J Obstet Gynecol. 1982;1142:568-72.
43. Aflatoonian A, Haghighi F, Hoseini M, Haghdani S. Does the repeat dose of GnRHa trigger in PCOS improve IVF cycles outcome? A clinical trial study. Int J Reprod Biomed. 2020;18(7):485-90.
44. Deepika K, Baiju P, Gautham P, Suvarna R, Arveen V, Kamini R. Repeat dose of GnRHa trigger in PCOS undergoing IVF cycles provides a better cycle outcome- A proof of concept study. J Hum Reprod Sci. 2017;10(4):271-80.

45. Kummer NE, Feinn RS, Griffin DW, Nulsen JC, Benadiva CA, Engmann LL. Predicting successful induction of oocyte maturation after GnRHa trigger. Hum Reprod. 2013;28:152-9.
46. Humaidan P, Bredkjaer HE, Westergaard LG, Yding Andersen C. 1,500 IU hCG administered at oocyte retrieval rescues the luteal phase when GnRHa is used for ovulation induction: a prospective, randomised, controlled study. Fertil Steril. 2010;93(3):847-54.
47. Fatemi HM, Polyzos NP, van Vaerenbergh I, Bourgain C, Blockeel C, Alsbjerg B, et al. Early luteal phase endocrine profile is affected by the mode of triggering final oocyte maturation and the luteal phase support used in rec FSH-GnRH antagonist in IVF cycles. Fertil Steril. 2013;100(3):742-7.
48. Chen S, Ye DS, Chen X, Yang XH, Zheng HY, Tang Y, et al. Circulating LH level after triggering oocyte maturation with GnRHa may predict oocyte yield in flexible GnRH antagonist protocol. Hum Reprod. 2012;27(5);1351-6.
49. Dunne C, Shan A, Nakhuda G. Measurement of Luteinising hormone level after GnRH agonist trigger is not useful for predicting oocyte maturity. J Obstet Gynaecol Can. 2018;40(12):1618-22.
50. Abbara A, Clarke SA, Dhillo Waljit S. Novel concepts for inducing final oocyte maturation in IVF treatment. Endocr Rev. 2018;39(5):593-628.
51. Haas J, Zilberberg E, Dar S, Kedem A, Machtinger R, Orvieto R. Co-administration of GnRHa and hCG for final oocyte maturation (double trigger) in patients with low number of oocytes retrieved per number of preovulatory follicles-a preliminary report. J Ovarian Res. 2014;7:77.
52. Chung K, Fogle R, Bendikson K, Christenson K, Paulson R. Microdose GnRHa in the absence of exogenous gonadotropins is not sufficient to induce multiple follicle development. Fertil Steril. 2011;95(1):317-9.
53. El Hachem H, Poulain M, Le Parco S, Fanchin R, Frydman N, Grynberg M. GnRHa priming increases the number of in vitro matured (IVM) oocytes available for cryopreservation in cancer patients seeking urgent fertility preservation (FP). Fertil Steril. 2013;100(3):S118.
54. European Recombinant LH study group. Human recombinant luteinizing hormone is as effective as, but safer than, u-hCG in inducing final follicular maturation and ovulation in IVF procedures-result of multicenter double blind study. JCEM. 2001;86(6):2607-18.
55. Meczekalski B, Katulski K, Podfigurna-Stopa A, Czyzyk A, Genazzani AD. Spontaneous endogenous pulsatile release of kisspeptin is temporally coupled with LH in healthy women. Fertil Steril. 2016;105(5):1345-50.
56. Ruohonen ST, Poutanen M, Tena-Sempere M. Review-Role of Kisspeptins in the control of HPO axis: old dogmas and new challenges. Fertil Steril. 2020;114(3):465-74.
57. Jayasena CN, Abbara A, Comninos AN, Nijher GM, Christopoulos G, Narayanaswamy S, et al. Kisspeptin-54 triggers egg maturation in women undergoing in vitro fertilisation. J Clinic Invest. 2014;124(8):3667-77.
58. Abbara A, Clarke S, Islam R, Prague JK, Comninos AN, Narayanaswamy S, et al. A second dose of Kisspeptin-54 improves oocyte maturation in women at high risk for OHSS: a phase 2 randomised controlled trial. Hum Reprod. 2017;32(9);1915-24.

Chapter 11

Analog Trigger: Are We Missing the Target?

Yuval Atzmon, Einat Shalom-Paz

■ INTRODUCTION

The final step of assisted reproductive technology (ART) before oocyte pick-up (OPU) is triggering ovulation. Various approaches are used to achieve the optimal maturation rate. The most common way uses human chorionic gonadotropins (hCG) with very good results.[1] Gonadotropin-releasing hormone agonist (GnRHa) was first used for ovulation induction, with the objective of mimicking the natural surge of luteinizing hormone (LH) in the nonstimulated cycles.[2] Its use for ovulation induction in in vitro fertilization (IVF) treatments was enabled after GnRH antagonist was introduced to the field of ART and it was shown to be as effective as hCG for inducing ovulation, however, with lower pregnancy rates.[1,3-5] Later, different medical conditions forced the need for an alternative to hCG. GnRHa was introduced mainly to avoid ovarian hyperstimulation syndrome (OHSS).[4,5] The adequate stimulation results using GnRHa to provoke an LH surge and the understanding of OHSS pathophysiology[6,7] made GnRHa an alternative for triggering ovulation with comparable numbers of oocytes and mature oocytes collected.[1] Its use is well established for oocyte donation programs and cycles that require separation of the OPU from the embryo transfer (ET), which is known as "segmentation". However, its use in fresh ET cycles is still controversial.

■ PHYSIOLOGY

The endogenous GnRH is a decapeptide (pGlu-His-Trp-Ser-Tyr-Gly-Leu-Arg-Pro-Gly-NH2)[8] with a short half-life due to rapid cleavage of the bonds between amino acids 5–6, 6–7, and 9–10. Various GnRH agonist analogs are currently available. These GnRH agonists are synthetically built with specific modifications. Usually, double substitutions are made, typically in positions 6 (amino acid substitution), 9 (alkylation), and 10 (deletion). These substitutions inhibit rapid degradation. Agonists with two substitutions include leuprorelin, buserelin, histrelin, goserelin, and deslorelin. Nafarelin and triptorelin are agonists with single substitutions at position 6.[9] Two of the most frequently used are triptorelin (Decapeptyl® 0.1 mg) and nafarelin (Synarel®).

■ TRIGGER FOR OVULATION

Luteinizing hormone and hCG are fundamental glycoproteins for development and reproductive activity. Although they activate the same receptor, LH chorionic gonadotropin receptor (LHCGR) hCG and LH molecules are only 85% similar. Multiple signaling pathways are activated by several LHCGR interactors. It is well-known that LH and hCG induce simultaneous increases of the second messenger cyclic adenosine monophosphate (cAMP) and Ca^{2+} through the LHCGR and that hCG is about five times more potent than LH in inducing cAMP production. Moreover, both hormones activate different pathways that lead to counter responses; LH is more active in the pERK and pAKT pathways with proliferative reactions and antiapoptotic signals, while hCG is more in the cAMP/PKA pathway and improves steroidogenesis and stimulates proapoptotic potential.[10]

The endogenous LH surge trigger for ovulation occurs via positive feedback of estradiol (E2) with an increase in GnRH frequency and amplitude pulses.[11] In natural cycles, LH surge duration is 48.7 ± 9.27 hours. The total LH surge is divided into three phases: a short ascending phase (14 h), a peak plateau phase (14 h), and a long descending phase (20 h).[12]

Triggering for LH surge to achieve oocyte maturation can be done artificially using GnRHa or hCG. GnRHa generates a different LH surge wave compared to the pituitary, in which LH levels rapidly increase and reach a peak level 4 hours after GnRHa administration, rapidly decrease afterwards and return to baseline 24 hours after GnRh administration.[13]

Ovulation trigger by hCG is based on the biological similarity of the alpha subunit of hCG and LH.[14] For the last 40 years, exogenous hCG has been used for final oocyte maturation. The release of the oocyte from the follicle usually occurs 36–40 hours after the injection. The serum levels of hCG gradually increase and reach a peak 24 hours after administration. Thereafter, serum hCG levels decrease with half-life of 8 days and by day 12 after the injection, it is not detected in the blood.[13] The increased glycosylation of hCG results in prolonged bioactivity, which in combination with the sustained luteotropic activity could induce OHSS **(Fig. 1)**.

Some may argue that hCG administration for ovulation induction causes an absence of follicle-stimulating hormone (FSH) surge and stimulation of the corpus luteum during the early luteal phase, which asynchronously raises E2 and progesterone during the early luteal phase and may shift the window of implantation.[15] The optimal trigger for ovulation has not yet been determined.

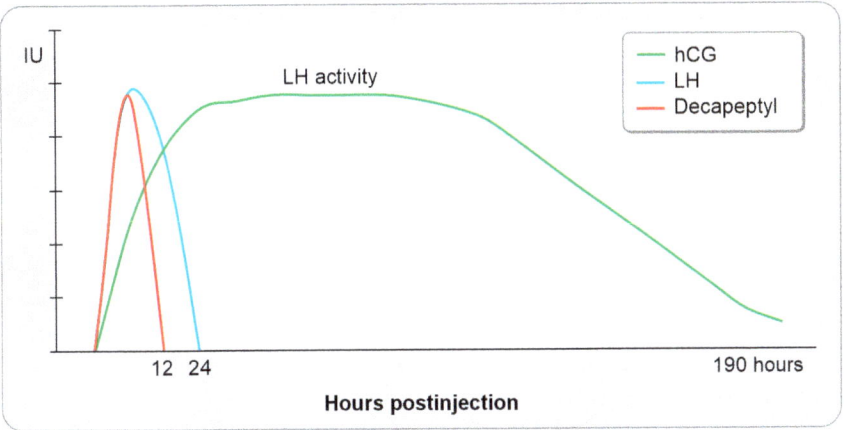

Fig. 1: The increased glycosylation of hCG.
(hCG: human chorionic gonadotropin; LH: luteinizing hormone)

CONTROVERSIES IN GnRHa TRIGGERING FOR OVULATION IN ASSISTED REPRODUCTIVE CYCLES

Due to luteal phase insufficiency, contributed by the low LH levels after GnRHa trigger,[16] low circulating progesterone concentrations were observed. This resulted in significantly lower implantation and pregnancy rates,[1,17] which restricted the use of GnRHa to cycles in which ET is not planned.

Pros of the GnRHa Trigger

It is well established that GnRHa triggers both FSH and LH surges, which expose the developed follicles to more physiologic hormonal changes, as compared to hCG and is sufficient to induce final oocyte maturation.[3,5] The use of GnRHa to trigger ovulation was expanded after GnRH antagonist was introduced to prevent premature ovulation due to suppression of the LH surge.[18,19]

A significant advantage of GnRHa triggering is based on the shorter LH activity, which leads to luteolysis and prevents OHSS by altering the vascular regulation mediators. This leads to lower production of vascular endothelial growth factor, which is the key factor in inducing vascular permeability of blood vessels.[6,7,20] The first study to show an alternative trigger for patients at high risk for OHSS was published in 1991, in a group of 38 women with E2 levels above 4,000 pg/mL. Using a GnRHa nasal spray, they had a pregnancy rate of 29% with no OHSS complications reported.[21] There is a consensus regarding the significant reduction and up to complete elimination of OHSS by using GnRHa as a trigger and avoiding hCG.[1,16,21] Only one rare case of OHSS was reported after GnRHa triggering[22] and this was probably related to mutation or polymorphisms of GnRH, FSH, or LH receptors.[23]

Along with the goal of eliminating OHSS, we must make sure that we do not compromise cycle outcomes. Several studies reported the use of GnRHa with comparable MII oocytes collected.[3,24] Some randomized controlled trials even demonstrated that more mature oocytes were obtained in the GnRHa group.[25-27] Oocyte and embryo quality was not adversely affected by GnRHa triggering, nor was the performance of thawed frozen embryos from fresh GnRHa trigger cycles, which demonstrated equivalent survival, implantation, clinical pregnancy, and ongoing pregnancy rates in the subsequent frozen ET cycle.[28] Studies evaluating donor oocytes triggered with GnRHa as compared to hCG showed comparable results in fertilization, pregnancy, and implantation rates.[29-31] Importantly, the euploidy rates of the embryos were comparable.[32]

Another advantage important to mention is that the patients reported less discomfort after GnRHa triggering, less bloating, and reduced ovarian volume,[33] which makes this trigger optimal for oocyte donors and any cycles that require segmentation between OPU and ET.

Drawbacks to the GnRHa Trigger

The various ovulation induction methods demonstrate significant differences in the physiological and clinical results in ART treatment. Several reports, including a Cochrane meta-analysis, summarized unfavorable outcomes, which resulted in limiting the use of GnRHa triggering.[1,34] Those studies pointed out several weaknesses of the GnRHa trigger. The main pitfall is the abnormal luteal phase. Consequently, lower pregnancy rates were achieved, with lower live birth rates and lower ongoing pregnancy rates (pregnancy beyond 12 weeks). Moreover, higher early miscarriage rates (before 12 weeks) were detected, as compared with patients treated with hCG trigger.[17] These findings are explained by the difference in the duration of activity of GnRHa compared with hCG and endogenous LH. Endogenous LH activity is shorter compared with hCG, which causes a luteolytic process due to reduced support in the corpus luteum. This primes impaired production of E2, progesterone, and inhibin A in the luteal phase.[4,13,35]

Failure of the GnRH Trigger

Several studies aimed to predict factors contributing to successful GnRHa stimulation[36] and the cause for suboptimal response to GnRHa.[37,38] A suboptimal LH surge was found to be the connecting link between cycles with suboptimal ovulation outcome, fewer oocytes collected, and lower mature oocyte rate.[37-40] Shapiro et al. reported a dramatic reduction in oocyte yield and maturity when LH levels were less than 12 IU/L 12 hours after GnRHa injection.[40] Kummer et al. found that peak E2 on the ovulation trigger day, post-trigger LH, LH rise, and progesterone were all correlated to total number of oocytes and mature oocytes retrieved. They also reported cases of triggering failure, with empty follicle syndrome. This occurred in patients with low levels of LH post-trigger (LH < 15 IU/L) and lower levels of progesterone (<3.5 ng/mL) 8-12 hours after GnRHa trigger.[37] Meyer et al. identified risk factors that cause a suboptimal response to GnRHa trigger. They also emphasized the impact of very low FSH and LH at the beginning of the cycle, as might be seen after a long duration of oral contraception use and low LH on the day of the trigger. The incidence of the suboptimal response to triggering with GnRHa only, when LH level was 0.1 IU/L and was compared to LH levels ≥0.5 IU/L decreased from 5.2 to 0.2%.[38]

Recently, the importance of LH levels at the beginning of stimulation was strengthened. GnRHa trigger in patients with LH levels <0.1 IU/L was susceptible to suboptimal responses, including empty follicle syndrome and fewer oocytes retrieved than expected. The response to GnRHa trigger improved as baseline LH levels increased. One of the parameters that could have contributed to this trigger failure was contraception use before the treatment cycle, resulting in downregulation of LH levels.[41]

VARIOUS APPROACHES TO OVERCOME LUTEAL PHASE INSUFFICIENCY

Once GnRHa is used to avoid OHSS, the segmentation approach is acceptable, to eliminate late OHSS if ET is accomplished.[42] However, there are situations in which we cannot avoid ET, such as low-quality embryos that are not suitable for vitrification. In these cases, we have to provide adequate luteal support to counteract the negative effect of the GnRHa trigger.[13,43] Two main approaches are discussed in the literature: intensive luteal phase support and low-dose hCG supplementation during the luteal phase.[17,25]

Intensive luteal phase support (iLPS) with higher estrogen and progesterone supplementation: A few studies reported comparable outcomes after GnRHa triggering in antagonist cycles, using intensive intramuscular progesterone support in terms of implantation rate, clinical pregnancy rate, and delivery rate.[33,44,45] A randomized controlled study by Engman et al. reported no significant differences in implantation, clinical pregnancy, and ongoing pregnancy rates between patients triggered with GnRHa in antagonist cycles to those triggered with hCG in agonist cycles. Both groups received intramuscular progesterone support and for the GnRHa trigger, estrogen doses were adjusted according to serum E2 levels.[33] Later, Imbar et al. compared the results of frozen thawed embryos and fresh ET conducted in GnRHa trigger cycle. The fresh ET was treated with iLPS including intramuscular progesterone and oral E_2 fresh ET cycle outcomes were compared to the fresh iLPS group. The implantation, clinical pregnancy, miscarriage, and live birth rates were comparable and most importantly, none of the patients in the fresh

ET group developed OHSS.[45] The best regimen for LPS was evaluated in a study that compared three groups. Group 1 received dual trigger (hCG with GnRHa) with standard luteal support, group 2 was triggered with GnRHa only and received the standard luteal support, and group 3 was triggered with GnRHa only and supplemented with iLPS. Significantly better results were achieved in the groups exposed to hCG or treated with iLPS. Comparable outcomes were seen in the iLPS and the standard luteal support groups with dual triggering.[46]

Studies that reported the effect of iLPS used intramuscular progesterone injections, which are inconvenient and painful. However, vaginal and oral progesterone supplementation has not been evaluated as part of iLPS in GnRHa trigger cycles. It is worth mentioning that several studies showed noninferior results in fresh and frozen ET using vaginal micronized progesterone, as well as oral dydrogesterone for luteal support.[47-49]

Most importantly, iLPS should be continued to 10 weeks of gestation in order to compensate for the early lysis of the corpus luteum after GnRHa triggering, compared to hCG triggering in which the corpus luteum lasts for a longer period.[35]

Human chorionic gonadotropin administration during the luteal phase: The rationale for supporting the secretions of the corpus luteum by hCG to rescue it from lysis was first given by Humaidan et al. at OPU as a proof of concept. They reported a 50% pregnancy rate and only one case of moderate OHSS.[50] Their subsequent prospective study on 305 IVF cycles that were triggered with 10,000 IU hCG or GnRHa supplemented with 1,500 IU hCG on the OPU day they reported no difference in biochemical pregnancy, ongoing pregnancy, early miscarriage, and delivery rates. They concluded that a small bolus of hCG in the GnRHa-triggered group secured the luteal phase and resulted in comparable reproductive outcomes.[51] Their next study aimed to personalize hCG support better. They categorized patients into four groups based on their risk of OHSS.[52] High-risk patients were randomized to receive either 1,500 IU or 5,000 IU of hCG supplementation on OPU day. Low-risk patients were randomized to receive either an additional injection of hCG 1,500 IU at OPU, with another dose of 1,500 IU or 5,000 IU hCG given at OPU +5 days. They concluded that GnRHa triggering followed by early luteal hCG support with one bolus of 1,500 IU hCG appears to reduce OHSS in at-risk patients. However, in the low-risk group, a second bolus of 1,500 IU hCG induced two cases of late-onset OHSS. However, in contrast to the above study by Humaidan,[52] Seyhan et al. reported that severe early OHSS can occur even after the GnRH agonist trigger and 1,500 IU hCG luteal rescue protocol.[53]

Low-dose hCG Support

A few studies evaluated the contribution of low-dose hCG for GnRHa trigger cycles, concomitantly with or separately from GnRHa trigger. In a retrospective study, Castillo et al. reported that the use of low doses of hCG in the luteal phase after agonist trigger was associated with normal pregnancy rates with no excess OHSS risk; although the overall rates of OHSS (moderate and severe) were 3.6% and 4.2%, respectively.[54]

Another study retrospectively evaluated patients at high risk for OHSS who were triggered with GnRHa and 500–1,000 IU hCG and another 300 IU given on day 6 after OPU, only when serum E_2 levels were below 800 pg/mL. No instances of OHSS were reported with this approach and the clinical and ongoing pregnancy rates were (48.5% vs. 17.4% and 46.9% vs. 17.4%, respectively) although not significantly different.[55]

Another retrospective study that compared GnRHa triggering alone to dual trigger with GnRHa and 1,000 IU of hCG reported significantly higher rates were observed in dual trigger group (52.9% vs. 30.9%; $p = 0.03$) with no difference in OHSS rate.[56]

So far, we believe there are inadequate data to safely recommend the addition of hCG to trigger oocyte maturation in patients at high risk for OHSS, regardless of the possible improvements in reproductive outcomes.

■ CONCLUSION

The discovery of analog trigger along with antagonist cycle has proven a beneficial concept for hyper-responder and PCOS patients. It had almost completely eliminated the risk of moderate to severe OHSS and an "OHSS-Free" clinic could be a reality. The drawback of inability to do fresh embryo transfer can be tackled by using dual trigger and intense luteal phase suppot with estrogen and progesterone along with low dose of hCG. analog trigger is more physiological as its not acting as a surrogate but causing real LH and FSH surge which proves beneficial to the quality of oocytes.

■ KEY POINTS

The dual aim of fertility treatments is the desire to succeed while minimizing the risk to patients. These two objectives do not always align. In order to achieve an OHSS-free clinic, the segmentation approach has gained more attention and hence is more focused on GnRHa triggering.

Unfortunately, the optimal protocol for luteal supplementation after GnRHa trigger has not yet been defined, which might compromise pregnancy rates in cases where fresh ET is deemed necessary.

Aside from that, using an antagonist protocol enables us to trigger ovulation safely and more physiologically. It resembles the natural LH surge, avoiding the prolonged action of hCG on steroidogenesis and permits lower hormonal levels that are closer to a natural cycle. Most importantly, GnRHa triggering helps eliminate OHSS due to the quick luteolysis that follows. This approach was shown not to compromise the number of mature oocytes achieved per cycle, and owing to the shorter life of the corpus luteum stimulated by the GnRHa, it enables a reduced treatment burden.

With the goal of eliminating OHSS and reducing the duration of E2 exposure after retrieval, all cases of oocyte donation as well as high-responder patients should be treated with antagonist protocols and GnRHa triggering. Fertility preservation for cancer patients also may benefit from a shorter luteal phase and lower hormonal levels after GnRHa triggering, without compromising the number of mature oocytes available for preservation.

Taken together, the concept of GnRHa triggering adds safety, efficacy, to modern IVF and is more patient friendly.

■ REFERENCES

1. Youssef MAFM, Van der Veen F, Al-Inany HG, Mochtar MH, Griesinger G, Nagi Mohesen M, et al. Gonadotropin-releasing hormone agonist versus HCG for oocyte triggering in antagonist-assisted reproductive technology. Cochrane Database Syst Rev. 2014;(10):CD008046.
2. Nakano R, Washio M, Kotsuji F, Mizuno T, Tojo S. Gonadotrophin response to synthetic luteinizing hormone releasing factor (LRF) in normal female and anovulatory patients. Endokrinologie. 1973;62(2):175-83.
3. Gonen Y, Balakier H, Powell W, Casper RF. Use of gonadotropin-releasing hormone agonist to trigger follicular maturation for in vitro fertilization. J Clin Endocrinol Metab. 1990;71(4):918-22.
4. Itskovitz J, Boldes R, Levron J, Erlik Y, Kahana L, Brandes JM. Induction of preovulatory luteinizing hormone surge and prevention of ovarian hyperstimulation syndrome by gonadotropin-releasing hormone agonist. Fertil Steril. 1991;56(2):213-20.
5. Segal S, Casper RF. Gonadotropin-releasing hormone agonist versus human chorionic gonadotropin for triggering follicular maturation in in vitro fertilization. Fertil Steril. 1992;57(6):1254-8.
6. Pellicer A, Albert C, Mercader A, Bonilla-Musoles F, Remohí J, Simón C. The pathogenesis of ovarian hyperstimulation syndrome: in vivo studies investigating the role of interleukin-1beta, interleukin-6, and vascular endothelial growth factor. Fertil Steril. 1999;71(3):482-9.
7. Wang T-H, Horng S-G, Chang C-L, Wu H-M, Tsai Y-J, Wang H-S, et al. Human chorionic gonadotropin-induced ovarian hyperstimulation syndrome is associated with up-regulation of vascular endothelial growth factor. J Clin Endocrinol Metab. 2002;87(7):3300-8.
8. Baba Y, Matsuo H, Schally AV. Structure of the porcine LH- and FSH-releasing hormone. II. Confirmation of the proposed structure by conventional sequential analyses. Biochem Biophys Res Commun. 1971;44(2):459-63.
9. Sealfon SC, Weinstein H, Millar RP. Molecular mechanisms of ligand interaction with the gonadotropin-releasing hormone receptor. Endocr Rev. 1997;18(2):180-205.
10. Casarini L, Santi D, Brigante G, Simoni M. Two Hormones for One Receptor: Evolution, Biochemistry, Actions, and Pathophysiology of LH and hCG. Endocr Rev. 2018;39(5):549-92.

11. Watanabe Y, Uenoyama Y, Suzuki J, Takase K, Suetomi Y, Ohkura S, et al. Oestrogen-induced activation of preoptic kisspeptin neurones may be involved in the luteinising hormone surge in male and female Japanese monkeys. J Neuroendocrinol. 2014;26(12):909-17.
12. Hoff JD, Quigley ME, Yen SS. Hormonal dynamics at midcycle: a reevaluation. J Clin Endocrinol Metab. 1983;57(4):792-6.
13. Fauser BC, de Jong D, Olivennes F, Wramsby H, Tay C, Itskovitz-Eldor J, et al. Endocrine profiles after triggering of final oocyte maturation with GnRH agonist after cotreatment with the GnRH antagonist ganirelix during ovarian hyperstimulation for in vitro fertilization. J Clin Endocrinol Metab. 2002;87(2):709-15.
14. Stenman UH, Tiitinen A, Alfthan H, Valmu L. The classification, functions and clinical use of different isoforms of HCG. Hum Reprod Update. 2006;12(6):769-84.
15. Yding Andersen C, Vilbour Andersen K. Improving the luteal phase after ovarian stimulation: reviewing new options. Reprod Biomed Online. 2014;28(5):552-9.
16. Engmann L, Benadiva C. GnRH agonist (buserelin) or HCG for ovulation induction in GnRH antagonist IVF/ICSI cycles: a prospective randomized study. Hum Reprod. 2005;20(11):3258-60.
17. Kolibianakis EM, Schultze-Mosgau A, Schroer A, van Steirteghem A, Devroey P, Diedrich K, et al. A lower ongoing pregnancy rate can be expected when GnRH agonist is used for triggering final oocyte maturation instead of HCG in patients undergoing IVF with GnRH antagonists. Hum Reprod. 2005;20(10):2887-92.
18. Fatemi HM, Platteau P, Albano C, Van Steirteghem A, Devroey P. Rescue IVF and coasting with the use of a GnRH antagonist after ovulation induction. Reprod Biomed Online. 2002;5(3):273-5.
19. Albano C, Smitz J, Camus M, Riethmüller-Winzen H, Van Steirteghem A, Devroey P. Comparison of different doses of gonadotropin-releasing hormone antagonist Cetrorelix during controlled ovarian hyperstimulation. Fertil Steril. 1997;67(5):917-22.
20. Cerrillo M, Rodríguez S, Mayoral M, Pacheco A, Martínez-Salazar J, Garcia-Velasco JA. Differential regulation of VEGF after final oocyte maturation with GnRH agonist versus hCG: a rationale for OHSS reduction. Fertil Steril. 2009;91(4 Suppl):1526-8.
21. Imoedemhe DA, Chan RC, Sigue AB, Pacpaco EL, Olazo AB. A new approach to the management of patients at risk of ovarian hyperstimulation in an in-vitro fertilization programme. Hum Reprod. 1991;6(8):1088-91.
22. Fatemi HM, Popovic-Todorovic B, Humaidan P, Kol S, Banker M, Devroey P, et al. Severe ovarian hyperstimulation syndrome after gonadotropin-releasing hormone (GnRH) agonist trigger and "freeze-all" approach in GnRH antagonist protocol. Fertil Steril. 2014;101(4):1008-11.
23. Qiao J, Han B. Diseases caused by mutations in luteinizing hormone/chorionic gonadotropin receptor. Prog Mol Biol Transl Sci. 2019;161:69-89.
24. Porter RN, Smith W, Craft IL, Abdulwahid NA, Jacobs HS. Induction of ovulation for in-vitro fertilisation using buserelin and gonadotropins. Lancet. 1984;2(8414):1284-5.
25. Humaidan P, Bredkjaer HE, Bungum L, Bungum M, Grøndahl ML, Westergaard L, et al. GnRH agonist (buserelin) or hCG for ovulation induction in GnRH

antagonist IVF/ICSI cycles: a prospective randomized study. Hum Reprod. 2005;20(5):1213-20.
26. Humaidan P, Kol S, Papanikolaou EG, Copenhagen GnRH Agonist Triggering Workshop Group. GnRH agonist for triggering of final oocyte maturation: time for a change of practice? Hum Reprod Update. 2011;17(4):510-24.
27. Krishna D, Dhoble S, Praneesh G, Rathore S, Upadhaya A, Rao K. Gonadotropin-releasing hormone agonist trigger is a better alternative than human chorionic gonadotropin in PCOS undergoing IVF cycles for an OHSS Free Clinic: A Randomized control trial. J Hum Reprod Sci. 2016;9(3):164-72.
28. Eldar-Geva T, Zylber-Haran E, Babayof R, Halevy-Shalem T, Ben-Chetrit A, Tsafrir A, et al. Similar outcome for cryopreserved embryo transfer following GnRH-antagonist/GnRH-agonist, GnRH-antagonist/HCG or long protocol ovarian stimulation. Reprod Biomed Online. 2007;14(2):148-54.
29. Acevedo B, Gomez-Palomares JL, Ricciarelli E, Hernández ER. Triggering ovulation with gonadotropin-releasing hormone agonists does not compromise embryo implantation rates. Fertil Steril. 2006;86(6):1682-7.
30. Galindo A, Bodri D, Guillén JJ, Colodrón M, Vernaeve V, Coll O. Triggering with HCG or GnRH agonist in GnRH antagonist treated oocyte donation cycles: a randomised clinical trial. Gynecol Endocrinol. 2009;25(1):60-6.
31. Erb TM, Vitek W, Wakim ANG. Gonadotropin-releasing hormone agonist or human chorionic gonadotropin for final oocyte maturation in an oocyte donor program. Fertil Steril. 2010;93(2):374-8.
32. Thorne J, Loza A, Kaye L, Nulsen J, Benadiva C, Grow D, et al. Euploidy rates between cycles triggered with gonadotropin-releasing hormone agonist and human chorionic gonadotropin. Fertil Steril. 2019;112(2):258-65.
33. Engmann L, DiLuigi A, Schmidt D, Nulsen J, Maier D, Benadiva C. The use of gonadotropin-releasing hormone (GnRH) agonist to induce oocyte maturation after cotreatment with GnRH antagonist in high-risk patients undergoing in vitro fertilization prevents the risk of ovarian hyperstimulation syndrome: a prospective randomized controlled study. Fertil Steril. 2008;89(1):84-91.
34. Griesinger G, Berndt H, Schultz L, Depenbusch M, Schultze-Mosgau A. Cumulative live birth rates after GnRH-agonist triggering of final oocyte maturation in patients at risk of OHSS: a prospective, clinical cohort study. Eur J Obstet Gynecol Reprod Biol. 2010;149(2):190-4.
35. Nevo O, Eldar-Geva T, Kol S, Itskovitz-Eldor J. Lower levels of inhibin A and pro-alphaC during the luteal phase after triggering oocyte maturation with a gonadotropin-releasing hormone agonist versus human chorionic gonadotropin. Fertil Steril. 2003;79(5):1123-8.
36. Castillo JC, Garcia-Velasco J, Humaidan P. Empty follicle syndrome after GnRHa triggering versus hCG triggering in COS. J Assist Reprod Genet. 2012;29(3):249-53.
37. Kummer NE, Feinn RS, Griffin DW, Nulsen JC, Benadiva CA, Engmann LL. Predicting successful induction of oocyte maturation after gonadotropin-releasing hormone agonist (GnRHa) trigger. Hum Reprod. 2013;28(1):152-9.
38. Meyer L, Murphy LA, Gumer A, Reichman DE, Rosenwaks Z, Cholst IN. Risk factors for a suboptimal response to gonadotropin-releasing hormone agonist trigger during in vitro fertilization cycles. Fertil Steril. 2015;104(3):637-42.

39. Asada Y, Itoi F, Honnma H, Takiguchi S, Fukunaga N, Hashiba Y, et al. Failure of GnRH agonist-triggered oocyte maturation: its cause and management. J Assist Reprod Genet. 2013;30(4):581-5.
40. Shapiro BS, Daneshmand ST, Restrepo H, Garner FC, Aguirre M, Hudson C. Efficacy of induced luteinizing hormone surge after "trigger" with gonadotropin-releasing hormone agonist. Fertil Steril. 2011;95(2):826-8.
41. Popovic-Todorovic B, Santos-Ribeiro S, Drakopoulos P, De Vos M, Racca A, Mackens S, et al. Predicting suboptimal oocyte yield following GnRH agonist trigger by measuring serum LH at the start of ovarian stimulation. Hum Reprod. 2019;34(10):2027-35.
42. Mathur RS, Akande AV, Keay SD, Hunt LP, Jenkins JM. Distinction between early and late ovarian hyperstimulation syndrome. Fertil Steril. 2000;73(5):901-7.
43. Beckers NGM, Macklon NS, Eijkemans MJ, Ludwig M, Felberbaum RE, Diedrich K, et al. Nonsupplemented luteal phase characteristics after the administration of recombinant human chorionic gonadotropin, recombinant luteinizing hormone, or gonadotropin-releasing hormone (GnRH) agonist to induce final oocyte maturation in in vitro fertilization patients after ovarian stimulation with recombinant follicle-stimulating hormone and GnRH antagonist cotreatment. J Clin Endocrinol Metab. 2003;88(9):4186-92.
44. Engmann L, Siano L, Schmidt D, Nulsen J, Maier D, Benadiva C. GnRH agonist to induce oocyte maturation during IVF in patients at high risk of OHSS. Reprod Biomed Online. 2006;13(5):639-44.
45. Imbar T, Kol S, Lossos F, Bdolah Y, Hurwitz A, Haimov-Kochman R. Reproductive outcome of fresh or frozen-thawed embryo transfer is similar in high-risk patients for ovarian hyperstimulation syndrome using GnRH agonist for final oocyte maturation and intensive luteal support. Hum Reprod. 2012;27(3):753-9.
46. Shapiro BS, Daneshmand ST, Garner FC, Aguirre M, Hudson C. Comparison of "triggers" using leuprolide acetate alone or in combination with low-dose human chorionic gonadotropin. Fertil Steril. 2011;95(8):2715-7.
47. Tournaye H, Sukhikh GT, Kahler E, Griesinger G. A Phase III randomized controlled trial comparing the efficacy, safety and tolerability of oral dydrogesterone versus micronized vaginal progesterone for luteal support in in vitro fertilization. Hum Reprod. 2017;32(5):1019-27.
48. Griesinger G, Blockeel C, Sukhikh GT, Patki A, Dhorepatil B, Yang D-Z, et al. Oral dydrogesterone versus intravaginal micronized progesterone gel for luteal phase support in IVF: a randomized clinical trial. Hum Reprod. 2018;33(12):2212-21.
49. Griesinger G, Blockeel C, Tournaye H. Oral dydrogesterone for luteal phase support in fresh in vitro fertilization cycles: a new standard? Fertil Steril. 2018;109(5):756-62.
50. Humaidan P. Luteal phase rescue in high-risk OHSS patients by GnRHa triggering in combination with low-dose HCG: a pilot study. Reprod Biomed Online. 2009;18(5):630-4.
51. Humaidan P, Ejdrup Bredkjaer H, Westergaard LG, Yding Andersen C. 1,500 IU human chorionic gonadotropin administered at oocyte retrieval rescues the luteal phase when gonadotropin-releasing hormone agonist is used for ovulation induction: a prospective, randomized, controlled study. Fertil Steril. 2010;93(3):847-54.

52. Humaidan P, Polyzos NP, Alsbjerg B, Erb K, Mikkelsen AL, Elbaek HO, et al. GnRHa trigger and individualized luteal phase hCG support according to ovarian response to stimulation: two prospective randomized controlled multicentre studies in IVF patients. Hum Reprod. 2013;28(9):2511-21.
53. Seyhan A, Ata B, Polat M, Son W-Y, Yarali H, Dahan MH. Severe early ovarian hyperstimulation syndrome following GnRH agonist trigger with the addition of 1500 IU hCG. Hum Reprod. 2013;28(9):2522-8.
54. Castillo JC, Dolz M, Bienvenido E, Abad L, Casañ EM, Bonilla-Musoles F. Cycles triggered with GnRH agonist: exploring low-dose HCG for luteal support. Reprod Biomed Online. 2010;20(2):175-81.
55. Huang C-Y, Shieh M-L, Li H-Y. The benefit of individualized low-dose hCG support for high responders in GnRHa-triggered IVF/ICSI cycles. J Chin Med Assoc. 2016;79(7):387-93.
56. Griffin D, Benadiva C, Kummer N, Budinetz T, Nulsen J, Engmann L. Dual trigger of oocyte maturation with gonadotropin-releasing hormone agonist and low-dose human chorionic gonadotropin to optimize live birth rates in high responders. Fertil Steril. 2012;97(6):1316-20.

Dual Trigger: It Works!

Rachana Sameer Deshpande, Padma Rekha Jirge

■ INTRODUCTION

The major contributors to improving safety and success rate in in vitro fertilization (IVF) have been the utilization of individualized ovarian stimulation protocols and the progress in laboratory science and technology. Ovarian reserve markers have contributed to identifying normal/hyper/poor responders before women go through the first cycle of IVF.[1] Identifying different types of responses to ovarian stimulation has certainly improved the safety of treatment.[2] This is achieved through a better choice of protocol, starting dose of gonadotropins, use of gonadotropin-releasing hormone agonists (GnRHa) for oocyte maturation, and selective "freeze all" strategy in those at high risk of developing ovarian hyperstimulation syndrome (OHSS). Introduction of the concept of women with low prognosis by the Poseidon group has drawn attention to the problem of suboptimal response in "normoresponders".[3] Progress in the understanding of luteal phase physiology and deficiencies has led to tailored luteal phase support based on the clinical scenario.[4] None of the above deliberations and interventions address the possible causative role of trigger in situations of suboptimal response, poor yield of mature oocytes, or genuine empty follicle syndrome (EFS).

It is evident that the efforts to improve clinical outcomes have concentrated on the follicular and luteal phase events. Explorations regarding the impact of ovulation trigger on IVF outcomes are limited. In the recent years, attempts have been made to address situations with suboptimal outcomes in normoresponders by modifying the trigger strategy.[5] In addition, embryo transfer during a fresh cycle may be considered without increasing the risk of OHSS even in hyper-responders in selected scenarios.[4] This review aims to provide a concurrent evidence-based view of the modifications in standard ovulation trigger and their possible place in IVF cycles.

■ SEARCH STRATEGY

An electronic search was performed in Medline (1966–2021) with search terms "ovulation trigger in IVF", "hCG trigger in IVF", "GnRHa trigger for IVF",

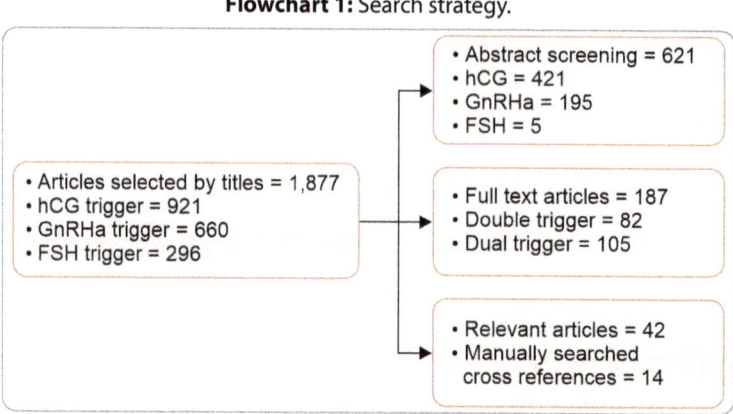

Flowchart 1: Search strategy.

(FSH: follicle-stimulating hormone; GnRHa: gonadotropin-releasing hormone agonist; hCG: human chorionic gonadotropin)

"dual or double trigger in IVF", and "FSH trigger in IVF". Total number of manuscripts in English retrieved were 1877. Appropriate cross-references were manually searched. The details of search strategy are shown in **Flowchart 1**.

■ OVULATION TRIGGER AND ITS IMPACT ON IVF OUTCOMES

Ovulation involves both luteinizing hormone (LH) and a more subdued follicle-stimulating hormone (FSH) surges in a natural cycle. This is considered necessary for oocyte maturation and follicular rupture. However, an understanding of the role of FSH in the surge is limited. Current understanding suggests that it promotes LH receptor formation in luteinizing granulosa cells, nuclear maturation, and cumulus expansion.[6-9] Evidence from IVF indicates a role for FSH in separation of cumulus-oocyte complex from the follicle wall and an association between intrafollicular FSH levels and oocyte recovery.[10] Evidence from animal studies suggests that FSH maintains the functional coupling between the oocyte and cumulus cells for a longer period and influences the functioning of signaling pathways.[11] However, FSH alone may not be able to sustain luteal function.[12] Endogenous LH surge has similar actions to FSH surge. In addition, it influences extracellular events encouraging granulosa cell proliferation.[13]

Human Chorionic Gonadotropin as Ovulation Trigger

Human chorionic gonadotropin (hCG) is used as a surrogate molecule for LH to induce luteinization of granulosa cells, and oocyte nuclear maturation in IVF. It is the most widely used ovulation trigger with an assumption that its actions are very similar to endogenous LH surge. It has a longer duration of action in comparison to endogenous LH. Even though both act on the same receptor, there are certain differences in their actions. Exogenous hCG encourages intracellular cyclic adenosine monophosphate (cAMP) accumulation and progesterone synthesis while endogenous LH has preferentially extracellular actions.[13]

Gonadotropin-releasing Hormone Agonist as Ovulation Trigger

Gonadotropin-releasing hormone agonist binds to GnRH receptor and induces both LH and FSH surge similar to that seen in a natural cycle. The surge is of a shorter duration compared to hCG and is complete within 24 hours.[14] It is now the preferred alternative to hCG in hyper-responders at a high risk of developing OHSS in IVF.[15-17] It has been noted that GnRHa-induced surge is associated with a better MII oocytes numbers and fertilization rate but with a lower implantation and clinical pregnancy rate compared to hCG.[18-20] Adverse impact on implantation and pregnancy is primarily due to its luteolytic effect. This has encouraged the practice of freezing all embryos when GnRHa is used as the ovulation trigger. Considering its safety, its use has been extended to oocyte donors and those undergoing IVF for fertility preservation where luteal phase disturbances are not of clinical concern.

Different preparations at different doses are in use to induce the necessary actions. Leuprolide (0.5–4 mg), triptorelin (0.2–0.4 mg), and buserelin (0.5 mg) are the GnRHa preparations commonly used in IVF.

■ DUAL TRIGGER

The term "dual trigger" refers to the use of GnRHa as the trigger to induce an endogenous FSH and LH surge while hCG is administered concomitantly to rescue the luteal phase. This is to allow embryo transfer in a fresh cycle, without an increase in the risk of early onset OHSS and at the same time overcome the negative impact of GnRHa on luteal function. Administration of hCG has been attempted at various doses:

- *In those at high risk of OHSS:* GnRHa trigger along with concomitant administration of 1,500 IU of hCG has shown improved oocyte maturation and good clinical outcomes with a low incidence of severe OHSS.[21-23]
- *In those not at risk of OHSS:* In women with normal response who have a low follicular output ratio with low number oocytes from dominant follicles or those with a high proportion of immature oocytes, concomitant administration of GnRHa and a standard dose of hCG may be beneficial. It is shown to increase number of oocytes, mature oocytes, better quality embryos, and higher clinical pregnancy rate.[24-27] However, such benefits have not been replicated universally.[28,29]

The most recent randomized controlled trials (RCTs) support the findings of the previous smaller studies and report a better live birth rate with dual trigger in normal responders.[30,31] Dual trigger is also found to be beneficial in normal responders with previous poor fertilization (<20%).[32] Dual trigger may increase oocyte maturity, fertilization, clinical pregnancy, and live birth rates in patients with a history of poor fertilization after standard hCG trigger alone.[33]

- *In poor responders:* Using a standard dose of hCG with a GnRHa trigger has been associated with an improved numbers of oocytes and mature oocytes, higher clinical pregnancies and live birth rates with dual trigger compared to conventional hCG trigger.[34-36] While an increase in the number of mature oocytes may be achieved with dual trigger in poor responders, further benefits in terms of an improved pregnancy rate or reduced miscarriage rate may not always be evident with such an intervention.[37]

It is to be noted that in hyper-responders in whom GnRHa is used as a trigger but embryo transfer in a fresh cycle is contemplated, a small dose of hCG is given either at oocyte retrieval or 5 days after the trigger with a view to rescue the luteal phase. Such interventions are not dual trigger as they do not have any impact on the oocyte parameters. Current evidence suggests a high incidence of severe OHSS of 26% when hCG is given at oocyte retrieval to rescue luteal phase.[38-40] An alternative strategy has been administration of a bolus of 1,500 IU of hCG 5 days after the trigger. This strategy is used selectively in hyper-responders who do not have any signs of early OHSS so that they can undergo a day 3 embryo transfer with an intensive luteal support.[41,42]

FSH and hCG: There have been two RCTs using a bolus of FSH along with hCG as a dual trigger. This has the advantage of being applicable in cycles treated with long agonist downregulation and in patients with hypothalamic dysfunction where GnRHa triggers cannot be utilized.

An initial RCT reported a better fertilization, a better chance of retrieving an oocyte from a mature follicle, and a trend toward better pregnancy rate in FSH group than hCG alone.[43] However, a subsequent RCT did not find any difference in the outcome measures.[44] A single study comparing various triggers shows that a combination of FSH 450 IU with 1,500 IU of hCG resulted in lower incidence of OHSS compared to half dose hCG, GnRHa, or dual trigger, irrespective of the protocol used.[45]

DOUBLE TRIGGER

Double trigger refers to administration of standard doses of both GnRHa and hCG as triggers but at different times in relation to planned ovum pick-up (OPU), usually GnRHa at 40 hours and hCG 34 hours prior to OPU. The advantages are:

- The GnRHa trigger results in simultaneous induction of LH and FSH surge, as seen with dual trigger.
- A prolongation of the time between ovulation triggering and OPU
- Rescue of luteal phase with hCG in addition to its ovulation triggering role

Limited evidence shows that this strategy may improve reproductive outcomes in those women who have experienced genuine EFS,[46] low number of MII oocytes,[47] or low follicular output ratio (<50%).[48] These studies have reported an improvement in the quality of embryos and an improvement in pregnancy rates in the above-mentioned subpopulations.

■ DISCUSSION

The field of assisted reproduction continues to strive to improve the outcomes of IVF. There has been an attempt in the recent years to critically look at the ovulation trigger used in IVF. While hCG is considered as the ideal surrogate to endogenous LH surge, it cannot induce a simultaneous FSH surge. The risk of OHSS associated with hCG and introduction of antagonist protocols into routine clinical practice opened an opportunity for alternative trigger option. GnRHa trigger has certain advantages over hCG as has been evident clinically.[15-17] In addition, it modulates the pigment epithelium derived factor (PEDF) and vascular endothelial growth factor (VEGF) ratio in granulosa cells in a manner opposite to that seen with hCG which may be an important mechanism in reducing the risk of OHSS.[49]

It is important to distinguish the terminology of "dual trigger" from "double trigger". The former refers to a simultaneous administration of GnRHa and different doses of hCG as dual triggers. A reduced dose of hCG is used in those at risk of OHSS, but a standard dose is used in normal or poor responders.[21-34] While the data remains limited, evidence from two meta-analyses involving four RCTs have shown improvement in some oocyte parameters with no clear benefit to pregnancy outcomes. However, both have affirmed the equivalence of this strategy compared to hCG as trigger and highlighted the need for larger and robust data to draw meaningful conclusions.[50,51] It is reassuring to note that neither of the trigger options have a negative impact on the euploidy rates in the resultant embryos.[52]

Differential gene expression in granulosa cells upon different triggers may explain improved oocyte and embryo quality with double trigger.[53]

Further, a study of transcriptome of cumulus cells following dual trigger has shown that such a strategy supports oocyte maturation and extracellular matrix remodeling, attenuates VEGF, and provides antioxidant support to the follicles across the spectrum of ovarian response.[54]

Double trigger refers to administration of GnRHa at 40 hours and a standard dose of hCG at 36 hours prior to OPU. This strategy has been utilized in those with low follicular output ratio, and with low MII oocytes or EFS in a previous cycle. The beneficial effects of extending the lag period up to 37–38 hours in improving live births after a GnRHa trigger have been previously documented.[55] However, extending it beyond this has the risk of ovulation before the scheduled OPU. Considering the rarity of situations needing this strategy and the limited data available, such a strategy should only be applied in a highly selective clinical scenario.

Current evidence shows that dual trigger with a small dose of hCG rescues the luteal phase and allows fresh cycle transfer in hyper-responders.[21-23] Dual trigger with a standard dose of hCG may be of benefit even in normal responders but needs further data.[24-27] It is also found to improve reproductive outcomes in poor responders.[34-36] While such a strategy may improve the yield of mature oocytes, it may not translate to clinical outcomes of improved pregnancy and live birth rates.[28,29] There is limited evidence on the efficacy of dual trigger with FSH and hCG at present.[43,44] If proved beneficial, such an intervention can be used in protocols incorporating GnRHa for pituitary downregulation.

Double trigger on the other hand may be of benefit for those with low follicular output ratio, low MII oocytes, and those with EFS, to improve the mature oocyte yield.[56] Such a strategy should be offered in highly selected clinical scenario as listed above and not adopted as routine intervention.

■ CONCLUSION

Ovulation trigger in conventional IVF plays a vital role in achieving oocyte maturation. Even though hCG is considered the ideal trigger in normal responders, dual trigger and double trigger may prove to be beneficial in those who exhibit abnormal follicular dynamics. Dual trigger may allow embryo transfer in fresh cycles in hyper-responders with a low risk of OHSS. However, these strategies should be used in carefully chosen clinical situations and cannot be considered as mainstream interventions until further evidence becomes available.

■ KEY POINTS

- hCG is the most widely used ovulation trigger.
- GnRH agonist alone improves safety in hyper-responders at risk of OHSS, oocyte donors and those opting for fertility preservation.
- Dual trigger refers to the simultaneous use of GnRHa and hCG as the trigger to induce an endogenous FSH and LH surge and to rescue the luteal phase respectively.
- GnRH agonist with low dose of hCG allows better oocyte maturation, without increasing risk of OHSS in hyper-responders and also allows fresh transfer by rescuing the luteal phase.

- GnRH with standard dose of hCG has shown beneficial effects in normo-responders with low follicular output ratio, high immature oocytes and previous poor fertilization.
- GnRH with standard dose of hCG in poor responders, increases the number of mature oocytes with unclear benefits in improving pregnancy rates.
- Double trigger, implies administration of both GnRH agonist and hCG at different times. This may benefit those with genuine empty follicle syndrome, low follicle output ratio and lower mature oocytes.
- Thus, dual trigger and double trigger may be beneficial in those with abnormal follicular dynamics. However, these strategies should be used in carefully chosen clinical situations and cannot be considered as mainstream interventions until further evidence becomes available.

REFERENCES

1. Nelson SM, Klein BM, Arce JC. Comparison of anti-Müllerian hormone levels and antral follicle count as predictor of ovarian response to controlled ovarian stimulation in good-prognosis patients at individual fertility clinics in two multicenter trials. Fertil Steril. 2015;103(4):923-30.
2. Fauser BCJM. Patient-tailored ovarian stimulation for in vitro fertilization. Fertil Steril. 2017;108(4):585-91.
3. Humaidan P, Alviggi C, Fischer R, Esteves SC. The novel POSEIDON stratification of 'Low prognosis patients in Assisted Reproductive Technology' and its proposed marker of successful outcome. F1000Res. 2016;5:2911.
4. Engmann L, Benadiva C, Humaidan P. GnRH agonist trigger for the induction of oocyte maturation in GnRH antagonist IVF cycles: a SWOT analysis. Reprod Biomed Online. 2016;32(3):274-85.
5. Orvieto R. Triggering final follicular maturation: hCG, GnRH-agonist, or both, when and to whom? J Assist Reprod Genet. 2017;34(9):1231-2.
6. Eppig JJ. FSH stimulates hyaluronic acid synthesis by oocyte-cumulus complexes from mouse preovulatory follicle. Nature. 1979;281(5731):483-4.
7. Strickland S, Beers WH. Studies on the role of plasminogen activator in ovulation. In vitro response of granulosa cells to gonadotropins, cyclic nucleotides, and prostaglandins. J Biol Chem. 1976;251:5694-702.
8. Yding Andersen C. Effect of FSH and its different isoforms on maturation of oocytes from pre-ovulatory follicles. Reprod Biomed Online. 2002;5(3):232-9.
9. Zelinski-Wooten MB, Hutchison JS, Hess DL, Wolf DP, Stouffer RL. Follicle stimulating hormone alone supports follicle growth and oocyte development in gonadotrophin-releasing hormone antagonist-treated monkeys. Hum Reprod. 1995;10(7):1658-66.
10. Rosen MP, Zamah AM, Shen S, Dobson AT, McCulloch CE, Rinaudo PF, et al. The effect of follicular fluid hormones on oocyte recovery after ovarian stimulation: FSH level predicts oocyte recovery. Reprod Biol Endocrinol. 2009;7:35.
11. Atef A, Francois P, Christian V, Marc-Andre S. The potential role of gap junction communication between cumulus cells and bovine oocytes during in vitro maturation. Mol Reprod Dev. 2005;71(3):358-67.

12. Christenson LK, Stouffer RL. Follicle-stimulating hormone and luteinizing hormone/chorionic gonadotropin stimulation of vascular endothelial growth factor production by macaque granulosa cells from pre- and periovulatory follicles. J Clin Endocrinol Metab. 1997;82(7):2135-42.
13. Casarini L, Lispi M, Longobardi S, Milosa F, La Marca A, Tagliasacchi D, et al. LH and hCG action on the same receptor results in quantitatively and qualitatively different intracellular signalling. PLoS One. 2012;7(10):e46682.
14. Gonen Y, Balakier H, Powell W, Casper RF. Use of gonadotropin-releasing hormone agonist to trigger follicular maturation for in vitro fertilization. J Clin Endocrinol Metab. 1990;71(4):918-22.
15. Itskovitz-Eldor J, Kol S, Mannaerts B. Use of a single bolus of GnRH agonist triptorelin to trigger ovulation after GnRH antagonist ganirelix treatment in women undergoing ovarian stimulation for assisted reproduction, with special reference to the prevention of ovarian hyperstimulation syndrome: preliminary report: short communication. Hum Reprod. 2000;15(9):1965-8.
16. Orvieto R. Can we eliminate severe ovarian hyperstimulation syndrome? Hum Reprod. 2005;20(2):320-2.
17. Devroey P, Polyzos NP, Blockeel C. An OHSS-Free Clinic by segmentation of IVF treatment. Hum Reprod. 2011;26(10):2593-7.
18. Griesinger G, Diedrich K, Devroey P, Kolibianakis EM. GnRH agonist for triggering final oocyte maturation in the GnRH antagonist ovarian hyperstimulation protocol: a systematic review and meta-analysis. Hum Reprod Update. 2006;12(2):159-68.
19. Orvieto R, Rabinson J, Meltzer S, Zohav E, Anteby E, Homburg R. Substituting HCG with GnRH agonist to trigger final follicular maturation: a retrospective comparison of three different ovarian stimulation protocols. Reprod Biomed Online. 2006;13(2):198-201.
20. Youssef MAFM, Van der Veen F, Al-Inany HG, Mochtar MH, Griesinger G, Nagi Mohesen M, et al. Gonadotropin-releasing hormone agonist versus HCG for oocyte triggering in antagonist-assisted reproductive technology. Cochrane Database Syst Rev. 2014;(10):CD008046.
21. Shapiro BS, Daneshmand ST, Garner FC, Aguirr M, Thomas S. Gonadotropin-releasing hormone agonist combined with a reduced dose of human chorionic gonadotropin for final oocyte maturation in fresh autologous cycles of in vitro fertilization. Fertil Steril. 2008;90(1):231-3.
22. Humaidan P, Ejdrup Bredkjaer H, Westergaard LG, Yding Andersen C. 1,500 IU human chorionic gonadotropin administered at oocyte retrieval rescues the luteal phase when gonadotropin-releasing hormone agonist is used for ovulation induction: a prospective, randomized, controlled study. Fertil Steril. 2010;93(3):847-54.
23. Shapiro BS, Daneshmand ST, Garner FC, Aguirre M, Hudson C. Comparison of "triggers" using leuprolide acetate alone or in combination with low-dose human chorionic gonadotropin. Fertil Steril. 2011;95(8):2715-7.
24. Lin MH, Wu FS, Lee RK, Li SH, Lin SY, Hwu YM. Dual trigger with combination of gonadotropin-releasing hormone agonist and human chorionic gonadotropin significantly improves the live-birth rate for normal responders in GnRH-antagonist cycles. Fertil Steril. 2013;100(5):1296-302.

25. Decleer W, Osmanagaoglu K, Seynhave B, Kolibianakis S, Tarlatzis B, Devroey P. Comparison of hCG triggering versus hCG in combination with a GnRH agonist: a prospective randomized controlled trial. Facts Views Vis Obgyn. 2014;6(4):203-9.
26. Fabris AM, Cruz M, Legidos V, Iglesias C, Muñoz M, García-Velasco JA. Dual triggering with gonadotropin-releasing hormone agonist and standard dose human chorionic gonadotropin in patients with a high immature oocyte rate. Reprod Sci. 2017;24(8):1221-5.
27. Seval MM, Özmen B, Atabekoğlu C, Şükür YE, Şimşir C, Kan Ö, et al. Dual trigger with gonadotropin-releasing hormone agonist and recombinant human chorionic gonadotropin improves in vitro fertilization outcome in gonadotropin-releasing hormone antagonist cycles. J Obstet Gynaecol Res. 2016;42(9):1146-51.
28. Mahajan N, Sharma S, Arora PR, Gupta S, Rani K, Naidu P. Evaluation of dual trigger with gonadotropin-releasing hormone agonist and human chorionic gonadotropin in improving oocyte maturity rates: a prospective randomized study. J Hum Reprod Sci. 2016;9(2):101-6.
29. Eftekhar M, Mojtahedi MF, Miraj S, Omid M. Final follicular maturation by administration of GnRH agonist plus HCG versus HCG in normal responders in ART cycles: An RCT. Int J Reprod Biomed. 2017;15(7):429-34.
30. Haas J, Bassil R, Samara N, Zilberberg E, Mehta C, Orvieto R, et al. GnRH agonist and hCG (dual trigger) versus hCG trigger for final follicular maturation: a double-blinded, randomized controlled study. Hum Reprod. 2020;35(7):1648-54.
31. Ali SS, Elsenosy E, Sayed GH, Farghaly TA, Youssef AA, Badran E, et al. Dual trigger using recombinant HCG and gonadotropin-releasing hormone agonist improve oocyte maturity and embryo grading for normal responders in GnRH antagonist cycles: Randomized controlled trial. J Gynecol Obstet Hum Reprod. 2020;49(5):101728.
32. Ben-Haroush A, Sapir O, Salman L, Altman E, Garor R, Margalit T, et al. Does 'Dual Trigger' Increase Oocyte Maturation Rate? J Obstet Gynaecol. 2020;40(6):860-2.
33. Elias RT, Pereira N, Artusa L, Kelly AG, Pasternak M, Lekovich JP, et al. Combined GnRH-agonist and human chorionic gonadotropin trigger improves ICSI cycle outcomes in patients with history of poor fertilization. J Assist Reprod Genet. 2017;34(6):781-8.
34. Lin MH, Wu FS, Hwu YM, Lee RK, Li RS, Li SH. Dual trigger with gonadotropin releasing hormone agonist and human chorionic gonadotropin significantly improves live birth rate for women with diminished ovarian reserve. Reprod Biol Endocrinol. 2019;17(1):7.
35. Maged AM, Ragab MA, Shohayeb A, Saber W, Ekladious S, Hussein EA, et al. Comparative study between single versus dual trigger for poor responders in GnRH-antagonist ICSI cycles: A randomized controlled study. Int J Gynaecol Obstet. 2021;152(3):395-400.
36. Kim SJ, Kim TH, Park JK, Eum JH, Lee WS, Lyu SW. Effect of a dual trigger on oocyte maturation in young women with decreased ovarian reserve for the purpose of elective oocyte cryopreservation. Clin Exp Reprod Med. 2020;47(4):306-11.
37. Zhang J, Wang Y, Mao X, Chen Q, Hong Q, Cai R, et al. Dual trigger of final oocyte maturation in poor ovarian responders undergoing IVF/ICSI cycles. Reprod Biomed Online. 2017;35(6):701-7.

38. Humaidan P, Papanikolaou EG, Kyrou D, Alsbjerg B, Polyzos NP, Devroey P, et al. The luteal phase after GnRH-agonist triggering of ovulation: present and future perspectives. Reprod Biomed Online. 2012;24:134-41.
39. Seyhan A, Ata B, Polat M, Son WY, Yarali H, Dahan MH. Severe early ovarian hyperstimulation syndrome following GnRH agonist trigger with the addition of 1500 IU hCG. Hum Reprod. 2013;28(9):2522-8.
40. Engmann LL, Maslow BS, Kaye LA, Griffin DW, DiLuigi AJ, Schmidt DW, et al. Low dose human chorionic gonadotropin administration at the time of gonadotropin releasing-hormone agonist trigger versus 35 h later in women at high risk of developing ovarian hyperstimulation syndrome: a prospective randomized double-blind clinical trial. J Ovarian Res. 2019;12(1):8.
41. Orvieto R. Ovarian hyperstimulation syndrome: an optimal solution for an unresolved enigma. J Ovarian Res. 2013;6(1):77.
42. Haas J, Kedem A, Machtinger R, Dar S, Hourovitz A, Yerushalmi G, et al. HCG (1500 IU) administration on day 3 after oocytes retrieval, following GnRH-agonist trigger for final follicular maturation, results in high sufficient mid luteal progesterone levels—a proof of concept. J Ovarian Res. 2014;7:35.
43. Lamb JD, Shen S, McCulloch C, Jalalian L, Cedars MI, Rosen MP. Follicle-stimulating hormone administered at the time of human chorionic gonadotropin trigger improves oocyte developmental competence in in vitro fertilization cycles: a randomized, double-blind, placebo-controlled trial. Fertil Steril. 2011;95(5):1655-60.
44. Qiu Q, Huang J, Li Y, Chen X, Lin H, Li L, et al. Does an FSH surge at the time of hCG trigger improve IVF/ICSI outcomes? A randomized, double-blinded, placebo-controlled study. Hum Reprod. 2020;35(6):1411-20.
45. Anaya Y, Mata DA, Letourneau J, Cakmak H, Cedars MI, Rosen MP. A novel oocyte maturation trigger using 1500 IU of human chorionic gonadotropin plus 450 IU of follicle-stimulating hormone may decrease ovarian hyperstimulation syndrome across all in vitro fertilization stimulation protocols. J Assist Reprod Genet. 2018;35(2):297-307.
46. Beck-Fruchter R, Weiss A, Lavee M, Geslevich Y, Shalev E. Empty follicle syndrome: successful treatment in a recurrent case and review of the literature. Hum Reprod. 2012;27(5):1357-67.
47. Zilberberg E, Haas J, Dar S, Kedem A, Machtinger R, Orvieto R. Co-administration of GnRH-agonist and hCG for final oocyte maturation in patients with low proportion of mature oocytes. Gyn Endocrinol. 2015;31(2):145-7.
48. Haas J, Zilberberg E, Dar S, Kedem A, Machtinger R, Orvieto R. Co-administration of GnRH-agonist and hCG for final oocyte maturation (double trigger) in patients with low number of oocytes retrieved per number of preovulatory follicles: a preliminary report. J Ovarian Res. 2014;7:77.
49. Miller I, Chuderland D, Ron-El R, Shalgi R, Ben-Ami I. GnRH agonist triggering modulates PEDF to VEGF ratio inversely to hCG in granulosa cells. J Clin Endocrinol Metab. 2015;100(11):E1428-36.
50. Ding N, Liu X, Jian Q, Liang Z, Wang F. Dual trigger of final oocyte maturation with a combination of GnRH agonist and hCG versus a hCG alone trigger in GnRH antagonist cycle for in vitro fertilization: a systematic review and meta-analysis. Eur J Obstet Gynecol Reprod Biol. 2017;218:92-8.

51. Chen CH, Tzeng CR, Wang PH, Liu WM, Chang HY, Chen HH, et al. Dual triggering with GnRH agonist plus hCG versus triggering with hCG alone for IVF/ICSI outcome in GnRH antagonist cycles: a systematic review and meta-analysis. Arch Gynecol Obstet. 2018;298(1):17-26.
52. Thorne J, Loza A, Kaye L, Nulsen J, Benadiva C, Grow D, et al. Euploidy rates between cycles triggered with gonadotropin-releasing hormone agonist and human chorionic gonadotropin. Fertil Steril. 2019;112(2):258-5.
53. Haas J, Ophir L, Barzilay E, Machtinger R, Yung Y, Orvieto R, et al. Standard human chorionic gonadotropin versus double trigger for final oocyte maturation results in different granulosa cells gene expressions: a pilot study. Fertil Steril. 2016;106(3):653-9.
54. Fuchs Weizman N, Wyse BA, Gat I, Balakier H, Sangaralingam M, Caballero J, et al. Triggering method in assisted reproduction alters the cumulus cell transcriptome. Reprod Biomed Online. 2019;39(2):211-24.
55. Hershkop E, Khakshooy A, Simons J, Weiss A, Geslevich J, Goldman S, et al. Ideal lag time from ovulation to oocyte aspiration using a GnRH agonist trigger. J Gynecol Obstet Hum Reprod. 2021;50(7):102055.
56. Kasum M, Kurdija K, Orešković S, Čehić E, Pavičić-Baldani D, Škrgatić L. Combined ovulation triggering with GnRH agonist and hCG in IVF patients. Gynecol Endocrinol. 2016;32(11):861-5.

Section

6

Downregulate it Right

- **Gonadotropin-releasing Hormone Analogs: Agonist and Antagonist**
  Madhuri Patil
- **Pretreatment in In Vitro Fertilization Cycles: Does it Work?**
  Aleyamma TK, Treasa Joseph, Mohan Shashikant Kamath

Chapter 13

Gonadotropin-releasing Hormone Analogs: Agonist and Antagonist

Madhuri Patil

■ INTRODUCTION

The efficacy of assisted reproductive technique (ART) was revolutionized by the ability to prevent an endogenous luteinizing hormone (LH) surge in the 1980s with the use of gonadotropin-releasing hormone (GnRH) agonists. Prior to this, the cancellation rate for superovulated cycles was as high as 25% due to the occurrence of premature LH surge that resulted in severely compromised outcomes. GnRH agonists were used in either long, short, or ultrashort protocols. GnRH agonists result in an initial flare followed by downregulation of the pituitary and thus require a long pretreatment period prior to initiation of gonadotropin stimulation. Use of GnRH agonist is also associated with increased probability of cyst formation, estrogen-deprivation symptoms, and has an increased risk for occurrence of ovarian hyperstimulation syndrome (OHSS). GnRH antagonists were first registered for use in ART to prevent LH surge in 2001. Their ability to cause immediate suppression of gonadotropin secretion has dramatically shorten the total duration of a treatment cycle, requires lesser dose of gonadotropins and does not have the initial flare effect hence preventing cyst formation. Moreover, there is immediate recovery of gonadotropin secretion once the GnRH antagonist is stopped. The advantage is that it can be combined with oral ovulogens and has a lower risk of developing OHSS.[1] The pituitary remains responsive to GnRH stimulation during antagonist co-treatment so a bolus dose of agonist can be administered instead of human chorionic gonadotropin (hCG) to trigger final oocyte maturation, which further reduces the incidence of OHSS. GnRH agonist when used to trigger ovulation has a short endogenous LH surge induced as compared to prolonged exogenous LH action induced by administration of hCG.[2] Initial studies did show that the pregnancy rates were better with the use of GnRH agonist, and this was probably due to the learning curve. However, today GnRH antagonists are as efficient as GnRH agonists and have an advantage of increased safety due to reduction in the incidence of OHSS without reducing likelihood of achieving live birth. The main difference between the GnRH agonist and antagonist protocol is difference in synchronization of follicular recruitment and growth. GnRH antagonists are associated with asynchronous development of the follicles and this can probably be reduced with pretreatment with estrogen, progesterone, or oral contraceptive pills (OCPs). GnRH antagonist protocols are of benefit in patients with anticipated hyperovarian response [anti-Müllerian hormone (AMH) >3 ng/mL]. GnRH antagonist use reduces the cycle cancellation rate and treatment burden as compared to GnRH agonists in poor responders (AMH <0.8 ng/mL).

The initial systematic reviews that compared the GnRH agonist long protocol with GnRH antagonist fixed protocol showed a significant number of oocytes retrieved, reduced clinical pregnancy rates, ongoing pregnancy rates, and live birth rates.[3,4] Initial studies showed that the incidence of severe OHSS was not significantly different between the 2 treatment regimens, but the same author later showed that the incidence of severe OHSS was significantly lower in the GnRH antagonist group.[1,5] A number of systematic reviews have been published over the past decade[6-10] and the recent review concluded that use of GnRH antagonists does not compromise effectiveness (clinical pregnancy and live birth rates) but significantly reduce the occurrence of OHSS.[8]

When a subgroup analysis was performed, the clinical pregnancy rate was significantly lower with GnRH antagonist treatment than with GnRH agonist long protocol in normal responders but was not different in polycystic ovary syndrome (PCOS) women and poor responders.[9] Today that we use is AMH and antral follicle count (AFC) stratified treatment for choosing the GnRH analog and the dose of follicle-stimulating hormone (FSH) for generating customized individualized stimulation protocol.[10]

■ GONADOTROPIN-RELEASING HORMONE AGONISTS

Drugs available are:
- Buserelin
- Suprefact
- Goserelin
- Nafarelin
- Leuprolide
- Decapeptyl

Mechanism of Action

The GnRH agonists occupy gonadotropin receptors to cause initial stimulation, then result in internalization of receptors and downregulation with continuous use over a few days.[11]

Route of Administration

Nasal spray: 100–300 µg given up to 6 times a day or subcutaneous injection.

GnRH Agonist Protocols

The long protocol (starting in the midluteal phase of the preceding cycle) gives the best IVF results with regard to oocyte yield and pregnancy rates.

It results in profound suppression of endogenous release of gonadotropins during the early follicular phase, allowing the early antral follicles to grow coordinately in response to exogenous gonadotropins to accomplish simultaneous maturation. Basically, it results in extended widening of the FSH window, increased FSH requirement and in the end more mature follicles and retrieved oocytes.

Ultrashort or Flare-up Protocol

It utilizes the initial boost of endogenous FSH.[12]

Dose: 500 µg/day from D1 or 2 for 3 days of GnRH agonist followed by gonadotropins till trigger. GnRH antagonists are started from day when follicle size is 14 mm **(Fig. 1)**.

Short Protocol (Fig. 2)

It provides initial folliculogenesis boost while subsequently preventing the endogenous surge.

Dose: 250–300 µg/day from D2 till hCG injection along with gonadotropins.

Long Protocol (Fig. 3)

It results in initial flare effect followed by pituitary desensitization with reversible inhibition of GT secretion.

Dose: 500–600 µg/day from D21 of previous menstrual cycle till menses.
  Dose reduced to 100–300 µg/day after onset of menses till hCG injection along with gonadotropins.

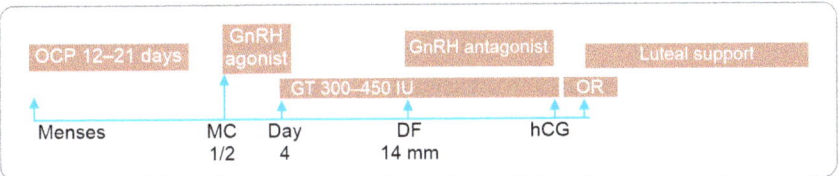

Fig. 1: Ultrashort or flare-up protocol. (GnRH: gonadotropin-releasing hormone; hCG: human chorionic gonadotropin; OCP: oral contraceptive pill)

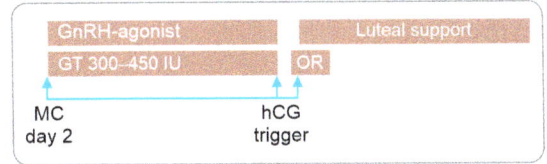

Fig. 2: Short protocol. (GnRH: gonadotropin-releasing hormone; hCG: human chorionic gonadotropin)

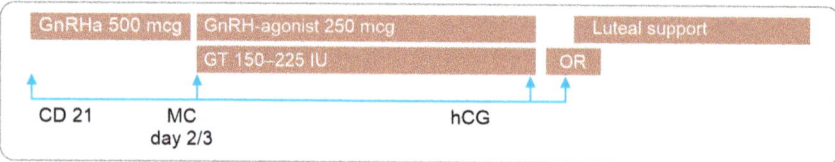

Fig. 3: Long protocol. (GnRH: gonadotropin-releasing hormone)

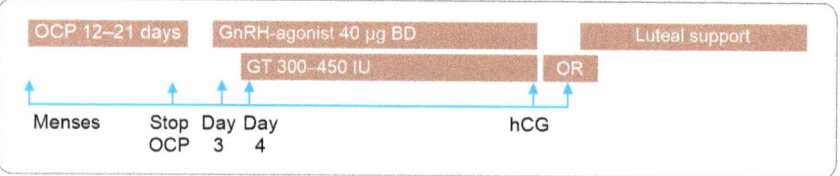

Fig. 4: Microdose flare protocol. (GnRH: gonadotropin-releasing hormone)

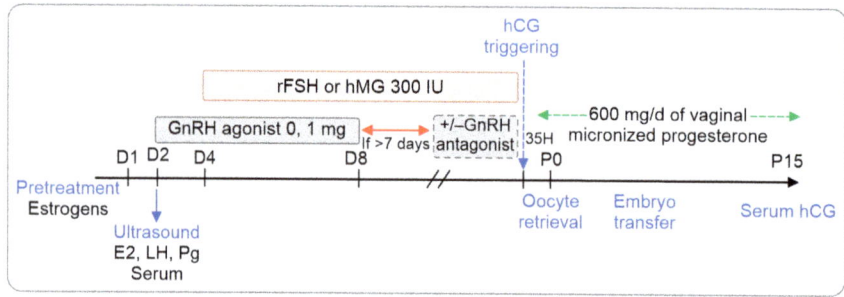

Fig. 5: Short agonist stop (SAS) protocol. (FSH: follicle-stimulating hormone; GnRH: gonadotropin-releasing hormone; hCG: human chorionic gonadotropin)

The long protocol gives significantly greater follicular recruitment, oocyte recovery, and fertilization rate, greater numbers of embryos for transfer.[13]

Microdose Flare Protocol

The GnRH agonist is initiated in the dose of 40 μg twice daily on the third day after stopping oral contraceptives. Two days after initiation of GnRH agonist, gonadotropins are initiated and both then continued till the day of hCG **(Fig. 4)**.[14]

Short Agonist Stop Protocol

The "short agonist stop" (SAS) stimulation protocol uses a double stimulation [flare up effect with the gonadotropin-releasing hormone (GnRH) agonist (GnRH-a) then gonadotropins] associated with a less strenuous blockage (discontinuation of GnRH-a) to favor follicular recruitment in order to obtain a better ovarian response **(Fig. 5)**.[15]

The SAS protocol uses GnRH-a at first for the flare up effect at the beginning of the cycle for 7 days in total then stopped, enabling pituitary desensitization in order to prevent a premature LH surge, associated with a controlled ovarian stimulation with gonadotropins at maximum dosage (300 IU/d).

Advantages of GnRH Agonist

- Eliminates LH surge
- Controls basal LH secretion
- Oocyte recovery programmed
- Enhances intrafollicular growth and recovery of better quality oocytes
- Widens the window of uterine implantation thus increasing pregnancy rates
- Reduced incidence of cancellation of cycles

Disadvantages of GnRHa

- 50% more GTs required
- Results in luteal phase defects, ovarian cyst formation, and has higher incidence of OHSS
- Atypical response
- Poor response
- Symptoms of estrogen deprivation

■ GONADOTROPIN-RELEASING HORMONE ANTAGONIST

Two different compounds available are cetrorelix and ganirelix. Cetrorelix seems to have highest suppressive rate/mg peptide of all other antagonist.[16]

Mechanism of Action

Immediately suppress gonadotropins by blocking GnRH receptor, restricting treatment only to those days when LH surge is likely to occur.[17] The inhibitory effect of GnRH antagonist is dose-dependent, and depends on equilibrium between endogenous GnRH and antagonist concentration.[18]

Once administered they immediately block the GnRH receptor in a competitive fashion and hence reduce LH and FSH secretion within a period of 8 hours. The inhibition of LH secretion is more pronounced than that of FSH.

In the GnRH antagonist protocol as against GnRH agonist protocol, endogenous FSH levels are not suppressed during the early follicular phase. The luteofollicular transition induces FSH levels above the threshold for a short period until hormonal feedback occurs, leading to the initiation of follicular growth of a few leading follicles. After exogenous FSH administration, FSH levels rise above threshold again and will initiate several additional follicles to grow. As soon as the leading follicles meet the hCG criteria, several other follicles will be of smaller sizes and may not be sensitive to hCG yet. Such an asynchronized cohort may therefore result in less oocytes retrieved, compared to the long agonist protocol.

Though the stimulation period is shorter with less gonadotropin units being required, the number of oocytes retrieved is less when compared with the long GnRH agonist protocol.

The GnRH antagonists bind to GnRH gonadotrope receptors and compete successfully with GnRH agonist molecule (endogenous) for receptor occupancy. Hence, there is immediate gonadotropin secretion arrest. Both agonist and antagonist are used to prevent LH surge, major difference is that flare up occurs only with agonists.[19]

GnRH Antagonist Protocols

Multiple-dose Protocol

The GnRH antagonist is given in the doses 0.25 mg subcutaneously in the mid-follicular phase (D Albano et al., 1997;[20] The Ganirelix Dose-Finding Study Group, 1998[21]). One can use either the fixed protocol (Borm and Mannaerts, 2000;[22] European Middle East Orgalutran Study Group, 2001;[23] Huirne et al., 2005),[24] where the GnRH antagonists are started on day 6 of stimulation or the flexible protocol, where they are started when the dominant follicle is 14 mm (Hohmann et al., 2003[25]).

Fixed GnRH antagonist regimens started the antagonist relatively late in the follicular phase, mostly stimulation day 6. Normally, the luteofollicular transitory rise of endogenous FSH starts the stimulation of a cohort of follicles that vary in stage of development as there is a decrease in FSH concentration just before exogenous FSH is started. Start of exogenous FSH allows further development of a few leading large follicles and several smaller follicles. Further there is again a small fall in the level of FSH, when the antagonist is started. As the criteria for administration of hCG are based on the size of the leading largest follicles, there are several immature follicles at that time. Though the stimulation period will be shorter with less FSH required, the number of mature oocytes obtained is definitely less compared to long GnRH agonist protocol (**Figs. 6 and 7**).

Thus, GnRH antagonist regimens result in less synchronization of the follicular cohort as compared to a long GnRH agonist cycle with lesser mature and more immature follicles.

Patients randomized to treatment with GnRH antagonist started ovarian stimulation with recombinant FSH on day 2 or 3 of menstrual cycle with a once daily subcutaneous injection. The GnRH antagonist was started on stimulation day 6 by daily subcutaneous administration up to and including day of human chorionic gonadotropin administration in fixed protocol and depending on follicular size in flexible protocol. In fixed protocol, GnRH

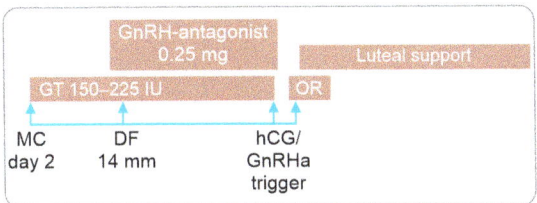

Fig. 6: Multiple dose flexible start protocol. (GnRH: gonadotropin-releasing hormone)

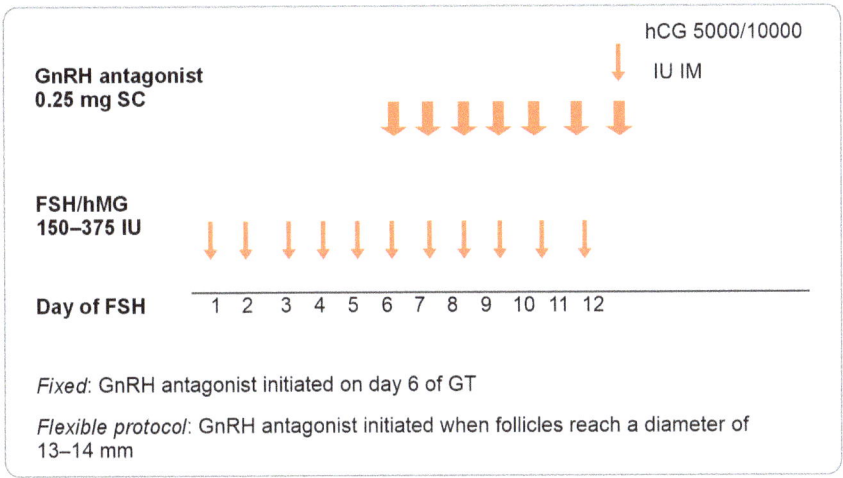

Fig. 7: Multiple dose protocols. (FSH: follicle-stimulating hormone; GnRH: gonadotropin-releasing hormone; hCG: human chorionic gonadotropin; hMG: human menopausal gonadotropin)

antagonist was started on day 6 of FSH treatment regardless of follicle size. This protocol was used by 7 included studies. In the flexible protocol GnRH antagonist is administered according to the follicle size and not cycle date nor the day of FSH administration. This protocol was identified in 13 included studies.[26]

Single Dose Protocol

One 3 mg dose is administered on day 6 of ovarian stimulation. If the criteria for triggering ovulation were not reached within 4 days, additional doses of cetrorelix (0.25 mg) were administered daily till the criteria for hCG administration were reached[27] **(Figs. 8 and 9).**

GnRH Antagonist: Early Administration

The problem of asynchronous development of follicles can be avoided by early suppression of FSH and LH by early GnRH antagonist administration (stimulation day 1) or by oral contraceptive (OC) pretreatment.

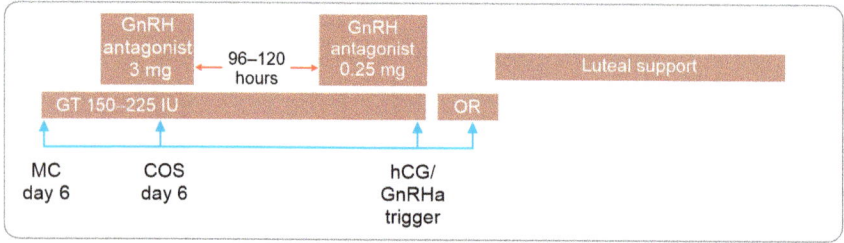

Fig. 8: Single dose fixed start. (COS: controlled ovarian stimulation; GnRH: gonadotropin-releasing hormone; hCG: human chorionic gonadotropin)

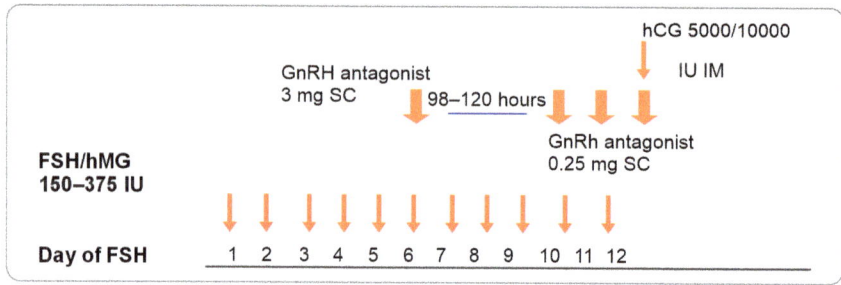

Fig. 9: Single dose protocols. (FSH: follicle-stimulating hormone; GnRH: gonadotropin-releasing hormone; hCG: human chorionic gonadotropin; hMG: human menopausal gonadotropin)

Oral contraceptive pills were started on day 2 of spontaneous menses of the cycle prior to the treatment cycle and were given for 21 days. GnRH antagonist started in the dose of 0.25 mg daily along with gonadotropins from day 2 of menstrual cycle (day 1 of stimulation) that followed the discontinuation of the OCP. Treatment with rFSH and GnRH antagonist continued daily thereafter, until and including the day of hCG administration **(Fig. 10)**.[28]

All GnRH antagonist protocols provide a shorter duration of treatment, lower GT consumption, lower risk of OHSS and ability to use bolus GnRH agonist to trigger midcycle LH surge. The implantation rate and pregnancy rates were similar to agonist.

An earlier start (cycle day 4 or 5) of GnRH antagonists is associated with improved pregnancy rates. So as per Koilibianakis, if we start GnRH antagonist on day 1 compared with day 6, there will be even further decrease in exposure to LH and estradiol during the early follicular phase and would be beneficial in PCOS women.[29] However, the pregnancy rates were similar. Additionally, this regimen will increase the cost due to the extended period of GnRH antagonist administration.

Similarly, another randomized control study done recently also concluded that fixed antagonist administration on day 5 of stimulation appears to achieve a comparable oocyte retrieved as with flexible antagonist administration, i.e., when follicular size is >14 mm.[30]

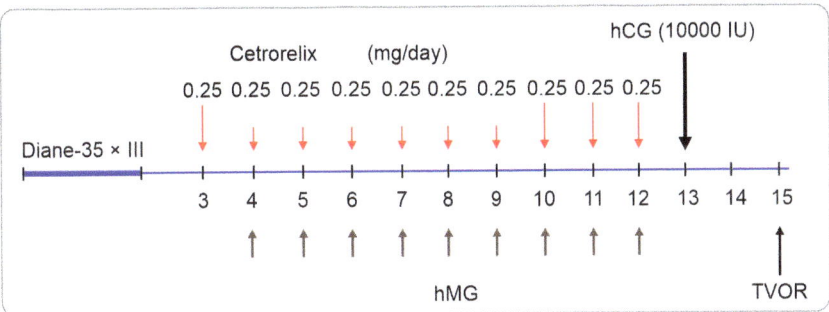

Fig. 10: GnRH antagonist—early administration protocol. (GnRH: gonadotropin-releasing hormone; hCG: human chorionic gonadotropin; hMG: human menopausal gonadotropin; TVOR: transvaginal oocyte retrieval)

■ GnRH AGONIST VERSUS ANTAGONIST
Endocrinological Profile
Difference between two GnRH Analogs

A progesterone rise during the late follicular phase has a negative predictive value for clinical outcome in both GnRH agonist and GnRH antagonist protocols. This is because high serum progesterone levels on the day of hCG administration induce both advanced endometrial histological maturation and differential endometrial gene expression which may have a negative effect on the implantation **(Table 1)**.

Premature progesterone rise during GnRH antagonist cycle of IVF is a frequent phenomenon and has been associated with lower pregnancy rates. The best available evidence supports the association between raised progesterone on day of hCG administration and the probability of clinical pregnancy in women undergoing ovarian stimulation with GnRH analog and gonadotropins for IVF. Significantly lower ongoing pregnancy rates are seen in patients with elevated progesterone at initiation of stimulation of GnRH antagonist, which is more common in a flexible protocol when the antagonists are initiated only after the dominant follicle is 14 mm.[31,32]

Though a previous meta-analysis failed to demonstrate any relationship between progesterone levels and clinical pregnancy rates data from large prospective randomized studies like the merit study[33] and a retrospective study of 4,000 cycles[34] consistently support that pregnancy rates are inversely related to progesterone levels on the day of hCG administration, when a threshold of 1.5 ng/mL is adopted.[35]

Luteinizing Hormone Supplementation

The increased pregnancy loss observed with low LH levels in GnRH agonist cycles and decreased probability of pregnancy associated with low LH levels, observed using high GnRH antagonist doses as a result of abrupt suppression

TABLE 1: Advantages and disadvantages for the use of GnRH agonist and antagonists in IVF.

Cycle parameter	Agonist	Antagonist
LH suppression timings	Longer 7–10 days	Shorter immediate
Profound LH suppression[36]	Yes	No
Duration of ovarian stimulation	Longer	Shorter
Dosage of gonadotropins	More	Lesser
Cost of cycle	More	Lesser
COC retrieved	More	Slightly lesser
Trigger choice	No (only hCG)	Yes (hCG, agonist, dual)
Luteal phase supplementation	Less	More
OHSS	More	Less
Cyst formation	Yes	No
Pregnancy rate	Slightly higher	Slightly lower
Hot flushes	Yes	No

(GnRH: gonadotropin-releasing hormone; IVF: in vitro fertilization; LH: luteinizing hormone; OHSS: ovarian hyperstimulation syndrome)

of endogenous LH by GnRH antagonist occurs in the mid-follicular phase, at a critical stage for follicular development. It was thus assumed that LH supplementation might improve pregnancy outcome in both groups, where one could add LH or increase the dose of LH in the form of recombinant LH or human menopausal gonadotropin (hMG).

As per Kolibianakis and colleagues, profound suppression of LH on day 8 of stimulation is associated with a significantly higher chance of achieving an ongoing pregnancy.[37,38] They also concluded that there was no indication that low endogenous levels after GnRH antagonist initiation are associated with decreased probability of pregnancy in IVF cycles.

On the basis of currently available data, it appears that LH supplementation in ovarian stimulation for IVF using GnRH antagonist cycles is not necessary and it does not improve the outcome.

Criteria for hCG Administration

There is a marked variation in the criteria used for triggering final oocyte maturation in IVF both in GnRH agonists and antagonist cycles. Recent data indicate that the timing of hCG administration might be important for the probability of pregnancy.[13] Prolongation of the follicular phase and luteal phase deficiency was shown to be associated with decreased pregnancy rates in GnRH antagonist cycle with GnRH agonist trigger.

Ovarian Hyperstimulation Syndrome

The incidence of OHSS associated with hospital admission was significantly lower in the antagonist group than in the agonist group. The incidence of grade I and II OHSS did not differ significantly between the two GnRH analogs but was in favor of GnRH-antagonist group, in which the incidence of OHSS was lower.[39]

Efficacy of GnRH Analogs in IVF

In the meta-analysis of randomized comparative trials between GnRH analogs, the absolute treatment effect of clinical pregnancy rate on an intention-to-treat basis was 5% in favor of the GnRH agonists. But recent studies did not show any significant difference in the live birth rates, suggesting that both GnRH analogs result in comparable pregnancy rates.[40]

The two phenomena that play an important role to facilitate optimal IVF results when GnRH analogs are used are:
1. Stable and low LH and progesterone levels throughout the stimulation phase to achieve optimal conditions for implantation.
   As per Saadat et al., no significant difference exists between serial progesterone levels and luteal phase endometrial histology between cycles utilizing agonist or antagonists.[41]
2. Sustained low levels of FSH before stimulation are started to allow optimal synchronization of the follicular cohort.

Comparisons of GnRH Antagonist versus GnRH Agonist Protocol in Poor Ovarian Responders Undergoing IVF

Various treatment regimens and interventions have been investigated in an effort to improve ovarian response and IVF outcome in poor responders. In women with age >40 with abnormal FSH levels, similar pregnancy rates were found with minimal stimulation protocol as with standard protocol and it was cost-effective too.[42] Other studies include the use of high doses of gonadotropins, the change to a "flare-up" protocol with OC pretreatment and the use of growth hormone or growth hormone-releasing factor or aspirin as adjunct therapies. The availability of GnRH antagonists has offered an alternative protocol for poor responders as GnRH-agonist long protocol may cause oversuppression of endogenous gonadotropin secretion at the stage of follicular recruitment. However, most of these interventions have only limited success in poor responders.[43-46]

Although the results of GnRH-antagonist in COS protocols offer a number of potential advantages compared with the conventional long GnRH-agonist protocol, the efficacy of GnRH-antagonist and GnRH-agonist in poor responder IVF patients is still controversial and further controlled randomized study is required.[47,48]

Cochrane review published in 2010 and a meta-analysis published in 2011 showed that the duration of stimulation was significantly lower in GnRH-antagonist protocols than long GnRH-agonist protocols in poor responder, no improvements were found in the number of oocytes and mature oocytes retrieved, the CCR and CPR with the use of GnRH-antagonist. GnRH antagonist resulted in a LH surge in 9% of poor responders, which was a cause for concern.[40]

In couples with poor responders, GnRH antagonists do not compromise ongoing pregnancy rates and are associated with less OHSS and, therefore, could be considered as standard treatment.[49]

Comparisons of GnRH Antagonist versus GnRH Agonist Protocol in Hyper-responders Undergoing IVF

The antagonist protocol eliminated the need for complete cryopreservation of embryos due to excessive response, coupled with significant reductions in the incidence of hospitalizations owing to the development of OHSS.

The antagonist protocol, in high responders, was also associated with higher fresh-cycle clinical pregnancy rates, required fewer days of FSH stimulation and was associated with lower egg yields compared with the agonist protocol these patients with low egg yields achieved pregnancy rates comparable with those with normal or high egg yields. Patients with AMH serum concentrations >40 pmol/L still remain at risk of developing an excessive response and OHSS despite the use of a "mild" antagonist protocol with hCG trigger.

Hence, conventional GnRH antagonist protocols represent a safer and more cost-effective treatment of choice for PCOS women undergoing IVF/ICSI cycles than long agonist protocol without compromising clinical outcomes.[50]

Oocyte Donation Cycles

Oocyte donation (OD) cycles, both the short GnRH agonist and antagonist protocols, appear to be similar in ovarian response and embryo quality and comparable in terms of recipients' pregnancy and implantation rates. The GnRH antagonist protocol could be the protocol of choice for ovarian stimulation in OD cycles, as the risk of OHSS could be reduced by the triggering of ovulation with a GnRH agonist.[51,52]

Oral Contraceptive Pill Pretreatment in Ovarian Stimulation with GnRH Antagonists and Agonist

The use of OCP has been advocated for programming IVF cycles using GnRH antagonists and improved synchronization of the recruitable cohort of ovarian follicles as against a GnRH agonist cycle, where it is used to prevent ovulation, which in turn will reduce the cyst formation after initiation of the agonist in a long protocol. But it was also observed that pretreatment with OCP has been associated with a longer duration of treatment and increased gonadotropin requirement.

The OC pretreatment using GnRH antagonists protocol with subsequent starting of FSH 2 or 3 days after the last OC intake is associated with deep suppression of LH and FSH levels and improved synchronization of the follicular cohort development compared with GnRH antagonist only protocols. This effect is not seen when FSH stimulation was started on day 5 after the last OCP. Apparently, timing the start of exogenous gonadotropin administration after OCP pretreatment affects follicular development.

As per Cochrane 2017, OCP pretreatment was found to be deleterious in terms of live birth rate and ongoing pregnancy rate in women undergoing IVF with antagonist protocol. Study did not comment about the effect of pretreatment on long agonist protocol.[53]

As per meta-analysis done in 2019 by Soo Yon Song on PCOS women, they found pretreatment with OCP in IVF may have adverse effect on clinical outcome.[54]

As per recent study by Pedro et al. published in 2020, use of OCP pretreatment for 12-30 days does not compromise live birth rate and cumulative live birth rate in IVF cycle.[55]

A comparison of pretreatment with OC pills, estradiol valerate versus no pretreatment prior to GnRH antagonist cycle was done and it was found that neither of these pretreatment could improve the fresh IVF embryo transfer outcome in an antagonist cycle.[56]

■ GnRH ANALOGS IN OVARIAN STIMULATION FOR IUI

Cochrane review 2021 says gonadotropins probably improve cumulative live birth rate compared with oral ovulogens.[57] LH surge is an absolute requirement for luteinization, final maturation of the oocyte, and follicle rupture. Premature LH surge occurs in 25-30% of stimulated intrauterine insemination (IUI) cycles and may interfere with timing of IUI or result in cancellation of IUI cycle and more treatment failures with IUI. Strategies to improve treatment outcome might focus on preventing premature LH surge.[58] Treatment with ganirelix effectively prevents premature LH rises, luteinization in subjects undergoing stimulated IUI.[59] So, we need to see whether use of GnRH agonist or antagonist in IUI cycles is cost-effective and helps in improving the outcome.

■ GnRH AGONISTS IN OVARIAN STIMULATION FOR IUI

There seems to be no role for GnRH-agonists in IUI programs as they increase cost as the dose of gonadotropins is increased tremendously. Its use also increases the incidence of multiple pregnancy without increasing the probability of conception. Thus, use of GnRH agonists with gonadotropins should be carefully considered in an IUI program.[60]

■ GnRH ANTAGONISTS IN OVARIAN STIMULATION FOR IUI

Gonadotropin-releasing hormone antagonist affectively reduces the premature luteinization rate in PCOS.[61] In addition, they may be helpful in cycle programming, timing ovulation, and avoidance of inseminations during weekends.[62]

Conversion of high-response gonadotropin–IUI cycles to "rescue" IVF using a GnRH antagonist is a cost-effective strategy that produces better results than regular IVF with relatively minimal morbidity, and shorter duration to achieve pregnancy. Implantation and ongoing clinical pregnancy rates tend to be higher than those from hyper-responder regular IVF patients.

Whether or not GnRH-antagonists are going to play a role in mild ovarian hyperstimulation/IUI programs need to be determined in future trials.[63] GnRH antagonist resulted in more monofollicular development, less premature luteinization, and less cycle cancellation in IUI cycles of patients with PCOS; however, the cost of stimulation increased. Evidence to support its use to improve clinical pregnancy outcome in PCOS patients undergoing COS in IUI treatment is inefficient.

Patients with a previous cancelled cycle because of premature luteinization are candidates for this treatment. GnRH agonists might be used as an alternative option instead of hCG for trigger in IUI cycle.[64]

■ CONCLUSION

The achievement of a simple, safe, and cost-effective treatment protocol in controlled ovarian hyperstimulation (COH) is of paramount importance to improve the quality of care in assisted reproduction. Both GnRH agonist and antagonist co-treatments during ovarian hyperstimulation for IVF are effective in preventing an undesirable premature rise in serum LH. When using GnRH antagonist, the daily low-dose protocol should be preferred over a single high-dose regimen. GnRH antagonist could produce a more physiological follicular selection than the long luteal GnRH agonist protocol, recruiting a smaller number of follicles and thus reducing OHSS risk.

Initial publications suggested that OCP pretreatment in GnRH antagonist cycles reduced the pregnancy rates but the clinical evidence generated recently suggests that OCP pretreatment can be used for planning IVF cycles.

In patients treated with FSH and GnRH analogs for IVF, the addition of rLH does not increase live birth rate or has any beneficial effect on secondary outcome variables. So, addition of LH from initiation of stimulation or from antagonist administration does not appear to be necessary. There is also no need to increase the starting dose of gonadotropins or to increase gonadotropin dose at antagonist initiation.

CHAPTER 13: Gonadotropin-releasing Hormone Analogs: Agonist...

The GnRH antagonist initiation on day 6 of stimulation appears to be superior to flexible initiation by a follicle of 14–16 mm, and probably initiation of GnRH antagonist earlier in the cycle if the estradiol levels are >200 pg/mL on day 5 of COS may prevent early rise of progesterone and, therefore, improve the pregnancy rates.

Today, the evidence suggests that the choice of GnRH analog for inhibiting the premature LH surge does not alter significantly the probability of live birth. But the OHSS rate in women receiving antagonist is significantly lower compared with the agonist protocols as hCG can be replaced by GnRH agonist for triggering final oocyte maturation. This may be associated with lower probability of pregnancy if a fresh transfer is done not using the modified luteal phase support protocol where hCG is given in the dose of 1,500 IU on the day of oocyte retrieval. The pregnancy rates remain same if all embryos are frozen and transferred in the subsequent cycle. GnRH antagonist protocol may be used for patients at high risk of developing OHSS to make the clinic an OHSS-free one.

Luteal phase supplementation is required following both GnRH agonist and antagonist co-treatment protocols with gonadotropins.

The GnRH antagonists may have a role in ovarian stimulation for IUI as well as their application in mild stimulation protocols for IVF. Use of GnRH agonist does not improve the outcome in IUI cycles.

This then has supported the use of individualization of COS in ART cycles (**Fig. 11**). Today, most protocols are selected on values of AMH and AFC.

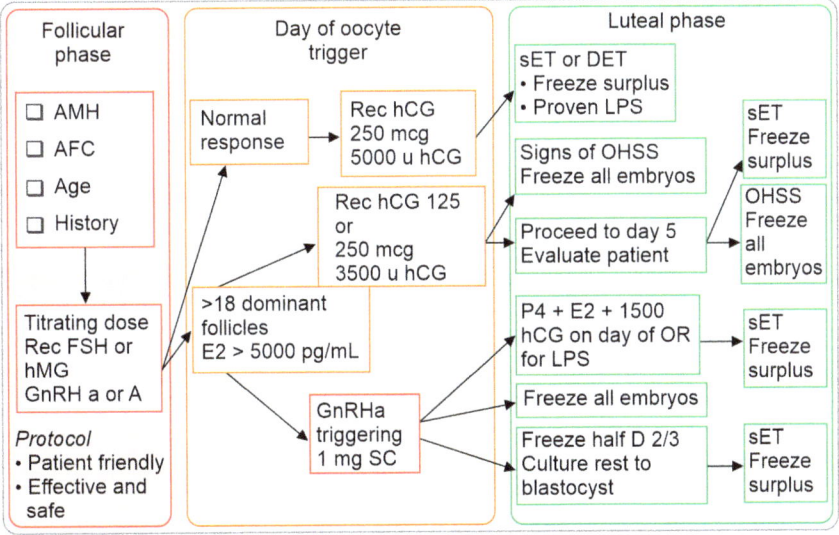

Fig. 11: Individualization of protocol. (AFC: antral follicle count; AMH: anti-Müllerian hormone; FSH: follicle-stimulating hormone; GnRH: gonadotropin-releasing hormone; hCG: human chorionic gonadotropin; hMG: human menopausal gonadotropin; OHSS: ovarian hyperstimulation syndrome)

This protocol enables the correct selection of the different GnRH analogs and the gonadotropin dose. The benefits of a personalized therapy are reduction in the risk of poor or hyper-response thus reducing the incidence of cancellation of the cycle and at the same time optimizing the outcome of ART.

■ KEY POINTS

- GnRH analogs have revolutionized the face of ART and had improved the oocytes yield.
- The increased gonadotropin requirements, occasional cyst formation and inability to use agonist trigger has made GnRH analog protocol less favorable.
- GnRH antagonist can be started later in the cycle as fixed or flexible protocol and acts immediately, reduces the dosage of gonadotropins, duration of stimulation, ability to use agonist trigger and makes OHSS free clinic a reality.
- Its equally responsive in hyper-responders, normoresponders, poor responders.
- An early day 5 start of antagonist is better in PCOS subpopulation.
- Pre-COCP treatment is deleterious for live birth rate in agonist as well as antagonist cycle, more in antagonist cycle.
- Oocyte yield, CPR, LBR are the same in both protocols.
- For all practical purposes antagonist protocol is safe and effective in every population.

■ REFERENCES

1. Al-Inany H, Aboulghar M. GnRH antagonist in assisted reproduction: a Cochrane review. Hum Reprod. 2002;17:874-85.
2. Youssef MA, Van der Veen F, Al-Inany HG, Mochtar MH, Griesinger G, Nagi Mohesen M, et al. Gonadotropin-releasing hormone agonist versus HCG for oocyte triggering in antagonist-assisted reproductive technology. Cochrane Database Syst Rev. 2014;(10):CD008046.
3. Kolibianakis EM, Collins J, Tarlatzis BC, Devroey P, Diedrich K, Griesinger G. Among patients treated for IVF with gonadotrophins and GnRH analogues, is the probability of live birth dependent on the type of analogue used? A systematic review and meta-analysis. Hum Reprod Update. 2006;12:651-71.
4. Orvieto R, Patrizio P. GnRH agonist versus GnRH antagonist in ovarian stimulation: an ongoing debate. Reprod Biomed Online. 2013;26:4-8.
5. Pundir J, Sunkara SK, El-Toukhy T, Khalaf Y. Meta-analysis of GnRH antagonist protocols: do they reduce the risk of OHSS in PCOS? Reprod Biomed Online. 2012;24:6-22.
6. Al-Inany HG, Abou-Setta AM, Aboulghar M. Gonadotrophin-releasing hormone antagonists for assisted conception: a Cochrane review. Reprod Biomed Online. 2007;14:640-9.

7. Al-Inany HG, Youssef MA, Aboulghar M, Broekmans F, Sterrenburg M, Smit J, et al. Gonadotrophin-releasing hormone antagonists for assisted reproductive technology. Cochrane Database Syst Rev. 2011;(5):CD001750.
8. Al-Inany HG, Youssef MA, Ayeleke RO, Brown J, Lam WS, Broekmans FJ. Gonadotrophin-releasing hormone antagonists for assisted reproductive technology. Cochrane Database Syst Rev. 2016;(4):CD001750.
9. Xiao JS, Su CM, Zeng XT. Comparisons of GnRH antagonist versus GnRH agonist protocol in supposed normal ovarian responders undergoing IVF: a systematic review and meta-analysis. PLoS One. 2014;9:e106854.
10. Nelson SM. Biomarkers of ovarian response: current and future applications. Fertil Steril. 2013;99(4):963-9.
11. Ortmann O, Weiss JM, Diedrich K. "Gonadotropin-releasing hormone (GnRH) and GnRH agonists: mechanisms of action." Reprod Biomed Online. 2002;5 Suppl 1:1-7.
12. Kahraman K, Berker B, Atabekoglu CS, Sonmezer M, Cetinkaya E, Aytac R, et al. Microdose gonadotropin-releasing hormone agonist flare-up protocol versus multiple dose gonadotropin-releasing hormone antagonist protocol in poor responders undergoing intracytoplasmic sperm injection-embryo transfer cycle. Fertil Steril. 2009;91(6):2437-44.
13. Tan SL, Kingsland C, Campbell S, Mills C, Bradfield J, Alexander N, et al. The long protocol of administration of gonadotropin-releasing hormone agonist is superior to the short protocol for ovarian stimulation for in vitro fertilization. Fertil Steril. 1992;57(4):810-4.
14. Surrey ES, Bower J, Hill DM, Ramsey J, Surrey MW. Clinical and endocrine effects of a microdose GnRH agonist flare regimen administered to poor responders who are undergoing in vitro fertilization. Fertil Steril. 1998;69(3):419-24.
15. Mauries C, Ranisavljevic N, Mollevi C, Brunet C, Hamamah S, Brouillet S, et al. "Short agonist stop" protocol, an ovarian stimulation for poor responders in in vitro fertilization (IVF): A pilot study. Front Endocrinol (Lausanne). 2022:13:1056520.
16. Klingmuller D, Schepke M, Enzweiler C, Bidlingmaier F. Hormonal responses to the new potent GnRH antagonist Cetrorelix. Acta Endocrinol (Copenh). 1993;128:15-8.
17. Bouchard P, Charbonnel B, Caraty A. The role of LHRH during the periovulatory period: a basis for the use of LHRH antagonists in ovulation induction. In: Filicori M, Flamigni C (Eds). Ovulation: Basic Science and Clinical Advances. Amsterdam: Excerpta Medica; 1994.
18. Reissmann T, Felberbaum R, Diedrich K, Engel J, Comaru-Schally AM, Schally AV. Development and applications of Luteinizing hormone-releasing antagonists in the treatment of infertility: an overview. Hum Reprod. 1995;10:1974-81.
19. Devroey P. GnRH antagonist. Fertil Steril. 2000;73(1):15-7.
20. Albano C, Felberbaum RE, Smitz J, Riethmuller-Winzen H, Engel J, Diedrich K, et al. Ovarian stimulation with HMG: results of a prospective randomized phase III European study comparing the luteinizing hormone-releasing hormone (LHRH)-antagonist cetrorelix and the LHRH-agonist buserelin. European Cetrorelix Study Group. Hum Reprod. 2000;15:526-53.
21. The Ganirelix Dose-Finding Study Group. A double-blind, randomized, dose finding study to assess the efficacy of the gonadotrophin-releasing hormone

antagonist ganirelix (Org 37462) to prevent premature luteinizing hormone surges in women undergoing ovarian stimulation with recombinant follicle stimulating hormone (Puregon). Hum Reprod. 1998;13:3023-31.

22. Borm G, Mannaerts B. Treatment with the gonadotrophin-releasing hormone antagonist ganirelix in women undergoing ovarian stimulation with recombinant follicle stimulating hormone is effective, safe and convenient: results of a controlled, randomized, multicentre trial. The European Orgalutran Study Group. Hum Reprod. 2000;15:1490-8.

23. European Middle East Orgalutran Study Group. Comparable clinical outcome using the GnRH antagonist ganirelix or a long protocol of the GnRH agonist triptorelin for the prevention of premature LH surges in women undergoing ovarian stimulation. Hum Reprod. 2001;16:644-51.

24. Huirne JA, van Loenen AC, Schats R, McDonnell J, Hompes PG, Schoemaker J, et al. Dose-finding study of daily GnRH antagonist for the prevention of premature LH surges in IVF/ICSI patients: optimal changes in LH and progesterone for clinical pregnancy. Hum Reprod. 2005;20:359-67.

25. Hohmann FP, Macklon NS, Flauser BC. A randomized comparison of two ovarian stimulation protocols with gonadotrophin-releasing hormone (GnRH) antagonist cotreatment for in vitro fertilization commencing recombinant follicle-stimulating hormone on cycle day 2 or 5 with the standard long GnRH agonist protocol. J Clin Endocrinol Metab. 2003;88:166-73.

26. Venetis CA, Storr A, Chua SJ, Mol BW, Longobardi S, Yin X, et al. What is the optimal GnRH antagonist protocol for ovarian stimulation during ART treatment? A systematic review and network meta-analysis. Hum Reprod Update. 2023;29(3):307-326.

27. Olivennes F, Fanchin R, Bouchard P, de Ziegler D, Taieb J, Selva J, et al. The single or dual administration of the gonadotrophin-releasing hormone antagonist Cetrorelix in an in vitro fertilization embryo transfer program. Fertil Steril. 1994;62:468-76.

28. Lainas TG, Petsas GK, Zorzovilis IZ, Iliadis GS, Lainas GT, Cazlaris HE, et al. Initiation of GnRH antagonist on Day 1 of stimulation as compared to the long agonist protocol in PCOS patients. A randomized controlled trial: effect on hormonal levels and follicular development. Hum Reprod. 2007;22(6):1540-6.

29. Kolibianakis EM, Albano C, Camus M, Tournaye H, Van Steirteghem AC, Devroey P. Initiation of gonadotrophin-releasing hormone antagonist on day 1 as compared to day 6 of stimulation: effect on hormonal levels and follicular development in in vitro fertilization cycles. J Clin Endocrinol Metab. 2003a;88:5632-7.

30. Luo X, Pei L, Li F, Li C, Huang G, Ye H. Fixed versus flexible antagonist protocol in women with predicted high ovarian response except PCOS: a randomized controlled trial. BMC Pregnancy Childbirth. 2021;21(1):348.

31. Van Vaerenbergh I, Fatemi HM, Blockeel C, Van Lommel L, In't Veld P, Schuit F, et al. Progesterone rise on HCG day in GnRH antagonist/rFSH stimulated cycles affects endometrial genes expression. Reprod Biomed Online. 2011;22:263-71.

32. Venetis CA, Kolibianakis EM, Papanikolaou E, Bontis J, Devroey P, Tarlatzis BC. Is progesterone elevation on the day of human chorionic gonadotrophin administration associated with the probability of pregnancy in in-vitro

fertilization? A systematic review and meta-analysis. Hum Reprod Update. 2007;13:343-55.
33. Andersen AN, Devroey P, Arce JC. Clinical outcome following stimulation with highly purified hMG or recombinant FSH in patients undergoing IVF: a randomized assessor-blind controlled trial. Hum Reprod. 2006;21(12):3217-27.
34. Bosch E, Labarta E, Crespo J, Simón C, Remohí J, Jenkins J, et al. Circulating progesterone levels and ongoing pregnancy rates in controlled ovarian stimulation cycles for in vitro fertilization: analysis of over 4000 cycles. Hum Reprod. 2010;25:2092-100.
35. Papanikolaou EG, Kolibianakis EM, Pozzobon C, Tank P, Tournaye H, Bourgain C, et al. Progesterone rise on the day of human chorionic gonadotrophin administration impairs pregnancy outcome in day 3 single-embryo transfer, while has no effect on day 5 single blastocyst transfer. Fertil Steril. 2009;91:949-52.
36. Kolibianakis EM, Zikopoulos K, Schiettecatte J, Smitz J, Tournaye H, Camus M, et al. Profound LH suppression after GnRH antagonist administration is associated with a significantly higher ongoing pregnancy rate in IVF. Hum Reprod. 2004;19(11):2490-6.
37. Kolibianakis EM, Collins J, Tarlatzis B, Papanikolaou E, Devroey P. Are endogenous LH levels during ovarian stimulation for IVF using GnRH analogues associated with the probability of ongoing pregnancy? A systematic review. Hum Reprod Update. 2006;12:3-12.
38. Hua L, Wang C. Recombinant-luteinzing hormone supplementation in women during IVF/ICSI cycles with GNRH-antagonist protocol: A systematic review and meta-analysis. Eur J Obstet Gynecol Reprod Biol. 2023;283:43-48.
39. Chen Y, Zhang Y, Hu M, Liu X, Qi H. Timing of human chorionic gonadotropin (hCG) hormone administration in IVF/ICSI protocols using GnRH agonist or antagonists: a systematic review and meta-analysis. Gynecol Endocrinol. 2014;30(6):431-7.
40. Lambalk CB, Banga FR, Huirne JA, Toftager M, Pinborg A, Homburg R, et al. GnRH antagonist versus long agonist protocols in IVF: a systematic review and meta-analysis accounting for patient type. Hum Reprod Update. 2017;23(5):560-79.
41. Saadat P, Boostanfar R, Slater CC, Tourgeman DE, Stanczyk FZ, Paulson RJ. Accelerated endometrial maturation in the luteal phase of cycles utilizing controlled ovarian hyperstimulation: impact of gonadotrophin-releasing hormone agonists versus antagonists. Fertil Steril. 2004;82:167-71.
42. Weghofer A, Margreiter M, Bassim S, Sevelda U, Beilhack E, Feichtinger W. Minimal stimulation using recombinant follicle-stimulating hormone and a gonadotrophin-releasing hormone antagonist in women of advanced age. Fertil Steril. 2004;81:1002-6.
43. Keay SD, Liversedge NH, Mathur RS, Jenkins JM. Assisted conception following poor ovarian response to gonadotrophin stimulation. Br J Obstet Gynaecol. 1997;104:521-7.
44. Turhan NO. Poor response—the devil is in the definition. Fertil Steril. 2006; 86:777.
45. Mahutte NG, Arici A. Poor responders: does the protocol make a difference? Curr Opin Obstet Gynecol. 2002;14:275-81.
46. Howles CM, Loumaye E, Germond M, Yates R, Brinsden P, Healy D, et al. Does growth hormone-releasing factor assist follicular development in poor

responder patients undergoing ovarian stimulation for in-vitro fertilization? Hum Reprod. 1999;14:1939-43.
47. Lok IH, Yip SK, Cheung LP, Yin Leung PH, Haines CJ. Adjuvant low-dose aspirin therapy in poor responders undergoing in vitro fertilization: a prospective, randomized, double-blind, placebo-controlled trial. Fertil Steril. 2004;81:556-61.
48. Pandian Z, McTavish AR, Aucott L, Hamilton MP, Bhattacharya S. Interventions for 'poor responders' to controlled ovarian hyper stimulation (COH) in in-vitro fertilisation (IVF). Cochrane Database Syst Rev. 2010;(1):CD004379.
49. Kadoura S, Alhalabi M, Nattouf AH. Conventional GnRH antagonist protocols versus long GnRH agonist protocol in IVF/ICSI cycles of polycystic ovary syndrome women: a systematic review and meta-analysis. Sci Rep. 2022;12:4456.
50. Bodri D, Vernaeve V, Guillén JJ, Vidal R, Figueras F, Coll O. Comparison between a GnRH antagonist and a GnRH agonist flare-up protocol in oocyte donors: a randomized clinical trial. Hum Reprod. 2006;21(9):2246-51.
51. Bodri D, Guillen JJ, Galindo A, Mataro D, Pujol A, Coll O. Triggering with human chorionic gonadotrophin or a gonadotrophin-releasing hormone agonist in gonadotrophin-releasing hormone antagonist-treated oocyte donor cycles: findings of a large retrospective cohort study. Fertil Steril. 2009;91:365-71.
52. Huirne JA, van Loenen AC, Donnez J, Pirard C, Homburg R, Schats R, et al. Effect of an oral contraceptive pill on follicular development in IVF/ICSI patients receiving a GnRH antagonist: a randomized study. Reprod Biomed Online. 2006b;13:235-45.
53. Farquhar C, Rombauts L, Kremer JA, Lethaby A, Ayeleke RO. Oral contraceptive pill, progestogen or oestrogen pretreatment for ovarian stimulation protocols for women undergoing assisted reproductive techniques. Cochrane Database Syst Rev. 2017;5(5):CD006109.
54. Song SY, Yang JB, Song MS, Oh HY, Lee GW, Lee M, et al. Effect of pretreatment with combined oral contraceptives on outcomes of assisted reproductive technology for women with polycystic ovary syndrome: a meta-analysis. Arch Gynecol Obstet. 2019;300:737-50.
55. Montoya-Botero P, Martinez F, Rodríguez-Purata J, Rodríguez I, Coroleu B, Polyzos NP. The effect of type of oral contraceptive pill and duration of use on fresh and cumulative live birth rates in IVF/ICSI cycles. Hum Reprod. 2020;35(4):826-36.
56. Shahrokh Tehrani Nejad E, Bakhtiari Ghaleh F, Eslami B, Haghollahi F, Bagheri M, Masoumi M. Comparison of pre-treatment with OCPs or estradiol valerate vs. no pre-treatment prior to GnRH antagonist used for IVF cycles: An RCT. Int J Reprod Biomed. 2018;16(8):535-40.
57. Cantineau AE, Rutten AG, Cohlen BJ. Agents for ovarian stimulation for intrauterine insemination (IUI) in ovulatory women with infertility. Cochrane Database Syst Rev. 2021;11(11):CD005356.
58. Cantineau AE, Cohlen BJ; Dutch IUI Study Group. The prevalence and influence of luteinizing hormone surges in stimulated cycles combined with intrauterine insemination during a prospective cohort study. Fertil Steril. 2007;88:107-12.
59. Lambalk CB, Leader A, Olivennes F, Fluker MR, Andersen AN, Ingerslev J, et al. Treatment with the GnRH antagonist ganirelix prevents premature LH rises and luteinisation in stimulated intrauterine insemination: results of a double-blind, placebo-controlled, multicentre trial. Hum Reprod. 2006;21:632-9.

60. Gagliardi CL, Emmi AM, Weiss G, Schmidt CL. Gonadotropin-releasing hormone agonist improves the efficiency of controlled ovarian hyperstimulation/intrauterine insemination. Fertil Steril. 1991;55(5):939-44.
61. Ertunc D, Tok EC, Savas A, Ozturk I, Dilek S. Gonadotrophin-releasing hormone antagonist use in controlled ovarian stimulation and intrauterine insemination cycles in women with polycystic ovary syndrome. Fertil Steril. 2010;93(4):1179-84.
62. Gomez-Palomares JL, Julia B, Acevedo-Martin B, Martinez-Burgos M, Hernandez ER, Ricciarelli E. Timing ovulation for intrauterine insemination with a GnRH antagonist. Hum Reprod. 2005;20:368-72.
63. Ragni G, Alagna F, Brigante C, Riccaboni A, Colombo M, Somigliana E, et al. GnRH antagonists and mild ovarian stimulation for intrauterine insemination: a randomized study comparing different gonadotropin dosages. Hum Reprod. 2004;19:54-8.
64. Taheripanah R, Zamaniyan M, Moridi A, Taheripanah A, Malih N. Comparing the effect of gonadotropin-releasing hormone agonist and human chorionic gonadotropin on final oocytes for ovulation triggering among infertile women undergoing intrauterine insemination: An RCT. Int J Reprod Biomed. 2017;15(6):351-6.

Chapter 14

Pretreatment in In Vitro Fertilization Cycles: Does it Work?

Aleyamma TK, Treasa Joseph, Mohan Shashikant Kamath

■ INTRODUCTION

There has been a steady increase in the number of assisted reproductive technology (ART) treatment cycles being performed across the world.[1] However, the live birth rate (LBR) continues to be low, ranging between 20 and 25% per initiated cycle.[1,2] The high cost of in vitro fertilization (IVF) treatment and low success rate add to the psychological burden for the infertile couple. In their quest to improve the treatment success rate, the clinicians often end up offering many pre-IVF interventions in the hope that they may prove beneficial. The effectiveness of many of these pretreatment therapies is not proven while others may be harmful.[3] In this chapter, we have critically evaluated the role of commonly used pre-IVF interventions such as oral contraceptive (OC) pill, antioxidants for male and female partner, androgens, metformin, and screening hysteroscopy.

■ ORAL CONTRACEPTIVES

Pretreatment with OC pills in ART practice is common. The OC pills are given for multiple reasons such as better follicular synchronization, reducing cyst formation and the amount of gonadotropin-releasing hormone (GnRH) agonist required for hypothalamo-pituitary suppression.[4] It is also used for IVF cycle programming in contemporary practice. Cycle programming helps in distributing IVF-related workload and avoid weekend procedures, hence ensures optimization of care. Reliance on OC pills for cycle programming is more for units performing IVF in batches. Estrogen component of OC pills inhibits the follicle-stimulating hormone (FSH) secretion while the progesterone component suppresses the luteinizing hormone (LH) through a negative feedback mechanism.

There is paucity of data from randomized controlled trials (RCTs) comparing effectiveness of OC pill in GnRH agonist cycles. One small RCT ($n = 54$) reported comparable pregnancy rates following OC pill pretreatment with depot GnRH agonist for downregulation compared to control group who did not receive OC pills (9% vs. 11%).[5] An RCT performed to evaluate the effectiveness of OC pill pretreatment in GnRH antagonist cycles versus no pretreatment reported a nonsignificant difference in ongoing pregnancy rates between the two groups [22.9% vs. 27.5%; 95% confidence interval (CI) −3.7% to +12.8%].[6] However, the pregnancy loss was significantly higher with OC pill pretreatment (36.4% vs. 21.6%; 95% CI of the difference −28.4% to 2.3%). In another RCT ($n = 228$), outcomes following GnRH antagonist cycle with OC pill pretreatment were compared with GnRH agonist without any pretreatment. The women received OC pill for 12-14 days and had a washout period of 5 days. The LBRs [44.3% vs. 47%; odds ratio (OR) 0.9, 95% CI 0.5-1.5] did not differ significantly between the two groups.[7]

An updated meta-analysis which included six RCTs showed statistically significant reduction of ongoing pregnancy with OC pill pretreatment [risk ratio (RR) 0.80, 95% CI: 0.66-0.97] compared to no pretreatment with a pill-free interval between 2 and 5 days prior to initiation of ovarian stimulation. There was no significant statistical heterogenicity noted when the six studies were pooled.[8] All the trials in the meta-analysis used 30 μg ethinyl estradiol and 150 μg levonorgestrel/desogestrel for 14-28 days. The suggested explanation for reduced pregnancy rates was negative impact of progestogen on endometrial receptivity and low endogenous LH levels due to suppressive effect which may affect oocyte competence or endometrial receptivity. However, it is unclear if addition of LH to counter low endogenous LH in a OC pill pretreated GnRH antagonist cycle will improve the outcome. An earlier study reported that following OC pill suppression, the endogenous gonadotropin levels returned to presuppression levels comparable to natural cycle after 5 days of stopping OC pill.[9] So, a pill-free washout period of 5 days is suggested prior to initiating ovarian stimulation. The OC pill pretreatment is associated with increased gonadotropin dose and duration of stimulation.[8] Endometrial biopsies obtained from young women undergoing oocyte donation cycles who underwent ovarian stimulation using GnRH antagonist cycle with and without OCP pretreatment did not show any significant difference in endometrial gene expression related to endometrial receptivity during the window of implantation.[10]

A Cochrane review after pooling six RCTs reported that there is moderate-quality evidence of lower LBR and ongoing pregnancy rate in OC pill pretreatment group (OR 0.74, 95% CI 0.58-0.95) in GnRH antagonist cycles. There was insufficient evidence to conclude if the pregnancy loss rates differed between the groups (OR 1.36, 95% CI 0.82-2.26). When OC pill pretreatment in GnRH antagonist cycle was compared with no pretreatment in GnRH agonist cycles, moderate-quality evidence from four RCTs suggested no difference in live birth or ongoing pregnancy rates (OR 0.89, 95% CI 0.64-1.25) but there were fewer pregnancy losses in OC pill pretreatment group (OR 0.40, 95% CI 0.22-0.72).[4] A retrospective cohort study evaluated effect of OC pill pretreatment in normo-ovulatory women undergoing IVF with GnRH agonist and GnRH antagonist protocols. The study reported lower following fresh transfer LBR in women using OC pill compared to those not using them (42.6% vs. 52.8%; $p < 0.001$). However, the LBRs following frozen embryo transfer cycles were similar (42.7% vs. 41.1%; p 0.54). The cumulative LBR was significantly lower in women using OC pill (62.8% vs. 67.6%; $p < 0.01$).[11]

In practice, there is some concern that delaying stimulation following OC pill may lead to asynchrony in GnRH antagonist cycles which may further lead to lower oocyte yield. An earlier study reported that synchronized ovarian stimulation with first follicle wave emergence in women using GnRH antagonist protocol (initiation of ovarian stimulation on day 1 versus day 4 of menstrual cycle) resulted in an increase in number of dominant follicles in the day 1 group but implantation rates and clinical pregnancy rates did not differ between the two groups.[12]

To summarize, OC pills pretreatment may lead to lower live birth in GnRH antagonist cycles following fresh transfer while the current evidence suggests no such negative impact on GnRH agonist cycle. However, the benefits of OC pill pretreatment in optimizing IVF workload have to be carefully considered against the possible negative impact on LBRs following IVF.

Progesterone Alone

Synthetic progestogen such as norethisterone has been used for IVF cycle programming and has a suppressive effect on pituitary LH secretion which helps in reducing incidence of ovarian cysts following GnRH flare effect.[9,13,14] In the agonist protocol, progestogen can be initiated at least 1 or 2 days prior to initiating GnRH agonist and can be continued for 5 days.[14] The GnRH agonist suppression is continued for 7–10 days and downregulation is confirmed before initiating controlled ovarian hyperstimulation (COH). Progesterone (e.g., norethisterone 10 mg/day) can be started from day 15 of the preceding cycle and given for 10–15 days for IVF programming purpose in an antagonist protocol.[9] After stopping progestogen, a 5-day pill washout period is advised before initiating COH with gonadotropin. Endocrinological profiling studies have suggested more synchronized growth of follicles following 5-day washout period following progesterone pretreatment.[9]

In a Cochrane review, pooled results from two RCTs did not show any significant difference in the live birth or ongoing pregnancy rates (OR 1.35, 95% CI 0.69–2.65) between progestogen pretreatment versus no pretreatment when agonist protocol was used.[4] Similarly, data from only one RCT showed that the LBR did not differ between progestogen pretreatment and control arm when an antagonist protocol was used (OR 0.67, 95% CI 0.18–2.54) and quality of evidence was low.

To summarize, progestogen alone can be used for cycle programming for both GnRH agonist and antagonist protocols as there is no evidence of any negative impact on ART treatment outcomes. Progestogen can be used as an alternative to the OC pill for cycle programming in agonist cycle. However, it can be a useful option in antagonist protocol since OC pill pretreatment has been associated with lower success rates.[4]

Estrogen Alone

Estrogen alone in the form of micronized 17-β estradiol can be used for IVF cycle programming at the dose of 2 mg per day.[9,15] It can be started in the mid luteal phase or 5 days prior to the expected onset of menses and continued for a maximum of 10 days.[16] When estrogen is used as pretreatment for cycle programming, the return of endogenous gonadotropin secretion (mainly FSH) to normal level occurs in 2-3 days as opposed to 5 days following pretreatment with progestogen or OC pills, hence a shorter pill-free washout period of one-two days is advised.[9]

In a Cochrane review, pooled results from two RCTs did not show any significant difference in the live birth (OR 0.79, 95% CI 0.53-1.17) or clinical pregnancy rates (OR 0.91, 95% CI 0.66-1.24) between estrogen pretreatment versus no pretreatment in antagonist cycles.[4]

To summarize, estrogen alone can be used as an alternative to OC pills for cycle programming in GnRH antagonist cycle, but with a shortened 1-2 days pill washout period. However, use of estrogen may increase the gonadotropin requirement and prolong stimulation duration.[15]

■ ANTIOXIDANTS

Oxidative stress is found to have a profound effect on both male and female infertility.[17,18] The balance between reactive oxygen species (ROS) and endogenous antioxidants is crucial for maintaining normal reproductive physiology.[19,20] While infertility itself is associated with higher levels of ROS, ART may contribute further to the oxidative stress.[17,21] The in vitro handling of the male and female gametes combined with the loss of follicular fluid and seminal plasma containing physiological antioxidants may cause inadvertent exposure of the gametes and embryo to higher levels of ROS.[21,22] Antioxidants are substances which inhibit the oxidation of biological molecules either by free radical scavenging or chelation.[23] It has been proposed that pretreatment with antioxidants may prove beneficial in both male and female infertility, especially prior to ART treatment.

Antioxidants (Female)

Changes in the ratio of ROS antioxidant concentrations are found to affect key events in the female reproductive physiology. It affects maturation of the oocyte, mainly meiosis I and II.[18] Additionally, increased ROS levels may cause DNA damage, membrane lipid peroxidation, and protein oxidation, thereby, affecting embryo quality and implantation directly.[24] The possible mechanisms by which antioxidants improve outcomes are by improving endometrial vascularity, reducing hyperandrogenism and insulin resistance, and influencing ovulation and cervical mucus.[25-27] Common antioxidants administered include myoinositol, vitamin C, D, E, arginine, and N-acetyl cysteine.[25,26,28]

The Cochrane review update published compared the effects of antioxidants on treatment outcomes in female infertility. Out of the 63 trials, pooled results from 18 trials (2,341 women) that compared antioxidants with either placebo, no treatment or standard treatment in women undergoing ART reported no significant difference in clinical pregnancy rates following pretreatment with antioxidants (OR 1.15, 95% CI 0.95–1.40). LBRs were reported by nine trials (806 women) and no significant difference was reported between the two groups (OR 1.36, 95% CI 0.96–1.93). Comparison antioxidants constituted mainly single agents comprising L-arginine, vitamin E, B, C, D, myo-inositol, and coenzyme Q10. The duration of administration was also variable, ranging from 2 weeks to 3 months prior to ART.[28]

To summarize, there was no clear evidence of any benefit when antioxidants were administered as pretreatment in infertile women prior to ART.

Antioxidants (Male)

It has been suggested that sperm damage caused by increased ROS levels may contribute to almost four-fifths of the cases of male infertility.[21] Mature spermatozoa are more vulnerable to ROS-mediated damage owing to the polyunsaturated fatty acid (PUFA)-rich sperm membrane combined with the lack of cytoplasm which is rich in antioxidants.[29] Oxidative stress mainly damages the sperm membrane and sperm DNA, causing decreased motility, fertilization, embryo development, and early pregnancy loss.[30-32] A number of studies have reported increased seminal levels of ROS and decreased antioxidants in infertile men.[19,33] It has been proposed that antioxidant supplementation in men with abnormal semen parameters may lead to improvement in semen parameters, especially in motility and concentration.[34,35] Additionally, some investigators have found that antioxidant administration may also benefit by reducing sperm DNA fragmentation.[36] These findings have predisposed the use of antioxidants as an adjuvant in ART.

The Cochrane review evaluating the role of antioxidant supplementation in male infertility included four trials in couples undergoing ART. Out of these, only two trials reported LBR, which was found to be significantly higher after pretreatment with antioxidants (Peto OR 3.61, 95% CI 1.27–10.29) as compared to placebo or no treatment. However, the clinical pregnancy rate was found to be comparable in both the groups (Peto OR 2.64, 95% CI 0.94–7.41).

The evidence was graded as low quality due to the heterogeneous study population and the varying types and duration of antioxidants used.[37] Another systematic review, which included observational studies and randomized trials, evaluated the effects of antioxidant pretreatment on semen parameters, sperm function, and ART outcomes in couples with male factor infertility. The reviewers analyzed three prospective trials in addition to the RCTs included in the Cochrane review.[38] While two of these reported improved fertilization rates following intracytoplasmic sperm injection (ICSI),[39,40] the third reported no difference in fertilization rates with antioxidant supplementation prior to ART.[41] Pregnancy rates and LBRs were not reported limiting the clinical applicability of the review.

To summarize, the current evidence suggests a possible benefit of oral antioxidant pretreatment prior to ART in male infertility. However, it is unclear whether the benefit of antioxidants would be significant in a specific subgroup, for example men with documented DNA damage. Additionally, there is a large knowledge gap regarding the type and dosage of antioxidants and reporting of clinically relevant outcomes following ART.

■ ANDROGENS

Dehydroepiandrostenedione (DHEA) and testosterone are androgens produced in the adrenal zona reticularis and the ovarian theca cells.[42,43] It is hypothesized that these androgens play a crucial role in maintaining follicular steroidogenesis by their autocrine or paracrine effects.[44] It is postulated that androgens may improve follicular response in ART by upregulation of both FSH and androgen receptors in the preantral and antral follicles preventing follicular atresia and increasing oocyte yield, especially in women with diminished ovarian reserve.[45,46]

The DHEA has been used as an oral supplement at varying doses (40–75 mg/day for up to 6 months prior to ART). Testosterone is administered as an oral (testosterone undecanoate 40 mg/day) or transdermal preparation (testosterone gel 1–2% at 12.5 mg/day or testosterone patch 2.5 mg/day).[47-49] Currently, there is no consensus regarding the appropriate dose or duration of either of the drugs for improving follicular response in ART. These androgens may be associated with adverse effects which is a cause of concern. Exogenous administration of androgens in women may affect bone mineral density, muscle mass, adipose tissue distribution, mood and psychological well-being. Androgens have also been reported to be associated with increased hair growth and acne.[50] Notably, it is still unclear whether androgens have any effect on the developing embryo.[51]

A Cochrane review published in 2015 investigated the role of pretreatment with dehydroepiandrosterone sulfate (DHEAS) or testosterone prior to ART. A total of 12 randomized trials compared DHEAS with either placebo or no treatment prior to ART. The dosage varied from 40 to 75 mg per day for 2–26 weeks. Pooled evidence from eight trials suggested significantly higher LBRs following pretreatment with DHEAS (OR 1.88, 95% CI 1.30–2.7), and the quality of evidence was moderate. Similarly, testosterone transdermal (patches/gel) was compared with placebo or no treatment at varying doses of 2.5 mg/day to 12.5 mg/day for a period of 5–28 days. Pooled results from four trials showed that LBRs were significantly higher with testosterone (OR 2.60, 95% CI 1.30–5.20) which was moderate-quality evidence. Although the study population mostly included women with documented poor response in the previous ART cycle, many studies were at high risk of performance bias. On excluding these studies from the analysis, the effect size reduced and the results were no longer significant for either DHEAS or testosterone. The data on adverse effects of either of the drugs was sparse and evidence was inconclusive to suggest any effect. The reviewers, therefore, concluded that there may be some benefit of pretreatment with DHEAS or testosterone in poor responders; however, there was a need for robust evidence.[52]

To summarize, testosterone and DHEAS may be considered for pretreatment in women with previous poor response in ART. However, it should be offered with caution since there is little information about its possible adverse effects in ART and early pregnancy.

■ METFORMIN

Metformin is an oral biguanide used commonly for treating type 2 diabetes mellitus. Due to its insulin suppressive effect, it may have a beneficial role in infertile polycystic ovarian syndrome (PCOS) women by improving ovulation rate and pregnancy outcomes.[53] Metformin is, however, associated with gastrointestinal side effects and in rare cases, it leads to lactic acidosis.[54] Metformin has been advised prior to or during ART treatment with doses ranging between 1,000 and 2,000 mg daily in women with PCOS for improving LBR and reducing ovarian hyperstimulation syndrome (OHSS).[55]

In a double-blinded, placebo-controlled RCT, the investigators evaluated whether metformin reduces the risk of OHSS in high-risk PCOS women ($n = 120$) undergoing ART.[56] The pituitary suppression was achieved using the long agonist protocol and women underwent fresh embryo transfers. Metformin or the placebo was initiated along with GnRH suppression. The OHSS rate was significantly reduced with metformin (8.3 vs. 30%; RR 0.28, 95% CI 0.11–0.67) compared to the placebo. However, there was no difference in the LBRs between the two arms (48.3 vs. 45%). A placebo-controlled RCT evaluated the role of metformin in reducing OHSS in PCOS women undergoing IVF with GnRH antagonist protocol.[57] No reduction in moderate–severe OHSS was noted in the metformin arm (16 vs. 12.2%) but significantly lower clinical pregnancy and LBRs were observed in the metformin arm compared to placebo.

A Cochrane review examined the role of metformin in PCOS women undergoing IVF and included nine RCTs ($n = 816$).[55] Pooled results from five trials did not find any significant difference in LBRs following metformin versus placebo (OR 1.39, 95% CI 0.81–2.40). However, the clinical pregnancy rate was higher in the metformin arm (OR 1.52, 95% CI 1.07–2.15; 8 RCTs) and the quality of evidence was moderate. Moderate-quality evidence suggested that there was a significantly lower risk of OHSS (OR 0.29, 95% CI 0.18–0.49) after metformin therapy compared to placebo. In eight of the nine included trials in the review, GnRH agonist protocol was used while the GnRH antagonist protocol was used in the remaining trials. In contemporary practice, GnRH antagonist is the preferred protocol for PCOS women undergoing ART due to significant reduction in OHSS risk. The risk of OHSS is further reduced by the use of GnRH trigger and "freeze all strategy", hence the applicability of the Cochrane review results may be limited in current IVF practice.[58,59]

The European Society of Human Reproduction and Embryology (ESHRE) guidelines on ovarian stimulation do not recommend routine use of metformin as an adjuvant, before or during ART when the GnRH antagonist is used in PCOS women.[59] To summarize, the role of metformin as an adjuvant prior or during ART can be considered only in PCOS women when the GnRH agonist protocol is being used for pituitary suppression for reduction of OHSS risk. However, the GnRH antagonist protocol with GnRH trigger with or without freeze all strategy is the recommended method for prevention of OHSS in contemporary IVF practice.[59]

■ PRE-IVF HYSTEROSCOPY

Hysteroscopy is a common gynecological procedure in contemporary practice. It is performed to detect intracavitary pathology in the uterus and can be carried out in an outpatient facility. Hysteroscopy provides the option of diagnosing and treating intracavitary uterine pathology in the same sitting.[60] Screening hysteroscopy is performed in an asymptomatic woman with no obvious intracavitary lesion detected on routine pelvic imaging. In symptomatic women or in those, who have a diagnosed intracavitary uterine pathology on pelvic imaging, an operative hysteroscopy is performed which involves detection and treatment of the lesion in the same sitting.[60,61]

Prior to ART, a transvaginal ultrasound is performed routinely to screen for any pelvic pathology and the assessment includes a closer scrutiny of the uterine cavity for undiagnosed lesions such as polyps, septum, or intrauterine adhesions. In clinical scenarios such as repeated IVF failures, suspected intracavitary uterine pathologies, or cervical stenosis, a pre-IVF hysteroscopy is often considered to "improve" the success rate of subsequent ART treatment.[61-64] However, it is unclear if invasive procedures such as pre-IVF hysteroscopy indeed improve the ART success. The suggested mechanisms for the perceived "benefit" are treatment of incidentally detected intracavitary pathologies, cervical dilatation which may facilitate subsequent embryo transfer and local endometrial injury leading to release of cytokines, which may help in the implantation process.[61,63,65]

There is a paucity of data from RCTs evaluating role of operative hysteroscopy in women with suspected intracavitary uterine pathology prior to ART.[60] Data from observational studies which evaluated the impact of hysteroscopic polypectomy in women undergoing IVF reported no clear benefit of removal of endometrial polyp (<2 cm in size) compared with expectant management.[66-68] In a retrospective cohort study ($n = 83$), women in whom endometrial polyp of <2 cm was detected during IVF were included.[68] One of the cohorts continued with IVF ($n = 49$) while the other group ($n = 34$) underwent hysteroscopic polypectomy following oocyte retrieval and embryos were frozen and transferred in subsequent cycles. The pregnancy rates were similar in both the groups (22.4 vs. 23.4%). A Cochrane review which reported lack of RCTs investigating effectiveness of hysteroscopic removal of polyp, septum, or adhesion suggested more trials to establish the role of operative hysteroscopy prior to IVF.[60] However, it is unlikely that such RCTs comparing operative versus diagnostic hysteroscopic intervention will be feasible due to ethical challenges and recruitment issues.[69]

In a large multicenter RCT from the Netherlands, women undergoing their first IVF were randomized to pre-IVF hysteroscopy ($n = 373$) versus direct IVF ($n = 377$) arms.[70] The LBR did not improve with pre-IVF hysteroscopy following first IVF [27 vs. 30%; relative risk (RR) 0.90; 95% CI 0.71–1.14]. The authors concluded that women with a normal ultrasound should not be offered routine pre-IVF hysteroscopy. Another large multicenter trial from Europe evaluated the role of pre-IVF hysteroscopy in women with recurrent implantation failure.[71] A total of 350 and 352 women were randomized to pre-IVF hysteroscopy and direct IVF arms, respectively. There was no significant difference between LBRs between the two arms (29 vs. 29%; RR 1.0, 95% CI 0.79–1.25). 85 women in the hysteroscopy arm had abnormal findings and the live birth (30%) did not differ compared to the control group (RR 1.06, 95% CI 0.74–1.51). A Cochrane review, which included ten RCTs ($n = 3,750$), evaluated the role of screening hysteroscopy in women undergoing ART.[61] The pooled result from six trials suggested improvement in the LBR after hysteroscopy (RR 1.26, 95% CI 1.11–1.43) when compared to no hysteroscopy and the quality of evidence was low. Similarly, the clinical pregnancy rate was also higher in the hysteroscopy arm (RR 1.32, 95% CI 1.20–1.45; 10 RCTs) but the quality of evidence was low. The majority of the trials did not provide sufficient study method details and the statistical heterogeneity was high. There was insufficient information regarding safety of hysteroscopy.

The reported prevalence of hysteroscopic abnormalities prior to IVF has been found to be highly variable, ranging between 12 and 45%.[62,70-72] The possible reason for the variation could be differences in population screened, detection rate which is operator dependent, and criteria for defining abnormal findings on hysteroscopy. These factors could also impact the studies evaluating the effectiveness of screening hysteroscopy prior to IVF.

CONCLUSION

To summarize, it is a prudent approach to offer operative hysteroscopy to women undergoing IVF who are symptomatic and/or have been diagnosed with intracavitary uterine pathology such as a large endometrial polyp, submucous fibroid, adhesions, or septum on pelvic imaging. However, for women who are asymptomatic and pelvic imaging is normal, the role of routine screening hysteroscopy is limited. The screening hysteroscopy can be considered in women with a history of difficult embryo transfer, cervical stenosis, or where intracavitary abnormality cannot be ruled out with pelvic imaging.

KEY POINTS

- Benefits of cycle programming with OC pill pretreatment are better follicular synchronization and optimization of IVF workload which has to be carefully weighed against possible negative impact on LBR in GnRH antagonist fresh cycles.
- The OC pill pretreatment is associated with increase in gonadotropin requitement and duration of stimulation.
- When OC pill is considered for cycle programming, a shorter duration of pretreatment and 5 day pill-free washout should be considered before initiating ovarian stimulation in IVF.
- Progestogen alone can be used for IVF cycle programming with a pill washout period of 5 days for women undergoing IVF with GnRH antagonist protocol.
- Estrogen alone can be used for IVF cycle programming with a pill washout period of 1–2 days for women undergoing IVF with GnRH antagonist protocol.
- Oral antioxidants for male partner can be considered as an adjuvant prior to ART in male infertility. However, it is unclear whether the effects are more profound for men with documented DNA damage. Furthermore, there is no clarity on the optimal dose and duration of antioxidant therapy in male partner.
- Antioxidant treatment does not seem to provide any additional benefit in infertile females prior to ART.
- Androgens may be offered as pretreatment in poor responders after careful consideration of possible adverse reactions and effects on early pregnancy.

- Metformin can be offered pre-IVF therapy in women at high risk of OHSS undergoing IVF and where as GnRH agonist protocol has been planned for achieving downregulation.
- Routine pre-IVF hysteroscopy should be avoided in women with normal pelvic imaging. Screening hysteroscopy can be offered in asymptomatic women undergoing IVF with a history of difficult embryo transfer, cervical stenosis, or where intracavitary abnormality cannot be ruled out with pelvic imaging.

REFERENCES

1. de Mouzon J, Chambers G, Zegers-Hochschild F, Mansour R, Ishihara O, Banker M, et al. International Committee for Monitoring Assisted Reproductive Technologies world report: assisted reproductive technology 2012. Hum Reprod. 2020;35(8):1900-13.
2. De Geyter C, Calhaz-Jorge C, Kupka M, Wyns C, Mocanu E, Motrenko T, et al. ART in Europe, 2015: results generated from European registries by ESHRE. Hum Reprod Open. 2020;2020(1):hoz038.
3. Kamath M, Mascarenhas M, Franik S, Liu E, Sunkara S. Clinical adjuncts in in vitro fertilization: a growing list. Fertil Steril. 2019;112(6):978-86.
4. Farquhar C, Rombauts L, Kremer J, Lethaby A, Ayeleke R. Oral contraceptive pill, progestogen or oestrogen pretreatment for ovarian stimulation protocols for women undergoing assisted reproductive techniques. Cochrane Database Syst Rev. 2017;5(5):CD006109.
5. Raoofi Z, Aflatoonian A. Ovarian cysts formation during depot formulation of GnRH-a therapy and the effect of pretreatment with oral contraceptive pills on subsequent implantation and pregnancy rate in ART cycles. Iran J Pharm Res. 2008;7:109-13.
6. Kolibianakis E, Papanikolaou E, Camus M, Tournaye H, Van Steirteghem A, Devroey P. Effect of oral contraceptive pill pretreatment on ongoing pregnancy rates in patients stimulated with GnRH antagonists and recombinant FSH for IVF. A randomized controlled trial. Hum Reprod. 2005;21(2):352-7.
7. Garcia-Velasco J, Bermejo A, Ruiz F, Martinez-Salazar J, Requena A, Pellicer A. Cycle scheduling with oral contraceptive pills in the GnRH antagonist protocol vs the long protocol: a randomized, controlled trial. Fertil Steril. 2011;96(3):590-3.
8. Griesinger G, Kolibianakis E, Venetis C, Diedrich K, Tarlatzis B. Oral contraceptive pretreatment significantly reduces ongoing pregnancy likelihood in gonadotropin-releasing hormone antagonist cycles: an updated meta-analysis. Fertil Steril. 2010;94(6):2382-4.
9. Cédrin-Durnerin I, Bständig B, Parneix I, Bied-Damon V, Avril C, Decanter C, et al. Effects of oral contraceptive, synthetic progestogen or natural estrogen pre-treatments on the hormonal profile and the antral follicle cohort before GnRH antagonist protocol. Hum Reprod. 2007;22(1):109-16.
10. Bermejo A, Iglesias C, Ruiz-Alonso M, Blesa D, Simón C, Pellicer A, et al. The impact of using the combined oral contraceptive pill for cycle scheduling on gene expression related to endometrial receptivity. Hum Reprod. 2014;29:1271-8.

11. Lu Y, Wang Y, Zhang T, Wang G, He Y, Lindheim S, et al. Effect of pretreatment oral contraceptives on fresh and cumulative live birth in vitro fertilization outcomes in ovulatory women. Fertil Steril. 2020;114(4):779-86.
12. Baerwald A, Anderson P, Yuzpe A, Case A, Fluker M. Synchronization of ovarian stimulation with follicle wave emergence in patients undergoing in vitro fertilization with a prior suboptimal response: a randomized, controlled trial. Fertil Steril. 2012;98(4):881-7.e2.
13. Anderson R, Stein A, Paulson R, Stanczyk F, Vijod A, Lobo R. Effects of norethindrone on gonadotropin and ovarian steroid secretion when used for cycle programming during in vitro fertilization. Fertil Steril. 1990;54(1):96-101.
14. Engmann L, Maconochie N, Bekir J, Tan S. Progestogen therapy during pituitary desensitization with gonadotropin-releasing hormone agonist prevents functional ovarian cyst formation: A prospective, randomized study. Am J Obstet Gynecol. 1999;181(3):576-82.
15. Cédrin-Durnerin I, Guivarc'h-Levêque A, Hugues J. Pretreatment with estrogen does not affect IVF-ICSI cycle outcome compared with no pretreatment in GnRH antagonist protocol: a prospective randomized trial. Fertil Steril. 2012;97(6):1359-64.e1.
16. Saple S, Agrawal M, Kawar S. Precycle estradiol in synchronization and scheduling of antagonist cycles. J Obstet Gynecol India. 2016;66(4):295-9.
17. Aitken R, Clarkson J. Cellular basis of defective sperm function and its association with the genesis of reactive oxygen species by human spermatozoa. Reproduction. 1987;81(2):459-69.
18. Behrman H, Kodaman P, Preston S, Gao S. Oxidative stress and the ovary. J Soc Gynecol Investig. 2001;8(Suppl 1):S40-2.
19. Agarwal A, Saleh R, Bedaiwy M. Role of reactive oxygen species in the pathophysiology of human reproduction. Fertil Steril. 2003;79(4):829-43.
20. Ford W. Regulation of sperm function by reactive oxygen species. Hum Reprod Update. 2004;10(5):387-99.
21. Agarwal A, Said T, Bedaiwy M, Banerjee J, Alvarez J. Oxidative stress in an assisted reproductive techniques setting. Fertil Steril. 2006;86(3):503-12.
22. du Plessis S, Makker K, Desai N, Agarwal A. Impact of oxidative stress on IVF. Expert Rev Obstet Gynecol. 2008;3(4):539-54.
23. Adewoyin M, Ibrahim M, Roszaman R, Isa M, Alewi N, Rafa A, et al. Male infertility: The effect of natural antioxidants and phytocompounds on seminal oxidative stress. Diseases. 2017;5(1):9.
24. Agarwal A, Aponte-Mellado A, Premkumar B, Shaman A, Gupta S. The effects of oxidative stress on female reproduction: a review. Reprod Biol Endocrinol. 2012;10(1):49.
25. Takasaki A, Tamura H, Taniguchi K, Asada H, Taketani T, Matsuoka A, et al. Luteal blood flow and luteal function. J Ovarian Res. 2009;2(1):1.
26. Thomson R, Spedding S, Buckley J. Vitamin D in the aetiology and management of polycystic ovary syndrome. Clin Endocrinol. 2012;77(3):343-50.
27. Badawy A, State O, Abdelgawad S. N-Acetyl cysteine and clomiphene citrate for induction of ovulation in polycystic ovary syndrome: a cross-over trial. Acta Obstet Gynecol Scand. 2007;86(2):218-22.
28. Showell M, Mackenzie-Proctor R, Jordan V, Hart R. Antioxidants for female subfertility. Cochrane Database Syst Rev. 2020;(8):CD007807.

29. Zini A, Lamirande E, Gagnon C. Reactive oxygen species in semen of infertile patients: levels of superoxide dismutase- and catalase-like activities in seminal plasma and spermatozoa. Int J Androl. 1993;16(3):183-8.
30. Robinson L, Gallos I, Conner S, Rajkhowa M, Miller D, Lewis S, et al. The effect of sperm DNA fragmentation on miscarriage rates: a systematic review and meta-analysis. Hum Reprod. 2012;27(10):2908-17.
31. Simon L, Murphy K, Shamsi M, Liu L, Emery B, Aston K, et al. Paternal influence of sperm DNA integrity on early embryonic development. Hum Reprod. 2014;29(11):2402-12.
32. Shimura T, Toyoshima M, Taga M, Shiraishi K, Uematsu N, Inoue M, et al. The Novel Surveillance Mechanism of the Trp53-Dependent S-Phase Checkpoint Ensures Chromosome Damage Repair and Preimplantation-Stage Development of Mouse Embryos Fertilized with X-Irradiated Sperm. Radiat Res. 2002;158(6):735-42.
33. Bykova M, Athayde K, Sharma R, Jha R, Sabanegh E, Agarwal A. Defining the reference value of seminal reactive oxygen species in a population of infertile men and normal healthy volunteers. Fertil Steril. 2007;88:S305.
34. Balercia G, Buldreghini E, Vignini A, Tiano L, Paggi F, Amoroso S, et al. Coenzyme Q10 treatment in infertile men with idiopathic asthenozoospermia: a placebo-controlled, double-blind randomized trial. Fertil Steril. 2009;91(5):1785-92.
35. Omu A, Al-Azemi M, Kehinde E, Anim J, Oriowo M, Mathew T. Indications of the mechanisms involved in improved sperm parameters by zinc therapy. Med Princ Pract. 2008;17(2):108-16.
36. Greco E. Reduction of the Incidence of Sperm DNA Fragmentation by Oral Antioxidant Treatment. J Androl. 2005;26(3):349-53.
37. Smits R, Mackenzie-Proctor R, Yazdani A, Stankiewicz M, Jordan V, Showell M. Antioxidants for male subfertility. Cochrane Database Syst Rev. 2019;3(3):CD007411.
38. Majzoub A, Agarwal A. Systematic review of antioxidant types and doses in male infertility: Benefits on semen parameters, advanced sperm function, assisted reproduction and live-birth rate. Arab J Urol. 2018;16(1):113-24.
39. Lewin A, Lavon H. The effect of coenzyme Q10 on sperm motility and function. Mol Aspects Med. 1997;18:213-9.
40. Geva E, Bartoov B, Zabludovsky N, Lessing J, Lerner-Geva L, Amit A. The effect of antioxidant treatment on human spermatozoa and fertilization rate in an in vitro fertilization program. Fertil Steril. 1996;66(3):430-4.
41. Greco E, Romano S, Iacobelli M, Ferrero S, Baroni E, Minasi M, et al. ICSI in cases of sperm DNA damage: beneficial effect of oral antioxidant treatment. Hum Reprod. 2005;20(9):2590-4.
42. Buvat J. Androgen therapy with dehydroepiandrosterone. World J Urol. 2003;21(5):346-55.
43. Davison S, Bell R, Donath S, Montalto J, Davis S. Androgen levels in adult females: Changes with age, menopause, and oophorectomy. J Clin Endocrinol Metab. 2005;90(7):3847-53.
44. Ryan K, Petro Z, Kaiser J. Steroid formation by isolated and recombined ovarian granulosa and thecal cells. J Clin Endocrinol Metab. 1968;28(3):355-8.
45. Garcia-Velasco J, Moreno L, Pacheco A, Guillén A, Duque L, Requena A, et al. The aromatase inhibitor letrozole increases the concentration of intraovarian

androgens and improves in vitro fertilization outcome in low responder patients: A pilot study. Fertil Steril. 2005;84(1):82-7.
46. Nielsen M, Rasmussen I, Kristensen S, Christensen S, Mollgard K, Wreford Andersen E, et al. In human granulosa cells from small antral follicles, androgen receptor mRNA and androgen levels in follicular fluid correlate with FSH receptor mRNA. Mol Hum Reprod. 2010;17(1):63-70.
47. Barad D, Brill H, Gleicher N. Update on the use of dehydroepiandrosterone supplementation among women with diminished ovarian function. J Assist Reprod Genet. 2007;24(12):629-34.
48. Balasch J, Fábregues F, Peñarrubia J, Carmona F, Casamitjana R, Creus M, et al. Pretreatment with transdermal testosterone may improve ovarian response to gonadotrophins in poor-responder IVF patients with normal basal concentrations of FSH. Hum Reprod. 2006;21(7):1884-93.
49. Kim C, Ahn J, Nah H, Kim S, Chae H, Kang B. Ovarian features after 2 weeks, 3 weeks and 4 weeks transdermal testosterone gel treatment and their associated effect on IVF/ICSI outcome in low responders. Fertil Steril. 2010;94(4): S155-6.
50. Somboonporn W, Bell R, Davis S. Testosterone for peri and postmenopausal women. Cochrane Database Syst Rev. 2005;(4):CD004509.
51. Sir-Petermann T, Maliqueo M, Angel B, Lara HE, PérezBravo F, Recabarren SE. Maternal serum androgens in pregnant women with polycystic ovarian syndrome: possible implications in prenatal androgenization. Hum Reprod. 2002;17(10):2573-9.
52. Nagels HE, Rishworth JR, Siristatidis CS, Kroon B. Androgens (dehydroepiandrosterone or testosterone) for women undergoing assisted reproduction. Cochrane Database Syst Rev. 2015;(11):CD009749.
53. Nestler J, Stovall D, Akhter N, Iuorno M, Jakubowicz D. Strategies for the use of insulin-sensitizing drugs to treat infertility in women with polycystic ovary syndrome. Fertil Steril. 2002;77(2):209-15.
54. Scheen A, Paquot N. Metformin revisited: A critical review of the benefit-risk balance in at-risk patients with type 2 diabetes. Diabetes Metab. 2013;39(3):179-90.
55. Tso LO, Costello MF, Albuquerque LE, Andriolo RB, Macedo CR. Metformin treatment before and during IVF or ICSI in women with polycystic ovary syndrome. Cochrane Database Syst Rev. 2014;2014(11):CD006105.
56. Palomba S, Falbo A, Carrillo L, Villani M, Orio F, Russo T, et al. Metformin reduces risk of ovarian hyperstimulation syndrome in patients with polycystic ovary syndrome during gonadotropin-stimulated in vitro fertilization cycles: a randomized, controlled trial. Fertil Steril. 2011;96(6):1384-90.e4.
57. Jacob S, Brewer C, Tang T, Picton H, Barth J, Balen A. A short course of metformin does not reduce OHSS in a GnRH antagonist cycle for women with PCOS undergoing IVF: a randomised placebo-controlled trial. Hum Reprod. 2016;31(12):2756-64.
58. Humaidan P, Polyzos N, Alsbjerg B, Erb K, Mikkelsen A, Elbaek H, et al. GnRHa trigger and individualized luteal phase hCG support according to ovarian response to stimulation: two prospective randomized controlled multi-centre studies in IVF patients. Hum Reprod. 2013;28(9):2511-21.

59. Ovarian Stimulation TEGGO, Bosch E, Broer S, Griesinger G, Grynberg M, Humaidan P, et al. ESHRE guideline: ovarian stimulation for IVF/ICSI. Hum Reprod Open. 2020;2020(2):hoaa009.
60. Bosteels J, van Wessel S, Weyers S, Broekmans FJ, D'Hooghe TM, Bongers MY, et al. Hysteroscopy for treating subfertility associated with suspected major uterine cavity abnormalities. Cochrane Database Syst Rev. 2018;12(12): CD009461.
61. Kamath M, Bosteels J, D'Hooghe T, Seshadri S, Weyers S, Mol B, et al. Screening hysteroscopy in subfertile women and women undergoing assisted reproduction. Cochrane Database Syst Rev. 2019;4(4):CD012856.
62. Oliveira F, Abdelmassih V, Diamond M, Dozortsev D, Nagy Z, Abdelmassih R. Uterine cavity findings and hysteroscopic interventions in patients undergoing in vitro fertilization–embryo transfer who repeatedly cannot conceive. Fertil Steril. 2003;80(6):1371-5.
63. Rama Raju G, Shashi Kumari G, Krishna K, Prakash G, Madan K. Assessment of uterine cavity by hysteroscopy in assisted reproduction programme and its influence on pregnancy outcome. Arch Gynecol Obstet. 2006;274(3):160-4.
64. Pritts E, Parker W, Olive D. Fibroids and infertility: an updated systematic review of the evidence. Fertil Steril. 2009;91(4):1215-23.
65. Barash A, Dekel N, Fieldust S, Segal I, Schechtman E, Granot I. Local injury to the endometrium doubles the incidence of successful pregnancies in patients undergoing in vitro fertilization. Fertil Steril. 2003;79(6):1317-22.
66. Isikoglu M, Berkkanoglu M, Senturk Z, Coetzee K, Ozgur K. Endometrial polyps smaller than 1.5 cm do not affect ICSI outcome. Reprod Biomed Online. 2006;12(2):199-204.
67. Ghaffari F, Arabipoor A, Bagheri Lankarani N, Hosseini F, Bahmanabadi A. Hysteroscopic polypectomy without cycle cancellation in IVF/ICSI cycles: a cross-sectional study. Eur J Obstet Gynecol Reprod Biol. 2016;205:37-42.
68. Lass A, Williams G, Abusheikha N, Brinsden P. The effect of endometrial polyps on outcomes of in vitro fertilization (IVF) cycles. J Assist Reprod Genet. 1999;16(8):410-5.
69. Wartolowska K, Collins G, Hopewell S, Judge A, Dean B, Rombach I, et al. Feasibility of surgical randomised controlled trials with a placebo arm: a systematic review. BMJ Open. 2016;6(3):e010194.
70. Smit J, Kasius J, Eijkemans M, Koks C, van Golde R, Nap A, et al. Hysteroscopy before in-vitro fertilisation (inSIGHT): a multicentre, randomised controlled trial. The Lancet. 2016;387(10038):2622-9.
71. El-Toukhy T, Campo R, Khalaf Y, Tabanelli C, Gianaroli L, Gordts S, et al. Hysteroscopy in recurrent in-vitro fertilisation failure (TROPHY): a multicentre, randomised controlled trial. Lancet. 2016;387(10038):2614-21.
72. Cenksoy P, Ficicioglu C, Yıldırım G, Yesiladali M. Hysteroscopic findings in women with recurrent IVF failures and the effect of correction of hysteroscopic findings on subsequent pregnancy rates. Arch Gynecol Obstet. 2012;287(2): 357-60.

Section

7

Determinants of an Optimal Protocol

- **Determinants of an Optimal Protocol**
  Seema Pandey, Shreya Gowni, Vidhu Modgil

Determinants of an Optimal Protocol

Seema Pandey, Shreya Gowni, Vidhu Modgil

■ INTRODUCTION

Though >2.5 million in vitro fertilization (IVF) cycles are being performed worldwide and it has been more than 4 decades since the birth of our first IVF baby, our success rate in terms of take-home baby rate has not increased beyond a certain percentage and has become stagnant. To improve the success of individual cycles, the knowledge of the patient's potential ovarian reserve and response can help clinicians individualize the medication dosage, which may reduce the adverse effects of an excessive ovarian response, decrease the rate of cancelled cycles, and ultimately, increase the pregnancy rate.

Even though each marker, as a stand-alone, may have some predictive value, they are not reliable across all patient groups consistently. Hence, combining facts, figures, and clinical judgment is essential **(Fig. 1)**.

■ PATIENT FACTORS

Reproductive Age: Biological versus Chronological Age

The patient's age is recognized as an independent negative prognostic factor and first marker of ovarian reserve. Age has a negative impact on both the number and quality of oocytes but the reproductive potential varies

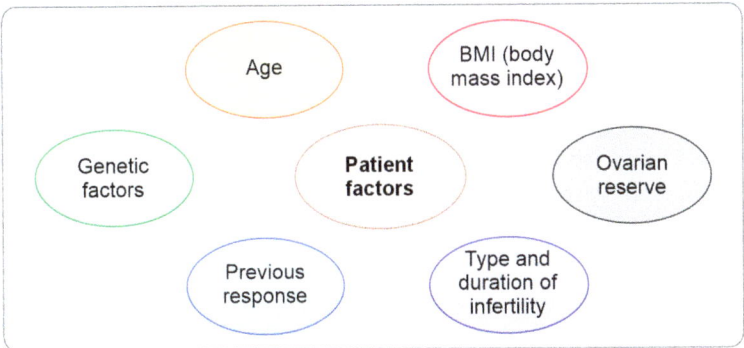

Fig. 1: Patients factors impacting the outcome in ART. (ART: assisted reproductive technology)

drastically among women of similar age; therefore, combining it with hormonal and functional tests gives a better prediction of her reproductive potential.[1]

The results of the study by Yan et al. showed that older women had a weaker response during controlled ovarian hyperstimulation (COH), fewer retrieved eggs, low-oocyte fertilization rate, low-quality embryo rates, low embryo implantation rate, low delivery, high abortion, and high preterm delivery.[2]

As age increases, the rate of aneuploidy has been shown to increase, and hence decreasing her chance of a live birth rate (LBR).[2]

Women older than 35 years experience a dramatic increase in embryo aneuploidy rate from a 30% baseline production up to 90% in their late 40s prior to the menopause.

Ovarian Reserve

Ovarian response to stimulation and reproductive potential can be different in women of similar age, according to the individual's ovarian reserve. Ovarian reserve tests have predictive value for ovarian response to gonadotropin stimulation. But their prediction of childbirth during assisted reproductive technology (ART) cycles is limited. Anti-Müllerian hormone (AMH), antral follicle count (AFC), and baseline follicle-stimulating hormone (FSH) are the most commonly tests used to evaluate ovarian reserve.

Anti-Müllerian Hormone

Anti-Müllerian hormone is produced by the granulosa cells surrounding the preantral and small antral follicles. Additionally, AMH is independent of FSH, and, therefore, its levels are a direct measure of the follicular pool production. The serum levels of AMH decrease throughout reproductive life and are undetectable in the postmenopausal period.

An association was observed between AMH level and the number of follicles in the ovary, which will indirectly predict the number of oocytes and live pregnancy rate.

Antral Follicle Count

The AFC is defined as the sum of follicles between 2 and 6 mm in both ovaries on a transvaginal ultrasound. It is one of the most common and most used parameters to predict the ovarian reserve and the patient response to ovarian stimulation. However, there is significant variation among different authors in the limits used to classify antral follicles.[3-6]

A study in Indonesia has shown that an AMH level of 1.40 µg/mL and AFC at 7 are the cut-off values used to predict good response and ovarian condition.[7]

Follicle-stimulating Hormone

Although AMH and AFC are more informative biomarkers of ovarian reserve and response baseline FSH level is still one of the commonly used tests for daily practices. It is generally accepted that the ovarian reserve is low when the FSH level exceeds 10–12 IU/L.[8] High FSH levels are associated with a low oocyte yield and high cycle cancellation rates.[8-12] In a previous meta-analysis, the baseline FSH level, female age, infertility duration, and oocyte number were predictors of IVF outcomes.[13] Elevated baseline FSH level is one of the used criteria for diagnosis of diminished ovarian reserve (DOR) in clinical practice.[14]

Factors Affecting the Ovarian Reserve (Figs. 2 and 3 and Flowchart 1)

- *Endometriosis:* There is a serious controversy as to whether endometriosis per se can affect the reproductive outcomes of women undergoing ARTs. Several authors have found that endometriosis has a negative impact,[15-17]

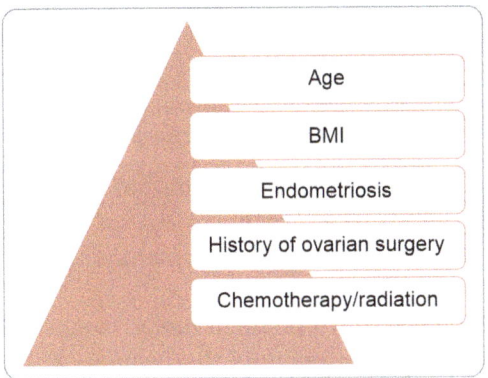

Fig. 2: Factors affecting the ovarian reserve. (BMI: body mass index)

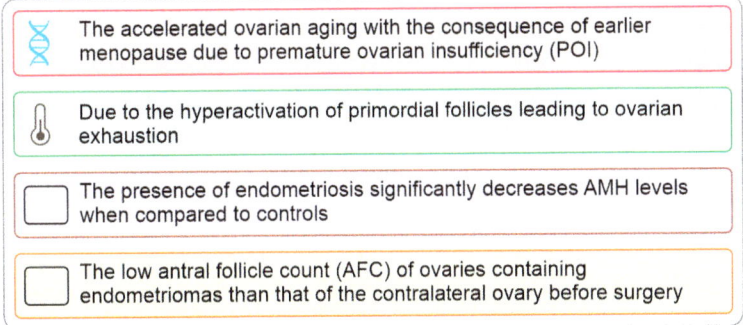

Fig. 3: Accelerated aging in endometriosis causes and impact. (AMH: anti-Müllerian hormone)

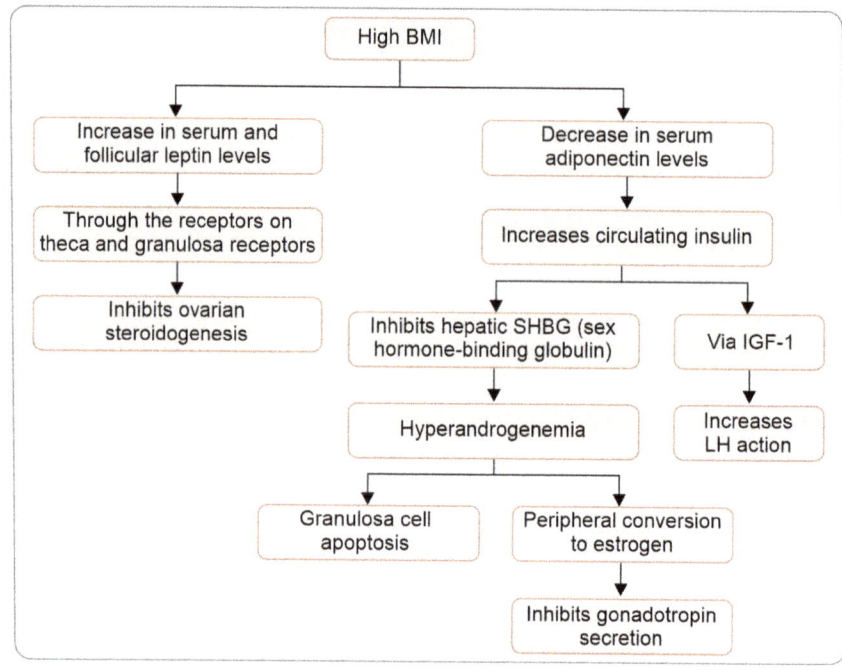

Flowchart 1: Impact of BMI on HPG axis.

(BMI: body mass index; HPG: hypothalamic-pituitary-gonadal; IGF: insulin-like growth factor; LH: luteinizing hormone)

while others have not found such association.[18-20] Severe endometriosis negatively affects ovarian response, oocyte quality, and embryos. However, fertilization rate is not different among the various stages of endometriosis.[21]

Endometriosis, especially endometriomas, compromises the ovarian reserve. It has been documented that women with endometriomas experience faster decline in serum AMH levels compared to their age-matched counterparts.

There are multiple reasons why endometriomas decrease ovarian reserve and give compromised response to ovarian stimulation in terms of reduced number of oocytes and MII oocytes retrieved when compared to women without endometriosis, no other differences in reproductive outcomes are observed. This leads to the belief that IVF/intracytoplasmic sperm injection (ICSI) is a beneficial ART approach for women with endometrioma.[22]

Why does endometrioma decrease ovarian reserve?
1. Mechanical stretch due to the size of cyst
2. Increased ROS-induced damage due to toxic substance present in the cyst
3. Increased fibrosis

4. Loss of cortex-specific stroma and smooth cell metaplasia
   5. Injury by iron content of the cyst seeping through the cyst wall
   6. Inadvertent surgical damage
- *History of ovarian surgery:* Due to vascular injury, infection after surgery, and micro-thromboembolism
- *Chemotherapy and radiotherapy:* For any ovarian or other malignancies compromise the reserve and the response to stimulation
- *Polycystic ovarian disease (PCOD):* Factors associated with a hyper-response and an increased risk of ovarian hyperstimulation syndrome (OHSS) include patient history,[23] the presence of polycystic ovary syndrome (PCOS), younger age, and lower body mass index (BMI).[24]
  The most predictive factor to identify women who may be susceptible for OHSS is antral follicle number. The study of Papanikolaou et al. (2006) also found high levels of E_2 to be unreliable in predicting risk of OHSS, but found follicle number to be significantly better ($p = 0.001$).[25]
  Studies of endocrine and ovarian reserve tests to predict hyper-response have not yielded consistent results.
  Among dynamic tests, neither the exogenous FSH ovarian reserve test (EFORT) nor the clomiphene citrate challenge test (CCCT) is adequate alone to predict hyper-response.[26]
- *Miscellaneous factors:*
  - Thyroid disorders
  - Hyperprolactinemia
  - Autoimmune disorders and connective tissue disorders
  - Other tuboperitoneal disease
  - Diabetes mellitus
  - It has been demonstrated that the cause of infertility plays a role in determining poor or intermediate outcomes.

Body mass index: High BMI works at two levels, by increasing serum and intrafollicular leptin levels it inhibits steroidogenesis and by decreasing serum adiponectin levels it mediates hyperinsulinemia pathway leading to decreased gonadotropin secretion and granulosa cell apoptosis.[27]

Decreased fertility is attributed to various parameters in obese women, such as endocrine and metabolic dysfunctions, which sequentially may affect follicular proliferation, implantation, and the growth of clinical pregnancy.

Obesity almost compromises all the parameters of a stimulated cycle starting from increased dosage of gonadotropins to the LBR, our penultimate determinant of success **(Table 1)**.

Psychological Factors (Fig. 4)

Psychological disturbances due to infertility can lead to depression, nervousness, distress, and poor quality of life. Nearly 32% of women in the early stages of infertility treatment are at risk of mental disorders.[28]

TABLE 1: Impact of obesity on ART outcome.

Impact of obesity	
Gonadotropin requirement	Increased
Response to stimulation	Poorer
Oocyte number	Reduced
Oocyte quality	Unchanged
Fertilization	Decreased
Embryo quality	Poorer in some studies
Cycle cancellation	Insufficient evidence
OHSS	Insufficient evidence
Pregnancy rate	Reduced in some studies
Miscarriage rate	Increased
Live birth	Insufficient evidence

(ART: assisted reproductive technology; OHSS: ovarian hyperstimulation syndrome)

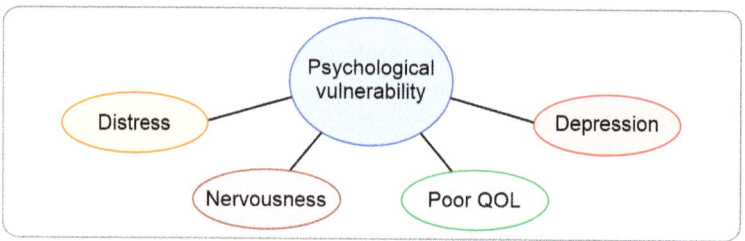

Fig. 4: Impact of psychological stress on life. (QOL: Quality of life)

Several psychological pathways may play a role that may affect her fertility or may disrupt infertility treatment success. These pathways include the hypothalamic-pituitary-adrenal (HPA) axis, which plays a role in stress response regulation, and the hypothalamic-pituitary-gonadal axis (HPG), which regulates reproduction.[29] Various mechanisms have been proposed about the impact of psychological factors on infertility, including impaired gonadotropin secretion, local effect of catecholamine on the uterus and fallopian tubes, and impaired immune processes involved in maintaining fertility.[30]

Genetic Factors

Single-nucleotide polymorphisms (SNPs) affecting in vitro fertilization outcome:
- Effects of different SNPs on various aspects of human reproduction include recurrent miscarriage, infertility, and fetal implant failure.
- The association of SNPs in various genes, including *MTHFR*, Leiden factor V, progesterone receptor, FSH receptor, plasminogen activating factor (*PAI-1*), prothrombin, and estrogen receptor gene, with different aspects of fertility has been observed **(Table 2)**.

TABLE 2: Effect of various gene mutations.

Genes	Mutation/polymorphism	Effect
MTHFR	CT genotype of *MTHFR* in nucleotide 677 of the mother	• Increases the chances of getting pregnant with IVF treatment[29] • Higher percentage of good-quality embryos
Leiden factor V	Leiden factor V genetic mutations	Have generally been shown to lead to failure of ART[31]
Progesterone receptor	PROGINS is a complex which includes a 306 bp Alu element in intron 7, a missense SNP in exon 4 and a silence SNP in exon 5, all of which are in complete linkage disequilibrium[32]	• For PGR, a functional SNP of PGR, PROGINS, was reported to be associated with adverse reproductive outcomes, including unexplained infertility and repeated IVF implantation failure (Su et al. 2011)[30] • Though PROGINS has been found to be associated with endometriosis-associated infertility, Gimenes et al. (2010) and Pisarska et al. (2003) found an increase in the prevalence of PROGINS mutations among women with idiopathic infertility[30]
FSH receptor	Mutations in the FSHR are associated with primary amenorrhea (Doherty et al., 2002; Meduri et al., 2003), and a common SNP in the *FSHR* gene (rs6166, causing a change from an asparagine (A) to a serine (S) residue at codon position 680; p.S680N) is associated with a different sensitivity to both exogenous (Perez Mayorga et al., 2000) and endogenous (Greb et al., 2005) FSH[32]	As a group, women with the S/S genotype have a higher FSH threshold than those with the A/A genotype (Sudo et al., 2002; Greb et al., 2005; de Koning et al., 2006) and may benefit from a higher dose of FSH when undergoing multifollicular stimulation (Behre et al., 2005; Jun et al., 2006)
P53	Prevalence of the codon 72 polymorphism in the *P53* gene[31]	Has a significant effect on implantation rejection rate in IVF cycles[32]
Prothrombin	Prothrombin G20210A mutations	Have generally been shown to lead to failure of ART[31]

Contd...

Contd...

Genes	Mutation/polymorphism	Effect
Estrogen receptor	• Rod et al. (2014) have reported that the FSHR variant p. Ser680Ser is associated with poor response to FSH stimulation • Rs6165, which causes an amino acid change of threonine to alanine, is located within the transmembrane region of FSHR protein (Yan et al. 2013) and hence is proposed to be involved in the hormone-binding ability of FSHR and FSH-mediated signal transduction during ovarian stimulation (Kene et al. 2004; Agrawal and Dighe 2009) • Other predictive markers of ovarian response are polymorphisms of the alpha gene of ESR (ESR1); rs2234693, also known as the PvuII restriction polymorphism, and rs9340799, also known as the XbaI restriction polymorphism[33]	Both these polymorphisms have been reported to be associated with the risk of infertility (Anagnostou et al. 2013). For the third SNP, the microsatellite length polymorphism ESR1 (TA)n, the longer ESR1 (TA)n microsatellite repeat polymorphism has been reported to be associated with an improved ovarian response to FSH[33]
Solute carrier gene (SLC)	Haggarty et al.[29] *SLC19A1* c.80G>A polymorphism increased homocysteine (Hcy) concentration	Higher concentrations of homocysteine usually lead to detrimental effects on IVF outcomes
LHB	Trp8Arg, Ile15Thr, and Gly102Ser polymorphisms	Polymorphisms lead to menstrual irregularities, infertility, and recurrent miscarriages[30]
GDF-9	GDF-9 and BMP15 polymorphisms in these genes (*GDF9*: c.546G>A, *BMP15*: c.2673C>T, c.29C>G, IVS1+905A>G)	Also associated with fertility success rates and increased occurrence of dizygotic twins[31]
CYP-19-A1	Tetranucleotide repeat polymorphism (TTTA) n in intron 4 of the *CYP19A1* gene leads to aromatase hyperactivity	Women with fewer (TTTA) repeats in this gene show lower estrogen concentrations which result in susceptibility to unexplained infertility[32]

(ART: assisted reproductive technology; FSH: follicle-stimulating hormone; IVF: in vitro fertilization; PGR: progesterone receptor; MTHFR: methylenetetrahydrofolate reductase; SNP: single-nucleotide polymorphism)

TYPE OF STIMULATION PROTOCOL

The method of ovarian stimulation may impact egg/embryo quality. The potential for the eggs to undergo maturation, successful fertilization, and subsequent progression to good-quality embryos that can produce a healthy offspring is thought to be genetically determined. However, the expression of such potential is susceptible to numerous extrinsic influences, especially to intraovarian hormonal changes during the preovulatory phase of the cycle. Gonadotropin-releasing hormone (GnRH) analogs are widely used in stimulation protocols either to downregulate the cycle or to prevent the premature luteinizing hormone (LH) surge. Antagonist protocol is the most used and preferred protocol worldwide for both hyper- and normoresponders, due to its ease of usage, comparable efficacy, and patient safety.[34] For low responders, the choice of agonist or antagonist protocol yields the same results **(Table 3)**.

TABLE 3: Comparing protocols to their effect on cycle variables.

Variables	Agonist protocol	Antagonist protocol	PPOS protocol
Pretreatment	Long and requires more injections and costlier	Short or none does not require long suppression	Short or none
Dose and duration of stimulation	More	Lesser than agonist protocol	More than antagonist protocol
Synchronous growth	Yes Allows a greater number of oocytes to be retrieved	No Asynchronous growth, so the number of oocytes retrieved is less than agonist protocol	No Asynchronous growth, outcome like antagonist protocol
Trigger choices	No Only hCG trigger can be given, which increases the chance of OHSS	Yes hCG/agonist/dual based on the situation	Yes hCG/agonist/dual based on the situation
Application as per expected response	Cannot be applied in high responder situations like PCOD	Can be applied to low and high responders	Can be applied to low and high responders

(hCG: human chorionic gonadotropin; PPOS: progestin-primed ovarian stimulation; PCOD: polycystic ovarian disease)

■ TYPE OF STIMULATION DRUG AND DOSE

Gonadotropin regimens have been used for ovarian stimulation for many decades, but the lack of prospective, randomized trials in the beginning has meant that optimal starting doses have not been established.[35]

The optimum dose is a dose which balances the response, assessed by the number of oocytes retrieved and negates the chance of either OHSS or cycle cancellation due to poor response **(Fig. 5)**.

A clinically appropriate ovarian response may be defined as retrieval of 5–14 oocytes per patient.[35]

Individualizing the dose of FSH, for a woman based on standard factors such as the AFC or BMI, is common at the beginning of stimulation and further dose adjustments are, however, based solely on clinical judgment and experience. There is a lack of specific scientific evidence as there have been no well-designed, prospective, randomized trials.

The effect of increasing the dose after 5 days of stimulation was studied in two studies.[35] Both found that increasing the dose did not rectify the initial poor response and did not increase pregnancy rates.

Type of Drugs

In either protocols, the choice of drug does not seem to make a significant difference. According to studies like van Wely et al., there is not much difference between recombinant FSH, purified FSH, highly purified FSH, or human menopausal gonadotropin, and are all equally recommended.[37]

The addition of LH to agonist or antagonist protocol has not shown any improved result and is not recommended with regards to safety.

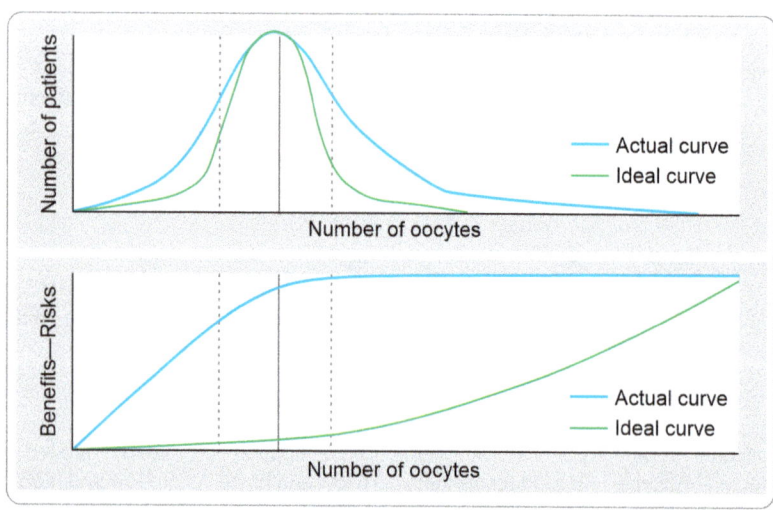

Fig. 5: Effect of gonadotropins dose of risk benefit ratio. Distribution of oocytes retrieved during multifollicular stimulation showing discrepancy between ideal and actual spread in a study by Popovic-Todorovic et al. (2003).[36]

■ ADJUVANTS

Adjuncts are supplements that may add additional value on top of standard fertility treatments.

- *Antioxidants:* Reactive oxygen species (ROS) can induce oxidative stress and lead to cell damage or death. Cells have antioxidant mechanisms which act to balance this process but it may often become unregulated. Initial evidence so far suggests that supplementation with CoQ-10 may reverse mitochondrial aging.[38] But there is still no data on dose and duration. Studies suggest that both excessive oxidative and antioxidative stress may be harmful and hence blind prescribing is not advocated.
- *Sildenafil* acts by potentiating the action of nitric oxide on vascular smooth muscle causing vasodilation. It has not shown to effect success rates and is not recommended.
- Routine use of metformin has not been shown to be beneficial in all PCOS population.
- *Dehydroepiandrosterone sulfate (DHEAS):* DHEA can enhance follicular function by increasing the production of insulin-like growth factor-1 (IGF-1) and increasing estradiol production in granulosa cells, acting as a precursor of androstenedione and testosterone in the ovarian theca cells **(Fig. 6)**.

  Many randomized controlled trials (RCTs) have indicated a positive outcome in poor responders, but these studies have been refuted by others. There is still no final consensus regarding its benefit.
- *Growth hormone:* Growth hormone acts by upregulating the local synthesis of IGF-1 which has a modulatory effect on FSH action. This further enhances the effect of gonadotropin action at the level of both the granulosa and theca cells.

  In a study by Norman RJ et al., the number of patients reaching an oocyte retrieval was significantly higher in the GH group; however, no differences were reported in the LBR.[39]

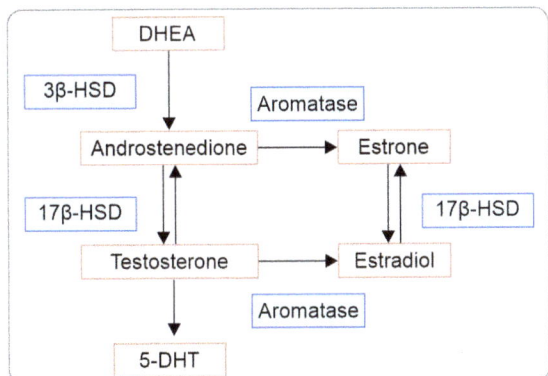

Fig. 6: Pathways showing estradiol conversion from DHEA.
(DHEA: dehydroepiandrosterone)

- *Testosterone gel:* According to T-TRANSPORT trial, pretreatment with 5.5 mg testosterone for 2 months prior to ovarian stimulation for IVF/ICSI does not increase clinical pregnancy rates as compared with placebo.[40]

■ TRIGGER FOR FINAL MATURATION

Unlike human chorionic gonadotropin (hCG) trigger, GnRH-a trigger stimulates FSH surge in addition to LH surge. FSH surge, in the mid-cycle, has a specific effect on oocyte maturation and leads to a further expansion of cumulus cells surrounding the oocyte and release of proteolytic enzymes involved in the process of ovulation.[41-44] This leads to better oocyte recovery rate and higher fertilization rates.

The level of LH surge following injection of hCG is slower than that following GnRH-a trigger,[45] and, therefore, GnRH-a trigger with effects of FSH along with the LH in the final follicular maturation may result a more physiological maturity.

The GnRH-a trigger significantly decreases the chance of OHSS making it the most widely used trigger for IVF cycles in clinics worldwide.

The most significant disadvantage of GnRH-a trigger is the severe luteal defect, which significantly decreases the success rate of a fresh embryo transfer.

In cases where a fresh transfer is planned for a normo- or poor responder, an hCG trigger is preferred over an agonist trigger as a fresh transfer is not recommended after an agonist trigger as shown by studies like Griesinger et al.[46]

Youssef et al. found no difference between rhCG or rhLH and uhCG for live birth or ongoing pregnancy rates or rates of OHSS. The same study showed that adding LH as a trigger is not recommended for final oocyte maturation.[47]

■ OVARIAN RESPONSE PREDICTION

Various studies have attempted to predict ovarian response with the help of parameters that may influence the outcome. Most noted are age, BMI, basal FSH, AMH, and AFC.

A study by Oliveira et al. attempted to use a simple index that was easy to use in daily practice and combined a small number of variables which together could accentuate the result of each individual variable in predicting ovarian response to stimulation and at the same time compensate for possible individual deficiencies.[1]

$$ORPI = \frac{AMH \times AFC}{Age\ of\ female\ partner}$$

The calculated value of the ovarian response prediction index (ORPI) in the study was not influenced by the protocol choice for the induction of ovulation or the doses of gonadotropin.

The regression analysis demonstrated significant ($p < 0.05$) positive correlations between the ORPI and the total number of oocytes collected ($r = 0.78$), total number of MII oocytes ($r = 0.70$), and the number of follicles ≥10 mm ($r = 0.82$), follicles ≥16 mm ($r = 0.67$) and follicles ≥18 mm ($r = 0.56$) on the hCG administration day with both agonist and antagonist protocol.

Another study by Jiang et al. included age, AMH, AFC, the diagnosis of endometriosis, decreased ovarian reserve, polycystic ovary syndrome, basal follicle-stimulating hormone, and basal luteinizing hormone. They developed a nomogram for calculating the predicted response with above factors **(Fig. 7)**. This study included around 1,944 patients.

The model was verified with 589 patients' data, which was consistent with the actual results, with a coincidence degree of 76.4%, and the consistency index of the model is 0.77.[48]

The follicular output rate (FORT) and follicle to oocyte index (FOI), qualitative markers of ovarian response, may reflect the follicular development dynamic in response to gonadotropins. Whether FOI and FORT may predict ovarian response as well and potential of embryo development is unknown. Morphological changes with the exact time-point of occurrence may be assessed by time-lapse imaging (TLI) and may be a valuable approach to evaluate the correlation between FORT and FOI and the competences of developing embryos. The objective of this study was to investigate if there are any effects of FORT and FOI on embryos morphokinetics.[49]

An increased time to complete morphokinetic events was observed among embryos derived from cycles with low-FORT, followed by those with medium-FORT. Embryos derived from cycles with high-FORT presented

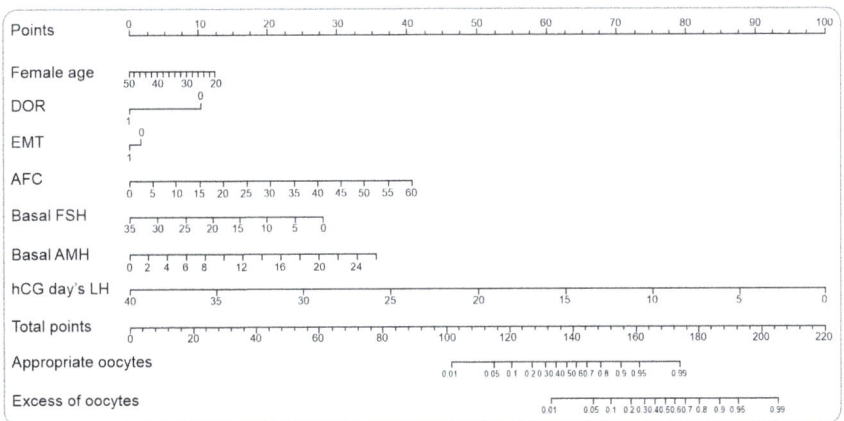

Fig. 7: Nomogram showing predicted response under multiple variables. (AFC: antral follicle count; AMH: anti-Müllerian hormone; EMT: endometriosis; DOR: diminished ovarian reserve; FSH: follicle-stimulating hormone; hCG: human chorionic gonadotropin; LH: luteinizing hormone)

a higher Kid-Score, followed by those from cycles with medium-FORT. Significantly higher rates of blastocyst formation and implantation were observed in embryos derived from cycles with high-FORT, followed by those with medium-FORT.[49]

◼ CONCLUSION

It is a challenge to predict responses and variability between patients. Further research into predictive factors and application of these factors into models that could be easily and consistently reproduced across clinics would be the first step toward evidence-based individualized treatments.

Predictive power will probably be more specific if individual genetic factors could be identified and introduced into prediction models. This identification requires extensive research and trials before it can be applied to general population.

◼ KEY POINTS

- Various factors influence the response to ovarian stimulation, which include patient factors such as age, BMI, ovarian reserve, previous response to stimulation, co-existing health issues like PCO and endometriosis, among many others.
- Certain factors still need research and investigating such as genetic factors, drugs, ideal dosages and the potential to include them to predict ovarian response.
- Type of drug, dose of the drug and adjuvants have not shown to be of any huge influence. More studies are required to evaluate their effects and find the individualized standard that may elicit a response which balances the risk-benefit ratio.
- Ovarian response predictor nomograms are few and difficult to apply in regular practice. Their effectiveness and accuracy in predicting response is an area of further research.

◼ REFERENCES

1. Oliveira JBA, Baruffi RL, Petersen CG, Mauri AL, Nascimento AM, Vagnini L, et al. A new ovarian response prediction index (ORPI): implications for individualised controlled ovarian stimulation. Reprod Biol Endocrinol. 2012;10:94.
2. Liu D, Li L, Sun N, Zhang X, Yin P, Zhang W, et al. Effects of body mass index on IVF outcomes in different age groups. BMC Womens Health. 2023;23:416.
3. Broekmans FJ, Kwee J, Hendriks DJ, Mol BW, Lambalk CB. A systematic review of tests predicting ovarian reserve and IVF outcome. Hum Reprod Update. 2006;12:685-718.
4. Chang MY, Chiang CH, Chiu TH, Hsieh TT, Soong YK. The antral follicle count predicts the outcome of pregnancy in a controlled ovarian hyperstimulation/intrauterine insemination program. J Assist Reprod Genet. 1998;15:12-7.

5. Broer SL, Dolleman M, Opmeer BC, Fauser BC, Mol BW, Broekmans FJ. AMH and AFC as predictors of excessive response in controlled ovarian hyperstimulation: a meta-analysis. Hum Reprod Update. 2011;17:46-54.
6. Muttukrishna S, McGarrigle H, Wakim R, Khadum I, Ranieri DM, Serhal P. Antral follicle count, anti-mullerian hormone and inhibin B: predictors of ovarian response in assisted reproductive technology? BJOG. 2005;112:1384-90.
7. Wiweko B, Afdi QF, Harzif AK, Pratama G, Sumapradja K, Muharam R, et al. Analysis of factors associated with ovarian reserve in a group of poor responders to in vitro fertilization: A cross-sectional study. Int J Reprod Biomed. 2020;18(12):1065-72.
8. Fang T, Su Z, Wang L, Yuan P, Li R, Ouyang N, et al. Predictive value of age-specific FSH levels for IVF-ET outcome in women with normal ovarian function. Reprod Biol Endocrinol. 2015;13:63.
9. Chang Y, Li J, Li X, Liu H, Liang X. Egg quality and pregnancy outcome in young infertile women with diminished ovarian reserve. Med Sci Monit. 2018;24:7279-84.
10. Chuang CC, Chen CD, Chao KH, Chen SU, Ho HN, Yang YS. Age is a better predictor of pregnancy potential than basel follicle-stimulating hormone levels in women undergoing in vitro fertilization. Fertil Steril. 2003;79:63-8.
11. Creus M, Peñarrubia J, Fábregues F, Vidal E, Carmona F, Casamitjana R, et al. Day 3 serum inhibin-B and FSH and age as predictors of assisted reproduction treatment outcome. Hum Reprod. 2000;15:2341-6.
12. Gingold JA, Lee JA, Whitehouse MC, Rodriguez-Purata J, Sandler B, Grunfeld L, et al. Maximum baseline FSH predicts reproductive outcome better than cycle-specific baseline FSH levels: waiting for a "better" month conveys limited retrieval benefits. Reprod Biol Endocrinol. 2015;13:91.
13. Van Loendersloot LL, Van Wely M, Limpens J, Bossuyt PM, Repping S, Van Der Veen F. Predictive factors in in vitro fertilization (IVF): a systematic review and meta-analysis. Hum Reprod Update. 2010;16:577-89.
14. Pastore LM, Christianson MS, Stelling J, Kearns WG, Segars JH. Reproductive ovarian testing and the alphabet soup of diagnoses: DOR, POI, POF, POR, and FOR. J Assist Reprod Genet. 2018;35:17-23.
15. Lin XN, Wei ML, Tong XM, Xu WH, Zhou F, Huang QX, et al. Outcome of in vitro fertilization in endometriosis-associated infertility: a 5-year database cohort study. Chin Med J (Engl). 2012;125(15):2688-93.
16. Kuivasaari P, Hippeläinen M, Anttila M, Heinonen S. Effect of endometriosis on IVF/ICSI outcome: stage III/IV endometriosis worsens cumulative pregnancy and live-born rates. Hum Reprod. 2005;20(11):3130-5.
17. Pellicer A, Oliveira N, Ruiz A, Remohí J, Simón C. Exploring the mechanism(s) of endometriosis-related infertility: an analysis of embryo development and implantation in assisted reproduction. Hum Reprod. 1995;10(Suppl 2):91-7.
18. Bongioanni F, Revelli A, Gennarelli G, Guidetti D, Delle Piane LD, Holte J. Ovarian endometriomas and IVF: a retrospective case-control study. Reprod Biol Endocrinol. 2011;9:81.
19. Ashrafi M, Fakheri T, Kiani K, Sadeghi M, Akhoond MR. Impact of the endometrioma on ovarian response and pregnancy rate in in vitro fertilization cycles. Int J Fertil Steril. 2014;8(1):29-34.
20. Suzuki T, Izumi S, Matsubayashi H, Awaji H, Yoshikata K, Makino T. Impact of ovarian endometrioma on oocytes and pregnancy outcome in in vitro fertilization. Fertil Steril. 2005;83(4):908-13.

21. Esmaeilzadeh S, Ghorbani M, Abdolahzadeh M, Chehrazi M, Jorsaraei SG, Mirabi P. Stages of endometriosis: Does it affect oocyte quality, embryo development and fertilization rate? JBRA Assist Reprod. 2022;26(4):620-6.
22. Zeng C, Lu R, Li X, Kuai Y, Wang S, Xue Q. The presence of ovarian endometrioma adversely affect ovarian reserve and response to stimulation but not oocyte quality or IVF/ICSI outcomes: a retrospective cohort study. J Ovarian Res. 2022;15:116.
23. Fiedler K, Ezcurra D. Predicting and preventing ovarian hyperstimulation syndrome (OHSS): the need for individualized not standardized treatment. Reprod Biol Endocrinol. 2012;10:32.
24. Enskog A, Henriksson M, Unander M, Nilsson L, Brannstrom M. Prospective study of the clinical and laboratory parameters of patients in whom ovarian hyperstimulation syndrome developed during controlled ovarian hyperstimulation for in vitro fertilization. Fertil Steril. 1999;71:808-14.
25. Papanikolaou EG, Pozzobon C, Kolibianakis EM, Camus M, Tournaye H, Fatemi HM, et al. Incidence and prediction of ovarian hyperstimulation syndrome in women undergoing gonadotropin-releasing hormone antagonist in vitro fertilization cycles. Fertil Steril. 2006;85:112-20.
26. Kwee J, Elting ME, Schats R, McDonnell J, Lambalk CB. Ovarian volume and antral follicle count for the prediction of low and hyper responders with in vitro fertilization. Reprod Biol Endocrinol. 2007;5:9-10.
27. Goldsammler M, Merhi Z, Buyuk E. Role of hormonal and inflammatory alterations in obesity-related reproductive dysfunction at the level of the hypothalamic-pituitary-ovarian axis. Reprod Biol Endocrinol. 2018;16:45.
28. Pozza A, Dettore D, Coccia ME. Depression and anxiety in pathways of medically assisted reproduction: the role of infertility stress dimensions. Clin Pract Epidemiol Ment Health. 2019;15:101-9.
29. Haggarty P, McCallum H, McBain H, Andrews K, Duthie S, McNeill G, et al. Effect of B vitamins and genetics on success of in-vitro fertilisation: prospective cohort study. Lancet. 2006;367(9521):1513-9.
30. Su MT, Lee IW, Chen YC, Kuo PL. Association of progesterone receptor polymorphism with idiopathic recurrent pregnancy loss in Taiwanese Han population. J Assist Reprod Genet. 2011;28(3):239-43.
31. Patounakis G, Bergh E, Forman EJ, Tao X, Lonczak A, Franasiak JM, et al. Multiple thrombophilic single nucleotide polymorphisms lack a significant effect on outcomes in fresh IVF cycles: an analysis of 1717 patients. J Assist Reprod Genet. 2016;33(1):67-73.
32. Kang HJ, Feng Z, Sun Y, Atwal G, Murphy ME, Rebbeck TR, et al. Single-nucleotide polymorphisms in the p53 pathway regulate fertility in humans. Proc Natl Acad Sci USA. 2009;106(24):9761-6.
33. Ganesh V, Venkatesan V, Koshy T, Reddy SN, Muthumuthiah S, Paul SFD. Association of estrogen, progesterone and follicle stimulating hormone receptor polymorphisms with in vitro fertilization outcomes. Syst Biol Reprod Med. 2018;64(4):260-5.
34. Lambalk CB, Banga FR, Huirne JA, Toftager M, Pinborg A, Homburg R, et al. GnRH antagonist versus long agonist protocols in IVF: a systematic review and meta-analysis accounting for patient type. Hum Reprod Update. 2017;23(5):560-79.

35. Fauser BCJM, Diedrich K, Devroey P, on behalf of the Evian Annual Reproduction (EVAR) Workshop Group 2007. Predictors of ovarian response: progress towards individualized treatment in ovulation induction and ovarian stimulation. Hum Reprod Update. 2008;14(1):1-14.
36. Popovic-Todorovic B, Loft A, Lindhard A, Bangsboll S, Andersson AM, Andersen AN. A prospective study of predictive factors of ovarian response in 'standard' IVF/ICSI patients treated with recombinant FSH. A suggestion for a recombinant FSH dosage normogram. Hum Reprod. 2003;18(4):781-7.
37. van Wely M, Kwan I, Burt AL, Thomas J, Vail A, Van der Veen F, et al. Recombinant versus urinary gonadotrophin for ovarian stimulation in assisted reproductive technology cycles. Cochrane Database Syst Rev. 2011;2011(2):CD005354.
38. Ben-Meir A, Burstein E, Borrego-Alvarez A, Chong J, Wong E, Yavorska T, et al. Coenzyme Q10 restores oocyte mitochondrial function and fertility during reproductive aging. Aging Cell. 2015;14:887-95.
39. Norman RJ, Alvino H, Hull LM, Mol BW, Hart RJ, Kelly TL, et al. Human growth hormone for poor responders: a randomized placebo-controlled trial provides no evidence for improved live birth rate. Reprod Biomed Online. 2019;38:908-15.
40. Polyzos NP, Martinez F, Blockeel C, Gosalvez A, De la Fuente L, Pinborg A, et al. O-066 Transdermal testosterone prior to ovarian stimulation for in vitro fertilization in women with poor ovarian response. A multicenter multinational double-blind placebo-controlled randomized trial (The T-TRANSPORT). Hum Reprod. 2023;38(Supplement_1):dead093.080.
41. Andersen CY. Effect of FSH and its different isoforms on maturation of oocytes from pre-ovulatory follicles. Reprod Biomed Online. 2002;5:232-9.
42. Karakji EG, Tsang BK. Regulation of rat granulosa cell plasminogen activator system: influence of interleukin-1 beta and ovarian follicular development. Biol Reprod. 1995;53:1302-10.
43. Richards JS, Hernandez-Gonzalez I, Gonzalez-Robayna I, Teuling E, Lo Y, Boerboom D, et al. Regulated expression of ADAMTS family members in follicles and cumulus oocyte complexes: evidence for specific and redundant patterns during ovulation. Biol Reprod. 2005;72:1241-55.
44. Eppig JJ. FSH stimulates hyaluronic acid synthesis by oocyte–cumulus cell complexes from mouse preovulatory follicles. Nature. 1979;281:483-4.
45. Shapiro BS, Andersen CY. Major drawbacks and additional benefits of agonist trigger-not ovarian hyperstimulation syndrome related. Fertil Steril. 2015;103:874-8.
46. Griesinger G, Diedrich K, Devroey P, Kolibianakis E. GnRH agonist for triggering final oocyte maturation in the GnRH antagonist ovarian hyperstimulation protocol: a systematic review and meta-analysis. Hum Reprod Update. 2006;12:159-68.
47. Youssef MA, Abou-Setta AM, Lam WS. Recombinant versus urinary human chorionic gonadotropin for final oocyte maturation triggering in IVF and ICSI cycles. Cochrane Database Syst Rev. 2011;(4):CD003719.
48. Jiang W, Zheng B, Liao X, Chen X, Zhu S, Li R, et al. Analysis of relative factors and prediction model for optimal ovarian response with gonadotropin-releasing hormone antagonist protocol. Front Endocrinol (Lausanne). 2022;13:1030201.
49. de Almeida Ferreira Braga DP, Setti AS, Guilherme P, Iaconelli A Jr, Borges E Jr. Understanding the implications of follicular output rate (FORT) and follicle to oocyte index (FOI) on embryo morphokinetics. Fertil Steril. 2023;120(4):E235.

Section 8

Ovarian Stimulation Protocols for IUI Cycle

- ❏ **Ovarian Stimulation Protocols in Intrauterine Insemination**
  Sunita Tandulwadkar, Bushra Khan, Rashmika Gandhi
- ❏ **Ovarian Stimulation Protocols for Normoresponders**
  Laurel Stadtmauer, Xuaochong Liu, Jayapriya Jayakumaran
- ❏ **Ovarian Stimulation Protocols for Hyper-responders**
  Seema Pandey, Sini Venugopal
- ❏ **Ovarian Stimulation Protocols for Poor Responders**
  Gautam Khastgir, Utpala Sen
- ❏ **Stimulation Protocols for Fertility Preservation**
  Kamal Ojha, Biswanath Ghosh Dastidar

Chapter 16: Ovarian Stimulation Protocols in Intrauterine Insemination

Sunita Tandulwadkar, Bushra Khan, Rashmika Gandhi

■ INTRODUCTION

Infertility has impacted millions worldwide, National Health Service (NHS) UK in 2021 estimated that one in every couple is suffering from inability or difficulty in conceiving. Infertility is commonly defined as the inability of a couple to conceive after 12 months of regular, unprotected intercourse in women <35 years of age, and after 6 months in women 35 years and older.[1]

■ OVARIAN STIMULATION AND INTRAUTERINE INSEMINATION

Intrauterine insemination (IUI) stands as one of the most performed procedures in assisted reproductive technology for treating infertility. Controlled ovarian hyperstimulation (COH) serves as a crucial initial step in the process of IUI.

Intrauterine insemination can be conducted in either the natural cycle or in conjunction with COH. The objective of IUI is to enhance pregnancy rates by increasing the number of dominant follicles per cycle, achieved through elevating serum follicle-stimulating hormone (FSH) levels, and increasing the number of sperms reaching the fallopian tubes and successfully resulting in higher fertilization. Agents that boost FSH serum levels to stimulate ovary encompass oral ovulogens such as clomiphene citrate (CC), letrozole, and exogenous gonadotropins. Historically, these above-mentioned drugs were developed and utilized to induce follicular growth and ovulation in anovulatory women or in patients with irregular cycles. However, more recently like from the mid-90s evidence developed that ovulation induction is recommended in ovulatory patients as well, especially in unexplained infertility. Cochrane library in 2021 republished their review on drugs used for ovulation induction in IUI since there was no clear consensus from innumerable research conducted on the above topic.[2] The review considered various combinations with clomiphene, letrozole, and gonadotropins alone and in combination, they also considered multifollicular growth versus monofollicular growth in IUI cycles, a fair consideration was emphasized in chances of multiple gestation when different protocols were used and main focus was laid on the fact that cycles were cancelled when more than three follicles developed. Although in vitro fertilization (IVF) per-cycle pregnancy rate is higher than in IUI, however, it is also the most expensive and invasive treatment.[3] A randomized controlled trial (RCT) conducted by Bensdorp and colleagues showed that live birth rates (LBRs) between three cycles of IVF with single embryo transfer and six cycles of IUI with ovarian stimulation were similar, and, therefore, IUI-OS should be advised as the treatment of first choice before IVF.[4]

■ DEVELOPMENT OF OVARIAN STIMULATING AGENTS

In early 20th century, scientists noticed that patients with pituitary lesions had atrophy of gonads, which resulted in discovery of pituitary gonadotropins, previously known as Prolan A and Prolan B by Fevold et al. in 1931.[5] Thereafter, FSH and luteinizing hormone (LH) were both isolated and purified initially from animal serum and later from urine of postmenopausal women which led to the discovery of human menopausal gonadotropin (hMG). Second important discovery was when the first estrogen antagonist tested in cancer patients also induced ovulation.

Different types of ovulation inducing drugs:
- *Oral:*
    - Clomiphene citrate
    - Letrozole
    - Anastrozole
    - Tamoxifen
- *Injectable:*
    - HP-hMG (highly purified human menopausal gonadotropin)
    - RecFSH (recombinant FSH)

■ CLOMIPHENE CITRATE

Clomiphene citrate belongs to selective estrogen receptor modulators (SERMs) group. They interact with estrogen receptors (ERs) within a target organ. However, CC structurally is a nonsteroidal derivative of triphenylchloroethylene. CC is very similar to estrogen hence it attaches to the ERs easily. Commercially, CC is available as a racemic mixture comprising two isomers: 38% zuclomiphene and 62% enclomiphene.[6]

Mechanism of Action

Clomiphene citrate binds to ERs in the hypothalamus, blocking the estrogen feedback loop and leading to increased levels of GnRH (gonadotropin-releasing hormone), which in turn stimulates pituitary gonadotropin secretion and promotes follicular development in the ovaries. CC also exerts direct effects on both the pituitary gland and the ovaries. However, its antiestrogenic effects at the level of the endometrium or cervix can occasionally have adverse effects on fertility in a minority of individuals.[7]

Indications for using CC in IUI patients:
- Anovulatory polycystic ovary syndrome (PCOS)
- Unexplained infertility
- Mild male factor for superovulation

Treatment Protocols

Standard Protocol

A baseline transvaginal ultrasound (TVS) should be performed between day 1 and 3 of the menstrual cycle to confirm the absence of any large follicles or cysts from the previous cycle before initiating treatment. CC therapy is typically initiated between day 2 and 5 of the cycle, starting on the day of spontaneous or induced bleeding, and administered for a total of 5 days. Initiating clomiphene earlier may stimulate the maturation of multiple follicles. The initial dose is usually 50 mg daily for 5 days. Studies have shown that the pregnancy rate remains consistent whether starting at 50 mg or 100 mg per day.[8] Side effects begin at the 50 mg dose, with potentially more serious reactions at 100 mg. Approximately, 50% of patients conceive with the 50 mg dose, and an additional 20% conceive with 100 mg.[9]

Ultrasound monitoring begins from day 9 of the menstrual cycle to track follicular growth and endometrial thickness. This monitoring serves to assess treatment progress and can help differentiate between CC failure (failure to conceive despite successful ovulation) and clomiphene resistance (failure to induce ovulation). If ovulation is not achieved, the dosage is increased incrementally by 50 mg up to a maximum of 150 mg daily for 5 days, although the FDA recommends a maximum daily dose of 100 mg. The highest dosage is typically maintained for 3-4 months before considering the patient unresponsive to CC. Most experts advise against exceeding 150 mg per day due to concerns about efficacy and safety.[7]

Mature follicle is expected to occur 5-10 days after the last day of therapy. When dominant follicle develops, hCG 5,000-10,000 IUI or recombinant hCG 250 μg is given to induce final follicular maturation and to ensure that ovulation is timed optimally with respect to follicular growth and IUI.

Stair-step Protocol

Traditionally stair-step protocol is used in patients where only 5 days of CC has not worked and instead of cancelling the cycle, one can step up the CC dose and monitor after another 5 days. Studies revealed similar LBR as standard CC protocol. Stair-step protocol may be available as an alternative for PCOS patients.

Side Effects of Clomiphene Citrate

- Antiestrogenic effects on cervical mucus and endometrial lining can affect the quality of cervical mucus, making it less favorable for sperm transport, reducing its implantation potential.
- Other causes of infertility also associated with ovulatory dysfunction such as tubal factors, severe endometriosis, and male factor infertility.
- *Lack of persistence:* Successful conception with CC often requires consistent timing of intercourse or IUI around ovulation. Lack of persistence in timing attempts to conceive during the fertile window can contribute to lower pregnancy rates despite ovulation induction.[10]

These factors highlight the complexity of achieving pregnancy with CC and underscore the importance of comprehensive evaluation and management tailored to individual patient needs in infertility treatment.

Side effects:
- Vasomotor flushes—10%
- Abdominal distention, bloating, soreness, pain—5.5%
- Breast discomfort—2%
- Nausea, vomiting—2.2%
- Headache—1.3%
- Visual symptoms 1.5%—CC should be promptly discontinued
- Dryness or loss of hair—0.3%
- Ovarian enlargement—5%; delay in next cycle treatment
- Increased risk of ectopic pregnancy
- Multiple pregnancy 5–8%
- Ovarian hyperstimulation syndrome (OHSS)

■ TAMOXIFEN

Tamoxifen is another SERM and has similar actions like CC without its side effects on cervical mucus and endometrium. It is administered at a dosage of 40 mg daily for 5 days starting between day 2 and 5.

■ LETROZOLE

Letrozole, as an aromatase inhibitor, functions similarly to CC in initiating gonadotropin release but through a different mechanism. Unlike CC, which blocks ERs to create an apparent estrogen-deficient state in the pituitary, letrozole works by reducing blood estrogen levels through inhibition of aromatase, the enzyme responsible for converting androgens to estrogens. This reduction in estrogen levels leads to a more pronounced initial release of FSH compared to CC.[11]

Moreover, letrozole offers additional benefits. Despite inducing an estrogen-deficient environment, it does not adversely affect the endometrium or cervical mucus due to its short half-life (approximately 45 hours). In contrast, CC's ER-blocking action persists for about 2 weeks, resulting in an estrogen-deficient state despite adequate estrogen levels in the bloodstream. This difference can impact endometrial receptivity and cervical mucus quality, potentially affecting embryo implantation.

Furthermore, letrozole may enhance follicular sensitivity to FSH by increasing the expression of FSH receptor genes peripherally. This mechanism contributes to improved follicular growth and development, which are crucial for successful ovulation and subsequent embryo implantation.

Overall, compared to CC, letrozole offers superior outcomes in terms of follicular growth, endometrial development, and potentially higher pregnancy rates. These advantages make letrozole a preferred choice for ovulation induction in certain patient populations, particularly those where optimizing endometrial conditions is critical for achieving pregnancy.[11]

Advantages

- *Monofollicular ovulation:* Aromatase inhibitors promote the development of a single dominant follicle, reducing the likelihood of multiple pregnancies compared to agents like gonadotropins. This also lowers the risk of severe OHSS.
- *No antiestrogenic effects on endometrium or cervix:* Unlike CC, aromatase inhibitors do not exert antiestrogenic effects on the endometrium or cervical mucus, potentially improving endometrial receptivity for implantation.
- *High safety profile:* Aromatase inhibitors have a short half-life and are associated with fewer adverse effects compared to other ovulation induction agents. This makes them generally well-tolerated by patients.
- *Higher pregnancy rates:* Studies have shown that aromatase inhibitors may offer higher pregnancy rates compared to CC, particularly in certain patient populations such as those with PCOS.

Treatment Protocol

Standard Protocol

The commonly practiced protocol for letrozole involves a daily dosage of 5 mg taken once daily for 5 consecutive days, typically administered from day 3 to 7 of the menstrual cycle. This regimen was initially adapted from a similar approach used with CC. Cochrane 2022[10] analysis showed that letrozole appears to improve LBRs in infertile women when used in comparison with CC. There is no difference in miscarriage rates and multiple pregnancy rates. Many studies have stated that letrozole and CC have similar pregnancy rates whereas there have been few which say that letrozole has better pregnancy rates.[11,12]

Extended Protocol

A longer administration protocol, where letrozole is taken from day 1 to 10 of the cycle at a lower dose of 2.5 mg daily, has been proposed. Comparative studies have shown that this extended 10-day regimen leads to significantly greater numbers of mature follicles and higher pregnancy rates compared to the standard 5-day protocol. Specifically, research indicates an average of 6.7 follicles with the 10-day regimen versus 3.9 follicles with the 5-day regimen. Pregnancy rates also show improvement, with 17.4% achieved with the 10-day protocol compared to 12.4% with the 5-day regimen.[13]

The potential mechanism behind these findings suggests that the longer duration of letrozole treatment allows for more follicular growth and maturation, thereby enhancing the chances of successful ovulation and subsequent pregnancy. This extended protocol may be particularly beneficial for patients who have not responded optimally to the standard 5-day regimen or who require a more robust follicular response.[14]

In clinical practice, the choice between the 5-day and 10-day letrozole protocols should consider individual patient factors, treatment goals, and the need for balancing efficacy with safety.

Aromatase Inhibitors Combined with Gonadotropins in Ovarian Stimulation for IUI

In a sequential regime, letrozole 2.5 mg was given from cycle days 3 to 7 and FSH was added on cycle day 6 and day 8 and ovulation triggered with hCG. The FSH dose required was 50% lower than with standard regimens. In addition, the pregnancy rate with a combination of aromatase inhibitor and FSH was equivalent to FSH alone, and almost twice the level seen with CC and FSH treatment.[15]

Another study[16] compared two groups, a combination of letrozole and FSH or FSH only. The number of growing follicles, the E2 level, and the endometrial thickness were lower in the letrozole group. The pregnancy rates were similar between the two groups, but the multiple pregnancy rate was lower in the combination group ($p < 0.05$).

Gómez et al.[17] randomized patients to undergo treatment with CC/FSH or letrozole/rFSH. Although there was a significantly lower peak serum E level in letrozole/rFSH compared with CC/rFSH (914 ± 187 vs. 1,207 ± 309 pg/mL, respectively; $p < 0.007$), there were no differences in the number of mature (>16 mm) preovulatory follicles. A significantly higher endometrial thickness was observed in the letrozole/FSH group (9.5 ± 1.5 mm vs. 7.3 ± 1.1 mm; $p = 0001$). The clinical pregnancy rates were similar between two groups (23.8% vs. 20%, respectively).

The risk for multiple pregnancy is about 3-7% overall, and there is no robust evidence proving any teratogenic effects of letrozole as compared with CC.

■ ANASTROZOLE

Many studies have suggested similar mechanism of action and clinical pregnancy rates as letrozole.[18]

■ GONADOTROPINS

Gonadotropins were introduced a century ago, a lot of advancement and discovery has been made in last 25 years. Currently, we have the highly purified and rFSH and hMG. Three major gonadotropins are similar in structure as in they are all glycoprotein with similar alpha chain and variable beta chains. Various milestones are described in the **Figure 1**.

Types of Gonadotropins (Table 1)

- *Urinary-derived gonadotropins (uFSH):* These include hMGs, which contain both FSH and LH, and purified FSH (uFSH), extracted from the urine of postmenopausal women.
- *Highly purified human menopausal gonadotropins (HP-hMG):* These are highly purified forms of hMG, with a higher FSH to LH ratio compared to traditional hMG.
- *Highly purified FSH*
- *Recombinant gonadotropins (rFSH):* Produced through recombinant DNA technology, these include recombinant FSH (rFSH) and recombinant LH (rLH).

In Cochrane Database Systematic Review,[19] in which 43 trials involving 3,957 women were included, author concluded that gonadotropins might be more effective in follicular growth during ovarian stimulation in IUI cycles. This review also stated that low dose of gonadotropins was safer especially in PCOS patients, whereas pregnancy rates were not different in low-dose or high-dose gonadotropin cycles.

Comparative Effectiveness of Gonadotropins

Recent studies have provided insights into the comparative effectiveness of various combinations.[2]
- *Gonadotropins versus antiestrogens (13 studies):* For live birth, the results of five studies were pooled and showed improvement in the cumulative LBR for gonadotropins compared to antiestrogens [odds ratio (OR) 1.37, 95% confidence interval (CI) 1.05-1.79; $I^2 = 30\%$]. Although gonadotropins lead to a higher multiple pregnancy rate compared with antiestrogens (OR 1.58, 95% CI 0.60-4.17; $I^2 = 58\%$; 7 studies, 2,139 participants).

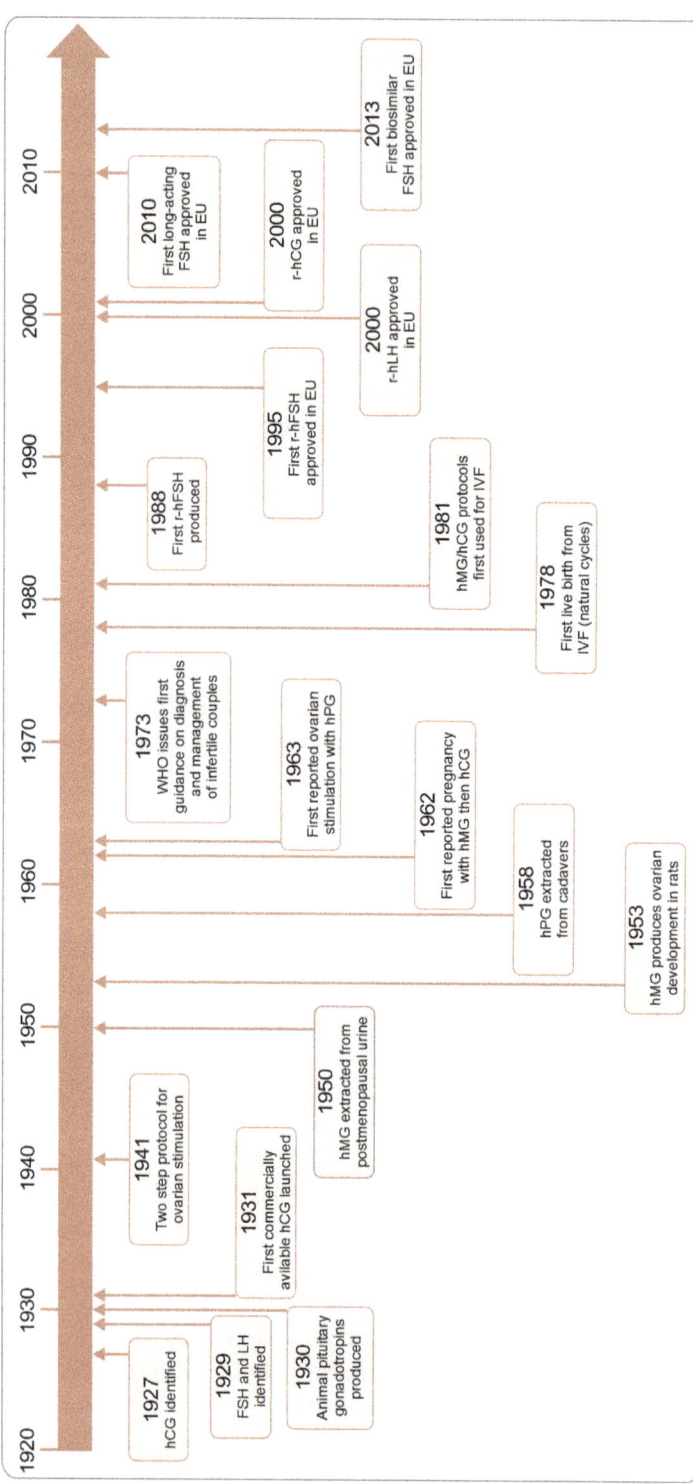

Fig. 1: Milestones in the development of gonadotropin preparations. (FSH: follicle-stimulating hormone; hCG: human chorionic gonadotropin; hMG: human menopausal gonadotropin; IVF: in vitro fertilization; LH: luteinizing hormone)
Source: Leão Rde B, Esteves SC. Gonadotropin therapy in assisted reproduction: an evolutionary perspective from biologics to biotech. Clinics (Sao Paulo). 2014;69(4):279-93.

TABLE 1: Differences between gonadotropin formulations.

	Purity (gonadotropin content)	Mean specific activity (IU/mg protein)	LH activity (IU/vial)	Injected protein per 75 IU (µg)
hMG	<5%	~100	75	~750
HP-hMG	<70%	2,000–2,500	75	~33
Rec-hFSH				
Follitropin beta	>99%	7,000–10,000	0	8.1
Follitropin alpha	>99%	13,645	0	6.1
Lutropin alpha (rec-hLH)	>99%	22,000	75	3.7

(FSH: follicle-stimulating hormone; hMG: human menopausal gonadotropin; LH: luteinizing hormone)
Source: Leão Rde B, Esteves SC. Gonadotropin therapy in assisted reproduction: An evolutionary perspective from biologics to biotech. Clinics (Sao Paulo). 2014;69(4):279-93.

- *Aromatase inhibitors versus antiestrogens (8 studies):* Both the drugs have shown similar pregnancy rates.
- *Gonadotropins with GnRH (gonadotropin-releasing hormone) agonist versus gonadotropins alone (4 studies):* Two studies revealed that we are uncertain whether gonadotropins with GnRH agonist lead to a higher multiple pregnancy rate compared to gonadotropins alone (OR 2.53, 95% CI 0.82–7.86; I^2 = 0; 2 studies, 264 participants).
- *Gonadotropins with GnRH antagonist versus gonadotropins alone (14 studies):* Three studies reported LBR per couple, but it is uncertain whether gonadotropins with GnRH antagonist improve LBR compared to gonadotropins (OR 1.5, 95% CI 0.52–4.39; I^2 = 81%; 3 studies, 419 participants).
- *Gonadotropins with antiestrogens versus gonadotropins alone (2 studies):* Neither of the studies reported data for LBR. It is uncertain whether gonadotropins combined with antiestrogens lead to a higher multiple pregnancy rate compared with gonadotropins alone, based on one study (OR 3.03, 95% CI 0.12–75.1; 1 study, 230 participants; low-certainty evidence).
- *Aromatase inhibitors versus gonadotropins (6 studies):* Two studies revealed that aromatase inhibitors may decrease LBR compared with gonadotropins (OR 0.49, 95% CI 0.34–0.71; I^2 = 0%; 2 studies, 651 participants; low-certainty evidence).

Rationale for Gonadotropin Use

Gonadotropins are used to directly stimulate the ovaries, promoting the development of multiple follicles. This increases the chances of achieving a successful pregnancy in IUI cycles. The goal is to produce one or two dominant follicles while minimizing the risk of multiple pregnancies and OHSS.

There are two primary protocols for ovulation induction: the step-up and step-down protocols. Treatment begins shortly after spontaneous or progesterone-induced bleeding. A baseline vaginal ultrasound scan should be performed to check for ovarian cysts and measure endometrial thickness.

- *Step-up protocol:* After the baseline transvaginal sonography on day 2 of menstrual cycle, gonadotropin at a dose of 37.5–75 U is started depending upon the patients weight for 5 days and it is then stepped up by another 37.5 U. Every 5 days dose can be increased till the time sufficient response is achieved. The gonadotropin dose should not increase above 225 IU/day. A dominant follicle greater than 10 mm is considered an adequate response, and the treatment is continued at the same dose until the day of hCG injection to trigger ovulation.
- *Step-down protocol:* The step-down protocol simulates a natural menstrual cycle. The goal is to quickly achieve an FSH threshold to stimulate a dominant follicle. It begins with 150 IU/day from day 2 of menses until a dominant follicle is observed (>10 mm). The gonadotropin dose is then reduced to 112.5 IU/day, and after 3 days, it is further reduced to 75 IU/day, continuing until the follicle reaches a mature size. If a dominant follicle is not seen after 3–5 days of treatment, the dose is increased by 37.5 IU/day. This protocol typically requires a shorter treatment period but demands strict monitoring.
- *Combination protocols:* Gonadotropins can be used in combination with other agents such as clomiphene or letrozole to enhance follicular development while potentially reducing the amount of gonadotropin required. In such protocols, clomiphene or letrozole is typically administered from cycle days 3–7, followed by gonadotropin injections starting on day 7–9 until the desired follicular response is achieved.[20]

Individualization of Protocol

Foremost point is that indication of ovulation induction should be kept in mind along with duration of infertility, age of female partner, BMI, and serum anti-Mullerian hormone (AMH) levels.

Monitoring

The standard method of monitoring is through vaginal ultrasound scanning (TVS), which is safe, accurate, and effective for evaluating follicular development to be done on day 2 followed by day 7–8 further till the time of trigger by alternate days.

Timing of Intrauterine Insemination

Ovulation is triggered when at least one follicle or more, measuring ≥18–20 mm, is seen on a transvaginal scan, using either 250 µg of r-hCG or 10,000 IU of urinary hCG. IUI is performed 36–40 hours later and this is done while keeping in mind that the oocyte remains fertilizable for a brief period of time (12–16) hours after ovulation.[21]

Luteal Phase Support

A meta-analysis stated that progesterone luteal phase support improved the chance of a clinical pregnancy after a single OS-IUI cycle in the gonadotropins subgroup [RR 1.56, 95% CI (1.06, 2.31); I^2 = 0%; 6 RCTs, 965 participants; moderate-quality evidence], but not in the gonadotropins + CC [RR 1.39, 95% CI (0.12, 16.33); I^2 = 0%; 2 RCTs, 319 participants].[22]

When to Cancel the Cycle?

A cycle is typically cancelled if more than three follicles have reached a mature size (>16 mm) or if more than four follicles are greater than 12 mm. In such cases, the couple is advised to avoid sexual intercourse. Alternatively, excess follicles can be aspirated, or the cycle can be converted to in vitro fertilization (IVF).

Complications and Side Effects

- Multiple pregnancies
- *Ovarian hyperstimulation syndrome (OHSS):* Usually mild to moderate in IUI cycles

Pregnancy Rates

Pregnancy rates depend on various factors. With gonadotropin stimulation, the pregnancy rate per cycle ranges from 4 to 40%, with a cumulative pregnancy rate of 30–60% in patients under 40 years old after approximately three cycles of IUI. In women under 40, superovulation with gonadotropin and IUI results in a pregnancy rate per cycle of 12.6%, with 11% twin pregnancies and 1.1% triplet pregnancies. For women over 40, the pregnancy rate per cycle is 7.4%, with 4.9% twin pregnancies and 0.7% triplet pregnancies. The number of motile sperm for insemination is also crucial, with the generally accepted cutoff being 1 million motile sperm in the insemination sample.[23]

How Many Cycles Should be done?

In the context of assisted reproductive technologies, we recommend only three cycles of superovulation and IUI. Considerations include cost-effectiveness and the psychological burden of repeated failures to achieve pregnancy.

Predictive Factors for Successful IUI

- Evidence suggests prewash semen sample of about >5 million and postwash at least 1 million.
- Advanced maternal and paternal age have negative impact on IUI results.[24]
- High DNA fragmentation is not always the cause of fail IUI.
- High BMI can also result in failed cycles.

■ CONCLUSION

Ovulation induction is a cornerstone of fertility treatment, offering various protocols and medications to optimize outcomes for patients undergoing IUI. Overall, the choice of ovulation induction agent and protocol should be individualized based on the patient's specific clinical scenario, underlying conditions, and response to previous treatments. Advancements in understanding the pharmacodynamics and optimizing the use of these agents continue to improve outcomes, offering hope to many couples struggling with infertility.

■ KEY POINTS

- Clomiphene citrate has been a long-standing first-line treatment due to its ease of use and favorable cost profile. However, its potential antiestrogenic effects on the endometrium and cervical mucus can sometimes limit its efficacy.
- Letrozole, an aromatase inhibitor, has emerged as an effective alternative, particularly for patients with PCOS. It offers a favorable side effect profile and higher LBRs compared to clomiphene, making it a valuable tool in the fertility specialist's arsenal.
- Gonadotropins provide a more direct stimulation of the ovaries, resulting in higher pregnancy rates, albeit with an increased risk of multiple pregnancies OHSS. Careful monitoring and individualized dosing protocols, such as the step-up and step-down approaches, are essential to mitigate these risks.
- The introduction of GnRH antagonists has further refined ovulation induction protocols. Their use can enhance the number of mature follicles and improve pregnancy rates, as evidenced by recent studies. However, the associated risk of multiple gestations necessitates careful consideration and patient counseling.

■ REFERENCES

1. Practice Committee of the American Society for Reproductive Medicine. Definitions of infertility and recurrent pregnancy loss: A committee opinion. Fertil Steril 2020;113(3):533-5.

2. Cantineau AEP, Rutten AGH, Cohlen BJ. Agents for ovarian stimulation for intrauterine insemination (IUI) in ovulatory women with infertility. Cochrane Database Syst Rev. 2021;(11):CD005356.
3. Tjon-Kon-Fat RI, Bensdorp AJ, Bossuyt PM, Koks C, Oosterhuis GJ, Hoek A, et al. Is IVF - served two different ways - more cost-effective than IUI with controlled ovarian hyperstimulation? Hum Reprod. 2015;30(10):2331-9.
4. Bensdorp AJ, Tjon-Kon-Fat RI, Bossuyt PM, Koks CA, Oosterhuis GJ, Hoek A, et al. Prevention of multiple pregnancies in couples with unexplained or mild male subfertility: randomised controlled trial of in vitro fertilisation with single embryo transfer or in vitro fertilisation in modified natural cycle compared with intrauterine insemination with controlled ovarian hyperstimulation. BMJ. 2015;9(350):g7771.
5. Fevold SL, Hisaw FL, Leonard SL. The gonad-stimulating and the luteinizing hormones of the anterior lobe of the hypophysis. Am J Physiol. 1931;97:291-301.
6. Mbi Feh MK, Patel P, Wadhwa R. (2024). Clomiphene. [online] Available from https://www.ncbi.nlm.nih.gov/books/NBK559292/. [Last accessed August, 2024]
7. Brown J, Farquhar C. Clomiphene and other antioestrogens for ovulation induction in polycystic ovarian syndrome. Cochrane Database Syst Rev. 2016;(12):CD002249.
8. Speroff L, Fritz MA. Clinical Gynecologic Endocrinology and Infertility, 7th edition. Philadelphia: Lippincot Williams Wilkins; 2005.
9. Osmanlıoğlu Ş, Şükür YE, Tokgöz VY, Özmen B, Sönmezer M, Berker B, et al. Intrauterine insemination with ovarian stimulation is a successful step prior to assisted reproductive technology for couples with unexplained infertility. J Obstet Gynaecol. 2022;42(3):472-7.
10. Teede HJ, Tay CT, Laven JJE, Dokras A, Moran LJ, Piltonen TT, et al.; International PCOS Network. Recommendations from the 2023 international evidence-based guideline for the assessment and management of polycystic ovary syndrome. Eur J Endocrinol. 2023;189(2):G43-G64.
11. Franik S, Le Q-K, Kremer JAM, Kiesel L, Farquhar C. Aromatase inhibitors (letrozole) for ovulation induction in infertile women with polycystic ovary syndrome. Cochrane Database Syst Rev. 2022;(9):CD010287.
12. Peng G, Yan Z, Liu Y, Li J, Ma J, Tong N, et al. The effects of first-line pharmacological treatments for reproductive outcomes in infertile women with PCOS: A systematic review and network meta-analysis. Reprod Biol Endocrinol. 2023;21(1):24.
13. Legro RS, Brzyski RG, Diamond MP, Coutifaris C, Schlaff WD, Casson P, et al.; NICHD Reproductive Medicine Network. Letrozole versus clomiphene for infertility in the polycystic ovary syndrome. N Engl J Med. 2014;371(2):119-29.
14. Badawy A, Mosbah A, Tharwat A, Eid M. Extended letrozole therapy for ovulation induction in clomiphene-resistant women with polycystic ovary syndrome: a novel protocol. Fertil Steril. 2009;92:236-9.
15. Pavone ME, Bulun SE. Clinical review: The use of aromatase inhibitors for ovulation induction and superovulation. J Clin Endocrinol Metab. 2013;98(5):1838-44.
16. Nuojua-Huttunen S, Tomas C, Bloigu R, Tuomivaara L, Martikainen H. Intrauterine insemination treatment in subfertility: An analysis of factors affecting outcome. Hum Reprod. 1999;14(3):698-703.

17. Gómez-Palomares JL, Juliá B, Acevedo-Martín B, Martínez-Burgos M, Hernández ER, Ricciarelli E. Timing ovulation for intrauterine insemination with a GnRH antagonist. Hum Reprod. 2005;20(2):368-72.
18. van Wely M, Kwan I, Burt AL, Thomas J, Vail A, Van der Veen F, et al. Recombinant versus urinary gonadotrophin for ovarian stimulation in assisted reproductive technology cycles. Cochrane Database Syst Rev. 2011;(2):CD005354.
19. Weiss NS, Kostova E, Nahuis M, Mol BJ, van der Veen F, van Wely M. Gonadotrophins for ovulation induction in women with polycystic ovary syndrome. Cochrane Database Syst Rev. 2019;(1):CD010290.
20. Cabry-Goubet R, Scheffler F, Belhadri-Mansouri N, Belloc S, Lourdel E, Devaux A, et al. Effect of Gonadotropin Types and Indications on Homologous Intrauterine Insemination Success: A Study from 1251 Cycles and a Review of the Literature. Biomed Res Int. 2017;2017:3512784.
21. Firouz M, Noori N, Ghasemi M, Dashipour A, Keikha N. Comparing the Effectiveness of Doing Intra-uterine Insemination 36 and 42 Hours After Human Chorionic Gonadotropin (HCG) Injection on Pregnancy Rate: A Randomized Clinical Trial. J Family Reprod Health. 2020;14(3):173-9.
22. Casarramona G, Lalmahomed T, Lemmen CHC, Eijkemans MJC, Broekmans FJM, Cantineau AEP, et al. The efficacy and safety of luteal phase support with progesterone following ovarian stimulation and intrauterine insemination: A systematic review and meta-analysis. Front Endocrinol. 2022;13:960393.
23. Cicek OS, Demir M. The impact of gonadotropin type on controlled ovarian stimulation and intrauterine insemination cycle outcomes. J Hum Reprod Sci. 2022;15:51-7.
24. Starosta A, Gordon CE, Hornstein MD. Predictive factors for intrauterine insemination outcomes: A review. Fertil Res Pract. 2020;6(1):23.

Chapter 17
Ovarian Stimulation Protocols for Normoresponders

Laurel Stadtmauer, Xuaochong Liu, Jayapriya Jayakumaran

■ INTRODUCTION

A typical 28-day menstrual cycle begins with a rise in follicle-stimulating hormone (FSH) levels followed by a decrease as estrogen from the developing follicle provides negative feedback. Luteinizing hormone (LH) slowly increases over the follicular phase, but then spikes at midcycle, resulting in maturation of the oocyte and ovulation. Progesterone rises on the day of the LH surge and is produced by the corpus luteum throughout the luteal phase. Progesterone is essential for implantation. If implantation does not occur, both estrogen and progesterone levels drop with the demise of the corpus luteum. This causes the subsequent rise of FSH that begins the next menstrual cycle.[1]

Many clinics use some method to prospectively identify the type of ovarian response to stimulation. These include ovarian reserve biochemical testing mainly anti-Müllerian hormone (AMH), antral follicle count (AFC), and age. AMH and AFC are best in predicting the number of oocytes retrieved and poor or hyper-responders[2-4] **(Fig. 1)**.

The goal of controlled ovarian stimulation (COS) is to mimic natural physiology with a high initial FSH dose and often various step-down regimens. Women then can be characterized into normal responders, hyper-responders, and low responders. This was described as early as 1983 by Drs Garcia and Georgeana Jones.[5] A normal response to standard in vitro fertilization (IVF) stimulation indicates normal ovarian function and, generally, a good prognosis, although this is still limited by a woman's age. Some women are "hyper" responders and are at risk for ovarian hyperstimulation syndrome (OHSS). While certain characteristics, such as polycystic ovary syndrome (PCOS), high AMH/AFC, young age, and thin body habitus, do increase the risk for hyper-response, hyperstimulation generally cannot be predicted and vigilance is key. A low response can be predicted by low AMH and suggests "ovarian aging" common in women of advanced maternal age and may be associated with poor IVF outcome.[3]

There are three basic phases of stimulation for an IVF cycle: prestimulation, stimulation, and luteal support. In the prestimulation phase, ovarian

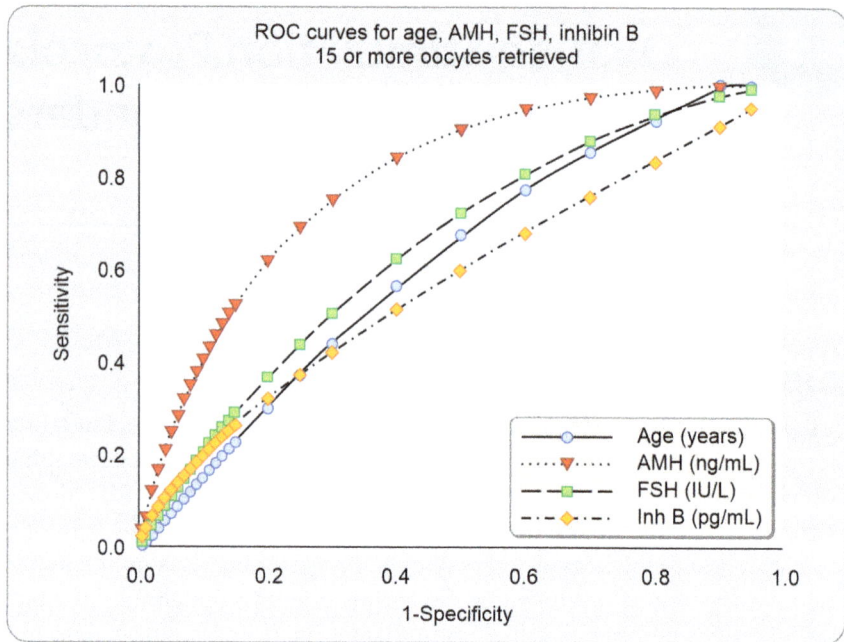

Fig. 1: ROC curves for age, AMH, FSH, inhibin B 15 or more oocytes retrieved. (AMH: anti-mullerian hormone; FSH: follicle-stimulating hormone; ROC: receiver operating characteristic)
Source: Riggs RM, Duran EH, Baker MW, Kimble TD, Hobeika E, Yin L, et al. Assessment of ovarian reserve with anti-Müllerian hormone: a comparison of the predictive value of anti-Müllerian hormone, follicle-stimulating hormone, inhibin B, and age. Am J Obstet Gynecol. 2008;199(2):202.e1-8.

activity is suppressed with leuprolide and/or with oral contraceptives in the previous cycle. The stimulation phase begins with the administration of gonadotropins to stimulate ovarian follicle growth; this is usually, but not always, during menses. Occasionally, a random start stimulation is also used, especially for fertility preservation. With a random start, gonadotropins can be initiated at any day in the cycle.

There are several choices of protocols including gonadotropin-releasing hormone (GnRH) agonists with "long" or "short" protocols versus GnRH antagonists, depending on the ovarian reserve. There are also choices in the type and preparation of medication: recombinant versus urinary gonadotropins, straight FSH versus a mixed protocol with FSH, and LH, human menopausal gonadotropin (hMG), or low-dose human chorionic gonadotropin (hCG).

Finally, there are various progesterone preparation options for luteal phase supplementation. Once optimum follicle size is reached, hCG is given and oocytes are retrieved 36 hours later. The support phase typically begins prior to embryo transfer using progesterone to provide hormonal support to the endometrium. These protocols will be discussed in the Chapter.

IN VITRO FERTILIZATION STIMULATION

The IVF ovarian stimulation goal is to induce ongoing maturation of multiple follicles for intrauterine insemination (IUI) or IVF to improve chances of pregnancy. Some of the same medications used for induction of ovulation are used for COS. COS is the deliberate and regulated production of a hormonal response intended to lead to the production of multiple eggs. In the context of assisted reproductive technology (ART), COS is one of the first steps involved in the IVF treatment process. The protocols for IVF are designed to create a balance between under- and overstimulation.

The goal is to achieve adequate numbers and quality of oocytes and number of euploid embryos leading to a normal singleton birth while maximizing the total reproductive potential of the cycle. The most serious complication that may arise from COS from IVF procedures is OHSS and this risk can be minimized with the protocol using low-dose gonadotropins and trigger with the GnRH agonist.[6]

The IVF stimulation protocols generally involve the use of three types of drugs. The purpose of the GnRH agonist (or antagonist) is to suppress release of LH from the woman's pituitary gland during the ovarian stimulation process. A woman's natural LH surge would cause premature ovulation of the eggs. GnRH agonists function by binding to and stimulating the GnRH receptors similar to native GnRH. Leuprolide acetate is the most common GnRH agonist used in ART cycles. With continuous administration of GnRH, first a "flare" results, which is an increased pituitary gonadotropin release in response to the excess GnRH signal. Following this, continued GnRH exposure results in desensitization of the pituitary, and gonadotropin release is suppressed. This provides complete control of the hypothalamic–pituitary–ovarian (HPO) axis for ART procedures.

A GnRH antagonist works to antagonize GnRH by binding and blocking GnRH receptors from signaling. Unlike the response to agonists that begins with a flare of FSH and LH release, the response to antagonists is the immediate suppression of gonadotropins. Two products are marketed for use in the United States: Cetrorelix and Ganirelix. GnRH antagonists have been used for all types of responders with some benefits. Antagonist protocols are shorter and may help reduce the dosage of FSH. They also prevent premature LH surges in women undergoing COS. Studies and meta-analysis of studies have shown equivalent outcomes with agonist and antagonist cycles with less injections, less days of stimulation, and lower levels of OHSS with the antagonist protocols.[7,8]

Follicle-stimulating hormone products stimulate development of multiple follicles in the ovaries by rescuing eggs that would normally undergo atresia in a natural cycle. hCG is used to cause final maturation of the eggs in the follicles and the number of follicles correlates with AMH.[9]

NORMAL RESPONDERS

The IVF stimulation protocol should be individualized to the patient. Good prognosis patients or normoresponders usually are patients with regular cycles, under the age of 40 years, have AMH of >1, AFC = 8–15, and average oocytes retrieved as 10–15. They do well with long stimulation with agonist or antagonist protocol with equivalent results. An example of a long-stimulation protocol for a normal responder is shown in **Figure 2**. Early studies had shown the long stimulation protocol to be superior for the live birth rates, but have increased length of stimulation and risk of ovarian hyperstimulation. This protocol has lower success in poor or hyper-responders.[10-12]

Oral contraceptives may be given during the prior cycle. Beginning after at least 6–7 days of oral contraceptives, leuprolide is given daily for prestimulation downregulation, and the dosage is decreased once menses begins (from 0.5 to 0.25 mg daily). After minimum of 1 week of oral contraceptive pills (OCPs), the recommendation is to overlap the leuprolide acetate with the last 5 days of OCPs. Once suppressed (estradiol levels <30 pg/mL) and with a bleed, gonadotropins are given daily. When monitoring indicates that follicles are ready with 3–4 follicles between 18 and 20 mm, hCG is administered, and oocyte retrieval is performed 36 hours later. Luteal phase support begins if a fresh transfer is planned. The starting dose of FSH is 225–300 IUs daily depending on the BMI.

Another type of stimulation protocol is the GnRH antagonist cycle, illustrated in **Figure 3**. An optional prestimulation suppression is achieved with oral contraceptives. Gonadotropins are initiated at least by day 2 or 3, of the cycle and the GnRH antagonist is started typically on day 6 of stimulation with a fixed protocol or a variable protocol based on follicle size >13 mm. It is continued until hCG is given.

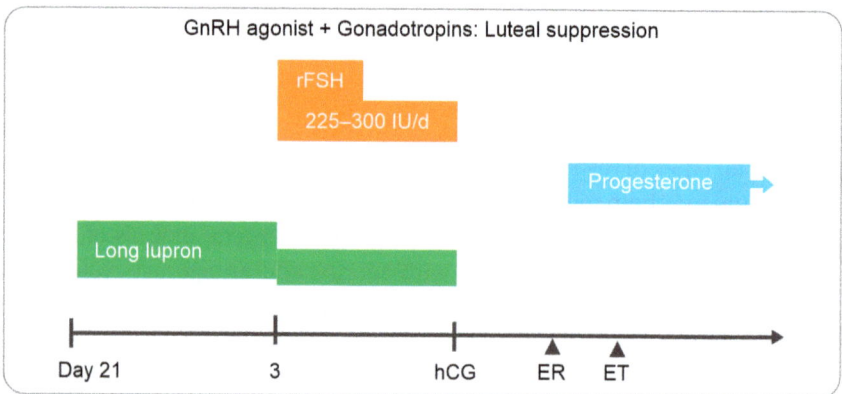

Fig. 2: GnRH agonist cycle for normal responders. (GnRH: gonadotropin-releasing hormone; hCG: human chorionic gonadotropin; rFSH: recombinant follicle-stimulating hormone)

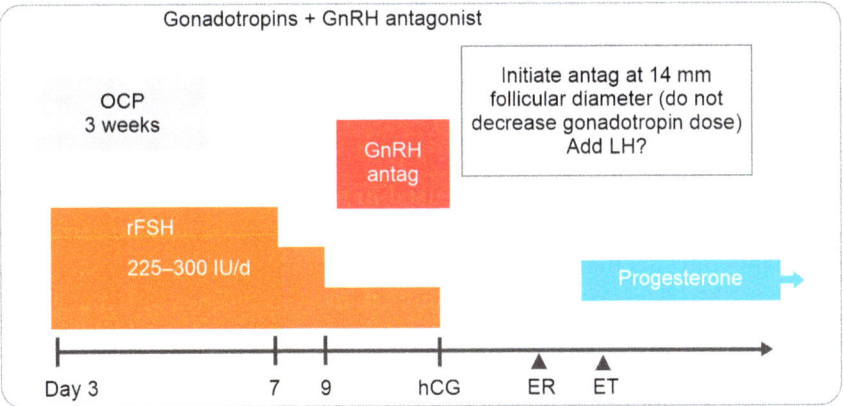

Fig. 3: IVF stimulation with GnRH antagonist flexible protocol. (GnRH: gonadotropin-releasing hormone; hCG: human chorionic gonadotropin; IVF: in vitro fertilization; LH: luteinizing hormone; rFSH: recombinant follicle-stimulating hormone)

FREEZE-ALL VERSUS FRESH TRANSFER IN NORMAL RESPONDERS

In a subset of women, the ovarian stimulation response may be associated with an endometrial advancement following endometrial histology evaluation on the day of oocyte retrieval using the Noyes criteria. The progesterone levels on day of trigger have been shown to be a predictor of patients who may have lower pregnancy rates in fresh cycles. In one study, all of the patients with endometrial advancement over 3 days were present in the group that had a $P_4 \geq 1.5$ ng/mL on the trigger day. The mean number of retrieved oocytes in this group of patients was 15.[13] In the normal responders with progesterone levels <1.5 ng/mL, fresh transfers provide equal success to the freeze-all cycles, suggesting that there was no interference that resulted from ovarian stimulation over the endometrium in this group of patients. Polyzos and Sunkara showed that the benefit of performing the freeze-all policy, particularly as it pertained to implantation potential, was only observed in the group of patients with the higher ovarian response (10-15 oocytes). This group of patients benefited from the freeze-all strategy. In suboptimal response group (4-9 oocytes), regardless of the strategy (fresh embryo transfer vs. freeze-all) used, the IVF outcomes were the same unless oral agents were used. The combination of recombinant follicle stimulating hormone (r-FSH) and hMG may be superior to r-FSH alone.[14]

The meta-analysis from Al-Inany et al. showed a better outcome in terms of the live birth rate when highly purified hMG was used for ovarian stimulation compared with r-FSH in the GnRH agonist long protocol. One of the most efficient stimulation protocols is the use of a combined protocol of human derived urinary FSH (uFSH) and rFSH. Combined protocol has resulted in a significant increase in the proportion of mature metaphase II oocytes and grade 1 embryos when compared to either rFSH or uFSH alone. A significantly higher delivery rate was achieved in rFSH + uFSH compared to the other protocols in poor and normal responders.[15]

■ MILD STIMULATION

Mild stimulation protocols can be used in normal responders as a way to reduce the cost but will produce less total number of oocytes. However, the pregnancy rates per transfer are not affected. It is an option for poor responders with low AMH who do not produce more than a few follicles with maximum stimulation as seen in **Figure 4**.[16-19] Stimulation can be initiated with either clomiphene citrate or letrozole for 5 days followed by gonadotropins, or with low-dose gonadotropins alone as seen in **Figure 5**. The GnRH antagonist is used to prevent premature ovulation. "Freeze-all" cycles are recommended on all mild stimulation cases, as the oral medications can affect the receptivity of the endometrium.[20-23]

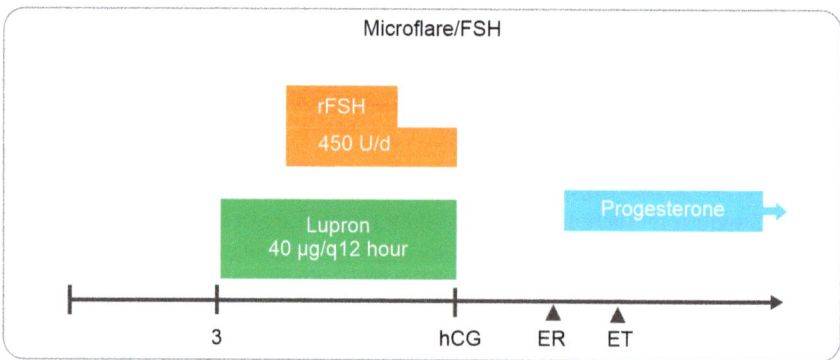

Fig. 4: Protocol for poor responders—microflare. (hCG: human chorionic gonadotropin; rFSH: recombinant follicle-stimulating hormone)

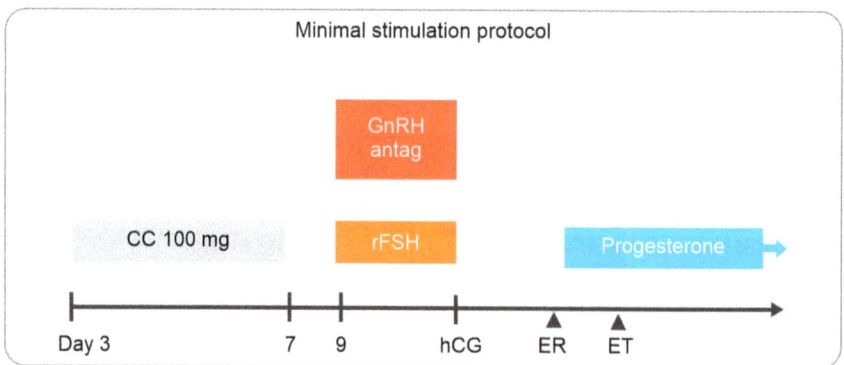

Fig. 5: Protocol for poor responders—minimal stimulation protocol. (GnRH: gonadotropin-releasing hormone; hCG: human chorionic gonadotropin; rFSH: recombinant follicle-stimulating hormone)

ROLE OF LUTEINIZING HORMONE

Recombinant LH, if available, is produced in the same fashion as recombinant FSH, by a transfected Chinese hamster ovary cell line. In most women, endogenous LH production is sufficient to provide adequate LH support during COS. Studies have shown no statistical difference in pregnancy outcomes when recombinant LH and recombinant FSH are co-administered, compared with using recombinant FSH alone in COS cycles.[24-26] Filicori treated women with secondary hypo/hypo with HP FSH or FSH and low-dose hCG.[25] They found that half the treatment cycle duration and less FSH was needed to achieve follicle growth with low-dose hCG addition. In addition, GnRH agonist and antagonist cycles can suppress LH profoundly in 10-15% in agonist and antagonist cycles. These patients have higher incidence of early pregnancy loss.[27,28] In addition, LH is needed in those patients who do not produce endogenous LH, such as those with hypothalamic amenorrhea or hypopituitarism.[29] As discussed above, the addition of recombinant LH may be beneficial in women who are poor responders.[22] The use of LH or GnRH-a as an ovulation trigger has been suggested, but not proven, to prevent OHSS.[30-32]

TRIGGER TIMING

The mean follicle diameter is determined by two perpendicular dimensions. Medication dosage is adjusted to avoid over- or understimulating the patient. The ideal follicle size for administering the hCG trigger is >12 mm with the largest three follicles at least 17 mm in diameter. The endometrium is measured in the sagittal plane from outer border of endometrium to the outer endometrial border at the thickest point. If a mild stimulation protocol is used with clomiphene citrate or letrozole, the optimal trigger size is at least three follicles at 20 mm or greater in diameter.

Only advanced stage antral follicles that are FSH dependent will grow with secondary recruitment and primary follicles are not affected by ovarian stimulation. Software is available using 3-dimensional technology that provides automated assessment of follicle volume and may save time in monitoring. Follicle diameters and volumes are calculated automatically and color-coded. **Figure 6** shows the comparisons of 2D with the 3D automated measurements.[33]

LUTEAL SUPPLEMENTATION

As early as the 1970s, it was known that ovarian stimulation leads to disruption of luteal phase and abnormal luteal phase in IVF cycles. This is due to elevated progesterone and luteal phase shortening with gonadotropins. This could be rescued by hCG but there is an increase in OHSS. When follicles have reached optimum size, hCG is administered as a trigger for ovulation to occur

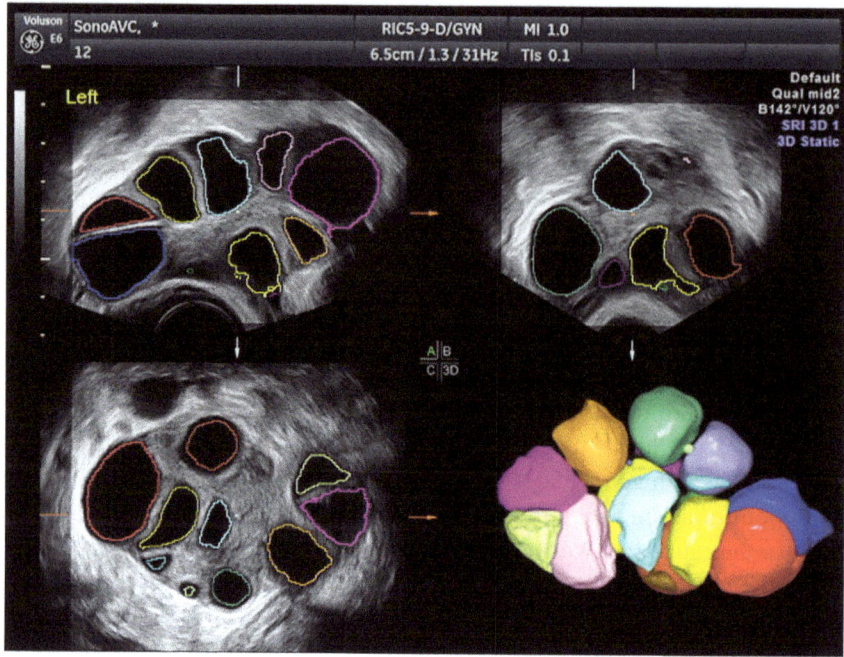

Fig. 6: SonoAVC follicle monitoring in 3D.
(SonoAVC: sonography-based automated volume count)

38–40 hours later. The usual dosage is 5,000–10,000 units. For IVF cycles, oocyte retrieval is thus scheduled in a tight time window before ovulation occurs to maximize the number of mature oocytes, usually about 36 hours after trigger. hCG also supports the function of the corpus luteum. As noted previously, if a GnRH agonist has not been used in the cycle, it may be given as the trigger to lessen the risk of ovarian hyperstimulation. Once ovulation is triggered, nearly all women in COS cycles require luteal phase support. High-dose GnRH agonists in IVF may create an induced luteal phase deficiency.

Progesterone is an essential hormone to aid in implantation and decrease uterine irritability. Progesterone has been shown to be effective when given intramuscularly or vaginally. The effectiveness of oral progesterone is not as clear.[34-36]

Alternatively, a supplemental dose of hCG 1 week after the ovulation trigger dose can assist in luteal phase support. Administration of 250 µg of recombinant hCG subcutaneously or 2,500–5,000 IU of hCG intramuscularly may be repeated 1 week after the initial trigger dose. This therapy ideally uses the patient's ovaries to produce the added progesterone.

Meta-analysis data demonstrate that hCG and progesterone are both effective in providing luteal phase support.[37] However, hCG increases the risk for ovarian hyperstimulation and thus is used infrequently in the United States. Progesterone may be administered in several ways: progesterone in oil, 50 mg IM daily; vaginal micronized progesterone, 600 mg daily; 8% progesterone vaginal gel, 90 mg daily; or micronized natural progesterone in vaginal tablets, 300 mg daily. Side effects of intramuscular progesterone include pain and allergic reaction. Also, the risk of allergic reaction is increased if peanut oil is used as a base for the hormone in oral or injectable forms. Localized irritation may also occur. While controversial, some groups add estradiol to their progesterone regimen.[38]

Generally, progesterone in any form is better than no luteal support. However, data do not show that one route is clearly better than others. A meta-analysis of randomized studies showed IM progesterone was better than the oral or vaginal route.[39] A Cochrane review demonstrated that progesterone after IVF increases the pregnancy rate and that the optimal route of progesterone has not been established.[40]

CONCLUSION

Normoresponder group is one of the best prognosis group where any protocol like long agonist, antagonist or mild stimulation protocol bring excellent results. As our results improve if we get 8–15 oocytes generally we follow conventional protocols. The advantage of antagonist is decrease gonadotropin requirement, flexibility of choosing a trigger and prevention of OHSS the long protocol gives us better and synchronus cohort and few extra oocytes. One has to remember that increasing the gonadotropin dosage brings out aneuploidy and displaced endometrial receptivity. So the treatment for each and every individual should be tailor made.

KEY POINTS

- These are some crucial points comparing agonist and antagonist protocols for normal responders.
- Generally, antagonists provide significant advantages to patients in terms of fewer injections, shorter stimulation days, and less suppression.
- Pregnancy rates for both treatments need to be continually monitored, but recent studies have shown equivalence.
- The incidence of OHSS is less with antagonists with an option to use an agonist as hCG trigger.
- The day the antagonist is started can be fixed or flexible based on follicle size. Some women need a mixed protocol to avoid a drop in estrogen on initiation of antagonist.

REFERENCES

1. Baerwald AR, Adams GP, Pierson RA. Ovarian antral folliculogenesis during the human menstrual cycle: a review. Hum Reprod Update. 2012;18(1):73-91.
2. Riggs RM, Duran EH, Baker MW, Kimble TD, Hobeika E, Yin L, et al. Assessment of ovarian reserve with anti-Müllerian hormone: a comparison of the predictive

value of anti-Müllerian hormone, follicle-stimulating hormone, inhibin B, and age. Am J Obstet Gynecol. 2008;199(2):202.e1-8.
3. Riggs R, Kimble T, Oehninger S, Bocca S, Zhao Y, Leader B, et al. Anti-Müllerian hormone serum levels predict response to controlled ovarian hyperstimulation but not embryo quality or pregnancy outcome in oocyte donation. Fertil Steril. 2011;95(1):410-2.
4. Steward RG, Lan L, Shah AA, Yeh JS, Price TM, Goldfarb JM, et al. Oocyte number as a predictor for ovarian hyperstimulation syndrome and live birth: an analysis of 256,381 in vitro fertilization cycles. Fertil Steril. 2014;101(4):967-73.
5. Garcia JE, Jones GS, Acosta AA, Wright G. Human menopausal gonadotropin/human chorionic gonadotropin follicular maturation for oocyte aspiration: Phase I, 1981. Fertil Steril. 1983;39(2):167-73.
6. Youssef MA, Van der Veen F, Al-Inany HG, Griesinger G, Mochtar MH, Aboulfoutouh I, et al. Gonadotropin-releasing hormone agonist versus HCG for oocyte triggering in antagonist assisted reproductive technology cycles. Cochrane Database Syst Rev. 2011(1):CD008046.
7. Fatemi HM, Doody K, Griesinger G, Witjes H, Mannaerts B. High ovarian response does not jeopardize ongoing pregnancy rates and increases cumulative pregnancy rates in a GnRH-antagonist protocol. Hum Reprod. 2013;28(2):442-52.
8. Lambalk CB, Banga FR, Huirne JA, Toftager M, Pinborg A, Homburg R, et al. GnRH antagonist versus long agonist protocols in IVF: a systematic review and meta-analysis accounting for patient type. Hum Reprod Update. 2017;23(5):560-79.
9. Arce JC, Andersen AN, Fernández-Sánchez M, Visnova H, Bosch E, García-Velasco JA, et al. Ovarian response to recombinant human follicle-stimulating hormone: a randomized, antimüllerian hormone-stratified, dose-response trial in women undergoing in vitro fertilization/intracytoplasmic sperm injection. Fertil Steril. 2014;102(6):1633-40.e5.
10. Pabuccu R, Onalan G, Kaya C. GnRH agonist and antagonist protocols for stage I-II endometriosis and endometrioma in in vitro fertilization/intracytoplasmic sperm injection cycles. Fertil Steril. 2007;88(4):832-9.
11. Prapas Y, Petousis S, Dagklis T, Panagiotidis Y, Papatheodorou A, Assunta I, et al. GnRH antagonist versus long GnRH agonist protocol in poor IVF responders: a randomized clinical trial. Eur J Obstet Gynecol Reprod Biol. 2013;166(1):43-6.
12. Trenkić M, Popović J, Kopitović V, Bjelica A, Živadinović R, Pop-Trajković S. Flexible GnRH antagonist protocol vs. long GnRH agonist protocol in patients with polycystic ovary syndrome treated for IVF: comparison of clinical outcome and embryo quality. Ginekol Pol. 2016;87(4):265-70.
13. Lee C-I, Chen H-H, Huang C-C, Lin P-Y, Lee T-H, Lee M-S. Early progesterone change associated with pregnancy outcome after fresh embryo transfer in assisted reproduction technology cycles with progesterone level of >1.5 ng/ml on human chorionic gonadotropin trigger day. Front Endocrinol (Lausanne). 2020;11:653.
14. Polyzos NP, Sunkara SK. Sub-optimal responders following controlled ovarian stimulation: an overlooked group? Hum Reprod. 2015;30(9):2005-8.
15. Al-Inany HG, Abou-Setta AM, Aboulghar MA, Mansour RT, Serour GI. Highly purified hMG achieves better pregnancy rates in IVF cycles but not ICSI cycles compared with recombinant FSH: a meta-analysis. Gynecol Endocrinol. 2009;25(6):372-8.

16. Baker VL. Mild ovarian stimulation for in vitro fertilization: one perspective from the USA. J Assist Reprod Genet. 2013;30(2):197-202.
17. Akman MA, Erden HF, Tosun SB, Bayazit N, Aksoy E, Bahceci M. Comparison of agonistic flare-up-protocol and antagonistic multiple dose protocol in ovarian stimulation of poor responders: results of a prospective randomized trial. Hum Reprod. 2001;16(5):868-70.
18. Muasher SJ. Treatment of low responders. J Assist Reprod Genet. 1993;10(2):112-4.
19. Zhang Y, Zhang C, Shu J, Guo J, Chang H-M, Leung PCK, et al. Adjuvant treatment strategies in ovarian stimulation for poor responders undergoing IVF: a systematic review and network meta-analysis. Hum Reprod Update. 2020;26(2):247-63.
20. Baart EB, Martini E, Eijkemans MJ, Van Opstal D, Beckers NG, Verhoeff A, et al. Milder ovarian stimulation for in-vitro fertilization reduces aneuploidy in the human preimplantation embryo: a randomized controlled trial. Hum Reprod. 2007;22(4):980-8.
21. Heijnen EM, Eijkemans MJ, De Klerk C, Polinder S, Beckers NG, Klinkert ER, et al. A mild treatment strategy for in-vitro fertilisation: a randomised non-inferiority trial. Lancet. 2007;369(9563):743-9.
22. Arvis P, Massin N, Lehert P. Effect of recombinant LH supplementation on cumulative live birth rate compared with FSH alone in poor ovarian responders: a large, real-world study. Reprod Biomed Online. 2021;42(3):546-54.
23. Leijdekkers JA, Torrance HL, Schouten NE, van Tilborg TC, Oudshoorn SC, Mol BWJ, et al. Individualized ovarian stimulation in IVF/ICSI treatment: it is time to stop using high FSH doses in predicted low responders. Hum Reprod. 2020;35(9):1954-63.
24. Levi-Setti PE, Cavagna M, Bulletti C. Recombinant gonadotrophins associated with GnRH antagonist (cetrorelix) in ovarian stimulation for ICSI: comparison of r-FSH alone and in combination with r-LH. Eur J Obstet Gynecol Reprod Biol. 2006;126(2):212-6.
25. Filicori M, Cognigni GE. Ovulation induction with pulsatile gonadotropin releasing hormone: missing in action. Fertil Steril. 2018;109(4):621-2.
26. Mochtar MH, Van der Veen, Ziech M, van Wely M. Recombinant luteinizing hormone (rLH) for controlled ovarian hyperstimulation in assisted reproductive cycles. Cochrane Database Syst Rev. 2007;(2):CD005070.
27. Chen CD, Chiang YT, Yang PK, Chen MJ, Chang CH, Yang YS, et al. Frequency of low serum LH is associated with increased early pregnancy loss in IVF/ICSI cycles. Reprod Biomed Online. 2016;33(4):449-57.
28. Benmachiche A, Benbouhedja S, Zoghmar A, Humaidan P. Low LH Level on the day of GnRH agonist trigger is associated with reduced ongoing pregnancy and live birth rates and increased early miscarriage rates following IVF/ICSI treatment and fresh embryo transfer. Front Endocrinol (Lausanne). 2019;10:639.
29. Di Segni N, Busnelli A, Secchi M, Cirillo F, Levi-Setti PE. Luteinizing hormone supplementation in women with hypogonadotropic hypogonadism seeking fertility care: Insights from a narrative review. Front Endocrinol (Lausanne). 2022;13:907249.
30. Kok JD, Looman CW, Weima SM, te Velde ER. A high number of oocytes obtained after ovarian hyperstimulation for in vitro fertilization or intracytoplasmic

sperm injection is not associated with decreased pregnancy outcome. Fertil Steril. 2006;85(4):918-24.
31. Fatemi HM, Popovic-Todorovic B, Humaidan P, Kol S, Banker M, Devroey P, et al. Severe ovarian hyperstimulation syndrome after gonadotropin-releasing hormone (GnRH) agonist trigger and "freeze-all" approach in GnRH antagonist protocol. Fertil Steril. 2014;101(4):1008-11.
32. Engmann L, DiLuigi A, Schmidt D, Nulsen J, Maier D, Benadiva C. The use of gonadotropin-releasing hormone (GnRH) agonist to induce oocyte maturation after cotreatment with GnRH antagonist in high-risk patients undergoing in vitro fertilization prevents the risk of ovarian hyperstimulation syndrome: a prospective randomized controlled study. Fertil Steril. 2008;89(1):84-91.
33. Deutch TD, Joergner I, Matson DO, Oehninger S, Bocca S, Hoenigmann D, et al. Automated assessment of ovarian follicles using a novel three-dimensional ultrasound software. Fertil Steril. 2009;92(5):1562-8.
34. Nosarka S, Kruger T, Siebert I, Grové D. Luteal phase support in in vitro fertilization: meta-analysis of randomized trials. Gynecol Obstet Invest. 2005; 60(2):67-74.
35. Pritts EA, Atwood AK. Luteal phase support in infertility treatment: a meta-analysis of the randomized trials. Hum Reprod. 2002;17(9):2287-99.
36. Daya S, Gunby J. Luteal phase support in assisted reproduction cycles. Cochrane Database Syst Rev. 2004;(3):CD004830.
37. Mohammed A, Woad KJ, Mann GE, Craigon J, Raine-Fenning N, Robinson RS. Evaluation of progestogen supplementation for luteal phase support in fresh in vitro fertilization cycles. Fertil Steril. 2019;112(3):491-502.e3.
38. Çakar E, Tasan HA, Kumru P, Cogendez E, Usal NT, Kutlu HT, et al. Combined use of oestradiol and progesterone to support luteal phase in antagonist intracytoplasmic sperm injection cycles of normoresponder women: a case-control study. J Obstet Gynaecol. 2020;40(2):264-9.
39. Zarutskie PW, Phillips JA. A meta-analysis of the route of administration of luteal phase support in assisted reproductive technology: vaginal versus intramuscular progesterone. Fertil Steril. 2009;92(1):163-9.
40. van der Linden M, Buckingham K, Farquhar C, Kremer JA, Metwally M. Luteal phase support for assisted reproduction cycles. Cochrane Database Syst Rev. 2011(10):CD009154.

Chapter 18
Ovarian Stimulation Protocols for Hyper-responders

Seema Pandey, Sini Venugopal

■ INTRODUCTION

The success of in vitro fertilization (IVF) and other assisted reproductive technologies (ARTs) is critically dependent on optimizing ovarian stimulation protocols that aims to provide good-quality oocytes and embryos with a resultant good pregnancy rate. The strategies utilized must not only achieve excellent embryo implantation rates, but must also seek to minimize medical complications. To achieve these, it is crucial to individualize stimulation with respect to chronological age, ovarian reserve, and endocrine status. Therefore, it is important to identify and prospectively differentiate the poor responder from the high responder, and whenever possible to specifically tailor the stimulation protocol.

Controlled ovarian stimulation (COS) is the most instrumental, modifiable, and evolving event in the process of IVF which determines the quality and quantity of good oocyte retrieval which ultimately is one of the most important prognostic factors for a successful reproductive outcome. Several protocols have been studied in an attempt to find the one which would ensure the most favorable reproductive outcome with minimal risks to the women. The favorable outcomes being clinical pregnancy and live birth, minimal or no risk of ovarian hyperstimulation syndrome (OHSS), and minimal or no risk of cycle cancellation either due to poor response or hyper-response along with being affordable too. In recent years, there has been a shift in the concept and approach of "one size fits all" to "individualization" in IVF treatment protocols. Apart from achieving a favorable reproductive outcome, this approach would also reduce the overall treatment costs and dropout rates of patients, mainly due to physical, psychological, and financial burden.

The term "hyper-response" refers to the retrieval of >15 oocytes following a standard COS protocol. The prevalence of hyper-response in IVF cycles is approximately around 7%. Since the initial years of ART, patients have been classified as "poor", "normal", or "high/hyper" responders with reference to their response to COS. Although these terms are widely used in research and in daily clinical practice, their precise definitions are still not fully or clearly agreed upon.

TABLE 1: Various definitions of hyper-response.

Author	Definition of excessive response
Nelson et al.	≥21 oocytes
La Marca et al.	>16 oocytes
Ebner et al.	≥15 oocytes
Lee et al.	OHSS
Riggs et al.	>15 oocytes
Nardo et al.	≥20 oocytes, E2 >17,000 pmol/L
Aflatoonian et al.	≥15 oocytes, E2 >3,000 pg/mL
Van Rooij et al.	≥14 oocytes
Eldar Geva et al.	≥14 oocytes
Kwee et al.	>20 oocytes
Ng et al.	≥15 oocytes

(OHSS: ovarian hyperstimulation syndrome)

Different authors have defined ovarian hyper-response differently with reference to the number of oocytes retrieved **(Table 1)**.

The patient profiles which are suggestive of a high-ovarian response or hyper-response are:
- Young age
- Lower BMI
- Long menstrual cycle
- Polycystic ovarian syndrome
- Hyper-response in a previous IVF cycle

The strong predictors of hyper-response are AMH (anti-Müllerian hormone) and AFC (antral follicle count).[1] Serum AMH level > 3.5 ng/mL has been shown to have a good sensitivity and specificity. AFC of >16 has been shown to be the most appropriate cut-off value for hyper-response.[2]

The implications of hyper-response in IVF are:
- Increased risk of IVF cycle cancellation
- Increased risk of freeze all
- Increased risk of OHSS
- Reduced pregnancy rate, at least in fresh cycle

CAUSES OF HYPER-RESPONSE

- A large ovarian pool of preantral follicles is a significant risk factor.
- Increased ovarian sensitivity to gonadotropins.

Activating mutations in follicle-stimulating hormone (FSH) receptors have been reported and the mutant FSH receptors displayed abnormally high sensitivity to both FSH and human chorionic gonadotropin (hCG).

TABLE 2: Prestimulation risk factor assessment.		
Clinical	**Laboratory**	**Sonological**
Young age	AMH	AFC
Lower BMI		PCO-morphology
PCOS diagnosis		High baseline ovarian volume
Previous high response		
(AFC: antral follicle count; AMH: anti-Müllerian hormone; PCOS: polycystic ovary syndrome)		

The Asn/Ser allelic variant may reflect a higher FSH sensitivity of follicles, leading to a better and more rapid ovarian response compared to the other two SNP variants. BMP15, a member of the transforming growth factor-β family, inhibits FSH receptor expression. A single nucleotide polymorphism in BMP15 is associated with high response to ovarian stimulation.[3]

A clear separation should be made between risk factors for high-ovarian response and the actual response to stimulation.[4] So, chronological evaluation of high-ovarian response is very important **(Table 2)**.

ASSESSMENT DURING OVARIAN RESPONSE TO STIMULATION

- Number of recruited follicles
- Serum E2 concentration
- Number of oocytes retrieved
- Ovarian sensitivity index (OSI)

A retrospective comparative cohort study done on 2,150 women who underwent first IVF cycles showed that OSI appears to be a highly reliable index of ovarian responsiveness to recombinant FSH and can be useful to estimate the FSH dose. OSI was calculated by dividing the total administered recombinant follicle-stimulating hormone (rFSH) dose by the number of oocytes retrieved at oocyte pick-up (OPU) to obtain the FSH-to-retrieved oocyte ratio.[4,5]

Many different protocols have been studied and tried in hyper-responders in an attempt to achieve maximum reproductive outcome with minimal risks. There have been new protocols, modifications in existing protocols, modifications in gonadotropin doses, type of gonadotropins used, modifications in trigger dose and type of trigger, modifications in downregulation regimens, modifications in luteal phase support, and addition of drugs like insulin-sensitizing agents as pretreatment and co-treatment agents. All these different approaches aim to prevent hyper-response and to optimize the reproductive outcomes. Some of the important protocols and approaches in hyper-responders are discussed here.

VARIOUS PROTOCOLS FOR HYPER-RESPONDERS

There are stepwise measures, starting from low gonadotropin doses to addition of various downregulating regimens and change in trigger type to segmentation of IVF cycle. **Table 3** shows all the possible ways of handling hyper-response in poor responders.

Low-dose Gonadotropin Step-up Dose Protocol

Hyper-responders show an excessive response to gonadotropin, so it is rational to think of an approach where the initial starting dose of gonadotropin is low and is then gradually stepped up. The principle of low-dose step-up protocol is based on the concept of FSH threshold and can yield a certain number of follicles at the same level of development which leads to a satisfactory oocyte retrieval, yet at the same time minimize the risks of hyper-response.[6,7]

Gonadotropin Step-down Protocol

The step-down protocol theoretically appears to mimic the physiological response of FSH release.[8] It induces multiple follicular growth at the onset of stimulation with a higher dose followed by a gradual decrease in the number of follicles recruited with a lower dose later, similar to the normal ovulatory cycle. But there were studies later on which suggested that the theoretical value of the step-down protocol, which mimics the physiological FSH release,

TABLE 3: Various regimens to control hyper-response in hyper-responders.

Pretreatment	Downregulation	Adjusting the dose of GN	Adjusting trigger	Postponing fresh transfer
COCs pretreatment	Antagonist protocol	Step-up protocol	Agonist trigger	Segmented IVF protocol
Early start antagonist protocol	Progesterone primed stimulation protocol	Step-down protocol	Dual trigger	Freeze-all protocol
	Mild stimulation protocol	Selective cutback protocol	Low-dose hCG trigger	
	Long agonist protocol	Sequential step-up/step-down protocol	Sliding scale hCG trigger	
	Antagonist rescue protocol	Individualization of gonadotropin-dose protocol		
		CONSORT algorithm		

(hCG: human chorionic gonadotropin; IVF: in vitro fertilization; GN: gonadotropins; COCs: combined oral contraceptives) has little practical importance in patients with polycystic ovary syndrome (PCOS) and hyper-response. In essence, FSH stimulation using the step-down protocol is unpredictable. Sometimes, it is excessive and at times, it is inert. Unavoidably, at the time of hCG injection, a considerable discrepancy in the mean follicular size is observed.

Selective Cut-back Protocol

In the selective cut-back protocol, as the primary follicular cohort matures, by selectively cutting back FSH dose while maintaining adequate hCG activity, low hyperstimulation rates and excellent ongoing pregnancy rates can be achieved.[9]

Sequential Step-up/Step-down Protocol

The sequential step-up/step-down regimen utilizes the best of both the step-up and step-down protocols. It is based on the combined effectiveness of the two conventional step-up and step-down protocols to induce uniform homogeneous follicular growth which could presumably lead to higher pregnancy rates, lower risk of multiple pregnancies, and OHSS. It induces a cohort of maturing follicles which is sustained uniformly throughout the period of ovarian stimulation.[7,8]

Individualization of FSH Dose Protocol

Hyper-responders are actual group of patients who get benefitted tremendously by individualizing gonadotropin dose.[10] Individualization not only decreases the chances of moderate-to-severe OHSS, but also it does not affect the cumulative live birth as well.[11,12] FSH dose individualization is based on prior ovarian reserve markers, mainly AMH and AFC.[13] Individualized FSH dosing significantly reduces moderate/severe OHSS and results in similar cumulative live birth rates.[14]

The incidence of OHSS was less when a stimulation dose of <150 IU was used in hyper-responders. But no consensus has been reached on whether ORT (ovarian reserve test)-based FSH dosing improves effectiveness and safety in women with a predicted hyper-response. More research is warranted to reach a consensus with regards to the recommendation of the individualized FSH dosing protocol.[13]

CONSORT Algorithm

The CONSORT (CONsistency in rFSH Starting dOses for individualized tReatmenT) dosing algorithm individualizes recombinant human FSH (r-FSH) doses for assisted reproduction technologies, assigning 37.5 IU increments according to patient characteristics: basal FSH, body mass index, age, and antral follicle count that has been proven to accurately predict ovarian response to ovarian stimulation.[10] A prospective, uncontrolled, international, 18-centre, pilot study of normo-ovulatory women aged 18–34 years inclusive, undergoing a long agonist treatment protocol was performed. The choice of gonadotropin starting dose is an important parameter to prevent OHSS. The use of CONSORT algorithm achieved an adequate oocyte yield and good pregnancy rates in this preliminary study. Adjustment of the algorithm could reduce cancellation rates.

In another randomized, controlled, open-label, phase IV study, ovarian response after a follitropin-alpha starting dose determined by the CONSORT calculator was compared with a standard dose (150 IU). 200 normo-ovulatory women (aged 18–34 years) eligible for assisted reproductive techniques were recruited (23 centers: nine European countries and Chile) and randomized into CONSORT = 96 and standard dosing = 104 groups. Although the CONSORT calculator was statistically inferior to standard dosing in the number of oocytes retrieved, clinical pregnancy rates (fresh embryo transfers) were similar in both groups, and incidence of OHSS was lower in the CONSORT group.

Sliding Scale Protocol for hCG Trigger

The incidence of OHSS can be minimized by lowering the hCG trigger dose for high responders. Despite the shift in approach to use antagonist-based protocols with subsequent gonadotropin-releasing hormone agonist (GnRHa) trigger, some literature suggests reduced clinical pregnancy, delivery rates and increased miscarriage rates. Some studies also suggest that some women may have a suboptimal response to GnRH agonist trigger. This led to the concept of lowering the hCG trigger dose for hyper-responders to reduce the risk of OHSS while still maximizing the reproductive outcomes.

A retrospective cohort study of 10,427 IVF/intracytoplasmic sperm injection (ICSI) cycles, utilizing the sliding scale hCG protocol were included.[15] The sliding scale hCG protocol uses dose adjustment according to E2 levels at trigger: 10,000 IU of hCG for E2 <1,500 pg/mL, 5,000 IU for E2 1,501–2,500 pg/mL, 4,000 IU for E2 2,501–3,000 pg/mL, and 3,300 IU for E2 >3,000 pg/mL. A subgroup analysis specific to high responders (E2 >3,000 pg/mL) compared cycles triggered by low-dose hCG (3,300 IU) versus dual trigger (2 mg leuprolide acetate + 1,500 IU hCG). This group consisted of 1,223 IVF patients who met criteria of high responders (E2 levels >3,000 pg/mL). Low-dose hCG appeared independently and significantly to reduce the risk of early and severe OHSS, without compromising the final oocyte maturation, number of oocytes retrieved, the number of embryos available for transfer, or clinical pregnancy rates in women undergoing ICSI. The study shows that doses as low as 3,300 IU hCG alone or dual trigger with 1,500 IU hCG and GnRH agonist are sufficient to maximize the oocyte maturity in patients.

The lack of a control group and the small sample size limit the ability to make this conclusion as definitive.[16]

Further prospective randomized clinical trials are needed to corroborate these preliminary findings.

Double Suppression Protocol

Double suppression protocol was being used by some, where one cycle of oral contraceptive pretreatment was administered before putting these patients on long agonist protocol along with step-down regimen of gonadotropin dosing. These cycles reflected an improved (luteinizing hormone) LH:FSH ratio, decreased serum androgens (DHEAS particularly), lower LH, and lower E2 after 14 days of downregulation. This protocol was also said to decrease number of oocytes retrieved along with E2 on the day of trigger. Clinically, this protocol led to lower cancellation rate along and lower rate of OHSS with favorable clinical and ongoing pregnancy rates.[17]

A prospective, nonrandomized, single-center cohort study of primary or secondary infertile patients undergoing IVF/ICSI treatment was done with the aim to investigate whether such pretreatment could reduce the incidence of OHSS for patients with different ovarian responses in IVF/ICSI treatment.[18] One cycle of OC pretreatment before the pituitary downregulation with GnRH-agonist for suspected high responders could moderately reduce their ovarian response to gonadotropins and obviously lower the morbidity rate of both early and late OHSS as well as the severe OHSS. However, such pretreatment for suspected normal responders seemed to have no impact on the outcome of ovarian hyperstimulation and the morbidity of OHSS.

GnRH Antagonist Salvage Protocol

Looking at the limited options like cancellation of cycle and coasting for preventing OHSS in hyper-responders on long agonist protocol and its emotional and financial burden on couple, this GnRH antagonist protocol was devised. In this protocol, agonist which was being used for downregulation is stopped and antagonist injection is added mostly from day 6 of cycle if E2 levels are very high or the number of recruited follicles is >25 and it was seen that by doing this the chances of cycle cancellation and OHSS were very low, and at the same time, there was no compromise in expected clinical pregnancy outcome.[19]

GnRH Antagonist Protocol

One of the prime concerns in COS for IVF/ICSI cycles is the occurrence of premature LH surge which is a major cause for cycle cancellation. Premature luteinization exists in up to 15–20% of IVF cycles, which may lead to poor oocyte yield or quality and cycle cancellation. Traditionally, premature LH surge was prevented by GnRH agonist downregulation. But long-agonist downregulation was associated with more complexity of procedure, longer duration of treatment, higher cost of treatment, and more risk for OHSS. Subsequently, the advent of GnRH antagonist came as a sigh of relief as GnRH antagonist caused rapid and reversible suppression of LH with absence of the initial flare effect.

The GnRH-antagonist protocol is the most preferred, standard, and first-choice protocol for hyper-responders. The use of a gonadotropin-releasing hormone (GnRH) antagonist has advantages over traditional GnRH agonist protocols in terms of a lower requirement for gonadotropins, reduced length of treatment, and reduced incidence of moderate-to-severe OHSS.

The advantages of using GnRH antagonist protocol are:
- Reduced incidence of OHSS
- Lower dose requirement for gonadotropins
- Reduced length of treatment cycle
- Reduced incidence of cycle cancellation
- Reduced patient hospitalization
- Reduction in treatment cost
- Allows the option of using GnRH agonist as trigger

In a large randomized controlled trial (RCT) of 1,050 first IVF cycles where antagonist protocol was compared to agonist downregulation protocol, the following findings were observed, which have set the stage for GnRH antagonist becoming the preferred kid on the block[20] **(Table 4)**.

Another meta-analysis with 50 studies did a comparative analysis of the GnRH antagonist protocol and GnRH agonist protocol among general IVF patients, women with PCOS, and poor responders.[21] Out of 50 studies, 34 studies were on general IVF patients, 10 studies on PCOS patients, and 6 studies on poor responders. Both these and several other studies show that the GnRH antagonist protocol resulted in lower OHSS rates both in general IVF patients and in women with PCOS. In general IVF patients, the ongoing pregnancy rate was significantly lower in the antagonist group compared with the agonist group. In women with PCOS and in women with poor ovarian

TABLE 4: Comparative study of agonist and antagonist.

Variables	GnRH antagonist cycle	Long GnRH agonist cycle
Severe OHSS	5.1%	8.9%
Moderate OHSS	10.2%	15.6%
Live birth rates	22.8%	23.8%
Ongoing pregnancy rates	24.9%	26.2%
Pregnancy rates	Same	Same

(GnRH: gonadotropin-releasing hormone; OHSS: ovarian hyperstimulation syndrome)

response, there was no difference in oocyte yield, ongoing pregnancy rate, and clinical pregnancy rate between the antagonist group and the agonist group, but there was a significantly lower OHSS rate in the antagonist group. Based on this systematic review, one could consider that in women with PCOS and poor responders, as the use of the GnRH antagonist protocol significantly reduces the OHSS risk and also does not seem to compromise the pregnancy rates, it can be considered as the standard and first-choice treatment in hyper-responders.

GnRH Agonist Trigger in GnRH Antagonist Protocol

Human chorionic gonadotropin (hCG) has been traditionally used as a trigger for final oocyte maturation. Due to biological activity of hCG similar to LH, since the mid-1970s, exogenous hCG has been used to trigger the final oocyte maturation and ovulation. hCG has the same effect as LH with long half-life of >24 hours.[22] It has a long luteotrophic effect, which increases the risk of OHSS. In various subsequent studies, GnRH agonist was used and proposed in the mid-cycle for gonadotropin surge stimulation. It was observed that with GnRH agonist trigger, release of both gonadotropins (LH/FSH) was similar to that of natural cycle, and also, the shorter duration of LH surge avoids incidence of OHSS.

The advantages of using GnRH agonist as a trigger:
- GnRH agonist trigger stimulates FSH surge, in addition to LH surge, which is more physiological, leading to more physiological and better maturity of the oocytes.
- FSH surge in the mid-cycle has specific beneficial effects on oocyte maturation and leads to further expansion of cumulus cells surrounding the oocyte and release of proteolytic enzymes involved in the process of ovulation. Agonist trigger showed better recovery of oocytes and higher fertilization rates in IVF compared to hCG trigger.[23]
- Agonist trigger leads to more maturity of the nucleus and the resumption of meiosis and subsequently increase in the number of metaphase II oocytes.
- Agonist trigger is associated with faster LH surge leading to better maturity of oocytes compared to hCG trigger.
- Agonist trigger significantly reduces the risk of OHSS. This is the most important benefit of using GnRH agonist trigger in hyper-responders.[24]
- The most important clinical advantage of GnRHa trigger is the potential to induce a rapid and reversible luteolysis and therefore decreasing the risk of OHSS progression. This results in severe luteal phase defect resulting from a short period of the induced LH and FSH peak. GnRH agonist particularly inhibits the secretion of vasoactive products, especially vascular endothelial growth factor (VEGF), from the corpus luteum.

Analysis of various studies shows that GnRH agonist trigger is the first choice and standard trigger in hyper-responders. A small additional bolus dose of hCG can be given for trigger or a modified luteal phase support can be given to women who plan for a fresh embryo transfer.[25]
- By reducing the OHSS risk, the overall cost of treatment is also reduced.

In the past, agonist trigger was followed by a freeze-all embryo for subsequent transfer, owing to severe luteolysis following agonist trigger.[26] But now, by adding small amount of hCG activity along with agonist trigger (dual trigger), or by doing recent modifications of luteal phase after GnRH agonist trigger, one gets an opportunity to continue the cycle and plan for fresh embryo transfer for women at risk for OHSS and achieve a good outcome.[27]

Segmentation of IVF Cycle

Freezing of all oocytes or embryos after GnRH trigger and transferring the embryos in a subsequent cycle is called "segmentation of IVF cycle". This procedure is of great benefit in women who are hyper-responders.[28,29]

Many studies and meta-analyses support segmentation cycles to show that pregnancies resulting from frozen-thawed embryo transfer (FET) in IVF have better obstetric and perinatal outcomes than fresh embryo transfer.[30] Some researchers have conflicting reports regarding FET cycles though.

Early GnRH Antagonist Protocol

In this protocol, GnRH antagonists are started early in the stimulation period, that is from Day-2.[31] A physiological increase in the FSH level during the luteal–follicular transition phase (interphase), in the GnRH antagonist cycles, may result in heterogeneous follicular development, leading to slightly lower mature oocyte yield. The presence of such—an asynchronized follicular growth may result in decreased mature oocyte yield with subsequent few embryos being formed. Hence, option of selection of good-quality embryos may be limited. It is believed that the interphase peak FSH increase can be inhibited by early GnRH antagonist administration initiated from the beginning of the menstrual cycle and such an early suppression of endogenous FSH may be advantageous for achieving follicular synchronization. This in turn leads to increased mature oocyte yield. The modified early GnRH antagonist start protocol may constitute an attractive alternative to the conventional antagonist protocols. The modified early GnRH antagonist start protocol has additional advantages over the previously attempted pretreatment strategies. First, this protocol can be commenced during the current menstrual cycle without waiting for the next cycle or without needing induced withdrawal bleeding. Secondly, this protocol may improve the early follicular endocrine environment by lowering the LH level, and LH support is provided when it is needed by highly purified human menopausal gonadotropin (HP-hMG).

Third, early antagonist administration can prevent earlier LH surges in some select patients. This has been proven in a multicenter randomized parallel-group trial comparing three different protocols that incorporated different modes of GnRH analog administration:[32] the early antagonist, conventional antagonist, and the long luteal. Early administration of a GnRH antagonist may possibly yield benefits due to a reduction in the incidence of moderate-to-severe OHSS in high-risk subjects with a similar number of oocytes retrieved, as well as a better clinical pregnancy rate per embryo transfer. To clarify these issues, further studies with more sample size are required.

Progesterone-primed Ovarian Stimulation Protocol

Though use of antagonist in downregulated cycle has solved lots of practical problems in our IVF clinics, but still a varied proportion (0.34–38%) of patients using GnRH antagonist protocol have been observed to experience a premature LH surge. So, there was a need for better options to prevent premature LH surge with good efficacy and safety profile. Oral contraceptive pills (OCPs) and synthetic progestin sharply decrease both serum FSH and LH values, with recovery of normal basal levels after a 5-day washout period. Previously when IVF treatment relied on fresh embryo transfers, progesterone could not be used to prevent LH surge, as it had negative effects on endometrial receptivity. But with the current scenario and advanced vitrification techniques, progesterone for prevention of LH surge can be used in controlled ovarian stimulation (COS). Medroxyprogesterone acetate (MPA) is an effective oral alternative for preventing premature LH surge in women undergoing COS for IVF. Kuang et al. reported the first randomized study which provided first-time evidence that MPA is effective as an oral treatment for the prevention of premature LH surge in women undergoing controlled ovarian hyperstimulation (COH) for IVF.[33] Here, MPA was used due to its certain merits over other progestins such as:
- Moderate-to-strong progestational action
- Fewer androgenic properties
- Does not interfere with measurement of endogenous progesterone production.

How does it work?
Progesterone inhibits GnRH pulse frequency which inhibits the LH pulsatility. Progesterone blocks the estrogen (E2)-induced gonadotropin surge.

But it was the study by Wang et al., which was the first randomised controlled trial to examine the efficacy and safety of a novel progestin-primed ovarian stimulation protocol in patients with PCOS who were undergoing IVF treatment.[34]

The benefits of the novel progesterone-primed ovarian stimulation (PPOS) protocol in terms of better pregnancy outcomes in women with

PCOS can be attributed to the following modifications of the hormonal and follicular microenvironmental milieu:
- Progestins in early follicular phase inhibit the synthesis and secretion of LH by reducing GnRH pulse frequency, which may correct abnormally high LH levels and hyperandrogenism in intrafollicular milieu during folliculogenesis and follicular maturation in women with PCOS.
- Progesterone plays a crucial role in oocyte maturation, fertilization, and embryo development directly or indirectly.
- There is accelerated conversion of progesterone to androstenedione in theca cells of PCOS women, due to high LH stimulation. This leads to a deficiency of progesterone in the intrafollicular milieu. So, addition of a progestin in a COS protocol in PCOS women seems rational to improve the follicular milieu for better follicular development, oocyte maturity, and pregnancy outcomes.

This study indicated that progestin treatment might improve oocyte quality, thereby better ongoing pregnancy rate and live birth rate along with reduced incidence of OHSS compared with a GnRH antagonist during COS in these patients.

There were additional advantages of an oral administration route instead of repeated injections of GnRH antagonist, a lower drug price, and more control over LH levels, which can reduce the patients' discomfort and costs.[35]

In a prospective RCT with 257 patients divided into two treatment groups at a 1:1 ratio of PPOS (130 patients) or GnRHa long protocol (127 patients) followed by their first IVF/ICSI with fresh/frozen embryo transfer where the primary outcome was the number of oocytes retrieved, they found no significant difference in the number (mean ± SD) of oocytes retrieved (11.8 ± 6.5 for PPOS vs. 11.3 ± 5.6 for GnRHa long protocol) or viable embryos (4.5 ± 3.0 for PPOS vs. 4.2 ± 2.9 for GnRHa long protocol) between the groups.[36] No patient from either group experienced a premature LH surge but, there were three cases of moderate or severe OHSS in GnRHa group and none in PPOS group. They found no significant difference in the clinical pregnancy rate of the first embryos transfer cycle between the two groups. They concluded that PPOS in combination with embryo cryopreservation as an ovarian stimulation regimen was as effective as GnRHa long protocol in ART cycles under varied endocrinal mechanisms. PPOS could also achieve comparable embryological and clinical outcomes while reducing the incidence of moderate and severe OHSS and gonadotropin dosage. It can be an alternative of the treatments for infertile patients with normal ovarian reserve undergoing IVF as well as traditional protocols.

In a meta-analysis published in 2021, authors tried to evaluate PPOS as conventional protocol for ART cycles where the primary outcome was clinical pregnancy rate, live birth rate, and incidence of OHSS, while, secondary outcomes were duration of stimulation, dose of gonadotropin for injection, progestin values on trigger day (ng/mL), number of retrieved oocytes, number of MII oocytes, number of obtained embryos, total cycle cancelation, and endometrial thickness. And they found that the PPOS protocol produces more embryos for transfer and a thicker endometrium than the control protocol, with a lower rate of OHSS and an equal live birth rate. Their conclusion was that the PPOS protocol could be a safe option as a personalized protocol for infertile patients.[37]

There are some studies where the progestins are started later on in the GnRH antagonist cycle, around Day-6 or 7 in a flexible way when at least one follicle reached ≥14 mm size.[38] This novel flexible PPOS (fPPOS) protocol seems to yield oocytes with similar reproductive potential as oocytes from GnRH antagonist cycle. Recipients of fresh oocytes from fPPOS and GnRH antagonist cycles had similar cleavage, blastulation, implantation, and live birth rates/ongoing pregnancy rates (50% vs. 48.6%). fPPOS with MPA seems to be an effective choice for preventing premature ovulation in women undergoing ovarian stimulation without compromising oocyte quality.

Some studies have shown conflicting results regarding efficacy of PPOS protocols in women with PCOS.

The large-scale application of PPOS could be revolutionary for several reasons. With the growing use of IVF, it is preferable to make the treatment as convenient as possible for the patients, possibly converting the route of administration from subcutaneous to oral intake. The cost of progestins compared with GnRH analogs also seems extremely beneficial. However, further studies are needed, especially on reproductive, obstetric, and long-term neonatal outcomes, before this protocol can be introduced on a wider scale.

The PPOS protocol can be used in all those patients who do not contemplate a fresh transfer which includes anticipated hyper-responders.[39]

In addition, a trend to a lower risk of preterm birth was observed among patients treated with PPOS protocol. The rate of formation of euploid blastocysts per oocyte was also similar (21%) in both treatment groups.[40] Dydrogesterone has also been used in PPOS protocol. A comparison was made between hMG (human menopausal gonadotropin) with dydrogesterone and hMG with MPA groups. There was no significant difference in the number of oocytes retrieved or in the incidence of OHSS. The clinical pregnancy rates were also similar between the two groups.[41]

The PPOS protocol was found to be safe and to have similar congenital malformation risk profile compared to other conventional IVF protocols in a meta-analysis of four studies done on 9,274 live-born infants **(Table 5)**.[42]

Mild Stimulation Protocol

A reduced gonadotropin dose is recommended to decrease the risk of OHSS in predicted hyper-responders if agonist protocols are used.[1] This type of

TABLE 5: Advantages and disadvantages of PPOS.

Advantages	Disadvantages
Convenient	Fresh embryo transfer not possible
Cost-effective	Cost may go high due to freeze all
Patient friendly	Long-term neonatal outcome has to be observed
Good tolerability	
No adverse effect of oocyte or embryo	

(PPOS: progesterone-primed ovarian stimulation)

TABLE 6: Principal advantages and disadvantages of mild ovarian stimulation for IVF.

Advantages	Disadvantages
Less patient discomfort	Fewer embryos available for cryopreservation
Fewer injections	Lower live birth rate per cycle in some studies
Lower risk of OHSS	Probable lower cumulative live birth rate (Including fresh and frozen transfers from a single oocyte retrieval)
Possible improvement in endometrial receptivity (Not proven)	
Possible improvement in embryo quality (Not proven)	
Cost-effectiveness (Not proven)	

(IVF: in vitro fertilization; OHSS: ovarian hyperstimulation syndrome)

stimulation protocol involves reduced dosage of gonadotropins or reduced duration of stimulation. The American Society for Reproductive Medicine (ASRM) Practice Committee proposed a daily dose of ≤150 IU gonadotropin (with or without oral compounds) to be considered as "mild ovarian stimulation" **(Table 6)**.[43-45]

Clomiphene can be used in mild stimulation protocol either for 5 days starting from Day-2 or till day of trigger.[46]

Letrozole can also be used with gonadotropins (hMG) in mild stimulation protocol.[47]

CONCLUSION

The success of any COS protocol depends primarily on its efficacy and safety profile, both in terms of reproductive and perinatal outcomes. Prevention of hyper-response begins with tailoring an individual's ovarian stimulation protocol based on their risk profile, through individualized COS. Selecting one standardized preventative approach for all patients undergoing COS is challenging, because the benefits and risks associated with each strategy vary between individuals. Identification of hormonal, functional, and genetic markers of ovarian response will help to facilitate an individualized COS. Treatment protocol for hyper-responders should focus on regimens which would reduce excessive ovarian response and its complications such as OHSS or cycle cancellations, but at the same time, it does not compromise on positive outcomes such as pregnancy rates and live birth rates. Dealing with hyper-responders begins with the identification of the "high-risk" woman through to the woman who is "actually at risk" and subsequently initiating the appropriate therapies. Women undergoing IVF face immense physical, mental, emotional, and financial burden. Hyper-response in these women adds exponentially to their burden. "Hyper-responder women" are an avenue toward which further research initiatives should be directed in a bid to strengthen the preexisting evidence base for available protocols and therapies and to develop novel protocols and techniques to aid in the prevention of hyper-response.

■ KEY POINTS

- Hyper-respondent group of patients are those who are actually at risk of getting ART-related complications like OHSS and multiple fetal gestations.
- The choice of protocols used for hyper-responders are antagonist protocol will step up gonadotropins uses and agonist trigger or dual trigger with sliding SCG doses.
- PPOS protocol is the new kid on the block which holds very good promise to become an ideal protocol, where we are freezing all the embryos.
- Segmented IVF should be mandatory for hyper-responders patient until proven otherwise.

■ REFERENCES

1. Guideline of the European Society of Human Reproduction and Embryology, October 2019. Ovarian Stimulation for IVF/ICSI.
2. Broer SL, Dólleman M, Opmeer BC, Fauser BC, Mol BW, Broekmans FJM. AMH and AFC as predictors of excessive response in controlled ovarian hyperstimulation: a meta-analysis. Hum Reprod Update. 2011;17(1):46-54.
3. Čuš M, Vlaisavljević V, Repnik K, Potočnik U, Kovačič B. Could polymorphisms of some hormonal receptor genes, involved in folliculogenesis help in predicting patient response to controlled ovarian stimulation? J Assist Reprod Genet. 2019;36(1):47-55.
4. Huber M, Hadziosmanovic N, Berglund L, Holte J. Using the ovarian sensitivity index to define poor, normal, and high response after controlled ovarian hyperstimulation in the long gonadotropin-releasing hormone-agonist protocol: suggestions for a new principle to solve an old problem. Fertil Steril. 2013;100(5):1270-6.

5. Revelli A, Gennarelli G, Biasoni V, Chiadò A, Carosso A, Evangelista F, et al. The ovarian sensitivity index (OSI) significantly correlates with ovarian reserve biomarkers, is more predictive of clinical pregnancy than the total number of oocytes, and is consistent in consecutive IVF cycles. J Clin Med. 2020;9(6):1914.
6. Matsuzaki T, Iwasa T, Yanagihara R, Komasaka M, Yano K, Mayila Y, et al. Pilot study of the optimal protocol of low dose step-up follicle stimulating hormone therapy for infertile women. Reprod Med Biol. 2018;17(3):315-24.
7. Koundouros SN. A comparison study of a novel stimulation protocol and the conventional low dose step-up and step-down regimens in patients with polycystic ovary syndrome undergoing in vitro fertilization. Fertil Steril. 2008;90(3):569-75.
8. Hugues JN, Cédrin-Durnerin I, Avril C, Bulwa S, Hervé F, Uzan M. Sequential step-up and step-down dose regimen: an alternative method for ovulation induction with follicle-stimulating hormone in polycystic ovarian syndrome. Hum Reprod. 1996;11(12):2581-4.
9. Bush MR, Swanson MS, Stephan S, Albrecht BH. Selective cut-back protocol for in-vitro fertilization (IVF) ovarian stimulation in patients with polycystic ovary syndrome (PCOS). Fertil Steril. 2007;88(1):S293.
10. Pouly JL, Olivennes F, Massin N, Celle M, Caizergues N, Contard F, et al. Usability and utility of the CONSORT calculator for FSH starting doses: a prospective observational study. Reprod Biomed Online. 2015;31:347-55.
11. Papaleo E, Zaffagnini S, Munaretto M, Vanni VS, Rebonato G, Grisendi V, et al. Clinical application of a nomogram based on age, serum FSH and AMH to select the FSH starting dose in IVF/ICSI cycles: a retrospective two-centres study. Eur J Obstet Gynecol Reprod Biol. 2016;207:94-9.
12. Nyboe Andersen A, Nelson SM, Fauser BC, García-Velasco JA, Klein BM, Arce JC, et al. Individualized versus conventional ovarian stimulation for in vitro fertilization: a multicenter, randomized, controlled, assessor-blinded, phase 3 noninferiority trial. Fertil Steril. 2017;107:387-96.
13. Oudshoorn SC, van Tilborg TC, Eijkemans MJC, Oosterhuis GJE, Friederich J, van Hooff MHA, et al.; on behalf of OPTIMIST study group. Individualized versus standard FSH dosing in women starting IVF/ICSI: an RCT. Part 2: The predicted hyper-responder. Hum Reprod. 2017;32(12):2506-14.
14. Lensen SF, Wilkinson J, Leijdekkers JA, La Marca A, Mol BWJ, Marjoribanks J, et al. Individualised gonadotropin dose selection using markers of ovarian reserve for women undergoing in vitro fertilisation plus intracytoplasmic sperm injection (IVF/ICSI). Cochrane Database Syst Rev. 2018;2(2):CD012693.
15. Gunnala V, Melnick A, Irani M, Reichman D, Schattman G, Davis O, et al. Sliding scale hCG trigger yields equivalent pregnancy outcomes and reduces ovarian hyperstimulation syndrome. Analysis of 10,427 IVF-ICSI cycles. PLoS One. 2017;12(4):e0176019.
16. Kashyap S, Parker K, Cedars MI, Rosenwaks Z. Ovarian hyperstimulation syndrome prevention strategies: reducing the human chorionic gonadotropin trigger dose. Semin Reprod Med. 2010;28(6):475-85.
17. Damario MA. Ovarian hyperstimulation syndrome prevention strategies: oral contraceptive pills-dual gonadotropin-releasing hormone agonist suppression with step-down gonadotropin protocols. Semin Reprod Med. 2010;28(6):468-74.
18. Wang L, Zhao Y, Dong X, Huang K, Wang R, Ji L, et al. Could pretreatment with oral contraceptives before pituitary down regulation reduce the incidence of

ovarian hyperstimulation syndrome in the IVF/ICSI procedure? Int J Clin Exp Med. 2015;8(2):2711-8.
19. Gustofson RL, Larsen FW, Bush MR, Segars JH. Treatment with GnRH antagonist in women suppressed with GnRH agonist may avoid cycle cancellation in patients at risk for ovarian hyperstimulation syndrome. Fertil Steril. 2006;85(1):251-4.
20. Toftager M, Bogstad J, Byrndorf T, Loss K, Roskaer J, Holland T, et al. Risk of severe OHSS in GnRH Antagonist Versus GnRH Agonist protocol, RCT including 1050 first IVF/ICSI cycles. Hum Reprod. 2016;31(6):1253-64.
21. Lambalk CB, Banga FR, Huirne JA, Toftager M, Pinborg A, Homburg R, et al. GnRH antagonist versus long agonist protocols in IVF: a systematic review and meta-analysis accounting for patient type. Hum Reprod Update. 2017;23(5):560-79.
22. Alyasin A, Mehdinejadiani S, Ghasemi M. GnRH agonist trigger versus hCG trigger in GnRH antagonist in IVF/ICSI cycle: a review article. Int J Reprod Biomed. 2016;14(9):557-66.
23. Lamb JD, Shen S, McCulloch C, Jalalian L, Cedars MI, Rosen MP. Follicle-stimulating hormone administered at the time of human chorionic gonadotropin trigger improves oocyte developmental competence in in vitro fertilization cycles: a randomized, double-blind, placebo-controlled trial. Fertil Steril. 2011;95:1655-60.
24. Fatemi HM, Popovic-Todorovic B, Humaiden P, Kol S, Banker M, Devroey P, et al. Severe ovarian hyperstimulation syndrome after gonadotropin-releasing hormone (GnRH) agonist trigger and freeze-all approach in GnRH antagonist protocol. Fertil Steril. 2014;101(4):1008-11.
25. Iliodromiti S, Blockeel C, Tremellen KP, Fleming R, Toumaye H, Humaiden P, et al. Consistent high clinical pregnancy rates and low ovarian hyperstimulation syndrome rates in high risk patients after GnRH agonist triggering and modified luteal support: a retrospective multicentre study. Hum Reprod. 2013;28(9):2529-36.
26. Shapiro BS, Andersen CY. Major drawbacks and additional benefits of agonist trigger—not ovarian hyperstimulation related. Fertil Steril. 2015;103(4):874-8.
27. Humaiden P, Polyzos NP, Alsbjerg B, Erb K, Mikkelsen AL, Elbaek HO, et al. GnRHa trigger and individualized luteal phase hCG support according to ovarian response to stimulation: two prospective randomized controlled multi-centre studies in IVF patients. Hum Reprod. 2013;28(9):2511-21.
28. Devroey P, Polyzos NP, Blockeel C. An OHSS-Free Clinic by segmentation of IVF treatment. Hum Reprod. 2011;26(10):2593-7.
29. Garcia-Velasco JA. Agonist trigger: what is the best approach? Agonist trigger with vitrification of oocytes or embryos. Fertil Steril. 2012;97(3):527-8.
30. Maheshwari A, Pandey S, Shetty A, Hamilton M, Bhattacharya S. Obstetric and perinatal outcomes in singleton pregnancies resulting from the transfer of frozen-thawed versus fresh embryos generated through in vitro fertilization treatment: a systematic review and meta-analysis. Fertil Steril. 2012;98(2):368-77.e 1-9.
31. Park CW, Hwang YI, Koo HS, Kang IS, Yang KM, Song IO. Early gonadotropin-releasing hormone antagonist start improves follicular synchronization and pregnancy outcome as compared to the conventional antagonist protocol. Clin Exp Reprod Med. 2014;41(4):158-64.
32. Shin JJ, Park KE, Choi YM, Kim HO, Choi DH, Lee WS, et al. Early gonadotropin-releasing hormone antagonist protocol in women with polycystic ovary syndrome: a preliminary randomized trial. Clin Exp Reprod Med. 2018;45(3):135-42.

33. Kuang Y, Chen Q, Fu Y, Wang Y, Hong Q, Lyu Q, et al. Medroxyprogesterone acetate is an effective oral alternative for preventing premature luteinizing hormone surges in women undergoing controlled ovarian hyperstimulation for in vitro fertilization. Fertil Steril. 2015;104(1):62-70.e3.
34. Wang N, Zhu Q, Ma M, et al. Comparison of a progestin-primed ovarian stimulation protocol in patients with polycystic ovary syndrome who are participating in an IVF programme: study protocol for a randomized controlled trial. BMJ Open. 2020;10:e038153.
35. Xiao ZN, Peng JL, Yang J, Xu WM. Flexible GnRH Antagonist Protocol versus Progestin-primed Ovarian Stimulation (PPOS) Protocol in Patients with Polycystic Ovary Syndrome: Comparison of Clinical Outcomes and Ovarian Response. Curr Med Sci. 2019;39:431-6.
36. Xi Q, Tao Y, Qiu M, Wang Y, Kuang Y. Comparison between PPOS and GnRHa-long protocol in clinical outcome with the first IVF/ICSI cycle: a randomized clinical trial. Clin Epidemiol. 2020;12:261-72.
37. Cui L, Lin Y, Wang F, Chen C. Effectiveness of progesterone-primed ovarian stimulation in assisted reproductive technology: a systematic review and meta-analysis. Arch Gynecol Obstet. 2021;303(3):615-30.
38. Yildiz S, Turkgeldi E, Angun B, Eraslan A, Urman B, Ata B. Comparison of a novel flexible progestin primed ovarian stimulation protocol and the flexible gonadotropin-releasing hormone antagonist protocol for assisted reproductive technology. Fertil Steril. 2019;112(4):677-83.
39. Ata B, Capuzzo M, Turkgeldi E, Yildiz S, La Marca A. Progestins for pituitary suppression during ovarian stimulation for ART: a comprehensive and systematic review including meta-analyses. Hum Reprod Update. 2021;27(1):48-66.
40. La Marca A, Capuzzo M, Sacchi S, Imbrogno MG, Spinella F, Varricchio MT, et al. Comparison of euploidy rates of blastocysts in women treated with progestins or GnRH antagonist to prevent the luteinizing hormone surge during ovarian stimulation. Hum Reprod. 2020;35(6):1325-31.
41. Yu S, Long H, Chang HY, Liu Y, Gao H, Zhu J, et al. New application of dydrogesterone as a part of a progestin-primed ovarian stimulation protocol for IVF: a randomized controlled trial including 516 first IVF/ICSI cycles. Hum Reprod. 2018;33(2):229-37.
42. Zolfaroli I, Ferriol GA, Mora JH, Cano A. Impact of progestin ovarian stimulation on newborn outcomes: a meta-analysis. J Assist Reprod Genet. 2020;37:1203-12.
43. Practice Committee Documents of the American Society for Reproductive Medicine. Comparison of pregnancy rates for poor responders using IVF with mild ovarian stimulation versus conventional IVF: A Guideline (2018).
44. Datta AK, Maheshwari A, Felix N, Campbell S, Nargund G. Mild versus conventional ovarian stimulation for IVF in poor, normal and hyper-responders: a systematic review and meta-analysis. Hum Reprod Update. 2021;27(2):229-53.
45. Nargund G, Fauser BCJM. Mild ovarian stimulation for IVF is the smartest way forward. Reprod Biomed Online. 2020;41(4):569-71.
46. Teramoto S, Kato O. Minimal ovarian stimulation with clomiphene citrate: a large-scale retrospective study. Reprod Biomed Online. 2007;15(2):134-48.
47. D'Amato G, Caringella AM, Stanziano A, Cantatore C, Palini S, Caroppo E. Mild ovarian stimulation with letrozole plus fixed dose human menopausal gonadotropin prior to IVF/ICSI for infertile non-obese women with polycystic ovarian syndrome being pre-treated with metformin: a pilot study. Reprod Biol Endocrinol. 2018;16(1):89.

Chapter 19

Ovarian Stimulation Protocols for Poor Responders

Gautam Khastgir, Utpala Sen

■ INTRODUCTION

Poor ovarian response (POR) is a challenging clinical condition in the field of assisted reproduction. Up to one-fourth of patients undergoing ovarian stimulation for in vitro fertilization (IVF) show POR.[1] These patients encompass the most vulnerable group concerning treatment failure and eventual dropout. Etiopathology of POR is a complex immunobiochemical process, which is poorly understood till date. However, there are some established factors which are responsible for POR. Depletion of ovarian follicle is one of the most important factors in this regard. This depletion can be contributed by natural aging process, chromosomal and genetic disorder, endometriosis, autoimmune disease, ovarian surgery, and chemotherapy.

Poor response in IVF treatment was first reported by Garcia et al. in 1983.[2] Subsequently, numerous studies have been conducted on poor responders. In 2011, a systematic review by Polyzos and Devroey highlighted 41 different definitions of POR in 47 randomized trials.[3] Lack of a uniform definition of poor response in those days made it difficult to compare studies and therefore no universally accepted management strategy evolved. In the same year, European Society for Human Reproduction and Embryology (ESHRE) put forward Bologna criteria (BC)—the first standardized definition of POR.[4]

■ CLASSIFICATION OF POOR RESPONDERS

According to BC, poor response in IVF has been defined when at least two of the following three features are present: (1) advanced maternal age (≥40 years) or any other risk factor for POR, (2) a previous POR (less than three oocyte retrieved), and (3) an abnormal ovarian reserve test (ORT) [antral follicle count (AFC) <7 or anti-Müllerian hormone (AMH) <1.1 ng/mL].[4] In the absence of advanced maternal age or abnormal ORT, two episodes of POR after maximal stimulation should also be considered as poor response. Several studies[5-7] in 2014 and 2015 have reported low-birth rate of around 6%

after following the BC. Moreover, subsequent investigations have revealed a significant heterogenicity within the BC population, where younger subjects showed better clinical prognosis.[8]

Continued effort to standardize the diagnosis of POR and to overcome the shortcomings of the BC, in 2016, a modified definition of "impaired ovarian response" has been proposed by the POSEIDON (Patient-Oriented Strategies Encompassing Individualized Oocyte Number) Group.[9] This novel classification advocates a better stratification of the "low-prognosis patient". It proposes four subgroups based on (1) quantitative and qualitative parameters such as age and the expected aneuploidy rate; (2) ovarian reserve biomarkers (AFC and/or AMH); and (3) ovarian response—provided a previous stimulation cycle has been performed.[1] Depending on age, oocyte yield, and ovarian reserve, POSEIDON group has introduced two main categories. Group 1 and 2 consist of "unexpected" poor response, while group 3 and 4 comprises "expected" poor response[10] **(Table 1)**. Group 1 and 2 are divided in subgroups depending on number of AFC (1a < 4; 1b 4–9; 2a <4; 2b <4–9). Overall, patients in groups 2 and 4 are older and therefore the risk of embryo aneuploidy is higher. On the contrary, subjects belonging to group 1 and 2 are young and have better ORT with relatively low risk of aneuploidy.

Drakopoulos et al.[1] conducted a SWOT (strengths, weaknesses, opportunities, and threats) analysis of POSEIDON criteria to identify its advantages and disadvantages. Identified strength was inclusion of both quantitative and qualitative criteria, better stratification of low-prognosis patients, and more homogeneous subpopulation of low-prognosis women. This has further enhanced the global acceptance of this classification. POSEIDON criteria not only help clinicians to identify and classify patients who have potentially low prognosis in assisted reproductive technology (ART), but also assist clinicians to formulate individualized treatment plan to maximize success rate.

■ MANAGEMENT

The POSEIDON population constitutes 47% of patients referred for IVF treatment. 55% of the patients belong to group 4 and 10% in group 3.[11]

TABLE 1: Risk stratification of POR (POSEIDON criteria).

	Adequate ovarian reserve		Poor ovarian reserve	
	Group I	*Group II*	*Group III*	*Group IV*
Age (years)	<35	≥35	<35	≥35
AFC	≥5	≥5	<5	<5
AMH	≥1.2 ng/mL	≥1.2 ng/mL	<1.2 ng/mL	<1.2 ng/mL

(AFC: antral follicle count; AMH: anti-Müllerian hormone; POR: poor ovarian response)

Treatment Modalities

Pituitary Suppression Regimens (Prestimulation Treatment)

Follicular development and ovulation from puberty till menopause take place in waves. An intact hypothalamo-pituitary-ovarian axis is required for the maintenance of this process. A complex neuroendocrine and hormonal interaction is essential for a development of a dominant follicle.

In poor responders, increased luteal phase follicle-stimulating hormone (FSH) promotes early recruitment of dominant follicle, which suppresses the growth of other developing follicles. The suppression of endogenous FSH is required to achieve synchronized development of adequate number of follicles. This suppression may be achieved by using estrogen, progestogen, oral contraceptive pills (OCPs), and gonadotropin-releasing hormone (GnRH) antagonist.

The ESHRE recommendation for ovulation induction[12] does not endorse use of estrogen or progesterone as a pretreatment, due to paucity of strong evidence. However, increased number of retrieved oocytes were reported with estrogen therapy, compared to no treatment. Same authors reported insufficient evidence regarding number of oocytes and live birth rate (LBR) while using progesterone. No difference in LBR/ongoing pregnancy rate or number of oocytes was reported while using OCP.[12]

Maged et al. in 2015[13] showed significant increase in clinical pregnancy rate (CPR) up to 30% along with number of oocytes in a delayed start protocol. They used OCP and estrogen in an antagonist protocol. In contrast, Aflatoonian[14] in 2017 showed no difference in CPR or number of oocytes retrieved, compared to conventional GnRH antagonist protocol. Therefore, GnRH antagonist pretreatment in a delayed start gonadotropin protocol is not favored.

Types of Protocol with Gonadotropins

Gonadotropin-stimulated cycles are designed to amplify ovary's natural follicular recruitment and development. Role of various forms of gonadotropins in ovarian stimulation is well established. However, there is no robust evidence to suggest significant difference in efficacy of different types of gonadotropins in POR. Essentially, the selection of molecule is driven by institutional preference, ease of administration, and economic considerations. The literature, therefore, reflects results of permutation and combination of various molecules. Recombinant FSH (rFSH), purified FSH, highly purified FSH, long-acting FSH, and human menopausal gonadotropins (hMG) are equally recommended for agonist protocol in general.

There is some evidence that the addition of recombinant human luteinizing hormone (rhLH) to rFSH may have beneficial effects on outcomes in women with POR. This combination results in increased FSH receptor expression and growth, improved follicular recruitment, and a reduced rate of granulosa cell apoptosis.[9]

In a meta-analysis in 2017, no difference in LBR, CPR, and oocyte yield was reported while comparing long agonist protocol with anatogonist.[15] Xiao[16] also showed no difference in CPR while comparing antagonist protocol with short agonist. However, fewer oocytes were retrieved in antagonist protocol. On the contrary, increased CPR of 29% with short agonist protocol was reported by Schimberni[17] with no difference in the number of oocytes.

Patients with diminished ovarian reserve (DOR), who are also expected poor responders, have been analyzed in a retrospective study by Ming-Chao Huang et al.[18] They concluded that GnRH agonist long protocol was more effective than GnRH antagonist protocol in young patients with DOR. In agonist group, injection leuprolide acetate 0.5 mg daily was commenced from mid-luteal phase of their pretreatment cycle. hMG of 300 IU was started from Day-2 or Day-3 of menstruation. Same dose of gonadotropin used in antagonist protocol where antagonist Cetrorelix 0.25 mg daily started on 6th day of hMG stimulation. They found lower LBR in antagonist group, though it was not statistically significant.

In another study, Sunkara et al.[19] compared long agonist protocol with short agonist and antagonist regime. In long agonist protocol, 400 µg of GnRH agonist was used as nasal spray once daily for 2 weeks, which was commenced in the mid-luteal phase. The dose was reduced to 200 µg daily with the onset of ovarian stimulation with gonadotropin. For short protocol, they used 200 µg of GnRH agonist along with gonadotropins, which was started on Day-2 or Day-3 of menstruation. For antagonist protocol, dose of 0.25 mg daily was started when the lead follicle reached 14 mm. In all three arms, same gonadotropin has been used and continued until human chorionic gonadotropin (hCG) trigger. They concluded that short agonist protocol is associated with less oocyte retrieved, which is not desirable in poor responders. Poor oocyte yield could be explained by the elevated progesterone level during early follicular phase, which is responsible for impaired follicular recruitment. Similar inference is also documented in a recent retrospective study by Madani et al.[20]

A prospective randomized controlled trial (RCT)[21] conducted on poor responders compared long GnRH agonist protocol with GnRH agonist stop protocol. In the study group (stop protocol), GnRH agonist administration was stopped with the onset of menstruation while gonadotropins administration was same in the control and study group. It was determined that early cessation of GnRH analog is associated with significantly higher number of oocyte retrieval.

Another study in 2021[22] confirmed that combination of Stop GnRH analog, letrozole priming, and multiple-dose GnRH antagonist controlled ovarian hyperstimulation protocol results in significantly higher number of follicles

>13 mm on the day of hCG administration and higher number of oocytes as well. In this study, patients received GnRH agonist triptorelin 0.1 mg/day from mid-luteal phase which was stopped at the onset of menstruation. Ovarian suppression was confirmed by E_2 level and ultrasonography findings. Letrozole 5 mg/day was then started and continued for 5 days followed by higher dose of gonadotropins. Once the leading follicle reached 13 mm, co-treatment with antagonist 0.5 mg/day was commenced and continued until the day of hCG trigger. Increased number of follicles and oocyte yield was noted in this study. They specially focused on POSEIDON Group 4 which is the most difficult subset of patients for IVF treatment.

There are conflicting data emerging from multiple studies looking at comparison between agonist and antagonist protocol. Therefore, both agonist and antagonist protocols are recommended by ESHRE guideline.[23]

The dose of gonadotropin is generally 150–300 IU. Higher number of oocytes are retrieved when 300–450 are used. However, no significant difference was observed in CPR. There is no study about the reduced dose (<150 IU) of gonadotropin.

Natural Cycle IVF/Mild Stimulation

Natural cycle IVF was suggested by some authors to avoid embryonic aneuploidy rate in stimulated cycles. It, however, did not get popularity because of its extremely low LBR (2.6% per cycle).[24]

Mild stimulation for IVF is a relatively new advancement in artificial reproductive technology, emerging as an alternative to traditional IVF. It has evolved, based on the principle of reduction of dosage and duration of ovarian stimulation aimed at producing 3–5 high-quality oocytes per IVF cycle. There is now ample evidence in the literature to refute the initial concern that mild IVF may severely compromise pregnancy and LBRs.

Originally, mild stimulation protocols were proposed to combat some of the shortcomings of traditional IVF. In the recent years, evidence is emerging on the role of this protocol on a very challenging subset of patients—"the poor responders".

Mild stimulation protocol involves administration of lesser dose of exogenous gonadotropins in GnRH antagonist co-treated cycles, in combination with oral antiestrogens like clomiphene citrate (CC) or aromatase inhibitors.

Ragni et al.[25] in 2012 reported similar LBR while comparing CC with short agonist FSH protocol. On the contrary, significant reduction in CPR was also reported when CC was added, compared to non-CC group.

Numerous studies have investigated various stimulation approaches for poor responders, over the last decade; However, a universally agreed protocol, which is unequivocally effective, is yet to be established.

Alberto Revelli et al.[26] conducted a study on expected poor responders in 2014. They used CC 100 μg/day from day 2 of cycle for 5 days, followed by hMG 150 IU s/c from the last day of CC. GnRH antagonist 0.25 mg/day was then started from day 8 until the day of ovulation trigger. In this study, urinary human chorionic gonadotropin (uhCG) 10,000 s/c has been used for final maturation of oocyte before oocyte retrieval.

They concluded that low dose stimulation in an antagonist cycle with uhCG trigger in poor responders resulted in similar clinical outcome as compared to classical long protocol with high doses of gonadotropins.

Minimal stimulation has also been done with CC from day 2 to 6 in the dosage of 100 mg daily, along with rFSH 150 IU s/c daily. Injection Cetrorelix was then commenced when diameter of follicle reached more than 14 mm. This was continued till the day of hCG injection. This was compared with a control arm of conventional treatment protocol. CPR, LBR, and miscarriage rate were comparable in both arms, despite higher number of cumulous oophorous complex in the conventional stimulation group.[27] Another retrospective multicentric cohort study confirmed that lesser number of oocytes are retrieved following mild stimulation, without jeopardizing LBR.[28]

Letrozole, an aromatase inhibitor, found a place for treatment of women with POR. Though initial standalone reports showed promising results with this molecule, ESHRE guidelines published in 2019 do not recommend this agent in the treatment of poor responders.[23]

A multi-center randomized trial was done by Youssef et al.[29] in 2017, where they use only low-dose gonadotropin (FSH—150 IU/day) from day 5, without using oral ovulation inducing drugs with an antagonist protocol for mild stimulation group. The conventional treatment group received high-dose gonadotropins in an agonist cycle. They found no significant difference in ongoing pregnancy rate, though the duration of ovarian stimulation and requirement of gonadotropins were much less in mild stimulation group.

Dual Stimulation

Dual stimulation in the same ovarian cycle is a novel approach to ovarian stimulation, which is particularly beneficial for poor responders and patients with poor ovarian reserve. Combination of follicular and luteal phase stimulation (LPS) was first reported by *Kuang et al.*[30] in 2014. The first stimulation was started with CC 25 mg per day from day 3 until ovulation trigger, combined with aromatase inhibitor (Letrozole) 2.5 mg per day starting on day 3 for 4 days, and hMG 150 IU every other day starting on Day 6 until the ovulation trigger. The second stimulation was instituted after the first oocyte retrieval, provided two or more antral follicles were identified. Letrozole 2.5 mg and hMG 225 IU per day were commenced from the day of retrieval until second ovulation trigger. For both the stimulations, final oocyte maturation was induced by using GnRH agonist Triptorelin 0.1 mg when three or more follicles attain size of 18 mm or more in diameter. Premature LH surge was prevented by using short term use of nonsteroidal anti-inflammatory drugs (NSAIDs) (ibuprofen 600 mg) for 2 days starting from the day of ovulation trigger. No GnRH antagonist was used for prevention of premature LH surge. They reported at least 1–6 embryos after double ovarian stimulation in the same cycle.

Later in 2018, Vaiarelli et al.[31] reported the increased chance of obtaining at least one euploid blastocyst in a single ovarian cycle from 40 to 70%. In contrast to previous studies, they have used maximal dose of FSH and LH in an antagonist protocol in follicular phase stimulation (FPS) and LPS. This approach reduced the risk of cycle cancellation and maximized oocyte yield per stimulation. All patients in this study received luteal estradiol priming (4 mg/day) from day 21 of menstrual cycle, to synchronize the follicular development. FPS was started with FSH 300 IU along with LH 75 IU per day. GnRH antagonist was started once the dominant follicle reached size of more than 13–14 mm, until the ovulation trigger. Final maturation was obtained by GnRH agonist. Five days after the first retrieval, LPS was started with the same protocol. All patients underwent frozen-thawed embryo transfer. In this, higher mean number of oocytes retrieved following LPS than FPS. However, both the stimulations have comparable clinical outcome. More important, the rate of obtaining a single euploid blastocyst has increased from 42.3 to 65.5% following dual stimulation.

Adjuvant Therapy

Growth hormone: Use of growth hormone in poor responders has increased LBR and oocyte yield, reported by a systemic review and meta-analysis.[32] However, ESHRE guideline does not recommend growth hormone as an adjuvant therapy, as there is no significant difference in ongoing pregnancy rate or number of oocytes retrieved.

Testosterone: Testosterone is an important agent used for poor responders. It can be used as pretreatment and also during ovarian stimulation. It is generally available as gel or dermal patch for topical use. Pretreatment dose of gel ranges from 10 to 12 mg/day and is used for 15–21 days during pituitary suppression. Patches are used in the dosage of 2.5 mg daily for 5 days. A Cochrane meta-analysis reported improved LBR with testosterone pretreatment.[33] Same authors found no difference in LBR when results were analyzed with exclusion of studies at high-risk performance bias. Therefore, testosterone pretreatment is not universally accepted.

Dehydroepiandrosterone (DHEA): This molecule has been used in poor responders with a dose of 75 mg/day. A Cochrane meta-analysis reported increased CPR with the use of DHEA. However, there are some studies in the literature which refute this evidence and therefore uniform consensus is lacking.

Aspirin: There is paucity of evidence to favor the use of aspirin, though there are anecdotal reports of its use as adjunctive therapy for poor responders.

Sildenafil: Co-administration of sildenafil with other modes of ovarian stimulation has been reported in some studies with controversial outcome.

Individualized Treatment Protocols based on POSEIDON "Expected" and "Unexpected" Stratification

Poor responders have a very low prognosis in spite of giving maximal effort. It is, therefore, prudent to focus on group 1 and 2, who are unexpected poor responders. There are no universally accepted treatment guidelines for these groups.

Management of Group 1

These patients have superior prognosis because of their age group (<35 years), better ORT (AFC ≥ 5, AMH ≥ 1.2 ng/mL). The pathophysiology in this group has diversity, starting from FSH receptor polymorphism to the effect of beta subunit of LH. These patients require higher dose of gonadotropin due to their suboptimal stimulation.[34,35] A recent retrospective study in 2018 reported that increase in the starting dose of FSH would yield more oocytes in patients who had suboptimal response in previous treatment cycle.[9] Patients who have genetic variant of LH gene would benefit from recombinant LH supplementation. These patients showed increased oocyte yield and higher CPR in spite of having normal ORT or inadequate response in previous cycle.[36] Dual stimulation should also be considered in this group.[37] The use of adjuvant therapy with growth hormone and testosterone is still restricted in this group due to lack of evidence.

Management of Group 2

This group consists of patients who are ≥35 years with AMH value 1.2 ng/mL and AFC ≥ 5 with a history of unexpected poor response. The increase in aneuploidy and decrease in euploid embryos are associated with increased age in this group.

The right pituitary suppression regimen with ideal gonadotropin selection and optimization of dose is required to develop an euploid blastocyst for maximum implantation potential.

The long GnRH protocol is preferred to short GnRH agonist regimen in this group.[38] However, antagonist protocol can also be used. Increased dose of gonadotropin in the range of 150–225 IU daily for stimulation would benefit them with higher number of oocyte yield.[39] Presence of FSH or LH receptor polymorphism will dictate use of LH supplementation in this group.[40] Adjuvant therapy in this group is still under trial.

Management of Group 3 and 4

This group consists of patients with AMH value <1.2 ng/mL and AFC < 5. The patients present significant challenge in clinical management due to paucity of comparative study in this regard.

Recently, a predictive tool named ART calculator was introduced. This calculator measures the number of oocytes required to get at least one euploid blastocyst for transfer. On the basis of some important factors, for instance age, sperm quality, and number of mature metaphase II (MII) oocyte, the calculator can make two types of predictions automatically. First, by using pretreatment information, it calculates the minimum number of oocytes required for a single euploid blastocyst. Second, it can predict the probability of having euploid blastocyst based on the actual number of mature oocytes retrieved. A final logistic regression analysis model was developed based on the above predictors.[41]

Natural cycle IVF is not recommended, as the number of mature oocytes is extremely important in this group. Moreover, low LBR after natural cycle has been reported by many studies. Addition of rLH (150 IU) to higher dose of rFSH (300 IU) in long downregulation protocol is also a promising option.[42]

Pu D et al.[43] in 2011, in their study, concluded that CPR is similar while comparing long GnRH agonist downregulation protocol to the primed GnRH regimen. However, Sunkara[19] reported increased number of oocytes in long protocol. This may be related to good synchronization of the follicle during downregulation, which subsequently enhances the number of oocytes. They also reported that just on more oocytes would increase the LBR by approximately 5%.[44] A recent retrospective study concluded that higher LBR can be achieved by using in GnRH antagonist protocol in POSEIDON group 3. This effect, however, was not observed in group 4. In patients with reduced AFC (<4), combination of recombinant LH and recombinant FSH is superior to hMG with regard to CPR.[45]

Dual stimulation is also effective for this population. High ongoing pregnancy rate of 20.7% has been reported in the literature.[26]

Overall, individualization of stimulation protocol would reduce cycle cancellation and increase the number of good-quality oocyte to obtain euploid blastocyst. This is the key to success in optimizing LBR. Recombinant FSH alone or in combination with recombinant LH is the best choice in group 4. Here, hMG does not add any significant benefit with regard to CPR or LBR. Use of corifollitropin alfa, a long acting FSH, followed by hMG can hypothetically increase the cumulative LBR. Nevertheless, more statistically significant results are warranted in this regard.[46]

■ CONCLUSION

Poor ovarian response is one of the most challenging situations in ART. Though this difficult setting of patients was recognized decades ago, a universally accepted definition evolved much later, in 2011 with ESHRE publication of BC. Further standardization of risk stratification evolved through the POSEIDON classification. Standardized diagnostic criteria have led to significant progress toward the development of evidence-based management strategies for POR. The innovative technique of ART calculator now is in practice to predict the minimum number of metaphase II oocytes to obtain at least one euploid blastocyst for transfer in each patient. Nevertheless, overall outcome of ovarian stimulation and subsequent reproductive outcome of this subset of patients remain suboptimal till date.

■ KEY POINTS

- One-fourth of patients undergoing IVF treatment are poor ovarian responders (POR).
- First standardized definition of POR with classification—The Bologna criteria was established by ESHRE.
- POSIEDON—Another novel classification offers superior stratification of poor responders.
- Minimal stimulation protocol scores over the natural cycle IVF in poor responders.
- Both agonist and antagonist protocols are considered equally efficacious
- Role of adjuvant therapy is yet to be established.
- POSIEDON classification has opened up new avenues for individualization of treatment protocol.
- ART calculator is an innovative tool for prediction of treatment outcome.

■ REFERENCES

1. Drakopoulos P, Bardhi E, Boudry L, Vaiarelli A, Makrigiannakis A, Esteves SC, et al. Update on the management of poor ovarian response in IVF: the shift from Bologna criteria to the POSEIDON concept. Ther Adv Reprod Health. 2020;14:2633494120941480.
2. Garcia JE, Jones GS, Acosta AA, Wright G. HMG/hCG follicular maturation for oocytes aspiration: phase II, 1981. Fertil Steril. 1983;39:174-9.
3. Polyzos NP, Devroey P. A systematic review of randomized trials for the treatment of poor ovarian responders: is there any light at the end of the tunnel? Fertil Steril. 2011;96(5):1058-61.
4. Ferraretti AP, La Marca A, Fauser BC, Tarlatzis B, Nargund G, Gianaroli L; ESHRE Working Group on Poor Ovarian Response Definition. ESHRE consensus on the definition of 'poor response' to ovarian stimulation for in vitro fertilization: The Bologna criteria. Hum Reprod. 2011;26(7):1616-24.
5. Polyzos NP, Tournaye H. Poor ovarian responders: to meta-analyses or not, that is the question. Hum Reprod. 2014;29(3):634-5.

6. La Marca A, Grisendi V, Giulini S, Sighinolfi G, Tirelli A, Argento C, et al. Live birth rates in the different combinations of the Bologna criteria poor ovarian responders: a validation study. J Assist Reprod Genet. 2015;32(6):931-7.
7. Busnelli A, Papaleo E, Del Prato D, La Vecchia I, Iachini E, Paffoni A, et al. A retrospective evaluation of prognosis and cost-effectiveness of IVF in poor responders according to the Bologna criteria. Hum Reprod. 2015;30(2):315-22.
8. Xu B, Chen Y, Geerts D, Yue J, Li Z, Zhu G, et al. Cumulative live birth rates in more than 3,000 patients with poor ovarian response: a 15-year survey of final in vitro fertilization outcome. Fertil Steril. 2018;109(6):1051-9.
9. Alviggi C, Andersen CY, Buehler K, Conforti A, De Placido G, Esteves SC, et al. A new more detailed stratification of low responders to ovarian stimulation: from a poor ovarian response to a low prognosis concept. Fertil Steril. 2016;105(6):1452-3.
10. Esteves SC, Roque M, Bedoschi GM, Conforti A, Humaidan P, Alviggi C. Defining low prognosis patients undergoing assisted reproductive technology: POSEIDON Criteria-The Why. Front Endocrinol (Lausanne). 2018;9:461.
11. Haahr T, Dosouto C, Alviggi C, Esteves SC, Humaidan P. Management strategies for POSEIDON groups 3 and 4. Front Endocrinol (Lausanne). 2019;10:614.
12. Farquhar C, Rombauts L, Kremer JA, Lethaby A, Ayeleke RO. Oral contraceptive pill, progestogen or oestrogen pretreatment for ovarian stimulation protocols for women undergoing assisted reproductive techniques. Cochrane Database Syst Rev. 2017;(5):CD006109.
13. Maged A, Nada A, Abohamila F, Hashem A, Mostafa W, Elzayat A. Delayed Start Versus Conventional GnRH Antagonist Protocol in Poor Responders Pretreated With Estradiol in Luteal Phase: a Randomized Controlled Trial. Reprod Sci. 2015;22(12):1627-31.
14. Aflatoonian A, Hosseinisadat A, Baradaran R, Farid Mojtahedi M. Pregnancy outcome of "delayed start" GnRH antagonist protocol versus GnRH antagonist protocol in poor responders: A clinical trial study. Int J Reprod Biomed (Yazd, Iran). 2017;15:231-8.
15. Lambalk CB, Banga FR, Huirne JA, Toftager M, Pinborg A, Homburg R, et al. GnRH antagonist versus long agonist protocols in IVF: a systematic review and meta-analysis accounting for patient type. Hum Reprod Update. 2017;23(5):560-79.
16. Xiao J, Chang S, Chen S. The effectiveness of gonadotropin-releasing hormone antagonist in poor ovarian responders undergoing in vitro fertilization: a systematic review and meta-analysis. Fertil Steril. 2013;100:1594-601.e1-9.
17. Schimberni M, Ciardo F, Schimberni M, Giallonardo A, De Pratti V, Sbracia M. Short gonadotropin-releasing hormone agonist versus flexible antagonist versus clomiphene citrate regimens in poor responders undergoing in vitro fertilization: a randomized controlled trial. Eur Rev Med Pharmacol Sci. 2016;20:4354-61.
18. Huang MC, Tzeng SL, Lee CI, Chen HH, Huang CC, Lee TH, et al. GnRH agonist long protocol versus GnRH antagonist protocol for various aged patients with diminished ovarian reserve: A retrospective study. PLoS One. 2018;13(11):e0207081.
19. Sunkara SK, Coomarasamy A, Faris R, Braude P, Khalaf Y. Long gonadotropin-releasing hormone agonist versus short agonist versus antagonist regimens in poor responders undergoing in vitro fertilization: a randomized controlled trial. Fertil Steril. 2014;101(1):147-53.

20. Madani T, Ashrafi M, Yeganeh LM. Comparison of different stimulation protocols efficacy in poor responders undergoing IVF: a retrospective study. Gynecol Endocrinol. 2012;28(2):102-5.
21. Garcia-Velasco JA, Isaza V, Requena A, Martínez-Salazar FJ, Landazábal A, Remohí J, et al. High doses of gonadotrophins combined with stop versus non-stop protocol of GnRH analogue administration in low responder IVF patients: a prospective, randomized, controlled trial. Hum Reprod. 2000;15(11):2292-6.
22. Orvieto R, Nahum R, Aizer A, Haas J, Kirshenbaum M. A Novel Stimulation Protocol for Poor-Responder Patients: Combining the Stop GnRH-ag Protocol with Letrozole Priming and Multiple-Dose GnRH-ant: A Proof of Concept. Gynecol Obstet Invest. 2021;86:149-54.
23. ESHRE Reproductive Endocrinology Guideline Group. (2019). Ovarian stimulation for IVF/ICSI. Guideline of the European Society of Human Reproduction and Embryology. [online] Available from https://www.eshre.eu/Guidelines-and-Legal/Guidelines/Ovarian-Stimulation-in-IVF-ICSI. [Last accessed April, 2024]
24. Polyzos NP, Blockeel C, Verpoest W, De Vos M, Stoop D, Vloeberghs V, et al. Live birth rates following natural cycle IVF in women with poor ovarian response according to the Bologna criteria. Hum Reprod. 2012;27(12):3481-6.
25. Ragni G, Levi-Setti PE, Fadini R, Brigante C, Scarduelli C, Alagna F, et al. Clomiphene citrate versus high doses of gonadotropins for in vitro fertilisation in women with compromised ovarian reserve: a randomised controlled non-inferiority trial. Reprod Biol Endocrinol. 2012;10:114.
26. Revelli A, Chiado A, Dalmasso P, Stabile V, Evangelista F, Basso G, et al. Mild versus long protocol for controlled ovarian hyperstimulation in patients with expected poor ovarian responsiveness undergoing IVF; a large prospective randomized trial. J Assist Reprod Genet. 2014;31:809-15.
27. Siristatidis C, Salamalekis G, Dafopoulos K, Basios G, Vogiatzi P, Papantoniou N. Mild versus conventional ovarian stimulation for poor responders undergoing IVF/ICSI. In Vivo. 2017;31(2):231-7.
28. Cozzolino M, Cecchino GN, Bosch E, Garcia-Velasco JA, Garrido N. Minimal ovarian stimulation is an alternative to conventional protocols for older women according to Poseidon's stratification: a retrospective multicenter cohort study. J Assist Reprod Genet. 2021;38(7):1799-807.
29. Youssef MA, van Wely M, Al-Inany H, Madani T, Jahangiri N, Khodabakhshi S, et al. A mild ovarian stimulation strategy in women with poor ovarian reserve undergoing IVF: a multicenter randomized non-inferiority trial. Hum Reprod. 2017;32(1):112-8.
30. Kuang Y, Chen Q, Hong Q, Luy Q, AiA, Fu Y, et al. Double stimulation during the follicular and luteal phases of poor responder in IVF/ICSI programmes. Reprod Biomed Online. 2014;29(6):684-91.
31. Vaiarelli A, Cimadomo D, Trabucco E, Vallefuoco R, Buffo L, Dusi L, et al. Double Stimulation in the Same Ovarian Cycle (DuoStim) to Maximize the Number of Oocytes Retrieved From Poor Prognosis Patients: A Multicenter Experience and SWOT Analysis. Front Endocrinol (Lausanne). 2018;9:317.
32. Li XL, Wang L, Lv F, Huang XM, Wang LP, Pan Y, et al. The influence of different growth hormone addition protocols to poor ovarian responders on clinical outcomes in controlled ovary stimulation cycles: A systematic review and meta-analysis. Medicine. 2017;96:e6443.

33. Nagels HE, Rishworth JR, Siristatidis CS, Kroon B. Androgens (dehydroepiandrosterone or testosterone) for women undergoing assisted reproduction. Cochrane Database Syst Rev. 2015;(11):CD009749.
34. Alviggi C, Clarizia R, Pettersson K, Mollo A, Humaidan P, Strina I, et al. Suboptimal response to GnRHa long protocol is associated with a common LH polymorphism. Reprod Biomed Online. 2009;18:9-14.
35. Alviggi C, Pettersson K, Longobardi S, Andersen CY, Conforti A, De Rosa P, et al. A common polymorphic allele of the LH beta-subunit gene is associated with higher exogenous FSH consumption during controlled ovarian stimulation for assisted reproductive technology. Reprod Biol Endocrinol. 2013;11:51.
36. Papaleo E, Vanni VS, Vigano P, La Marca A, Pagliardini L, Vitrano R, et al. Recombinant LH administration in subsequent cycle after "unexpected" poor response to recombinant FSH monotherapy. Gynecol Endocrinol. 2014;30:813-6.
37. Ubaldi FM, Capalbo A, Vaiarelli A, Cimadomo D, Colamaria S, Alviggi C, et al. Follicular versus luteal phase ovarian stimulation during the same menstrual cycle (DuoStim) in a reduced ovarian reserve population results in a similar euploid blastocyst formation rate: new insight in ovarian reserve exploitation. Fertil Steril. 2016;105:1488-95.
38. Siristatidis CS, Gibreel A, Basios G, Maheshwari A, Bhattacharya S. Gonadotrophin-releasing hormone agonist protocols for pituitary suppression in assisted reproduction. Cochrane Database Syst Rev. 2015;(11):CD006919.
39. Lunenfeld B, Bilger W, Longobardi S, Kirsten J, D'Hooghe T, Sunkara SK. Decision points for individualized hormonal stimulation with recombinant gonadotropins for treatment of women with infertility. Gynecol Endocrinol. 2019;35:1027-36.
40. Alviggi C, Conforti A, Santi D, Esteves SC, Andersen CY, Humaidan P, et al. Clinical relevance of genetic variants of gonadotropins and their receptors in controlled ovarian stimulation: a systematic review and meta-analysis. Hum Reprod Update. 2018;24:599-614.
41. Esteves S, Carvalho J, Bento F, Santos J. A novel predictive model to estimate the number of mature oocytes required for obtaining at least one euploid blastocyst for transfer in couples undergoing in vitro fertilization/intracytoplasmic sperm injection: the ART calculator. Front Endocrinol. 2019;10:99.
42. Humaidan P, Chin W, Rogoff D, D'Hooghe T, Longobardi S, Hubbard J, et al. Efficacy and safety of follitropin alfa/lutropin alfa in ART: a randomized controlled trial in poor ovarian responders. Hum Reprod. 2017;32:544-55.
43. Pu D, Wu J, Liu J. Comparisons of GnRH antagonist versus GnRH agonist protocol in poor ovarian responders undergoing IVF. Hum Reprod. 2011;26:2742-9.
44. Sunkara SK, Rittenberg V, Raine-Fenning N, Bhattacharya S, Zamora J, Coomarasamy A. Association between the number of eggs and live birth in IVF treatment: an analysis of 400,135 treatment cycles. Hum Reprod. 2011;26:1768-74.
45. Mignini Renzini M, Brigante C, Coticchio G, Dal Canto M, Caliari I, Comi R, et al. Retrospective analysis of treatments with recombinant FSH and recombinant LH versus human menopausal gonadotropin in women with reduced ovarian reserve. J Assist Reprod Genet. 2017;34:1645-51.
46. Drakopoulos P, Vuong TNL, Ho NAV, Vaiarelli A, Ho MT, Blockeel C, et al. Corifollitropin alfa followed by highly purified HMG versus recombinant FSH in young poor ovarian responders: a multicentre randomized controlled clinical trial. Hum Reprod. 2017;32:2225.

Chapter 20

Stimulation Protocols for Fertility Preservation

Kamal Ojha, Biswanath Ghosh Dastidar

■ INTRODUCTION

The term "fertility preservation" is commonly used to refer to pre-emptive fertility treatment in couples or single woman who does not wish to, or cannot, opt for assisted conception at the time of presentation to the fertility clinic and anticipate a reduction in fertility at a later time when they may want a child. Such treatment commonly includes initiating one or more ovarian stimulation cycles resulting in transvaginal ultrasound-guided oocyte retrievals followed by freezing the eggs or embryos thus generated. Freezing oocytes is a relatively newer technology compared to embryo freezing and should be provided in centers with proven experience. A recent review has reported that freezing ovarian cortical tissue and future autotransplantation at a later date has also resulted in 87 live births, apart from more ongoing pregnancies so far.[1,2] However, it is a technologically advanced procedure and not routinely offered by all assisted reproductive technology (ART) units. Before menarche in pediatric patients, ovarian tissue cryopreservation may be the only option. Thus, it is of interest to discuss the ways in which ovarian stimulation protocols may be optimized for patients seeking preservation of future fertility.

■ INDICATIONS

The diagnosis of cancer and impending radiochemotherapy is perhaps the most common and important medical indication for initiation of ovarian stimulation with a view to freeze embryos, or eggs in the case of women who are unmarried or not in stable, long-term relationships. Both radiation and alkylating agents are known to have severe adverse impact on future fertility.[3] Thus, it has become common practice to proceed with one or two cycles of ovarian stimulation and egg retrievals in these women before exposing them to the detrimental effects of cancer therapy.

Moreover, certain other diseases and their treatment often result in ovarian damage. These include endometriosis; hematological diseases such as aplastic anemia, thalassemia, and sickle cell anemia; and autoimmune diseases unresponsive to immunosuppressive therapy such as systemic lupus erythematosus (SLE).[4,5] Before proceeding with the necessary treatment, it is preferred to explore the option of harvesting and freezing eggs from these women following one or more ovarian stimulation cycles.

Recent decades have also witnessed a growing number of women who wish to delay childbearing for social reasons such as career building, single relationship status, or other sociofinancial considerations.[6] Fertility preservation strategies are also appropriate modalities of intervention in these patient populations.

It may be worthwhile to highlight here that the approach to a fertility preservation in vitro fertilization (IVF) cycle before impending cancer therapy warrants a more urgent and fast-tracked approach compared to social freezing cycles and deserves consideration to be treated as an adjunct to a life-saving intervention. However, even for social freezing cycles, it is advisable not to waste too much time given the correct indications, particularly in women of advanced reproductive age where ovarian reserve often drops dramatically within a space of a few months.[7] In fact, there may be clinical situations where the ovarian reserve may be so low that fertility preservation should be actively discouraged and appropriate counseling provided.

■ ASSESSMENT OF OVARIAN RESERVE

Before starting a cycle of ovarian stimulation, it is necessary to assess the patient's ovarian reserve and predict likely response to controlled ovarian stimulation (COS) with exogenous gonadotropins and other agents. Such baseline evaluation is essential to determine starting dose of gonadotropin stimulation and optimize adequate yield of oocytes, as well as avoid ovarian hyperstimulation syndrome (OHSS). Where the ovarian reserve is low, counseling the patient about the expected low success rates and ensuring expectations are managed appropriately are essential.

Currently, the best predictors of ovarian response to hormonal stimulation are the patient's age, history of previous response to COS, and markers of ovarian reserve such as anti-Müllerian hormone (AMH) and antral follicle count (AFC).

Based on such evaluation, patients may be broadly classified as good responders/hyper-responders, and moderate to poor responders. Frank poor responders and patients diagnosed with premature ovarian insufficiency (POI) may be better suited for donor IVF cycles since the freeze-thaw process of embryos, and particularly oocytes, is associated with attrition in number available for future embryo transfer (ET), thereby defeating the purpose of proceeding with a stimulation cycle in the first place. Thus counseling and managing expectations are very helpful in the long term. Individualized cycle planning is required for polycystic ovary syndrome (PCOS) patients as ovarian stimulation in this subgroup is often challenging. In our experience, there are also patients who exhibit atypical or unexpected patterns of response to ovarian stimulation and are possibly better assigned to a fourth subcategory requiring individualized care.

■ CYCLE PLANNING

Gonadotropin-releasing hormone antagonist cycles with GnRH agonist trigger for final oocyte maturation prior to egg retrieval appear to be an appropriate strategy for freeze-all cycles. Starting dose of gonadotropins is determined based on evaluation of likely ovarian response, as previously discussed. Cycle monitoring is carried out by serial transvaginal ultrasonography (TV-USG) and serum estradiol (E2) measurements on alternate days from day 5 or 6 of stimulation and subsequent gonadotropin dose tailored accordingly. Daily antagonist is started when lead follicle measures 14 mm[8] and induction trigger given when at least 2–3 follicles measure 17–18 mm or more and egg retrieval performed 35–37 hours later.

Cycle planning assumes particular significance for poor ovarian responders (PORs). For this group of patients, it is necessary to critically plan starting stimulation dose and counsel the patient appropriately in order to set realistic expectations for cycle outcomes. This is particularly important for PORs of a lower age group and in some instances, the patient and provider may opt to proceed for donor IVF cycles, thereby completely altering the course of treatment. Hence, in the context of impending cancer treatment, it is important to achieve such clarity early.

For this purpose, it may be useful to use the ESHRE's Bologna criteria as a guideline to identify this cohort of women which defines PORs as women with any two of the following three criteria—advanced maternal age >40 years (or other risk factors); previous poor ovarian response (<3 oocytes with conventional stimulation, or a cancelled cycle); or an abnormal ovarian reserve test (ORT) as documented by AMH <0.5–1.1 ng/mL or total AFC < 5–7 follicles.[9]

In our clinical practice, we find it may be useful to group patients contemplating COS for a fertility preservation cycle based on expected ovarian response and set targets, tailor our stimulation regimen, and set expectations accordingly, as shown in **Table 1**.

TABLE 1: Follicle and oocyte targets per COS cycle for fertility preservation (GDIFR, local protocol).

Patient group	Follicles > 15 mm	Oocytes
Good responders	15–20	10–15
Moderate–poor responders	10–15	5–10
Hyper-responders	20–25	15–20

(COS: controlled ovarian stimulation)

COUNSELING

The authors of this monograph strongly feel that the role of counseling patients appropriately and adequately prior to a fertility preservation stimulation cycle cannot be overemphasized. A major proportion of patients considering such intervention are likely to find themselves in uniquely stressful situations—either grappling with the implications of cancer and its treatment; or faced with the prospect of diminishing childbearing potential at a stage of life when they are not yet prepared to start a family.

Such counseling should cover two distinct aspects. Firstly, it is important to provide general support and information to these patients. Secondly, it is important to explain the implications of undergoing such treatment, including a frank discussion of its limitations. These would include a detailed exchange about the processes of free-thaw and oocyte survival rates, the possibility of having few or no embryos to transfer, the possibility of the treatment culmination in a failure to achieve pregnancy, and evaluating the current literature on future impact on live-born babies.

Ideally, such counseling needs to be undertaken by a specialist independent of the team treating the patients, but with a background in fertility.

STIMULATION PROTOCOLS

Stimulation protocols for fertility preservation are best individualized according to patient group, as discussed above. For this purpose, in our clinical practice in India, we broadly divide patients into the following four categories based on ovarian reserve and history of response to ovarian hyperstimulation:
1. Good responders/hyper-responders
2. Moderate responders
3. PCOS patients
4. Patients demonstrating atypical or unexpected ovarian response patterns

Good Responders/Hyper-responders

It is reasonable to categorize patients as good responders if they are below the age of 32 with good ovarian reserve, and particularly if they have a history of good response to ovarian stimulation in the past. For egg-freezing cycles, the strategy should be to obtain a high yield of mature oocytes for vitrification. Thus, in selected patients, we may perform COS with a relatively high initial starting dose of recombinant follicle-stimulating hormone (FSH) as compared to fresh IVF cycles for similar patients. In most cases, we would use around 150 units of recombinant gonadotropins in an antagonist cycle with agonist trigger in order to achieve optimal outcome and balance the twin needs for high-oocyte yield and patient safety. It may be worthwhile to pre-screen this patient population for PCOS and body mass index (BMI) before proceeding with these cycles. In women with raised BMI, a higher dose of 225 units may be used.

Moderate Responders or Poor Responders

This group would include patients aged 32 and above with average to reasonable ovarian reserve and/or past response to COS. For egg-freezing cycles, it would be a reasonable strategy to pursue aggressive ovarian stimulation with high dose of recombinant FSH. A good rule of thumb may be to use 1–2 additional ampoules of rFSH than one would use for a conventional IVF cycle, which in many of these patients may be around 225 units. Antagonist cycle with serial follicle and E2 tracking would be performed and triggered with GnRH agonist when at least three or more follicles measure ≥18 mm.

Polycystic Ovary Syndrome Patients

As with any other fresh IVF cycle, COS for egg freezing in PCOS patients, whether with a cancer comorbidity or requesting a social freezing cycle, is challenging and requires careful individualization. It is highly desirable to pursue an aggressive course of management for PCOS for at least 3 months prior to COS in order to improve the metabolic profile of the patient in order to optimize cycle outcome. Pretreatment assessment of hormonal and metabolic profile is essential, both clinically and biochemically. Even a moderate reduction of body weight in obese PCOS patients prior to ovarian stimulation by exercise and diet has been shown to result in significantly better results. Besides, pretherapy with adjuvants such as inositol[10] or metformin[11] where indicated is also thought to improve cycle results.

All cycles in PCOS patients should preferably be antagonist cycles with agonist trigger. Additionally, it may be advisable to practice restrained COS in cases of frank PCOS, as documented by clinical, biochemical, or imaging studies. In these cases, it is important to counsel patients about possible low yield of oocytes for freezing.

The dose, however, again depends on the age and BMI. Recombinant FSH delivery systems available internationally with a pen have the advantage of delivering dose, which increase, at intervals of 12.5 units. It is useful to be able to titrate dosage from 150 to 300 units increasing at 12.5–25 units based on age, BMI, and previous response.

Atypical or Unexpected Ovarian Response Patterns

In patients who exhibit atypical or unexplained ovarian response patterns, it is important to critically review other factors such as role of advanced age, obesity, thyroid function, prolactin levels, receptor dysfunction, and undiagnosed PCOS. Moreover, past history of ovarian surgery has to be taken into consideration, as does the possibility of past or present undiagnosed pelvic and ovarian endometriosis. All these patients require careful, individualized care.

CONSIDERATIONS PRIOR TO FERTILITY PRESERVATION IN CANCER PATIENTS

Extent of the Problem

Over the last 20 years, cancer death rates have been dropping by around 1.5% annually due to early diagnosis and better treatment option.[12] Different treatment regimens pose risk of damage to ovarian function to different extents, although the detrimental impact of both alkylating agents and radiation is well recognized.[13] Combination chemotherapy is common in most patients and results in cumulative gonadotoxicity.[14] Most of these women are at risk of iatrogenic premature ovarian failure (POF).[15] Hence, there is a growing population of young female cancer survivors whose future fertility is of concern.

Cancer and Ovarian Stimulation Planning

Diminished ovarian response to stimulation has been documented in women who have undergone chemotherapy for cancer prior to oocyte retrieval,[17] thereby leading to consensus toward retrieving oocytes before commencing with cancer therapy **(Table 2)**. However, cancer being a predominantly catabolic state associated with weight loss, malnutrition, hypothalamic-pituitary-ovarian (HPO) axis dysfunction, and stress hormone-induced aberrations in prolactin secretion, there has also been legitimate concern about whether the disease process itself has a detrimental impact on results of ovarian stimulation.[18]

TABLE 2: Ovarian damage risk with different cancer therapy regimens.[16]

Degree of risk	Cancer therapy regimen
High risk (>80%)	HSCT, TBI, combination chemotherapy in women >40 years
Intermediate risk	Combination chemotherapy in women 30–39 years old
Low risk	Vincristine, methotrexate, and fluorouracil
Unknown risk	Taxanes and tyrosine kinase inhibitors

(HSCT: hematopoietic stem cell transplantation; TBI: total body irradiation)
Source: Modified from Lee SJ, Schover LR, Partridge AH, Patrizio P, Wallace WH, Hagerty K, et al. American Society of Clinical Oncology recommendations on fertility preservation in cancer patients. J Clin Oncol. 2006;24(18):2917-31.

However, a recent meta-analysis of retrospective cohort studies comparing differences in response to stimulation between women with cancer who are yet to start therapy and age-matched healthy controls has revealed no impact on number of oocytes retrieved, number of mature eggs obtained, number of 2 PN embryos generated, or fertilization rates.[19] In such women, AMH and AFC have been shown to be good indicators of ovarian response to exogenous stimulation prior to commencement of cancer therapy.[20] Moreover, such response appears to be similar irrespective of the type of cancer.[21]

At least two consecutive cycles may be considered in order to maximize oocyte yield for freezing as it has been shown that such a strategy results in higher egg numbers and embryos generated without significantly delaying time interval from surgery to chemotherapy.[22] Results have been demonstrated to be similar between standard early follicular phase stimulation and random start stimulation cycles which include mid-follicular phase or luteal phase start in terms of outcome measures such as oocyte yield, mature eggs obtained, and fertilization rates, thereby making flexible cycle scheduling possible in these patients where time is often of the essence.[23]

Letrozole alone or in combination with rFSH is preferred in estrogen-dependent cancers such as breast cancers for ovarian stimulation. Timing of letrozole in breast cancer patients undergoing COS has been shown to affect egg retrieval rates with better results when commenced after initial stimulation with gonadotropins.[24] Use of agonist trigger has been documented to result in yield of greater M-II oocyte as well as 2-PN embryos available for freezing compared to hCG trigger in cancer patients of similar demographics, both in only gonadotropin as well as gonadotropin plus letrozole stimulation cycles.[25]

■ CONCLUSION

The emergence of advanced chemoradiotherapy has led to an increasing population of young cancer survivors whose future fertility is of concern. Women electively opting for late childbearing and family completion are also at risk for age-related future subfertility. Fertility preservation strategies are thus useful for all these populations of patients. Freezing and autotransplantation of ovarian cortical tissue being a niche service not yet widely available, elective oocyte or embryo freezing remains the most viable strategy for fertility preservation for most patients who are likely to need such services.

While planning ovarian stimulation protocols for these patients, it is important to strive to maximize the yield of oocytes bearing in mind the natural attrition in numbers often seen following freeze-thaw cycles of oocyte cryopreservation. It is important to determine the initial starting

CHAPTER 20: Stimulation Protocols for Fertility Preservation

dose of gonadotropin after careful evaluation of the patient's likely response to ovarian stimulation based on age, past history, and ovarian reserve. Stratifying patients according to these markers is often a useful strategy. Current data suggests that antagonist cycles with agonist triggering for final oocyte maturation may be the most judicious approach to planning these cycles. PCOS patients need careful individualization of stimulation protocols. Multiple strategies are useful to optimize outcome for cancer patients undergoing stimulation cycles. These include random start stimulation, consecutive cycles to maximize yield, and use of letrozole in estrogen-dependent cancers.

■ KEY POINTS

- Fertility preservation refers to preemptive fertility treatment to offer a greater chance of future childbearing to women who wish to delay childbearing for socioprofessional reasons, are about to start gonadotoxic cancer therapy, or are undergoing treatment for other diseases with expected adverse impact on fertility.
- The current approach to fertility preservation is based on one or more ovarian stimulation cycles followed by freezing the embryos thus generated for future transfer. Oocyte freezing should be offered by centers with appropriate experience and ovarian tissue preservation and autotransplantation techniques may have a bigger role to play in the future.
- Prompt and aggressive commencement of cycles may be appropriate in patients with reducing ovarian reserves as well as those with cancer and about to start treatment. It is important to appropriately counsel patients in situations where donor IVF or adoption may be more suitable options.
- The role of counseling patients appropriately to set realistic expectations tailored to their particular situations cannot be overemphasized.
- Stimulation regimens need to be tailored to patients' situations and individualized according to age, BMI, past response to ovarian stimulation, ovarian reserve, and the presence of PCOS or other concomitant diseases which could potentially lead to atypical responses.

■ REFERENCES

1. Kristensen SG, Giorgione V, Humaidan P, Alsbjerg B, Bjørn AMB, Ernst E, et al. Fertility preservation and refreezing of transplanted ovarian tissue—a potential new way of managing patients with low risk of malignant cell recurrence. Fertil Steril. 2017;107(5):1206-13.
2. Jensen AK, Macklon KT, Fedder J, Ernst E, Humaidan P, Andersen CY. 86 successful births and 9 ongoing pregnancies worldwide in women transplanted with frozen-thawed ovarian tissue: Focus on birth and perinatal outcome in 40 of these children. J Assist Reprod Genet. 2017;34(3):325-36.

3. Thomas-Teinturier C, Allodji RS, Svetlova E, Frey MA, Oberlin O, Millischer AE, et al. Ovarian reserve after treatment with alkylating agents during childhood. Hum Reprod. 2015;30(6):1437-46.
4. Donnez J, Dolmans MM. Preservation of fertility in females with haematological malignancy. Br J Haematol. 2011;154(2):175-84.
5. Slavin S, Nagler A, Aker M, Shapira MY, Cividalli G, Or R. Non-myeloablative stem cell transplantation and donor lymphocyte infusion for the treatment of cancer and life-threatening non-malignant disorders. Rev Clin Exp Hematol. 2001;5(2):135-46.
6. Petropanagos A, Cattapan A, Baylis F, Leader A. Social egg freezing: Risk, benefits and other considerations. CMAJ. 2015;187(9):666-9.
7. Amanvermez R, Tosun M. An update on ovarian aging and ovarian reserve tests. Int J Fertil Steril. 2016;9(4):411-5. .
8. Ludwig M, Katalinic A, Banz C, Schröder AK, Löning M, Weiss JM, et al. Tailoring the GnRH antagonist cetrorelix acetate to individual patient's needs in ovarian stimulation for IVF: Results of a prospective, randomized study. Hum Reprod. 2002;17(11):2842-5.
9. Sallam HN, Ezzeldin F, Agameya AF, Abdel-Rahman AF, El-Garem Y. The definition of "poor response": Bologna criteria. Hum Reprod. 2012;27(2):626-7.
10. Vartanyan EV, Tsaturova KA, Devyatova EA, Mikhaylyukova AS, Levin VA, Petuhova NL, et al. Improvement in quality of oocytes in polycystic ovarian syndrome in programs of in vitro fertilization. Gynecol Endocrinol. 2017;33(sup1):8-11.
11. Tso LO, Costello MF, Albuquerque LET, Andriolo RB, Macedo CR. Metformin treatment before and during IVF or ICSI in women with polycystic ovary syndrome. Cochrane Database Syst Rev. 2020;12(12):CD006105.
12. Siegel RL, Miller KD, Jemal A. Cancer statistics, 2020. CA Cancer J Clin. 2020;70(1):7-30.
13. Meirow D, Assad G, Dor J, Rabinovici J. The GnRh antagonist cetrorelix reduces cyclophosphamide-induced ovarian follicular destruction in mice. Hum Reprod. 2004;19(6):1294-9.
14. Donnez J, Martinez-Madrid B, Jadoul P, Van Langendonckt A, Demylle D, Dolmans MM. Ovarian tissue cryopreservation and transplantation: A review. Hum Reprod Update. 2006;12(5):519-35.
15. Bray F, Jemal A, Grey N, Ferlay J, Forman D. Global cancer transitions according to the Human Development Index (2008-2030): A population-based study. Lancet Oncol. 2012;13(8):790-801.
16. Lee SJ, Schover LR, Partridge AH, Patrizio P, Wallace WH, Hagerty K, et al. American Society of Clinical Oncology recommendations on fertility preservation in cancer patients. J Clin Oncol. 2006;24(18):2917-31.
17. Ginsburg ES, Yanushpolsky EH, Jackson KV. In vitro fertilization for cancer patients and survivors. Fertil Steril. 2001;75(4):705-10.
18. Agarwal A, Said TM. Implications of systemic malignancies on human fertility. Reprod Biomed Online. 2004;9(5):673-9.
19. Turan V, Quinn MM, Dayioglu N, Rosen MP, Oktay K. The impact of malignancy on response to ovarian stimulation for fertility preservation: a meta-analysis. Fertil Steril. 2018;110(7):1347-55.

20. Arslan E, Karsy M, Moy F, Oktay K. The role of combined anti-mullerian hormone and antral follicle count assessment in predicting cycle outcomes in cancer patients undergoing controlled ovarian stimulation for fertility preservation. Fertil Steril. 2011;96(3):S201.
21. Creux H, Monnier P, Oliviero F, Son W, Buckett W. Influence of the type of cancer on ovarian stimulation response in a fertility preservation program. Fertil Steril. 2017;108(3):E33.
22. Turan V, Bedoschi G, Moy F, Oktay K. Safety and feasibility of performing two consecutive ovarian stimulation cycles with the use of letrozole-gonadotropin protocol for fertility preservation in breast cancer patients. Fertil Steril. 2013;100(6):1681-5.e1.
23. Cakmak H, Katz A, Cedars MI, Rosen MP. Effective method for emergency fertility preservation: Random-start controlled ovarian stimulation. Fertil Steril. 2013;100(6):1673-80.
24. Diaz-Garcia C, Domingo J, Romero A, Martinez M, Rubio JM, Garcia-Velasco JA, et al. The timing of administration of letrozole significantly affects the oocyte recovery rate in breast cancer patients undergoing controlled ovarian stimulation for fertility preservation. Fertil Steril. 2015;104(3):E327.
25. Pereira N, Kelly AG, Stone LD, Witzke JD, Lekovich JP, Elias RT, et al. Gonadotropin-releasing hormone agonist trigger increases the number of oocytes and embryos available for cryopreservation in cancer patients undergoing ovarian stimulation for fertility preservation. Fertil Steril. 2017;108(3):532-8.

Section 9

Adjuvants: Do they Work?

- **Adjuvants in Assisted Reproductive Technology**
  Nandita Palshetkar, Rohan Palshetkar
- **Insulin Sensitizers: Metformin and Inositols**
  N Sanjeeva Reddy, Radha Vembu

Chapter 21: Adjuvants in Assisted Reproductive Technology

Nandita Palshetkar, Rohan Palshetkar

■ INTRODUCTION

Infertility affects approximately 13–14% of reproductive-aged couples. It is defined as the inability to conceive after 1 year of properly timed, unprotected intercourse. The number and quality of a woman's oocytes decline with age. The decline in the number of oocytes begins at 20 weeks' gestation when the female fetus has approximately 6–7 million oogonia (largest lifetime endowment). The number of oocytes decreases to approximately 2–3 million at birth and decreases again to 300,000 by the time of puberty. In the recent era, parenthood has taken a step back. Pursuing one's education, career, and not finding the right partner are some of the reasons why childbearing may be delayed in some couples. But due to this declining oocyte reserve, there is difficulty in conceiving as a woman gets older. Besides this, as age increases, the quality of eggs continues to decline. Quality of eggs is an important factor for conception and a healthy pregnancy. This is irrespective of whether a couple is trying to conceive naturally or through fertility treatments. As age begins to increase, there is also a worry about chromosomal abnormalities in the offspring. This could lead to increased risk of miscarriage as well as birth defects.

▌POOR OOCYTE QUALITY AND CHROMOSOMAL ABNORMALITIES

Beyond the age of 40, the ability to get good-quality oocytes reduces. As maternal age continues to increase, the number of normal oocytes that is available is only 10–20%. One treatment modality that is available is oocyte donation, which will result in younger eggs with good quality. This treatment modality not only improves the quality of eggs but also diminishes the chances of chromosomal abnormalities in the offspring.

Another treatment modality is the nuclear transfer of an oocyte into the cytoplasm of another enucleated oocyte. Zhang et al. published a study in a patient with 2 failures. 8 out 12 patient oocytes were fertilized and 12 out of 15 donor oocytes were fertilized. The patient's pronuclei were transferred subzonally into an enucleated donor cytoplasm resulting in seven reconstructed zygotes. Five viable reconstructed embryos were transferred into the patient's uterus resulting in a triplet pregnancy with fetal heartbeats, normal karyotypes, and nuclear genetic fingerprinting matching the mother's genetic fingerprinting. Fetal mitochondrial DNA profiles were identical to those from donor cytoplasm with no detection of patient's mitochondrial DNA. This report suggests that a potentially viable pregnancy with normal karyotype can be achieved through pronuclear transfer. Ongoing work to establish the efficacy and safety of pronuclear transfer will result in its use as an aid for human reproduction.[1]

■ POOR OVARIAN RESERVE

It is the main factor to consider when considering women above the age of 40. There used to be a lack of universally accepted diagnostic criteria for poor ovarian reserve (POR). Various tests have been used to diagnose POR. One of the earliest ovarian reserve tests (ORTs) used was follicle-stimulating hormone (FSH). An elevated FSH level is associated with poor response; however, a normal FSH level did not exclude poor response. Also, elevation of FSH occurs quite late in women with decreasing ovarian reserve. Therefore, FSH is not an ideal test to identify poor responders.[2] Antral follicle count (AFC) and Anti-Müllerian hormone (AMH) are one of the most sensitive markers of ovarian reserve. Besides this, they are ideal to set out stimulation protocols for each patient individually. Both AFC and AMH provide a reliable and accurate prediction of ovarian response.

Earlier there used to be a lack of universally accepted diagnostic criteria for POR. To overcome this limitation, there was a consensus meeting of "ESHRE working group on POR discussion" in 2011.[3] They set out the Bologna criteria.

Bologna criteria recommend the presence of at least two of the following three features for diagnosis of POR:
1. Advanced maternal age (≥40 years) or any other risk factor for POR
2. A previous POR (≤3 oocytes with a conventional stimulation protocol)
3. An abnormal ORT (i.e., AFC, 5–7 follicles or AMH, 0.5–1.1 ng/mL)

Two episodes of POR after maximal stimulation are sufficient to define a patient as poor responder in the absence of advanced maternal age or abnormal ORT.

■ ADJUVANT THERAPY

Dehydroepiandrosterone and Testosterone

Androgen supplementation in the form of oral dehydroepiandrosterone (DHEA) or transdermal testosterone in poor responders has been explored as it is believed to improve the intrafollicular environment and follicular sensitivity to exogenous FSH. Meta-analysis by Naegels HE in 2015 suggested that pretreatment with DHEA may improve live birth rate (LBR) but, however, the quality of evidence was moderate and there was insufficient data to carry out a conclusion.[4] In patients with POR, pretreatment with testosterone gel prior to controlled ovarian stimulation (COS) resulted in higher number of oocytes, higher fertilization rate, more number of embryos, and better implantation rate.[5] Currently there is a T-TRANSPORT Trial underway to give us a more robust information about the effects of testosterone in poor ovarian responders.

Growth Hormone

Growth hormone (GH) is another adjuvant that may be used to improve the oocyte yield and pregnancy rates. A meta-analysis published in 2017 concluded that GH in controlled ovarian hyperstimulation (COH) reduced the duration of ovarian stimulation and also yielded in a larger number of oocytes; however, there was no evidence of increase in LBRs. Another meta-analysis published in July 2020 showed that GH supplementation improved LBR, clinical pregnancy rate (CPR), and retrieved oocytes number and reduced cancellation rates. However, both meta-analyses suggested that there need to be more randomized controlled trials (RCTs) with larger samples sizes to give robust conclusion about the efficacy of GH.[6,7]

Coenzyme Q10

Coenzyme Q10 (CoQ10) is another adjuvant that is available for use. It improves oocyte metabolism, corrects mitochondrial function and spindle alignment. Higher levels of CoQ10 have been associated with optimal embryo parameters and higher pregnancy rates.[8]

Melatonin

Recently, melatonin is being used as an adjunct for patients with POR. It regulates ovarian function by regulating gonadotropin release in hypothalamic–pituitary–ovarian (HPO) axis via its specific receptors. Besides this, it also protects the ovary from oxidative stress. Studies have shown that melatonin improves yield and quality of oocytes and also improves fertilization rates.[9-11]

■ PRETREATMENT

As a strategy to improve follicular synchronization, to prevent premature ovulation, and also as a measure to schedule cycles, oral contraceptive pills (OCPs), pretreatment with OCPs, progesterone, or estradiol may be used. Even though studies have shown that there is no difference in the pregnancy rates, the duration of stimulation may increase with the use OCPs.[12,13]

CONTROLLED OVARIAN STIMULATION FOR IN VITRO FERTILIZATION

In patients above the age of 40, due to the POR, high levels of gonadotropins (300–450 IU/day) may be required to get a higher oocyte yield. In order to improve oocyte quality and consequently embryo quality, luteinizing hormone (LH) may be added in the early follicular phase. But, the evidence available regarding the same is inconclusive.[14] Low-dose human chorionic gonadotropin (hCG) supplementation or addition of pure human menopausal gonadotropin (hMG) where hCG is the source of LH activity has shown some improvements in the oocyte yield.[15,16] Luteal start of FSH has been used to influence the recruitment of follicles without any reported clinical benefit.[17]

AGONISTS

In patients with POR, agonists are widely used to prevent endogenous LH surge. Long agonist protocol increases both duration of treatment and total dose of gonadotropins necessary to affect follicular development in poor responders. However, agonists due to their initial flare effect may help in recruitment of the follicles. Hence, short agonist protocol where agonist administration is initiated in the early follicular phase before gonadotropin administration is one of the most widely used agonist protocols in poor responders.[18] Some clinicians prefer microdose flare and ultrashort protocol in order to minimize the pituitary suppression; however, they have not shown to improve clinical outcomes.[19,20]

ANTAGONISTS

Over the last decade, the antagonist protocol has been popular in the management of women with POR. The antagonist protocol prevents the premature LH surge without increasing the duration of treatment. The antagonist protocol has similar pregnancy rates as the short agonist protocol. Two meta-analyses have not found any difference in the pregnancy rate between antagonist and short agonist protocols.[21,22]

NATURAL CYCLE IN VITRO FERTILIZATION

Clinicians sometimes use this method as an alternative to the high-dose gonadotropin regimens in patients with POR. It may have improvements in oocyte quality and may also reduce the financial burden of high-dose regimens.[23-25] Natural cycle in vitro fertilization (IVF) may be modified by the addition of antagonists and low doses of FSH.[26-29] Another modification that may be done is by minimal stimulation with either letrozole or clomiphene citrate with the addition of low doses of gonadotropins.[30] This may improve oocyte yield and quality at the time of oocyte retrieval. However, the cancellation rate for natural cycles is as high as 50%. The pregnancy rates reported in natural IVF cycles are 8–18%. This protocol provides an alternate protocol for patients with POR when high-dose FSH protocol is unsuccessful.[19,20]

■ OVARIAN REJUVENATION

In 2010, phosphatase and tensin homolog (PTEN) enzyme inhibitors and phosphatidylinositol-3 kinase activators were used to activate the AKT pathway in dormant follicles in murine and human ovaries.[31] This suggested that patients with POR with residual follicles could be activated to develop follicles for oocyte retrieval.[32] After removing the ovaries, the residual follicles were activated in the laboratory using AKT stimulators. Post activation, there was ovarian tissue autotransplantation. In 2016, Jun Zhai used the same protocol but improved the technique by grafting back fresh tissues. In six of the 14 patients (43%), a total of 15 follicle development waves were detected, and four patients had successful oocyte retrieval to yield six oocytes. For two patients showing no spontaneous follicle growth, human menopausal gonadotropin treatment induced follicle growth at 6–8 months after grafting. After vitro fertilization of oocyte retrieved, four early embryos were derived. Following embryo transfer, one patient became pregnant and delivered a healthy baby boy, with three other embryos under cryopreservation.[32]

Another modality used for ovarian rejuvenation is platelet-rich plasma (PRP). PRP includes a number of soluble mediators which orchestrate complex immune responses and tissue regeneration.[33] PRP orchestrates a regulatory interplay of cellular migration, extracellular matrix remodeling, cell proliferation, apoptosis, differentiation, and angiogenesis in response to widespread cell damage.[34] Following injury, platelets are among the first cells to arrive and following activation emit a multitude of biologically active mediators to rectify the injury.[35] The ovary is an organ which undergoes monthly injury and repair with each ovulation. A study published in 2018 by Scott Sills showed how intraovarian injection of autologous PRP affected ovarian reserve. PRP was obtained from four patients in patients with POR (mean age = 42 ± 4 years). 5-mL activated PRP was injected into the ovary. There was decreased FSH levels and increased AMH levels within 2 months. In each of the four patients, at least one blastocyst was formed which was suitable for cryopreservation.[36]

Clinical use of PRP is perhaps best known for managing thrombocytopenia to improve hemostasis. However, PRP also includes numerous soluble mediators which orchestrate complex immune responses and tissue regeneration.[1] Closely associated with inflammatory signaling, PRP figures prominently in tissue regeneration and orchestrates a regulatory interplay of cellular migration, extracellular matrix remodeling, cell proliferation, apoptosis, differentiation, and angiogenesis[2] in response to widespread cell damage. Following trauma or local ischemia as with myocardial infarction or stroke, platelets are among the first cells to arrive and, following activation, emit a multitude of biologically active mediators to rectify the tissue insult.[3] Notably, the human ovary is covered by an epithelial monolayer which sustains cyclic "injury" and local tissue repair with each ovulation. While resident stem cells have been thought crucial for the regeneration needed for hemostasis and organ integrity here, the identity and mode of action for these cells remain incompletely characterized. Although recent research has opened a doorway into ovarian stem cell biology,[4,5] clinical explorations in this field have thus far been limited.

Notwithstanding the now well-established surgical role of PRP in tissue repair, some researchers have suggested that platelets may contribute to overall organ function as well.[6] As a central problem in many clinical infertility presentations is ovarian senescence and an inexorable decline in oocyte endowment, it seems plausible to consider using autologous PRP in a reproductive context. Particularly since the concept of reduced (or entirely lost) fertility potential associated with ovarian failure is the focus of ongoing research, the possibility of PRP improving the ovarian microenvironment—and even interacting with putative ovarian germline stem cells (GSCs)—warrants serious consideration. Here, we report on autologous activated PRP as applied to human ovaries in an office setting, and provide the first clinical data on IVF cycle characteristics following this intervention.

CONCLUSION

Fertility after 40 is plagued by reduced size of primordial follicles, and the resulting oocytes that are formed are likely to be of suboptimal quality. An early recourse to artificial reproductive techniques seems to be the only option with a reasonable chance of achieving pregnancy in women above 40. Currently, there is no treatment besides egg donation to overcome the problem of poor oocyte quality. With newer interventions such as PRP and stem cells coming into forefront, there may be a way of overcoming this hurdle and give women an offspring with their own genetics.

KEY POINTS

- Infertility affects 17–18% of reproductive-aged couples.
- The number and quality of oocytes decline with age, impacting fertility.
- Dehydroepiandrosterone (DHEA), testosterone, growth hormone (GH), coenzyme Q10 (CoQ10) and melatonin have been used as adjuvants with mixed results.
- Ovarian rejuvenation through various techniques like in-vitro activation and intraovarian PRP provide new avenues into patients of POR.

REFERENCES

1. Zhang J, Zhuang G, Zeng Y, Grifo J, Acosta C, Shu Y, et al. Pregnancy derived from human zygote pronuclear transfer in a patient who had arrested embryos after IVF. Reprod Biomed Online. 2016;33(4):529-33.
2. Galey-Fontaine J, Cédrin-Durnerin I, Chaïbi R, Massin N, Hugues JN. Age and ovarian reserve are distinct predictive factors of cycle outcome in low responders. Reprod Biomed Online. 2005;10(1):94-9.
3. Ferraretti AP, La Marca A, Fauser BC, Tarlatzis B, Nargund G, Gianaroli L; ESHRE working group on Poor Ovarian Response Definition. ESHRE consensus on the definition of 'poor response' to ovarian stimulation for in vitro fertilization: the Bologna criteria. Hum Reprod. 2011;26(7):1616-24.
4. Nagels HE, Rishworth JR, Siristatidis CS, Kroon B. Androgens (dehydroepiandrosterone or testosterone) for women undergoing assisted reproduction. Cochrane Database Syst Rev. 2015;(11):CD009749.
5. Doan HT, Quan LH, Nguyen TT. The effectiveness of transdermal testosterone gel 1% (androgel) for poor responders undergoing in vitro fertilization. Gynecol Endocrinol. 2017;33(12):977-9.
6. Hart RJ, Rombauts L, Norman RJ. Growth hormone in IVF cycles: any hope? Curr Opin Obstet Gynecol. 2017;29(3):119-25.
7. Yang P, Wu R, Zhang H. The effect of growth hormone supplementation in poor ovarian responders undergoing IVF or ICSI: a meta-analysis of randomized controlled trials. Reprod Biol Endocrinol. 2020;18(1):76.
8. Akarsu S, Gode F, Isik AZ, Dikmen ZG, Tekindal MA. The association between coenzyme Q10 concentrations in follicular fluid with embryo morphokinetics and pregnancy rate in assisted reproductive techniques. J Assist Reprod Genet. 2017;34(5):599-605.
9. Nishihara T1, Hashimoto S, Ito K, Nakaoka Y, Matsumoto K, Hosoi Y, et al. Oral melatonin supplementation improves oocyte and embryo quality in women undergoing in vitro fertilization-embryo transfer. Gynecol Endocrinol. 2014;30(5):359-62.
10. Tamura H, Takasaki A, Miwa I, Taniguchi K, Maekawa R, Asada H, et al. Oxidative stress impairs oocyte quality and melatonin protects oocytes from free radical damage and improves fertilization rate. J Pineal Res. 2008;44(3):280-7.
11. Eryilmaz OG1, Devran A, Sarikaya E, Aksakal FN, Mollamahmutoğlu L, Cicek N. Melatonin improves the oocyte and the embryo in IVF patients with sleep disturbances, but does not improve the sleeping problems. J Assist Reprod Genet. 2011;28(9):815-20.
12. al-Mizyen E, Sabatini L, Lower AM, Wilson CM, al-Shawaf T, Grudzinskas JG. Does pretreatment with progestogen or oral contraceptive pills in low responders followed by the GnRHa flare protocol improve the outcome of IVF-ET? J Assist Reprod Genet. 2000;17:140-6.
13. Hauzman EE, Zapata A, Bermejo A, Iglesias C, Pellicer A, Garcia-Velasco JA. Cycle scheduling for *in vitro* fertilization with oral contraceptive pills versus oral estradiol valerate: A randomized, controlled trial. Reprod Biol Endocrinol. 2013;11:96.
14. Mochtar MH, Van der Veen, Ziech M, van Wely M. Recombinant luteinizing hormone (rLH) for controlled ovarian hyperstimulation in assisted reproductive cycles. Cochrane Database Syst Rev. 2007;18(2):CD005070.

15. Madani T, Mohammadi Yeganeh L, Khodabakhshi S, Akhoond MR, Hasani F. Efficacy of low dose hCG on oocyte maturity for ovarian stimulation in poor responder women undergoing intracytoplasmic sperm injection cycle: A randomized controlled trial. J Assist Reprod Genet. 2012;29:1213-20.
16. Polyzos NP, De Vos M, Corona R, Vloeberghs V, Ortega-Hrepich C, Stoop D, et al. Addition of highly purified HMG after corifollitropin alfa in antagonist-treated poor ovarian responders: A pilot study. Hum Reprod. 2013;28:1254-60.
17. Kansal Kalra S, Ratcliffe S, Gracia CR, Martino L, Coutifaris C, Barnhart KT. Randomized controlled pilot trial of luteal phase recombinant FSH stimulation in poor responders. Reprod Biomed Online. 2008;17:745-50.
18. Padilla SL, Dugan K, Maruschak V, Shalika S, Smith RD. Use of the flare-up protocol with high dose human follicle stimulating hormone and human menopausal gonadotropins for *in vitro* fertilization in poor responders. Fertil Steril. 1996;65:796-9.
19. Loutradis D, Drakakis P, Vomvolaki E, Antsaklis A. Different ovarian stimulation protocols for women with diminished ovarian reserve. J Assist Reprod Genet. 2007;24:597-611.
20. Ubaldi F, Vaiarelli A, D'Anna R, Rienzi L. Management of poor responders in IVF: Is there anything new? Biomed Res Int. 2014;2014:352098.
21. Griesinger G, Diedrich K, Tarlatzis BC, Kolibianakis EM. GnRH-antagonists in ovarian stimulation for IVF in patients with poor response to gonadotrophins, polycystic ovary syndrome, and risk of ovarian hyperstimulation: A meta-analysis. Reprod Biomed Online. 2006;13:628-38.
22. Pu D, Wu J, Liu J. Comparisons of GnRH antagonist versus GnRH agonist protocol in poor ovarian responders undergoing IVF. Hum Reprod. 2011;26:2742-9.
23. Feldman B, Seidman DS, Levron J, Bider D, Shulman A, Shine S, et al. *In vitro* fertilization following natural cycles in poor responders. Gynecol Endocrinol. 2001;15:328-34.
24. Schimberni M, Morgia F, Colabianchi J, Giallonardo A, Piscitelli C, Giannini P, et al. Natural-cycle *in vitro* fertilization in poor responder patients: A survey of 500 consecutive cycles. Fertil Steril. 2009;92:1297-301.
25. Polyzos NP, Blockeel C, Verpoest W, De Vos M, Stoop D, Vloeberghs V, et al. Live birth rates following natural cycle IVF in women with poor ovarian response according to the Bologna criteria. Hum Reprod. 2012;27:3481-6.
26. Elizur SE, Aslan D, Shulman A, Weisz B, Bider D, Dor J. Modified natural cycle using GnRH antagonist can be an optional treatment in poor responders undergoing IVF. J Assist Reprod Genet. 2005;22:75-9.
27. Kedem A, Tsur A, Haas J, Yerushalmi GM, Hourvitz A, Machtinger R, et al. Is the modified natural *in vitro* fertilization cycle justified in patients with "genuine" poor response to controlled ovarian hyperstimulation? Fertil Steril. 2014;101:1624-8.
28. Lainas TG, Sfontouris IA, Venetis CA, Lainas GT, Zorzovilis IZ, Tarlatzis BC, et al. Live birth rates after modified natural cycle compared with high-dose FSH stimulation using GnRH antagonists in poor responders. Hum Reprod. 2015;30:2321-30.
29. Polyzos NP, Drakopoulos P, Tournaye H. Modified natural cycle IVF for poor ovarian responders: Rethink before concluding. Hum Reprod. 2016;31:221-2.

30. Jovanovic VP, Kort DH, Guarnaccia MM, Sauer MV, Lobo RA. Does the addition of clomiphene citrate or letrazole to gonadotropin treatment enhance the oocyte yield in poor responders undergoing IVF? J Assist Reprod Genet. 2011;28:1067-72.
31. Li J, Kawamura K, Cheng Y, Liu S, Klein C, Liu S, et al. Activation of dormant ovarian follicles to generate mature eggs. Proc Natl Acad Sci U S A. 2010;107: 10280-4.
32. Zhai J, Yao G, Dong F, Bu Z, Cheng Y, Sato Y, et al. In vitro activation of follicles and fresh tissue auto-transplantation in primary ovarian insufficiency patients. J Clin Endocrinol Metab. 2016;101(11):4405-12.
33. Nurden AT. Platelets, inflammation and tissue regeneration. Thromb Haemost. 2011;105(Suppl.1):S13-S33.
34. Gurtner GC, Werner S, Barrandon Y, Longaker MT. Wound repair and regeneration. Nature. 2008;453:314-21.
35. Stellos K, Kopf S, Paul A, Marquardt JU, Gawaz M, Huard J, et al. Platelets in regeneration. Semin Thromb Hemost. 2010;36:175-84.
36. Sills ES, Rickers NS, Li X, Palermo GD. First data on in vitro fertilization and blastocyst formation after intraovarian injection of calcium gluconate-activated autologous platelet rich plasma. Gynecol Endocrinol. 2018;34(9):756-60.

Chapter 22

Insulin Sensitizers: Metformin and Inositols

N Sanjeeva Reddy, Radha Vembu

■ INTRODUCTION

Polycystic ovarian syndrome (PCOS) is characterized by oligo-ovulation or anovulation, clinical or biochemical evidence of hyperandrogenism, and ultrasound features of polycystic ovaries. It is seen in up to 13% of women in reproductive age group.[1] The pathogenesis of PCOS includes hyperandrogenemia, hyperinsulinemia, altered follicle-stimulating hormone (FSH) and luteinizing hormone (LH) ratio, metabolic aberrances, inflammation, advanced glycation end products, and endoplasmic reticulum stress.

■ HYPERINSULINEMIA

Insulin stimulates theca cell androgen production and suppresses hepatic production of sex hormone-binding globulin (SHBG). So, hyperinsulinemia leads to increased intraovarian androgens which disrupt folliculogenesis, cause premature follicular atresia and follicular arrest. The resulting anovulation leads to unopposed action of estrogen on endometrium leading to endometrial hyperplasia.

Overweight women are prone for insulin resistance (IR) which can lead to abnormal carbohydrate and lipid metabolism.[2] Moreover, hyperinsulinemia reduces the circulating level of SHBG and increases free testosterone, which inhibits follicular maturation with consequent menstrual irregularity and infertility[3] **(Fig. 1)**.

■ INSULIN RESISTANCE

Insulin resistance is defined as "state in which a greater than normal amount of insulin is required to elicit a quantitatively normal response" and maintain glucose levels in normal range.[4] Even though IR is not part of diagnostic criteria for PCOS, still along with hyperinsulinemia, it forms central to the pathophysiology of PCOS. It has been noted by standard clamp techniques and WHO criteria for IR, that 85% of women with PCOS diagnosed by Rotterdam criteria are affected (75% of lean and 95% of overweight and obese women).[5]

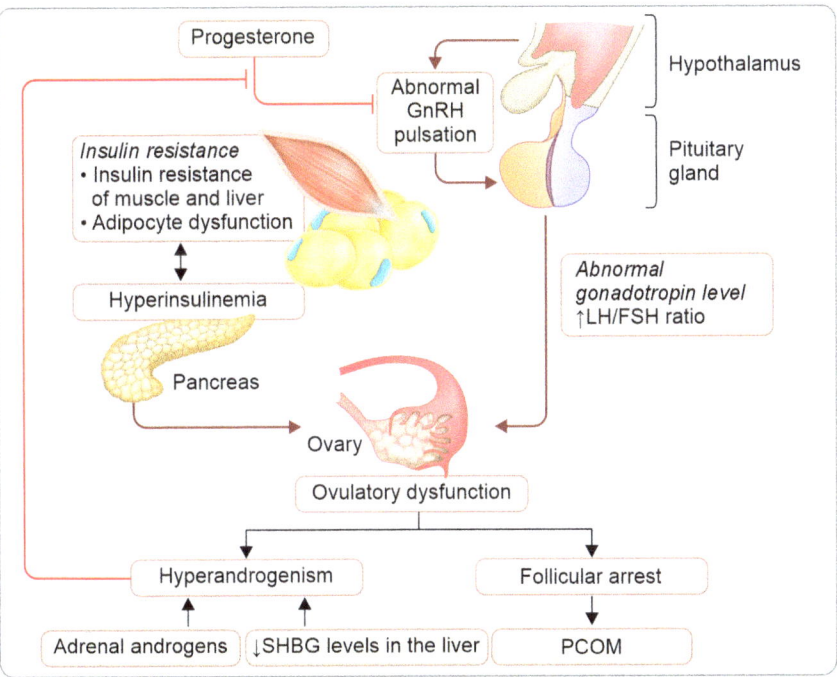

Fig. 1: Effect of hyperinsulinemia. (FSH: follicle-stimulating hormone; GnRH: gonadotropin-releasing hormone; LH: luteinizing hormone; PCOM: polycystic ovarian morphology; SHBG: sex hormone-binding globulin)

Insulin resistance in these PCOS women increases the risk of impaired glucose tolerance, type II diabetes mellitus (DM), dyslipidemia, and chronic subclinical inflammation **(Fig. 2)**.

The main treatment modalities for anovulatory PCOS women include:
- Lifestyle modification—diet and exercise
- Ovulation induction—oral ovulogens and gonadotropins
- Insulin sensitizers
- Laparoscopic ovarian drilling

■ INSULIN SENSITIZERS

Insulin sensitizers are being used since 1950s for the treatment of type II DM. These drugs are often used to reduce IR in obese patients with PCOS **(Box 1)**.

Among the insulin sensitizers, metformin has been extensively studied and evidence shows that it may have metabolic and reproductive benefits.[7]

Metformin

Metformin is a biguanide commonly used as an oral hypoglycemic agent to reduce IR in patients with type II DM. It is a category B drug used to treat

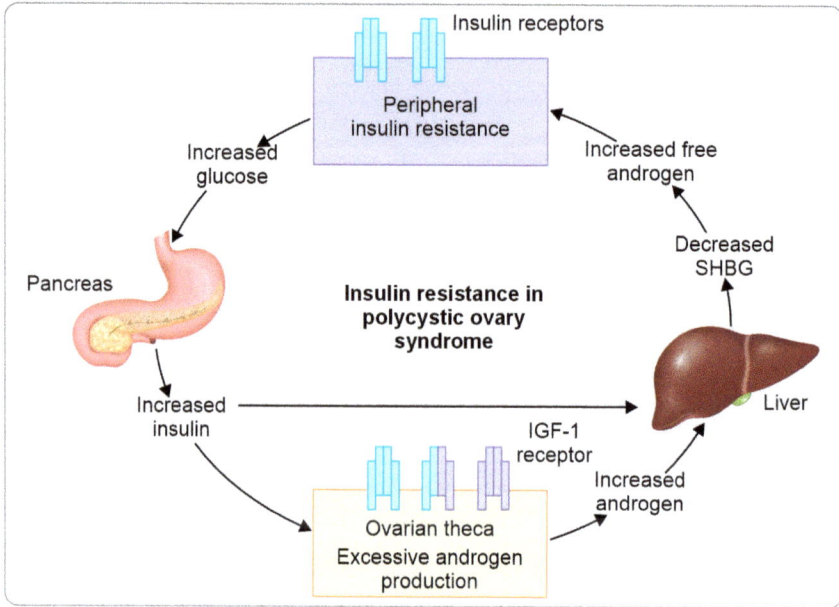

Fig. 2: Insulin resistance in PCOS women.[6] (IGF-1: insulin-like growth factor 1; PCOS: polycystic ovarian syndrome; SHBG: sex hormone-binding globulin)

> **BOX 1:** Insulin sensitizers.
>
> - Metformin
> - Glucagon-like peptide-1 (GLP-1) receptor agonists
> - Thiazolidinediones
> - Statins
> - α-lipoic acid

gestational DM in pregnancy. It does not affect insulin secretion but can improve insulin action.[8]

Mechanism of Action

It primarily inhibits hepatic glucose production, although it decreases intestinal glucose uptake and increases insulin sensitivity in peripheral tissues. The Diabetes Prevention Program has shown that metformin can delay the onset of DM in high-risk population and a decrease in hyperinsulinemia reduces androgen levels.

Metformin likely improves ovulation induction in PCOS women by:
- Reducing insulin levels and altering the effect of insulin on ovarian androgen biosynthesis, theca cell proliferation, improves menstrual cyclicity, corrects anovulation and endometrial growth
- Through a direct effect, it inhibits ovarian gluconeogenesis and thus reduces ovarian androgen production. Metformin has been shown to

inhibit gonadotropin-releasing hormone (GnRH) release by activation of hypothalamic AMPK, a crucial regulator of food intake in mammals, in a dose-dependent and time-dependent fashion[9] **(Box 2)**.

Role of genetic factor in metformin action: There is heterogeneity in the clinical response to metformin in PCOS and this might be mediated by the polymorphism in genes involved in metformin transport or action.

Indirectly metformin activates AMPK and results in mitochondrial biogenesis and glycolysis[11] **(Fig. 3)**.

BOX 2: Mechanism of action of metformin.

Metformin—mechanism of action:
- Reduce blood lipid levels
- Reduce liver glucose production
- Insulin-mediated glucose uptake—liver and skeletal muscles
- Reduce the utilization of gluconeogenic substrates

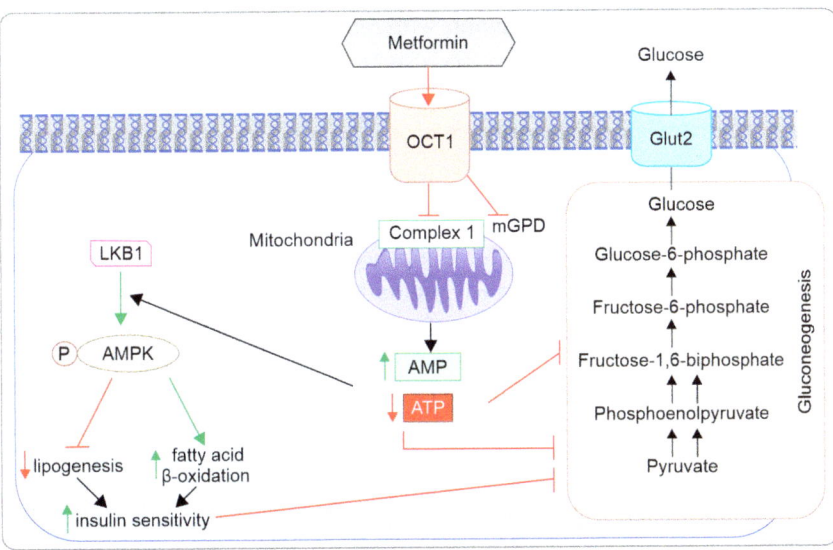

Fig. 3: Metformin-induced inhibition of mitochondrial complex I.[10] The direct inhibition of complex I by metformin decreases the production of ATP ensuing in increases in AMP. The increase in the [AMP] to [ATP] ratio signals energy resulting in inhibition of high-energy demanding gluconeogenesis process. This ratio leads to the activation of the AMPK complex leading to a decrease in lipogenesis, increase in fatty acid beta-oxidation with an improvement in insulin sensitivity which allows the restoration of gluconeogenesis. The inhibition of metformin on mGPD prevents the use of lactate or glycerol for gluconeogenesis. (AMP: adenosine monophosphate; ATP: adenosine triphosphate; OCT1: organic cation transporter 1; LKB1: liver kinase B1; Glut2: glucose transporter 2; mGPD: mitochondrial glycerol phosphate dehydrogenase)

Indications for Metformin

- PCOS women with documented IR or type II DM
- High-risk women—morbid obesity, metabolic syndrome without confirmed IR
- Clomiphene-resistant PCOS
- Prevention of ovarian hyperstimulation syndrome (OHSS) in PCOS women undergoing agonist protocol for controlled ovarian stimulation.

Dose and Side Effects of Metformin

It is usually started in the dose of 500 mg once daily and increased gradually up to 1,500 mg and a maximum dose of 2,000 mg/day. Some clinicians prefer to titrate up to the full dose over the initial first few weeks of therapy (500 mg/day for 1 week, 500 mg twice daily for 1 week, and 500 mg thrice daily) to minimize gastrointestinal side effects. The target dose is 500–850 mg thrice daily.

Nausea, vomiting, and diarrhea are the most common side effects. Most of the times, it resolves spontaneously and by titrating the increase of dose. Lactic acidosis can occur in patients with renal impairment. The use of long-acting preparations may reduce these gastrointestinal side effects. However, there is no consensus on the dose and duration of metformin therapy according to the latest Cochrane review.[12]

Metformin and Weight Loss

Even though previous studies have suggested that metformin therapy may help in weight reduction, recent systematic review and meta-analysis and Cochrane review showed that metformin has limited impact on weight loss when combined with lifestyle modification in obese PCOS women[13] or compared to placebo or no treatment.[12]

Metformin and Hyperandrogenism

In PCOS women with hyperandrogenism, metformin (1) reduces secretion of LH by the pituitary, (2) reduces ovarian and/or adrenal secretion of androgens, (3) increases liver levels of SHBG.[14] The reduction in insulin levels after metformin therapy in women with PCOS is closely correlated with an increase in insulin-like growth factor binding protein-1 (IGFBP-1) and a decrease in the IGF-1/IGFBP-1 ratio, indicating a reduction in IGF-1 availability in peripheral tissues.

Metformin increases the tyrosine activity of insulin receptors and decreases the androgen production. So, 6 months of metformin treatment in adolescent PCOS can reduce the Ferriman–Gallwey score significantly.[15]

Metformin and Hirsutism

According to Cochrane review 2020, metformin is less effective in improving hirsutism compared to oral contraceptive pill (OCP) in women with BMI 25–30 kg/m^2 and uncertain in women with BMI <25 kg/m^2 and >30 kg/m^2. Either metformin or OCP alone may be less effective in improving hirsutism compared to its combination.[16]

Adolescent PCOS

Metformin alone or in combination with OCP is recommended to manage weight and metabolic comorbidities. In adolescents with a clear diagnosis of PCOS, metformin can be considered in addition to lifestyle intervention. It is tried in the dose of 1,500–1,700 mg/day.[17]

Metformin and Ovulation Induction

Metformin alone: Various studies have shown contradictory results when metformin is compared with clomiphene citrate (CC) and letrozole alone.

American Society for Reproductive Medicine (ASRM) committee opinion: There is fair evidence that metformin alone is less effective than CC alone for achieving ovulation induction, clinical pregnancy rate (CPR), and live birth rate (LBR) in women with PCOS (Grade B). But there is insufficient evidence to suggest metformin alone increases pregnancy or LBR compared to letrozole alone (Grade C).[18]

Metformin in combination with other ovulation induction agents: Combination of CC and metformin is superior to metformin alone for ovulation, clinical pregnancy, and LBR. Furthermore, metformin does not improve the metabolic parameters such as fasting insulin, glucose, testosterone, and lipid profiles.[12] When CC plus metformin is compared with CC alone, there was no significant difference in ovulation rates, continuing pregnancy, or LBR.[19]

American Society of Assisted Reproduction committee opinion for metformin:
- There is good evidence that metformin in combination with CC improves ovulation and CPR but does not improve LBR compared with CC alone in PCOS women (Grade A).
- There is fair evidence that pretreatment with metformin for at least 3 months followed by addition of another ovulation inducing agent increases the LBR (Grade B).

Women with BMI >35 kg/m^2 and those with CC resistance showed benefit with combination of CC and metformin, although there is no evidence of a difference in LBR.[12,20] Combination of metformin with CC or letrozole has shown varying results. Addition of metformin to CC is more effective to achieve pregnancy than to letrozole.[21]

In a recent Cochrane review, authors have concluded that metformin may increase the LBR among women undergoing ovulation induction with gonadotropins and can be started before giving ovulation induction.[22]

As per the American Society of Assisted Reproduction committee opinion:[18] Metformin alone when compared with placebo increases the ovulation rate in PCOS women, but should not be the first line of treatment for anovulation as better drugs are available for ovulation induction. Metformin alone does not increase the miscarriage rates when stopped at initiation of pregnancy. There is insufficient evidence that metformin with other ovulation induction agents will increase the LBR.

Metformin and Assisted Reproductive Technology

In recent systematic review and meta-analysis, metformin treatment reduced the risk of OHSS but the overall CPR or LBR showed no association in PCOS women undergoing assisted reproductive technology (ART). So, metformin should be carefully considered in PCOS women undergoing ART and may be preferred in women with BMI >26 kg/m^2.[23]

It has been suggested that co-treatment with metformin may improve the outcome of ART. In a Cochrane review 2015, they observed that metformin before or during ART improved the CPR (OR 1.52, 95% CI 1.07–2.15) and there was no effect on miscarriage rate. However, there was a significant reduction in risk of OHSS in GnRH agonist long protocol when metformin was used. This might be probably by modulating the ovarian response to the stimulation.[24]

In GnRH agonist protocol with adjunct metformin therapy in PCOS women undergoing ART, metformin can be commenced at the start of GnRH agonist treatment to improve the CPR and reduce the risk of OHSS and stopped at the time of pregnancy confirmation. As GnRH antagonist protocol is recommended in patients at risk of OHSS, the role of metformin is unclear in antagonist protocol.[25]

Metformin and Pregnancy

Metformin is widely used among PCOS women. However, its association with ART outcome is controversial. In a Finnish study, metformin was administered 3 months prior to fertility treatment and continued up to 12 weeks of pregnancy. They observed increase in pregnancy rate with greatest benefit in obese women and LBR was also significantly more in metformin group. So, according to Cochrane review, miscarriage rates are more in obese women and metformin appears to reduce the miscarriage rate in these women[12] **(Box 3)**.

Women with PCOS are at increased risk of pregnancy-related complications, including gestational diabetes, pregnancy-induced hypertension,

CHAPTER 22: Insulin Sensitizers: Metformin and Inositols

BOX 3: Recommendations for use of metformin in PCOS.[29]

Recommendations:
- Metformin alone should not be used as first-line therapy for ovulation induction in women with PCOS, since ovulation induction agents such as CC or letrozole are more effective
- Metformin alone is not likely to increase LBR in women seeking pregnancy in the short term, utilizing metformin in individualized cases of PCOS with the goal of improving ovulation rates over the long-term may be of benefit
- In the context of increased ovulation rate and overall improved insulin resistance on metformin along with other ovulation-inducing agents may be beneficial in increasing pregnancy rates, although there is insufficient evidence of an increase in LBR

(CC: clomiphene citrate; LBR: live birth rate; PCOS: polycystic ovarian syndrome)

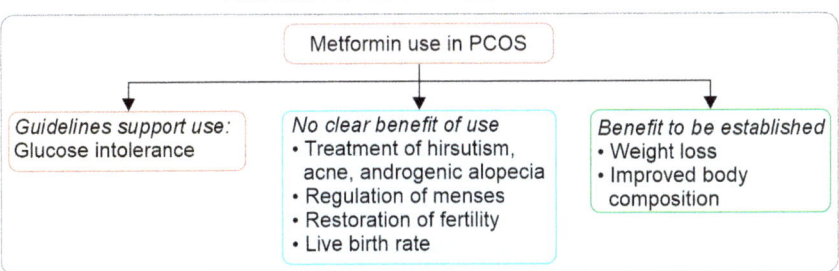

Flowchart 1: Metformin use in PCOS.[27,28]

(PCOS: polycystic ovarian syndrome)

preeclampsia, and neonatal morbidity.[26] Metformin has a good safety profile during pregnancy, belonging to Category B drug. As metformin has favorable effect on metabolic and cardiovascular events in diabetic population, it seemed to improve even in pregnancies in PCOS women. However, a large RCT showed no improvement if continued throughout pregnancy except for nonsignificant reduction in late miscarriages and preterm deliveries[27,28] **(Flowchart 1)**.

International evidence-based guidelines for metformin in PCOS are given in **Box 4**.

Thiazolidinediones

Thiazolidinediones such as troglitazone, rosiglitazone, and pioglitazone activate transcription of genes that affect glucose and lipid metabolism mediating decreased free fatty acid levels and decreased visceral fat mass.[30]

Liao et al. studied metformin alone versus metformin and rosiglitazone group for 6 months and observed a significant decrease in BMI in metformin group with no change in combination group, although six pregnancies were achieved in the combination group and only two in metformin alone group.[31]

BOX 4: International evidence-based guidelines for metformin in PCOS.[29]

Guidelines for metformin for ovulation induction in PCOS (2018):[29]
- Good evidence that metformin alone vs. placebo increases the ovulation rate in women with PCOS *(Grade A)*
- Insufficient evidence to suggest that metformin alone increases pregnancy rates or live birth rates compared with placebo or letrozole *(Grade C)*
- Fair evidence that metformin alone is less effective than CC alone for the achievement of ovulation induction, clinical pregnancy, and live birth in women with PCOS *(Grade B)*
- Good evidence that metformin in combination with CC improves ovulation and clinical pregnancy rates but does not improve live birth rates compared with CC alone in women with PCOS *(Grade A)*
- Fair evidence that pretreatment with metformin for at least 3 months followed by the addition of another ovulation-inducing drug increases live birth rate *(Grade B)*
- Fair evidence that CC–metformin improves ovulation and pregnancy rates compared with CC alone in CC-resistant PCOS women *(Grade B)*
- Fair evidence that overall pregnancy rates are not different with CC–metformin, CC–LOD, or LOD alone in women with CC-resistant PCOS *(Grade B)*.
- Insufficient evidence regarding pregnancy rate or live birth rate with the use of metformin alone compared with LOD for ovulation induction in CC-resistant PCOS patients *(Grade C)*
- Insufficient evidence to compare metformin plus CC to aromatase inhibitors alone or metformin plus aromatase inhibitors for ovulation induction in CC-resistant women *(Grade C)*
- Insufficient or conflicting evidence regarding metformin use combined with CC compared with gonadotropins for ovulation induction in women with CC-resistant PCOS *(Grade C)*
- Fair evidence that metformin used while attempting pregnancy and stopped at the initiation of pregnancy does not affect the rate of miscarriage *(Grade B)*
- Insufficient evidence to recommend metformin during pregnancy to reduce the chance of miscarriage *(Grade C)*
- Good evidence that metformin alone does not increase the rate of multiple pregnancy *(Grade A)*. While there is no evidence of an effect (either increase or decrease) on multiple pregnancy rates in cycles using combination CC plus metformin vs. CC alone, there remains insufficient data on this matter due to lack of adequate power to detect a difference *(Grade C)*
- Insufficient evidence of a reduced risk for multiple pregnancy with the addition of metformin to FSH compared with FSH alone *(Grade C)*
- Insufficient good-quality evidence to determine if metformin is more effective in nonobese or obese women with PCOS *(Grade C)*

(CC: clomiphene citrate; FSH: follicle-stimulating hormone; LOD: laparoscopic ovarian drilling; PCOS: polycystic ovary syndrome)

Mohsen et al. observed enhancement of ovulation along with insulin sensitivity with CC and rosiglitazone than with CC alone without any significant difference in cumulative pregnancy rates in both the groups.[32]

Both rosiglitazone and pioglitazone are category C drug and have very little short-term risk, even though no adverse congenital defects have been found, hence should be discontinued immediately after pregnancy is confirmed.

Even though troglitazone 400 mg/day for 12 weeks can improve ovulation, it is abandoned in view of hepatotoxicity. Rosiglitazone in the dose of 4 mg twice daily has been shown to enhance both spontaneous and clomiphene-induced ovulation in obese PCOS women. However, neither of them have been extensively evaluated for ovulation induction.

Glucagon-like Peptide-1

Newer insulin sensitizer such as glucagon-like peptide-1 (GLP-1) is a peptide hormone secreted by intestinal L cells that promote insulin secretion. It improves IR, inhibiting appetite and food intake, delaying gastric emptying, and reducing body weight. The currently licensed drugs for treatment of type II DM include exenatide and liraglutide, the latter for treatment of obesity as well[33] and they are tried in women with PCOS.

Glucagon-like peptide-1 receptor agonist directly inhibits the inflammatory pathway by reducing macrophage infiltration to increase the insulin sensitivity of fat, muscle, and liver tissues.[34] It also improves the IR indirectly by changing energy utilization efficiency, reducing fat synthesis and increasing lipolysis in the liver, obstructing a fructose-induced lipid metabolic disorder based on the parasympathetic nervous system, and inhibiting the excessive production of very low-density lipoprotein in the liver.[35]

In a systematic review and meta-analysis, GLP-1 receptor agonist was found to be superior to metformin for improving the insulin sensitivity and reducing the BMI and abdominal girth in PCOS women. They had similar effects on menstrual frequency, serum total testosterone, free androgen index (FAI), SHBG, dehydroepiandrosterone sulfate (DHEA-S), Ferriman–Gallwey scores, androstenedione, LH, fasting blood glucose, FINS, triglycerides, total cholesterol, and blood pressure when compared with metformin. However, the incidence of nausea and headache was higher than with metformin.[36]

In a study, 60 oligo-ovulatory PCOS women were randomized to receive metformin or exenatide or a combination of both. Even though all groups showed improvement in ovulation, endocrine and metabolic parameters, it was greatest in the combination group.[37]

Inositols

Among the inositols, myoinositol (MI) is extensively studied. MI is one of the nine stereoisomers of a sugar belonging to vitamin B complex group. It is converted to Di-chiro inositol (DCI) in cells and plays an important role in morphogenesis, cell growth, and lipid synthesis. It acts by a membrane-associated sodium-dependent inositol co-transporter GLUT4 as a post-receptor mediator (second messenger) of insulin signal and decreases hyperinsulinemia. MI improves ovarian function, decreases LH/FSH ratio, reduces serum androgens, increases SHBG, and decreases serum total and free testosterone.[38] The ideal dose of MI has not yet been defined and the studies have used 1–4 g per day in different settings[39,40] **(Fig. 4)**.

Myoinositol plays an important role in activating calcium channels and hence oocyte maturation. So, treatment with MI and folic acid reduces the number of germinal vesicles and degenerated oocytes at pickup without affecting the number of oocytes retrieved.[41]

As it acts at ovarian level, MI corrects the IR and oocyte quality. It also corrects hormonal disturbances at ovarian level like reduce hyperandrogenism and regulate menstrual cycles ovulation and hirsutism thus reducing the dose of gonadotropins and risk of OHSS in PCOS women during ovulation induction and in vitro fertilization (IVF).[40,42]

Administration of DCI in PCOS women causes a significant reduction in serum testosterone levels and clinical manifestation of hyperandrogenism, with improvement in metabolic parameters and ovulation.[43]

In an RCT, metformin (500 mg) along with MI (600 mg) thrice daily is compared with metformin (500 mg) thrice daily alone in PCOS women undergoing ovulation induction. They observed a significant improvement in menstrual cycle length ($p = 0.03$) and bleeding days ($p = 0.01$), homeostatic model assessment for insulin resistance (HOMA-IR) ($p = 0.03$), CPR (63.3% vs. 33.3%; $p = 0.001$), and LBR (55% vs. 26.67%; $p = 0.002$) in combination of metformin and MI group.[44] However, studies with larger sample size are required to confirm this finding as only 60 women were studied in both the groups. Administration of MI along with DCI in physiological plasma ratio of 40:1 in obese PCOS women might reduce the metabolic and clinical alteration of PCOS and can reduce the risk of metabolic syndrome.[45]

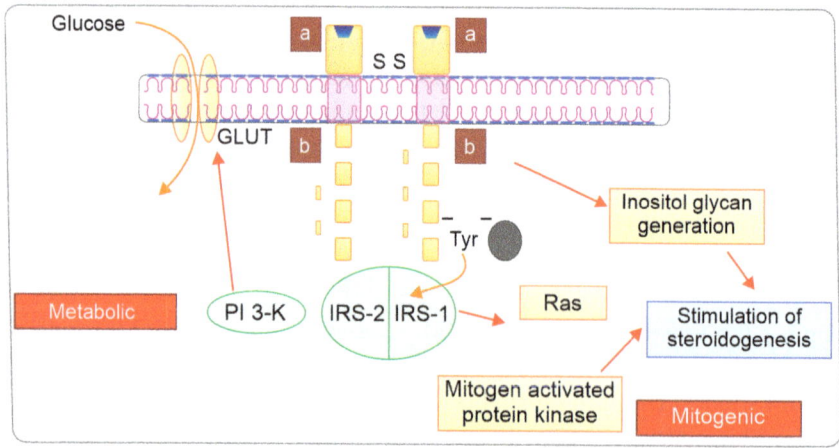

Fig. 4: Insulin also acts on the ovary through the inositol glycan system.[14]

Only a few cases of gastrointestinal discomfort such as nausea and diarrhea were reported with high doses (>18 g) so its use is considered safe for long-term therapy.

Myoinositol is converted into DCI by insulin-dependent epimerase. High DCI concentration is seen in liver, muscles, and fat that is responsible for glycogen synthesis and storage. This conversion is affected when there is IR. MI deficiency is related to poor oocyte quality, so supplementation with 4 g/day in PCOS women improves hormonal profile, restores ovulation, and induces regular menstrual cycle in both nonobese and obese PCOS.[38] It also improves oocyte quality and reduces the administration of FSH during IVF.[46]

Since MI and DCI regulate different biological processes, concomitant administration of both may be more beneficial in overweight PCOS women. So, DCI rapidly reduces peripheral hyperinsulinemia and MI improves the ovulatory function after 3 months of administration. MI can be combined with metformin and this synergistic action has significantly reduced the dose of the drugs without affecting the efficacy.[47,48]

Newer Treatments: Statins

In PCOS women, statins reduce the serum cholesterol from which sex steroids including androgens are synthesized. It can improve the hyperandrogenic profile and restore ovulation by reducing steroidogenesis. Statins have intrinsic antioxidant properties and exert control on cell proliferation and hence improving ovulatory function. Monacolin is a natural statin derived from red yeast rice.[14]

Alpha-Lipoic Acid

Obesity is associated with impaired reproductive potential. Oxidative stress, low-grade chronic inflammation, and mitochondrial dysfunctions seen in obesity can affect oocyte environment and function. In a pilot study, MI (2 g/day) and folic acid (400 µg/day) along with α-lipoic acid (800 mg/day) in obese infertile women might reduce the oxidative stress of the oocyte environment and can improve pregnancy rate.[49]

■ CONCLUSION

Various drugs that improve insulin sensitivity have been proposed and even though metformin is the most commonly used drug, it has a limited role in improving the reproductive outcome in women with PCOS. However, there may be benefit in certain specific groups like in obese PCOS women with CC resistance and women undergoing IVF/intracytoplasmic sperm injection (ICSI) with agonist protocol as it reduces the risk of OHSS. There is insufficient evidence to recommend other insulin sensitizers in the treatment of anovulatory PCOS women.

KEY POINTS

- PCOS is a common endocrine disorder and is a diagnosis of exclusion.
- It is associated with hyperandrogenism, hyperinsulinemia, altered FSH/LH ratio.
- Hyperinsulinemia can lead on to ovulatory dysfunction, follicular arrest and PCOM morphology.
- Metformin is the most commonly used insulin sensitizer
- Titrated dose of metformin is preferred to minimize the gastrointestinal side effects.
- Metformin is indicated in women with BMI >35 kg/m^2, CC resistance, agonist protocol to reduce the risk of OHSS.
- There is insufficient evidence to recommend other insulin sensitizers in the treatment of PCOS women.

REFERENCES

1. Bozdag G, Mumusoglu S, Zengin D, Karabulut E, Yildiz BO. The prevalence and phenotypic features of polycystic ovary syndrome: a systematic review and meta-analysis. Hum Reprod. 2016;31(12):2841-55.
2. Mahalingaiah S, Diamanti-Kandarakis E. Targets to treat metabolic syndrome in polycystic ovary syndrome. Expert Opin Ther Targets. 2015;19(11):1561-74.
3. Li Y, Chen C, Ma Y, Xiao J, Luo G, Li Y, et al. Multi-system reproductive metabolic disorder: significance for the pathogenesis and therapy of polycystic ovary syndrome (PCOS). Life Sci. 2019;228:167-75.
4. Mantzoros CS, Flier JS. Insulin resistance: the clinical spectrum. In: Mazzoferi E (Ed). Advances in Endocrinology and Metabolism, 6th edition. St. Louis: Mosby-Year Book; 1995. p. 193.
5. Stepto NK, Cassar S, Joham AE, Hutchison SK, Harrison CL, Goldstein RF, et al. Women with polycystic ovary syndrome have intrinsic insulin resistance on euglycaemic-hyperinsulaemic clamp. Hum Reprod. 2013;28:777-84.
6. Taylor HS, Pal L, Selvi E. Speroff's clinical Gynecologic Endocrinology and infertility, 9th edition. Philadelphia: Lippincott Williams and Wilkins; 2019. Chapter 11: Chronic Anovulation and the polycystic ovary syndrome; pp. 395-441.
7. Nardo LG, Rai R. Metformin therapy in the management of polycystic ovary syndrome: endocrine, metabolic and reproductive effects. Gynecol Endocrinol. 2001;15:373-80.
8. Moghetti P, Castello R, Negri C, Tosi F, Perrone F, Caputo M, et al. Metformin effects on clinical features, endocrine and metabolic profiles, and insulin sensitivity in polycystic ovary syndrome: a randomized, double-blind, placebo-controlled 6-month trial, followed by open, long-term clinical evaluation. J Clin Endocrinol Metab. 2000;85(1):139-46.
9. Coyral-Castel S, Tosca L, Ferreira G, Jeanpierre E, Rame C, Lomet D, et al. The effect of AMP-activated kinase activation on gonadotrophin-releasing hormone secretion in GT1-7 cells and its potential role in hypothalamic regulation of the oestrous cyclicity in rats. J Neuroendocrinol. 2008;20:335-46.

10. Foretz M, Hébrard S, Leclerc J, Zarrinpashneh E, Soty M, Mithieux G, et al. Metformin inhibits hepatic gluconeogenesis in mice independently of the LKB1/AMPK pathway via a decrease in hepatic energy state. J Clin Invest. 2010;120:2355-69.
11. Madiraju AK, Qiu Y, Perry RJ, Rahimi Y, Zhang X-M, Zhang D, et al. Metformin inhibits gluconeogenesis via a redox-dependent mechanism in vivo. Nat Med. 2018;24:1384-94.
12. Morley LC, Tang T, Yasmin EY, Lord JM, Norman RJ, Balen AH. Insulin-sensitising drugs (metformin, rosiglitazone, pioglitazone, D-chiro-inositol) for women with polycystic ovary syndrome, oligo amenorrhoea and subfertility. Cochrane Database Syst Rev. 2017;11(11):CD003053.
13. Naderpoor N, Shorakae S, de Courten B, Misso ML, Moran LJ, Teede HJ. Metformin and lifestyle modification in polycystic ovary syndrome: systematic review and meta-analysis. Hum Reprod Update. 2016;22:408-9.
14. Morgante G, Massaro MG, Di Sabatino A, Cappelli V, De Leo V. Therapeutic approach for metabolic disorders and infertility in women with PCOS. Gynecol Endocrinol. 2018;34(1):4-9.
15. De Leo V, Musacchio MC, Morgante G, Piomboni P, Petraglia F. Metformin treatment is effective in obese teenage girls with PCOS. Hum Reprod. 2006;21:2252-6.
16. Fraison E, Kostova E, Moran LJ, Bilal S, Ee CC, Venetis C, et al. Metformin versus the combined oral contraceptive pill for hirsutism, acne, and menstrual pattern in polycystic ovary syndrome (Review). Cochrane Database Syst Rev. 2020;(8):CD005552.
17. Peña AS, Witchel SF, Hoeger KM, Oberfield SE, Vogiatzi MG, Misso M, et al. Adolescent polycystic ovary syndrome according to the international evidence based guideline. BMC Med. 2020;18:72.
18. Practice Committee of the American Society for Reproductive Medicine. Role of metformin for ovulation induction in infertile patients with polycystic ovary syndrome (PCOS): a guideline. Fertil Steril. 2017;108(3):426-441.
19. Moll E, Bossuyt PM, Korevaar JC, Lambalk CB, van der Veen F. Effect of clomifene citrate plus metformin and clomifene citrate plus placebo on induction of ovulation in women with newly diagnosed polycystic ovary syndrome: randomised double blind clinical trial. BMJ. 2006;332:1485.
20. Legro RS, Barnhart HX, Schlaff WD, Carr BR, Diamond MP, Carson SA, et al.; Cooperative Multicenter Reproductive Medicine Network. Clomiphene, metformin, or both for infertility in the polycystic ovary syndrome. N Engl J Med. 2007;356:551-66.
21. Shrivastava U, Shrestha S, Dhakal R. Combined Clomiphene Citrate-Metformin Versus Letrozole-Metformin in Achieving Pregnancy among Women with Polycystic Ovary Syndrome. Gynecol Reprod Health. 2019;3(1):1-5.
22. Bordewijk EM, Nahuis M, Costello MF, Van der Veen F, Tso LO, Mol BW, et al. Metformin during ovulation induction with gonadotrophins followed by timed inter-course or intrauterine insemination for subfertility associated with polycystic ovary syndrome. Cochrane Database Syst Rev. 2017;1(1):CD009090.
23. Wu Y, Tu M, Huang Y, Liu Y, Zhang D. Association of Metformin with Pregnancy Outcomes with Polycystic Ovarian Syndrome Undergoing In Vitro Fertilization: A Systematic Review and Meta-analysis. JAMA Network Open. 2020;3(8):e2011995.

24. Tso LO, Costello MF, Albuquerque LET, Andriolo RB, Marjoribanks J, Macedo CR. Metformin treatment before and during in vitro fertilization or intracytoplasmic sperm injection in women with polycystic ovary syndrome: summary of a Cochrane review. Fertil Steril. 2015;104:542-4.
25. Balen AH, Morley LC, Misso M, Franks S, Legro RS, Wijeyaratne CN, et al. The management of anovulatory infertility in women with polycystic ovary syndrome: an analysis of the evidence to support the development of global WHO guidance. Hum Reprod Update. 2016;22:687-708.
26. Boomsma CM, Eijkemans MJ, Hughes EG, Visser GH, Fauser BC, Macklon NS. A meta-analysis of pregnancy outcomes in women with polycystic ovary syndrome. Hum Reprod Update. 2006;12:673-83.
27. Vanky E, Stridsklev S, Heimstad R, Romundstad P, Skogøy K, Kleggetveit O, et al. Metformin versus placebo from first trimester to delivery in polycystic ovary syndrome. J Clin Endocrinol Metab. 2010;95(12):E448-55.
28. Sam S, Ehrmann DA. Metformin therapy for the reproductive and metabolic consequences of polycystic ovary syndrome. Diabetologia. 2017;60(9):1656-61.
29. Teede H, Misso M, Costello M, Dokras A, Laven J, Moran L, et al. (2018). International evidence-based guideline for the assessment and management of polycystic ovary syndrome 2018. [online] Available from https://www.monash.edu/__data/assets/pdf_file/0004/1412644/PCOS_Evidence-Based-Guidelines_20181009.pdf. [Last accessed April, 2024].
30. Glintborg D, Andersen M. Thiazolinedione treatment in PCOS—an update. Gynecol Endocrinol. 2010;26(11):791-803.
31. Liao L, Tian YJ, Zhao JJ, Xin Y, Xing HY, Dong JJ. Metformin versus metformin plus rosiglitazone in women with polycystic ovary syndrome. Chin Med J. 2011;124(5):714-8.
32. Mohsen IA. A randomised controlled trial of the effect of rosiglitazone and clomiphene citrate versus clomiphene citrate alone in overweight/obese women with polycystic syndrome. Gynecol Endocrinol. 2012;28(4):269-72.
33. Conway G, Dewailly D, Diamanti-Kandarakis E, Escobar-Morreale HF, Franks S, Gambineri A, et al. The polycystic ovary syndrome: a position statement from the European Society of Endocrinology. Eur J Endocrinol. 2014;171:P1-29.
34. Lee YS, Park MS, Choung JS, Kim SS, Oh HH, Choi CS, et al. Glucagon-like peptide-1 inhibits adipose tissue macrophage infiltration and inflammation in an obese mouse model of diabetes. Diabetologia. 2012;55:2456-68.
35. Taher J, Baker CL, Cuizon C, Masoudpour H, Zhang R, Farr S, et al. GLP-1 receptor agonism ameliorates hepatic VLDL overproduction and de novo lipogenesis in insulin resistance. Mol Metab. 2014;3:823-33.
36. Han Y, Li Y, He B. GLP-1 receptor agonists versus metformin in PCOS: a systematic review and meta-analysis. Reprod Biomed Online. 2019;39(2):332-42.
37. Elkind-Hirsch K, Marrioneaux O, Bhushan M, Vernor D, Bhushan R. Comparison of single and combined treatment with exenatide and metformin on menstrual cyclicity in overweight women with polycystic ovary syndrome. J Clin Endocrinol Metab. 2008;93:2670-8.
38. Carlomagno G, Unfer V. Inositol safety: clinical evidences. Eur Rev Med Pharmacol Sci. 2011;15:931-6.
39. Chirania K, Misra S, Behera S. A randomised clinical trial comparing myoinositol & metformin in PCOS. Int J Reprod Contracept Obstet Gynecol. 2017;6:1814-20.

40. Artini PG, Di Berardino OM, Papini F, Genazzani AD, Simi G, Ruggiero M, et al. Endocrine and clinical effects of myo-inositol administration in polycystic ovary syndrome. A randomized study. Gynecol Endocrinol. 2013;29:375-9.
41. Ciotta L, Stracquadanio M, Pagano I, Carbonaro A, Palumbo M, Gulino F. Effects of myo-inositol supplementation on oocyte's quality in PCOS patients: a double blind trial. Eur Rev Med Pharmacol Sci. 2011;15:509-14.
42. Facchinetti F, Orru B, Grandi G, Unfer V. Short-term effects of metformin and myo-inositol in women with polycystic ovarian syndrome (PCOS): a meta-analysis of randomized clinical trials. Gynecol Endocrinol. 2019;35(3): 198-206.
43. Morgante G, Orvieto R, Di Sabatino A, Musacchio MC, De Leo V. The role of inositol supplementation in patients with polycystic ovary syndrome, with insulin resistance, undergoing the low-dose gonadotropin ovulation induction regimen. Fertil Steril. 2011;95:2642-4.
44. Agrawal A, Mahey R, Kachhawa G, Khadgawat R, Vanamail P, Kriplani A. Comparison of metformin plus myoinositol vs metformin alone in PCOS women undergoing ovulation induction cycles: randomized controlled trial. Gynecol Endocrinol. 2019;35(6):511-4.
45. Nordio M, Proietti E. The combined therapy with myo-inositol and D-Chiro-inositol reduces the risk of metabolic disease in PCOS overweight patients compared to myo-inositol supplementation alone. Eur Rev Med Pharmacol Sci. 2012;16:575-81.
46. Unfer V, Carlomagno G, Rizzo P, Raffone E, Roseff S. Myo-inositol rather than D-chiro-inositol is able to improve oocyte quality in intracytoplasmic sperm injection cycles. A prospective, controlled, randomized trial. Eur Rev Med Pharmacol Sci. 2011;15:452-7.
47. Nagaria T, Mohapatra A, Jaiswal J. Effect of Myoinositol and Metformin in combination on clinical and hormonal profile in patients of polycystic ovarian syndrome. Int J Reprod Contracept Obstet Gynecol. 2019;8(2):702-9.
48. Thakur SS, Anjum S, Siddiqui SS. Randomised controlled trial: comparing effects of metformin versus myoinositol versus metformin and myoinositol on ovarian functions and metabolic factors in polycystic ovarian syndrome. Int J Reprod Contracept Obstet Gynecol. 2020;9:2542-9.
49. Novielli C, Anelli GM, Lisso F, Marzorati A, Parrilla B, Oneta M, et al. Effects of α-lipoic acid and myo-inositol supplementation on the oocyte environment of infertile obese women: A preliminary study. Reprod Biol. 2020;20(4):541-6.

Section

Luteal Phase Support

- **Luteal Phase Support in Intrauterine Insemination Cycles**
  Bhavana Mittal, Chandana Bhat
- **Luteal Phase Support in Assisted Reproductive Technology Cycles: Fresh and Frozen Embryo Transfer**
  Anu Chawla, Manisha Nandi

Luteal Phase Support in Intrauterine Insemination Cycles

Bhavana Mittal, Chandana Bhat

■ INTRODUCTION

Intrauterine insemination (IUI) increases the probability of conception in couples who are subfertile. During a normal menstrual cycle, the luteinizing hormone (LH) surge causes ovulation and also stimulates the corpus luteal cells to produce progesterone, thus inducing the vascularization and the thickening of the endometrium to help in implantation. Following implantation, the placenta produces human chorionic gonadotropin (hCG), which stimulates the corpus luteum to produce many different hormones, among which *the sex steroid, progesterone*, is of primary importance because it is necessary and sufficient to transform the endometrium to a state that is receptive to blastocyst implantation and to maintain early pregnancy and the LH that is produced after the ovulation surge which maintains the progesterone production, decreases only when hCG from the growing trophoblast takes over.

In controlled ovarian hyperstimulation cycles, the increased levels of steroid inhibit the pituitary secretion of LH and this is thought to shorten the luteal phase and cause premature luteolysis, which is manifested by a shortened luteal phase with low concentrations of progesterone. Evidence states that 12% of women undergoing gonadotropin-stimulated ovulation induction experience luteal phase defects and 20% have shortened luteal phase.[1] This creates suboptimal environment for blastocysts implantation and maintenance of early pregnancy.

Why should luteal phase be supported in mild ovarian stimulation–IUI cycles?
Concept of luteal phase deficiency: Luteal phase deficiency is defined as a luteal phase shorter than 11 days, or a lag of >2 days in endometrial histological development, or low mid-luteal progesterone values <10 ng/mL. Jones and colleagues showed that the administration of exogenous progesterone could correct this luteal deficiency.[2]

In normal ovulatory cycles, two days following the LH surge, progesterone level increases and reaches its maximum to about 21 ng/mL on the 8th day of

LH surge, then starts to decline from day 9 reaching to about half level (11 ng/mL) on the 10th day. Finally, it returns to its baseline level 5 days later.

This pattern is different in controlled ovarian stimulation cycles, so that progesterone reaches its maximum level 6–8 days after hCG injection and then suddenly drops. If pregnancy does not occur, progesterone reaches its baseline level about 4 days later. Thus, luteal phase duration is 1–3 days shorter compared to spontaneous ovulatory cycles.

It has been reported by Hull et al.[3] that progesterone levels are raised by a factor of 1.5 after clomiphene use and Radwanska et al.[4] found that progesterone value increased from 9.0 ± 5.9 ng/mL to 27.3 ± 10.3 ng/mL in conception cycles following clomiphene citrate with or without hCG and in letrozole cycles, average midluteal progesterone levels were 12.8 ng/mL.

Causes of luteal phase deficiency: Suprahysiologic estradiol level → Low LH level → inhibition of the corpus luteum leading to asynchronicity of estradiol and progesterone production.

Effects of luteal phase deficiency: Suboptimal production of progesterone results in endometrial developmental failure and loss of synchronicity between the embryo and endometrium, which are essential in both implantation and maintenance of early pregnancy as nucleolar channel system in the endometrium, a marker for endometrial receptivity requires minimum progesterone level was 5 ng/mL.[5]

Evidence has shown that increased mid-luteal serum progesterone levels were not associated with a higher clinical pregnancy rate in women who underwent controlled ovarian stimulation with IUI. However, a lower mid-luteal progesterone level was proposed to be a predictor for treatment failure and this forms the basis for luteal phase support in IUI cycle.

What are the effects of drugs used for ovarian stimulation on corpus luteum (CL)?

- *Clomiphene citrate (CC):* There is a dose-responsive positive relationship between luteal phase estrogen (E) and progesterone (P) levels with CC administration. The potential for CC to increase CL function has led to its proposal as a treatment modality for patients with insufficient luteal phase endogenous P secretion and it has been documented that women using CC for ovarian stimulation, in comparison to spontaneous cycles, achieved higher serum progesterone levels during the mid-luteal phase.
- *Letrozole, a selective aromatase inhibitor:* Data regarding endometrial function in letrozole cycles is lacking. However, letrozole also increases the mid-luteal progesterone level.
- Gonadotropins stimulate the ovaries directly to produce E, which in turn results in negative feedback at the levels of the hypothalamus and pituitary. This impairs the normal pulsatile release of LH from the

pituitary and disrupts the P secretion from the corpus luteum. Following ovarian stimulation with gonadotropins, a shortened luteal phase has been demonstrated thus resulting in insufficient luteal phase serum P levels. Hence, there is biologic plausibility for the benefit of exogenous P for luteal support in gonadotropin–IUI cycles as there was a difference in live birth outcomes of ~4% with low mid-luteal progesterone in gonadotropin–IUI cycles.[6]

What is the effect of trigger on the luteal phase?
The half-life of hCG is relatively long, that if at least 5,000 IU are used for triggering ovulation, biologically significant amounts persist for at least 10 days by which time the embryo starts secreting hCG to support the corpus luteum.

Ovulation triggered by gonadotropin-releasing hormone (GnRH) agonist is known to negatively impact luteal function and endometrial receptivity. Ovulation triggered with GnRH agonist results in the release of endogenous LH, which has a significantly shorter half-life than hCG, 60 minutes versus 24 hours, which predisposes cycles triggered with GnRH agonist to luteal phase deficiency.

Luteal support—drugs, dosage, and route: Drugs—
1. Progesterone
2. Progesterone + estrogen
3. Human chorionic gonadotropin
4. Gonadotropin-releasing hormone agonist

1. *Progesterone:* This is the key hormone of luteal phase which can make or break a pregnancy and is the main luteal phase support given in the controlled ovarian stimulation–IUI cycles.
   - Progesterone preparations can be divided into two main groups: Natural progesterone with its derivatives and synthetic progesterone with its derivatives.
   - Natural progesterone is quickly inactivated when taken orally because of its rapid metabolism in liver and intestine resulting in poor oral bioavailability hence vaginal route of progesterone administration is widely used.
   - No consensus exists about the ideal dose and route of progesterone administration. Data from studies done on luteal phase support in in vitro fertilization (IVF) show no significant differences in pregnancy rates were observed when intramuscular or vaginal routes were used and also when vaginal progesterone gel and tablet forms were applied.[7,8] This is also supported by the Cochrane review that showed no significant difference between intramuscular and vaginal progesterone in terms of live birth rate and ongoing pregnancy rates in IVF cycles.[9]

- The dose of progesterone capsules mostly varies between 200 and 600 mg.
- The mean serum value of progesterone with a vaginal capsule dose of 400 mg is 14 ng/mL.[10] A recent study[11] concluded 300 mg dose was sufficient and was associated with similarly successful ongoing pregnancy rates as compared to 600 mg of progesterone.
- Though vaginal progesterone is a time-tested route of progesterone administration, study by Malhotra J and Krishnaprasad K[12] concluded that oral administration of natural micronized progesterone as sustained release (SR) preparation offers slow yet consistent systemic concentrations in the therapeutic range of ≥14 ng/mL for sustaining pregnancy while offering once a day dosage convenience for better patient compliance.
- In a recent study by Khosravi et al.,[13] vaginal progesterone capsules 400 mg/24 h, once daily, were compared with oral dydrogesterone (20 mg) in clomiphene citrate + recombinant follicle-stimulating hormone (rFSH)–IUI cycles. Although the results were not statistically significant, the mid-luteal progesterone level in the oral dydrogesterone arm was higher and, accordingly miscarriage rate was lower. Consequently, this study demonstrated that oral dydrogesterone could also be effective as luteal phase support in IUI cycles.

  As evident from the above trials, luteal phase progesterone supplement plays a significant role in improving the pregnancy rates in gonadotropin stimulated cycles, though few studies support this view and few do not. **Table 1** summarizes various studies using progesterone as luteal phase support in an IUI Cycle.

  Various routes and commonly used dosages of progesterone: **Tables 2 and 3** summarize the various advantages and disadvantages of various routes of progesterone administration and their preferred route and dosage as well.

2. *Progesterone with estrogen:* Not routinely indicated in all IUI cycles as luteal phase support. Indicated in cases of:
   - Hypogonadotropic hypogonadism
   - Hypothalamic amenorrhea
   - Treated with GnRH agonist pretreatment

   Formulation and dose: Estradiol valerate—2 mg oral, twice a day, however other routes like transdermal and vaginal can also be used.

3. *Human chorionic gonadotropin:* The shortened luteal phase in gonadotropin-stimulated cycles can be normalized by mid-luteal hCG administration, and also it can be used as a luteal phase support in GnRHa-triggered cycles as they result in a shorter duration of LH release in comparison to hCG-triggered cycles. It is usually given in the dose of 2,500 IU IM as single dose 35 hours to 5 days after GnRHa trigger.

CHAPTER 23: Luteal Phase Support in Intrauterine Insemination Cycles

TABLE 1: Studies supporting luteal phase support in different scenario.

RCT	Drug used for ovarian stimulation–IUI cycle	Luteal phase support	Clinical pregnancy rate (LPS vs. no support)
Erdem et al.,[14] 2009	rFSH	Vaginal progesterone gel, 90 mg/24 h, until 12th week	21.2% vs. 12.7% (0.028)
Kyrou et al.,[15] 2010	Clomiphene citrate	Vaginal progesterone suppositories, 200 mg/8 h, until 7th week	7.3% vs. 8.7% (NS)
Ebrahimi et al.,[16] 2010	Clomiphene citrate + hMG	Vaginal progesterone suppositories, 400 mg/24 h, until 10th week	11.5% vs. 10% (NS)
Maher,[17] 2011	rFSH	Vaginal progesterone gel, 90 mg/24 h, for 14 days	29.5% vs. 19.8% (0.07)
Agha-Hosseini et al.,[18] 2012	Clomiphene citrate, clomiphene citrate + hMG, letrozole, letrozole + hMG	Vaginal progesterone suppositories, 400 mg/24 h, until 12th week	24.3% vs. 14.1% (0.02)
Hossein Rashidi et al.,[19] 2014	Clomiphene citrate + hMG	Vaginal progesterone suppositories, 400 mg/12 h, until 8th week	15.8% vs. 12.7% (NS)

(hMG: human menopausal gonadotropin; IUI: intrauterine insemination; LPS: luteal phase support; RCT: randomized controlled trial; rFSH: recombinant follicle-stimulating hormone)

A randomized controlled trial (RCT) by Keenan et al.[20] who administered 2,500 IU hCG on 3rd, 6th, and 9th day after the ovulatory dose of 10,000 IU hCG found no significant differences in the pregnancy rates in hCG-supported versus unsupported cycles.

4. *GnRH agonist:* Luteal phase GnRHa administration can elevate the progesterone level and consequently the luteal phase duration, although studies have failed to prove statistically significant improvement in pregnancy rate in the GnRHa group. It is administered as 0.1 mg triptorelin—8 days after hCG administration or 6 days after ovulation—mid-luteal phase.[21]

In a study done by Azra et al.,[22] it was administered as 0.1 mg (triptorelin) subcutaneously 4 days after IUI. The mean serum level progesterone 10 days after IUI in vaginal progesterone group was 33.45 ± 18.12 ng/mL and in GnRHa group it was 32.50 ± 23.82 ng/mL. This study concluded that GnRH agonist showed comparable effect with vaginal progesterone on

TABLE 2: Advantages and disadvantages of various routes of progesterone administration.

	Progesterone		
Intramuscular	**Vaginal**	**Subcutaneous/oral**	
High-serum progesterone levels with adequate endometrial secretory changes with satisfactory pregnancy rates	Better steady state plasma progesterone level with avoidance of first pass metabolism	Better compliance *dydrogesterone has good oral bioavailability* compared to micronized oral progesterone	Once a day dosage with better patient tolerability compared to intramuscular route
Adverse effects: • Daily injections • Severe inflammation • Pain • Sterile abscesses	*Adverse effects*: • Discharge • Irritation • Local warmth	More trials needed to justify its use in IUI cycles	

(IUI: intrauterine insemination)

TABLE 3: Various doses of progesterone.

Route of administration	Formulation	Recommended regimens
Vaginal	Micronized progesterone capsules	200–600 mg/day
	Bioadhesive progesterone gel	90 mg once a day
	Vaginal ring releasing progesterone	Not yet available
Oral	Dydrogesterone tablets	10 mg once or twice a day
Intramuscular	Natural progesterone in oil ampoules	25–100 mg/day
Subcutaneous	Water-soluble progesterone-hydroxypropyl-β-cyclodextrin complex	25 mg/day

luteal phase supporting in patients with unexplained infertility. However, more studies are required to prove its role as a LPS.

When to start the luteal phase support and how long to give?
Progesterone supplementation is usually started on the day of IUI or the next day after IUI, though it can be started up to 2 days after IUI and continued up to urine pregnancy test.

In case of a positive pregnancy test, progesterone support can be supplemented throughout the first trimester though a strong evidence to support this is lacking.

EVIDENCE ABOUT LUTEAL PHASE SUPPORT IN IUI CYCLE IN A NUTSHELL

There is a lacuna in definitive evidence regarding luteal phase support in IUI cycles. However, studies by Erdem et al.[14] and Agha-Hosseini et al.[18] support the view that luteal phase LH levels are reduced in gonadotropin–IUI cycles and this might produce a luteal phase defect and hence support the use of luteal phase support in gonadotropin-stimulated IUI cycles mainly in cases of unexplained infertility as they improve pregnancy outcomes. This was also supported by clinical trial done by Alleyassin et al.[23] who concluded from their study that with the use of vaginal P as a luteal phase support, clinical pregnancy rates in controlled ovarian stimulation and IUI in patients with unexplained or mild male factor infertility significantly improved.

However, these are contradicted in trials by Burak Karadag et al.[24] and Peeraer et al.[25] who concluded that although in IUI cycles stimulated with gonadotropins, a trend toward a higher clinical pregnancy rate as well as live birth rate was observed in the luteal phase support group but was not statistically significant and hence not routinely recommended. This is also supported in a recent trial by Keskin et al.[26] who concluded that there is no significant benefit of luteal phase support in IUI cycles stimulated with gonadotropins.

In women with polycystic ovary syndrome (PCOS) stimulated with letrozole, Montville et al.[27] reported an improved clinical pregnancy rate with luteal phase progesterone support, although the results were on the contrary for women stimulated with clomiphene citrate.

Ragni et al.[28] compared the luteal phase profile in patients stimulated with gonadotropin with/without GnRH antagonist for IUI cycles and demonstrated that the progesterone level was similar in the luteal phase in both groups without the need for luteal phase supplementation in the antagonist group.

The recent meta-analysis and systemic review by Green et al.,[29] which evaluated 11 trials studying 2,842 patients undergoing 4,065 cycles, concluded that there was no benefit on clinical pregnancy with progesterone support for patients who underwent ovulation induction with clomiphene (RR 0.85, 95% CI 0.52–1.41) or clomiphene plus gonadotropins (RR 1.26, 95% CI 0.90–1.76) and progesterone luteal phase support is beneficial to patients undergoing ovulation induction with gonadotropins in IUI cycles.

CONCLUSION

It is well proven beyond doubt that stimulated IVF cycles require luteal phase support. Although luteal phase support in IUI cycles stimulated with gonadotropins is widely adopted with trials demonstrating improved outcomes, more RCTs are required to show absolute benefit.

KEY POINTS

- In mildly stimulated (1-2 follicles) IUI cycles, there is no biological or empirical evidence that treatment with progesterone in the luteal phase improves the pregnancy rate.
- Vaginal micronized progesterone is luteal phase support of choice, with oral dydrogesterone showing promising role.
- There is a need for further RCTs to evaluate the most effective route, dose, and duration of luteal phase support in stimulated IUI cycles.

REFERENCES

1. Olson JL, Rebar RW, Schreiber JR, Vaitukaitis JL. Shortened luteal phase after ovulation induction with human menopausal gonadotropin and human chorionic gonadotropin. Fertil Steril. 1983;39:284-91.
2. Jones GS. The luteal phase defect. Fertil Steril. 1976;27:351.
3. Hull MGR, Savage PE, Bromham DR, Ismail AA, Morris AF. The value of single serum progesterone measurement in the mid-luteal phase as a criterion of a potentially fertile cycle ("ovulation") derived from treated and untreated conception cycles. Fertil Steril. 1982;37:355-60.
4. Radwanska E, Hammond J, Smith P. Single midluteal progesterone assay in the management of ovulatory infertility. J Reprod Med. 1981;26;85-9.
5. Nejat EJ, Szmyga MJ, Zapantis G, Meier UT. Progesterone threshold determines nucleolar channel system formation in human endometrium. Reprod Sci. 2014;21:915-20.
6. Hansen KR, Eisenberg E, Baker V, Hill MJ, Chen S, Talken S, et al. Midluteal Progesterone: A Marker of Treatment Outcomes in Couples With Unexplained Infertility. J Clin Endocrinol Metab. 2018;103(7):2743-51.
7. Nosarka S, Kruger T, Siebert I, Grové D. Luteal phase support in in vitro fertilization: meta-analysis of randomized trials. Gynecol Obstet Invest. 2005;60:67-74.
8. Polyzos NP, Messini CI, Papanikolaou EG, Mauri D, Tzioras S, Badawy A, et al. Vaginal progesterone gel for luteal phase support in IVF/ICSI cycles: a meta-analysis. Fertil Steril. 2010;94:2083-7.
9. Child T, Leonard SA, Evans JS, Lass A. Systematic review of the clinical efficacy of vaginal progesterone for luteal phase support in assisted reproductive technology cycles. Reprod Biomed Online. 2018;36(6):630-45.
10. Aali BS, Ebrahimipour S, Medhdizadeh S. The effectiveness of luteal phase support with cyclogest in ovarian stimulated intrauterine insemination cycles: A randomized controlled trial. Iran J Reprod Med. 2013;11(4):309-14.
11. Biberoglu EH, Tanrıkulu F, Erdem M, Erdem A, Biberoglu KO. Luteal phase support in intrauterine insemination cycles: a prospective randomized study of 300 mg versus 600 mg intravaginal progesterone tablet. Gynecol Endocrinol. 2016;32(1):55-7.
12. Malhotra J, Krishnaprasad K. Open-label, Prospective, Investigator Initiated Study to Assess the Clinical Role of Oral Natural or Synthetic Progesterone During Stimulated IUI Cycles for Unexplained Infertility. J Clin Diagn Res. 2016;10(1):QC08-10.

13. Khosravi D, Taheripanah R, Taheripanah A, Tarighat Monfared V, Hosseini-Zijoud SM. Comparison of oral dydrogesterone with vaginal progesterone for luteal support in IUI cycles: a randomized clinical trial. Iran J Reprod Med. 2015;13:433-8.
14. Erdem A, Erdem M, Atmaca S, Guler I. Impact of luteal phase support on pregnancy rates in intrauterine insemination cycles: a prospective randomized study. Fertil Steril. 2009;91:2508-13.
15. Kyrou D, Fatemi HM, Tournaye H, Devroey P. Luteal phase support in normo-ovulatory women stimulated with clomiphene citrate for intrauterine insemination: need or habit? Hum Reprod. 2010;25:2501-6.
16. Ebrahimi M, Asbagh FA, Darvish S. The effect of luteal phase support on pregnancy rates of the stimulated intrauterine insemination cycles in couples with unexplained infertility. Int J Fertil Steril. 2010;4:51-6.
17. Maher MA. Luteal phase support may improve pregnancy outcomes during intrauterine insemination cycles. Eur J Obstet Gynecol Reprod Biol. 2011;157:57-62.
18. Agha-Hosseini M, Rahmani M, Alleyassin A, Safdarian L, Sarvi F. The effect of progesterone supplementation on pregnancy rates in controlled ovarian stimulation and intrauterine insemination cycles: a randomized prospective trial. Eur J Obstet Gynecol Reprod Biol. 2012;165:249-53.
19. Hossein Rashidi B, Davari Tanha F, Rahmanpour H, Ghazizadeh M. Luteal phase support in the intrauterine insemination (IUI) cycles: a randomized double blind, placebo controlled study. J Family Reprod Health. 2014;8:149-53.
20. Keenan JA, Moghissi KS. Luteal phase support with hCG does not improve fecundity rate in human menopausal gonadotropin-stimulated cycles. Obstet Gynecol. 1992;79(6):983-7.
21. Soliman BS. Impact of luteal phase injection by single dose gonadotropin-releasing hormone agonist in women undergoing intrauterine insemination. JFIV Reprod Med Genet. 2015;3:152.
22. Azmoodeh A, Mohamadpoor J, Asbagh FA, Ghaseminezhad A, Lorzadeh N, Forghani F. The comparison of GNRH agonist administration versus vaginal progesterone on serum progesterone in luteal phase in ovarian hyperstimulation and intrauterine insemination cycles in unexplained infertility. Int J Med Health Res. 2016;2(9):84-8.
23. Alleyassin A, Agha Hosseini M, Sarvi F, Safdarian L, Rahmanpour H, Kokab AA. The effect of progesterone supplementation on pregnancy rates in controlled ovarian stimulation and intrauterine insemination cycles: a randomized prospective trial. Fertil Steril. 2012;98(3):S197.
24. Karadag B, Dilbaz B, Karcaaltincaba D, Sahin EG, Ercan F, Karasu Y, et al. The effect of luteal-phase support with vaginal progesterone on pregnancy rates in gonadotropin and clomiphene citrate/intra-uterine insemination cycles in unexplained infertility: A prospective randomised study. J Obstet Gynaecol. 2016;36(6):794-9.
25. Peeraer K, D'Hooghe T, Laurent P, Pelckmans S, Delvigne A, Laenen A, et al. Impact of luteal phase support with vaginal progesterone on the clinical pregnancy rate in intrauterine insemination cycles stimulated with gonadotropins: a randomized multicenter study. Fertil Steril. 2016;106(6):1490-5.

26. Keskin M, Aytaç R. Does Luteal Phase Support Effect Pregnancy Rates in Intrauterine Insemination Cycles? A Prospective Randomised Controlled Study in a Tertiary Center. Obstet Gynecol Int. 2020;2020:6234070.
27. Montville C, Khabbaz M, Aubuchon M, Williams D, Thomas M. Luteal support with intravaginal progesterone increases clinical pregnancy rates in women with polycystic ovary syndrome using letrozole for ovulation induction. Fertil Steril. 2010;94:678-83.
28. Ragni G, Vegetti W, Baroni E, Colombo M, Arnoldi M, Lombroso G, et al. Comparison of luteal phase profile in gonadotrophin stimulated cycles with or without a gonadotrophin-releasing hormone antagonist. Hum Reprod. 2001;16:2258-62.
29. Green KA, Zolton JR, Schermerhorn SM, Lewis TD, Healy MW, Terry N, et al. Progesterone luteal support after ovulation induction and intrauterine insemination: an updated systematic review and meta-analysis. Fertil Steril. 2017;107(4):924-33.e5.

Chapter 24

Luteal Phase Support in Assisted Reproductive Technology Cycles: Fresh and Frozen Embryo Transfer

Anu Chawla, Manisha Nandi

■ INTRODUCTION

Luteal phase support (LPS) is a critical aspect of assisted reproductive technology (ART), particularly in the context of embryo transfer cycles. While fresh embryo transfer cycles benefit from the natural hormonal milieu, frozen embryo transfer (FET) cycles necessitate careful hormonal manipulation to ensure optimal endometrial receptivity and successful implantation. This chapter delves into the specific requirements and protocols for LPS in FET cycles, comparing natural, modified natural, and programmed endometrial preparation protocols. The physiological nuances and clinical outcomes of these approaches are examined to provide a comprehensive understanding of LPS in ART.[1]

■ RELEVANT ASPECTS OF A FROZEN EMBRYO TRANSFER: PERSPECTIVE OF REQUIRED LUTEAL SUPPORT

Frozen embryo transfer cycles offer a more physiological endometrial environment devoid of supraphysiological hormone levels. However, the synchronicity between endometrial and embryonic development remains an area of ongoing research. The presence of a corpus luteum is essential for its pulsatile secretion of progesterone and endogenous molecules like relaxin, which are pivotal for implantation. In hormone replacement therapy (HRT), FET cycles, where the corpus luteum is absent, robust exogenous steroid support is imperative for securing the implantation process. The preparation of the endometrium and the provision of optimal exogenous luteal support are of paramount importance.[2]

■ SALIENT FEATURES RELATED TO THE LUTEAL PHASE SUPPORT IN FET CYCLES

- *Clinical efficacy:* Clinical outcomes are generally comparable across natural, modified natural, and programmed endometrial preparation protocols.
- *Protocol variability:* Luteal phase support varies according to the chosen protocol for FET cycles.

- *Programmed FET-HRT cycles:* These cycles necessitate luteal phase support due to the absence of the corpus luteum.
- *Efficacy of additional LPS:* Current data suggests that additional luteal phase support does not significantly enhance outcomes in natural or modified natural FET cycles.
- *Consensus on LPS:* There is no consensus on the optimal type and duration of progesterone support in FET-HRT cycles. Both 180 mg/day vaginal progesterone gel and 50–100 mg/day intramuscular progesterone have shown similar efficacy.
- *Serum progesterone threshold:* A serum progesterone level exceeding 9–10 ng/mL during the mid-luteal phase in programmed FET cycles appears to improve reproductive outcomes.
- *Oral dydrogesterone:* Data on oral dydrogesterone for luteal support in FET cycles is currently insufficient.[3]

■ PROTOCOLS USED FOR ENDOMETRIAL PREPARATION

Endometrial preparation protocols for FET can be categorized into two types:

Natural and modified natural cycles:
1. *Natural cycle:* Utilizes the observation of a natural luteinizing hormone (LH) surge or the induction of ovulation to determine the timing of embryo thawing and transfer. Ideal for women with regular, ovulatory cycles, this protocol aims to synchronize the endometrium and embryo without exogenous hormones, targeting the physiologic implantation window (7–10 days postovulation).
2. *Modified natural cycle:* Involves triggering ovulation with LH or human chorionic gonadotropin (hCG) when the dominant follicle is >17 mm, endometrial thickness is >7 mm, and serum progesterone is <1.5 ng/mL. While luteal phase insufficiency is reported in about 8% of natural cycles, outcomes can vary.[4]
3. *Programmed FET-HRT cycles:*
   Aim: To replicate the follicular phase of the menstrual cycle with exogenous estradiol, followed by progesterone.
   Protocol: Endometrial proliferation is achieved through oral or transdermal estrogen, which also suppresses endogenous follicle development and upregulates progesterone receptors. Once sufficient proliferation is observed (up to 20 days), secretory transformation is induced with progesterone.
   Timing: FET is scheduled based on the embryo stage and progesterone timing, with a critical need for extensive luteal support due to the absence of the corpus luteum. Progesterone support is generally continued for 7–12 weeks of gestation, although higher levels of progesterone during weeks 5–8 of gestation correlate with better pregnancy outcomes.[5]

HYPERTENSIVE DISORDERS AND HIGHER ADVERSE PERINATAL OUTCOMES IN PROGRAMMED FET PREGNANCIES

Programmed FET pregnancies may exhibit reduced secretion of angiogenic molecules like relaxin and vascular endothelial growth factor (VEGF), which are crucial for implantation and vascular compliance. This deficiency is associated with an increased risk of hypertensive disorders of pregnancy, as evidenced by meta-analyses indicating a relative risk (RR) of 1.29 (95% CI 1.07–1.56) for such complications.[6-8]

SERUM PROGESTERONE LEVELS TO BE ACHIEVED

Key studies by: Yovich et al. (2015), Labarta et al. (2017), Cedrin-Durnein et al. (2018), Marre et al. (2019), and Volovsky et al. (2020) suggest that achieving a minimum serum progesterone level of 9–10 ng/mL during the mid-luteal phase in programmed FET-HRT cycles is crucial for optimal reproductive outcomes.[9,10]

CONCLUSION

Luteal phase support in FET cycles is essential for achieving successful implantation and pregnancy outcomes. While natural and modified natural cycles can benefit from minimal intervention, programmed FET cycles require rigorous hormonal support to compensate for the absence of a corpus luteum. Continued research and well-designed randomized controlled trials are necessary to refine these protocols and optimize patient care in ART.

KEY POINTS

Luteal phase support is critical in FET cycles, especially in the absence of a corpus luteum:
- Natural and modified natural cycles may require minimal luteal support, while programmed FET cycles necessitate extensive hormonal supplementation.
- Achieving a serum progesterone level >9–10 ng/mL during the mid-luteal phase in programmed FET cycles is crucial for optimal outcomes.
- Programmed FET cycles are associated with a higher risk of hypertensive disorders due to lower secretion of angiogenic molecules.
- Continued research is essential to establish consensus on the optimal type and duration of luteal support in FET cycles.

REFERENCES

1. Diagnosis and treatment of luteal phase deficiency: a committee opinion by the Practice Committees of the American Society for Reproductive Medicine

and the Society for Reproductive Endocrinology and Infertility. Fertil Steril. 2021;115(6):1416-23.
2. Wu H, Zhang S, Lin X, Wang S, Zhou P. Luteal phase support for in vitro fertilization/intracytoplasmic sperm injection fresh cycles: a systematic review and network meta-analysis. Reprod Biol Endocrinol. 2021;19(1):103.
3. Shoham G, Leong M, Weissman A. A 10-year follow-up on the practice of luteal phase support using worldwide web-based surveys. Reprod Biol Endocrinol. 2021;19(1):15.
4. Hoff JD, Quigley ME, Yen SS. Hormonal dynamics at midcycle: a reevaluation. J Clin Endocrinol Metab. 1983;57(4):792-6.
5. Itskovitz J, Boldes R, Levron J, Erlik Y, Kahana L, Brandes JM. Induction of preovulatory luteinizing hormone surge and prevention of ovarian hyperstimulation syndrome by gonadotropin-releasing hormone agonist. Fertil Steril. 1991;56(2):213-20.
6. Filicori M, Butler JP, Crowley WH. Neuroendocrine regulation of the corpus luteum in the human. Evidence for pulsatile progesterone secretion. J Clin Invest. 1984;73(6):1638-47.
7. Anckaert E, Jank A, Petzold J, Rohsmann F, Paris R, Renggli M, et al. Extensive monitoring of the natural menstrual cycle using the serum biomarkers estradiol, luteinizing hormone and progesterone. Pract Lab Med. 2021;25:e00211.
8. Leiva R, Bouchard T, Boehringer H, Abulla S, Ecochard R. Random serum progesterone threshold to confirm ovulation. Steroids. 2015:101:125-9.
9. Abbara A, Clarke SA, Dhillo WS. Novel concepts for inducing final oocyte maturation in in vitro fertilization treatment. Endocr Rev. 2018;39(5):593-628.
10. Duncan WC. The inadequate corpus luteum. Reprod Fertil. 2021;2(1):C1-C7.

Section

Complications of Ovarian Stimulation

❑ **Complications Encountered during Oocyte Retrieval**
   Ameet S Patki, Khyati R Pandya
❑ **Ovarian Hyperstimulation Syndrome: Prevention and Cure**
   Kedar Ganla, Rana Choudhary, Priyanka Harshavardhan Vora

Complications Encountered during Oocyte Retrieval

Chapter 25

Ameet S Patki, Khyati R Pandya

■ INTRODUCTION

Oocyte pick-up (OPU) involves aspirating the fluid-filled ovarian follicles that contain eggs through a needle adapted for transvaginal ultrasonography (TvUSG) probes. Whereas oocyte collection has been performed laparoscopically in the past, transvaginal ultrasound-guided oocyte aspiration under intravenous sedation is now the standard technique.[1] This procedure was first described by Wickland et al.[2] in 1985 and is widely used today in the practice of assisted reproductive techniques.[3,4] This simple, effective, and popular method represents the gold standard technique. The advantages of transvaginal OPU, in comparison with the transabdominal or laparoscopic approach, include:

- Better visualization and shorter distance of ovary from the transducer
- High recovery rate of good-quality oocytes with minimal discomfort for patients
- The use of local anesthesia with sedation instead of general anesthesia
- Decreased risk of intestinal trauma
- It can be easily learned.
- Decreased costs for patients
- Quick postinterventional recovery

However, in some patients, transabdominal ultrasound facilitated access when the ovaries were transposed or enlarged above the pelvic brim. Transabdominal-guided oocyte retrieval continues to be used at some centers for rare patients who have ovaries inaccessible by vaginal ultrasound.

■ BASIC PRINCIPLES OF THE OPU TECHNIQUE

Even though oocyte retrieval (OPU) comprises a relatively small proportion of the lengthy in vitro fertilization (IVF) treatment process, it is important to perform the procedure with the correct technique to maintain the maximum oocyte count and avoid potentially life-threatening complications. In this context, the OPU procedure is critical for successful IVF treatment outcomes. Nevertheless, despite the advantages, the aspiration needle may injure the adjacent pelvic organs leading to serious complications. Following are few complications related to OPU.

Pain

Patients tolerate the pain caused by the OPU well. The pain increases with the number of oocytes retrieved indicating the greater trauma with a higher number of oocytes. Taking into account that severe stimulation protocols are accompanied by major health risks, the increased pain underlines the necessity to keep ovarian stimulation as soft as possible.[5] However, a few patients experienced severe pain that sometimes even required hospital admission. 2 hours after the procedure, 16.9% of patients rated their pain to be medium and 3.1% to be severe or very severe. 2 days after the OPU, 7.6% of patients still experienced medium pain and 1.7% severe or very severe pain. In seven cases (0.7%), the patient's pain required a hospital admission.

Bleeding

The most common problem associated with OPU is minor vaginal hemorrhage that is seen in 2.8% of cases. Rarely severe intra-abdominal bleeding is observed. The only other prospective study on this topic observed a vaginal bleeding in 8.6% of OPUs.[6] However, in most cases, the blood loss was minor; in only 0.8% of OPUs, the bleeding exceeded 100 mL and in 1.0% application of local pressure was required. In 0.11% of OPUs, a severe intra-abdominal bleeding occurred. Retrospective studies have reported the incidence of severe intra-abdominal bleedings with 0.08–0.2%.[7] Bergh and Lundkvist interviewed 12 IVF centers about the complications of OPUs by a questionnaire.[8] They reported that vaginal bleeding (without further specification) occurred in 0.5% of procedures. Acute hemorrhage from the ovary, and bleeding or hematomas due to vascular damage in the uterus, ovary, and iliac vein are very rare (0.04–0.07%), but may require surgical intervention when they do occur.[7,9] Bleeding may be in the form of vaginal, intraperitoneal, or retroperitoneal bleeding. Acute intraperitoneal and retroperitoneal bleeding may be recognized during or immediately after TvUSG in the absence of any observable vaginal bleeding, and retroperitoneal bleeding in particular may develop gradually and be diagnosed by USG or other imaging methods after the development of bleeding-induced signs. For example, cases of retroperitoneal hematoma (i.e., the "Cullen finding"), which have a good course and manifest as periumbilical hematoma, have been reported in the literature.[10] Although massive hemorrhages are mostly due to ovarian, uterine, and iliac vessel injuries, cases of massive retroperitoneal hemorrhage due to injury to the middle sacral vein and cases of massive hematuria due to bladder pseudoaneurysm hemorrhage have also been reported.[8,11] Serious bleeding may occur due to clotting disorders.[8,11] In their studies, Battaglia et al. (2000) and El-Shawarby et al. (2004) reported severe bleeding in patients with Factor IX deficiency, and in patients with essential thrombocytopenia.[12,13] Severe bleeding can also occur as a consequence of bleeding disorders and medical problems influencing coagulation.

Infection

An infection can originate from the vaginal puncture during the OPU procedure where there is a contamination from vaginal bacteria into the intraperitoneal space.[14] The presence of pre-existent latent pelvic infection or pelvic endometriosis or teratoma may be another contributing factor. In some difficult cases, puncture of hydrosalpinx or an accidental puncture of an attached bowel loop during the procedure may occur, which may lead to severe septicemia.[15] The incidence of pelvic infections and tuboovarian abscesses reported in the literature is 0.3-0.6%. In a recent review, El-Shawarby et al. (2004) described three different pathways for such infections.[13] Direct inoculation of vaginal microorganisms may occur by puncture through the nonsterile vagina. The risk of pelvic infections after OPU seems also related to the history of pelvic inflammatory disease. Reinfection may occur through puncture of chronically infected ovaries. In a retrospective study, Dicker et al. (1993) described nine cases of tuboovarian and pelvic abscesses, all with a previous history of pelvic inflammatory disease.[7] Although least likely, infection may occur through direct puncture of the bowel with an inflammatory or infectious spillage. Bennett et al. (1993) found in their series a minor pelvic infection in 0.3% of cases defined by pyorexia and pelvic tenderness with no evidence of abscess formation on ultrasound.[6] All patients were treated with antibiotic therapy. More severe infections leading to an abscess also occurred in 0.3% of cases.[6] This incidence is in accordance with the retrospective analyses.[16] However, the preventive treatment with antibiotics does not seem to be helpful and is discussed to be a possible harm for the outcome of IVF cycles.

Pelvic Organ Injury

Pelvic structures may be inadvertently traumatized by the aspiration needle. Akman et al. and Roest et al. reported perforated appendicitis in two patients after OPU, and the needle hole was observed in these cases.[17,18] The risk of injury of the bowel appears to be more theoretical than actual. Ultrasound guidance allows visualization of the bowel. However, bowel injuries might also occur more frequently without being diagnosed and resolve spontaneously.[17,18] Intestinal injury is more likely to develop in patients with advanced endometriosis, previous surgery, or pelvic adhesions related to previous infections.[8] Ureteral injury or ureteral obstruction has also been reported. As per Miller et al., ureteral injuries are underreported, due to the anatomical position of the ureter anterolateral of the upper vaginal fornix.[19]

Paracervical Block

A transient leg paresis may develop, which usually disappears after 2-4 hours.

■ CHALLENGES FOR OPU

Endometriosis

A sizable fraction of endometriosis patients might need assisted reproductive technology. In addition to focusing solely on reproductive results, earlier research and meta-analyses on endometriosis have also drawn attention to the dearth of information regarding potential side effects of IVF treatment, particularly during the OPU procedure.[20] Given the possibility of ovarian endometriomas or pelvic adhesions linked to endometriosis, it is plausible to assume that OPU may be more difficult and complex to execute in endometriosis patients. However, further clinical research is needed in this area because the data that are now available are insufficient to predict the complication rates and difficulties related to the oocyte retrieval technique in patients with endometriosis. Additionally, the effects of endometriosis have not been thoroughly studied in the literature, particularly with regard to success rates and the difficulties and problems involved with oocyte retrieval techniques.

Endometriosis negatively impacts OPU processes and may negatively impact OPU procedures' performance (total number of oocytes retrieved per needle entry) during IVF/ICSI treatment. Since these patients are genuinely healthy people, oocyte retrieval procedures should be carried out with the utmost care and safety. The least amount of interference and complication rates together with an appropriate number of oocytes retrieved during the process determine the effectiveness and success of an oocyte retrieval technique. A greater number of oocytes might be extracted thanks to the straightforward and effective OPU process, which also improves the visibility of smaller follicles.[21] While OPU is widely acknowledged as a safe and uncomplicated procedure, defining specific difficulty metrics for evaluation is challenging due to the lack of distinct and well-defined characteristics for the surgical technique. In our study, we assessed the need for assistance as a difficulty parameter—a parameter that has never been assessed before. Assistance may be explored in endometriosis since access to the ovaries can be difficult due to greater rates of adnexal adhesions. Assistance was observed to be significantly needed when manual abdominal compression was required to correct the ovaries during OPU. No significant correlations were observed between the total number of oocytes extracted per needle entry and the prevalence of ovarian adhesions, which is used to estimate the requirement for assistance. According to a different study, the presence of attached ovaries may inhibit ovarian movement, making the OPU procedure simpler to carry out.[6] The simpler oocyte collection and reduced ovarian mobility may be explained by higher ovarian adhesion rates (p <0.001) in the endometriosis group. In endometriosis patients, limited ovarian mobility may have also lessened the requirement for manual ovarian fixation. Visible oocytes that are inaccessible and cannot be harvested due to ovarian endometrioma are a significant concern in endometriomas that has not yet been examined. In this instance, it is possible to assess the retrieved oocyte percentage (visualized follicles/retrieved oocyte number). We can analyze OPU performance, or the number of oocytes extracted per needle insertion, as an innovative approach. Compared to the endometriosis group, the control group's performance rates were greater. Nevertheless, there was no association (p = 0.68) between the diameters of ovarian endometriomas and the quantity of oocytes extracted. Punctures for endometriomas should not be promoted. Perioperative prophylactic antibiotic usage may also help lower the risk of infection, according to certain findings.[7] Follicular contamination with endometrioma content is uncommon but possible in the absence of endometrioma puncture. Because punctures might result in damage, it is important to limit the number of needle inserts and practice through visualization under ultrasound guidance. It has been proposed that infections or endometriosis-related pelvic adhesions may raise the chance of these injuries because of the deformed anatomy.

Obesity

It was shown that obesity is an additional risk that could make it difficult to access the ovaries. The fact that more needle penetrations occurred in patients with higher BMIs (>30 kg/m^2) further corroborated this finding. Furthermore, only a higher number of needle inserts could indicate that the process is difficult. Numerous elements were discovered to be in charge of the rise in needle entry, particularly in individuals who were fat.

In the event of internal bleeding or other organ damage in a patient who is hemodynamically unstable, the IVF center must have proactively developed rules on patient resuscitation and access to the operating room (safety standard).

The OPU video recording may be useful in determining the causes of issues and enhancing the OPU technique in terms of the kinds of maneuvers to be used during oocyte aspiration and the ultrasound settings for clear imaging.

■ FUTURE DEVELOPMENTS

Doppler studies can be useful to detect vascular areas in case of doubt in 2D ultrasound imaging. Doppler could differentiate from hypoechogenic areas that look alike as superficial follicles versus iliac or paraovarian vessels (position, content, and fluid movement). Further research is needed to answer whether this modality of imaging needs to be applied routinely during OPU.

Artificial intelligence, based on US features, patient profile, and biochemical metrics information, can be used as a predictor of how much the follicle grows in the next few days. Artificial intelligence here can be very useful when predicting the growth of poor responders' follicles and this can be a direction for future research. Another application could be to classify the follicles during the process of growth and use this information in OPU and embryo selection for transfer.

CONCLUSION

Oocyte pickup in an expert hands is a boon for those who can not conceive on their own. If done properly and with utmost care its a daycare procedure and totally safe. Mild pain and side effects like nausea and vomiting due to anesthesia are its commonest side effects. However, in obese patients sometime organ injury can take place and in rarest of rare a vascular injury. To learn the art one should thoroughly follow a structured hands on training program and be in constant touch with ones mentor for any kind of backup. We have to remember complications will occur but we should know to identify it and tackle it.

KEY POINTS

- Patient safety is of utmost importance as its not an emergency procedure.
- Before starting the stimulation localize the ovaries and its relation to the adjacent organs.
- The knowledge of proper pelvic anatomy is must.
- Complications happen very rarely but one should have high index of suspicion to tackle them.
- Keep a backup for power and equipment.

REFERENCES

1. Ditkoff EC, Plumb J, Selick A, Sauer MV. Anesthesia practices in the United States common to in vitro fertilization (IVF) centers. J Assist Reprod Genet. 1997;14(3):145-7.
2. Wickland M, Enk L, Hamberger L. Transvesical and Transvaginal Approaches for the Aspiration of Follicles by Use of Ultrasound. Ann N Y Acad Sci. 1985;442:182-94.
3. Wikland M, Enk L, Hammarberg K, Nilsson L. Use of a vaginal transducer for oocyte retrieval in an IVF/ET program. J Clin Ultrasound. 1987;15(4):245-51.
4. Hammarberg K, Enk L, Nilsson L, Wikland M. Oocyte retrieval under the guidance of a vaginal transducer: evaluation of patient acceptance. Hum Reprod. 1987;2(6):487-90.
5. Ludwig M, Tölg R, Richardt G, Katus HA, Diedrich K. Myocardial infarction associated with ovarian hyperstimulation syndrome. JAMA. 1999;282:632-3.
6. Bennett SJ, Waterstone JJ, Cheng WC, Parsons J. Complications of transvaginal ultrasound-directed follicle aspiration: a review of 2760 consecutive procedures. J Assist Reprod Genet. 1993;10:772-8.

7. Dicker D, Ashkenazi J, Feldberg D, Levy T, Dekel A, Ben Rafael Z. Severe abdominal complications after transvaginal ultrasonographically guided retrieval of oocytes for in vitro fertilization and embryo transfer. Fertil Steril. 1993;59:1313-5.
8. Bergh T, Lundkvist Ö. Clinical complications during in-vitro fertilization treatment. Hum Reprod. 1992;7:625-6.
9. Ragni G, Scarduelli C, Calanna G, Santi G, Benaglia L, Somigliana E. Blood loss during transvaginal oocyte retrieval. Gynecol Obstet Invest. 2009;67(1):32-5.
10. Bentov Y, Levitas E, Silberstein T, Potashnik G. Cullen's sign following ultrasound-guided transvaginal oocyte retrieval. Fertil Steril. 2006;85(1):227.
11. Jayakrishnan K, Raman VK, Vijayalakshmi VK, Baheti S, Nambiar D. Massive hematuria with hemodynamic instability - complication of oocyte retrieval. Fertil Steril. 2011;96(1):e22-4.
12. Battaglia C, Regnani G, Giulini S, Madgar L, Genazzani AD, Volpe A. Severe intraabdominal bleeding after transvaginal oocyte retrieval for IVF-ET and coagulation factor XI deficiency: a case report. J Assist Reprod Genet. 2001;18(3):178-81.
13. El-Shawarby SA, Margara RA, Trew GH, Laffan MA, Lavery SA. Thrombocythemia and hemoperitoneum after transvaginal oocyte retrieval for in vitro fertilization. Fertil Steril. 2004;82(3):735-7.
14. Kelada E, Ghani R. Bilateral ovarian abscesses following transvaginal oocyte retrieval for IVF: a case report and review of literature. J Assist Reprod Genet. 2007;24:143-5.
15. Amso NN. Potential health hazards of assisted reproduction. Problems facing the clinician. Hum Reprod. 1995;10:1628-30.
16. Ashkenazi J, Farhi J, Dicker D, Feldberg D, Shalev J, Ben Rafael Z. Acute pelvic inflammatory disease after oocyte retrieval: adverse effects on the results of implantation. Fertil Steril. 1994;61:526-8.
17. Akman MA, Katz E, Damewood MD, Ramzy AI, Garcia JE. Perforated appendicitis and ectopic pregnancy following in-vitro fertilization. Hum Reprod. 1995;10(12):3325-6.
18. Roest J, Mous HV, Zeilmaker GH, Verhoeff A. The incidence of major clinical complications in a Dutch transport IVF programme. Hum Reprod Update. 1996;2(4):345-53.
19. Miller PB. Acute ureteral obstruction following transvaginal oocyte retrieval for IVF: Case report. Hum Reprod. 2002;17(1):137-8.
20. Hamdan M, Dunselman G, Li TC, Cheong Y. The impact of endometrioma on IVF/ICSI outcomes: a systematic review and meta-analysis. Hum Reprod Update. 2015;21:809-25.
21. Sarhan A, Muasher SJ. Surgical complications of in vitro fertilization. Middle East Fertil Soc J. 2007;12:1-7.

Chapter 26: Ovarian Hyperstimulation Syndrome: Prevention and Cure

Kedar Ganla, Rana Choudhary, Priyanka Harshavardhan Vora

■ INTRODUCTION

Ovarian hyperstimulation syndrome (OHSS) is a broad spectrum of signs and symptoms that include abdominal distention and discomfort, enlarged ovaries, ascites, and other complications of enhanced vascular permeability. The incidence of moderate OHSS is estimated to be between 3 and 8%, but can reach up to 20%. Around 0.1–3% of women may end up with severe OHSS.[1,2]

The OHSS can be classified into **(Table 1)**:
- *Early OHSS:* It occurs within 7–8 days after the ovulation triggering injection of human chorionic gonadotropin (hCG) although elicited by hCG, is related to an exaggerated ovarian response to gonadotropin stimulation

TABLE 1: RCOG classification of severity of OHSS.	
Category	*Features*
Mild OHSS	• Abdominal bloating • Mild abdominal pain • Ovarian size usually <8 cm
Moderate OHSS	• Moderate abdominal pain • Nausea ± vomiting • Ultrasound evidence of ascites • Ovarian size usually 8–12 cm
Severe OHSS	• Clinical ascites (±hydrothorax) • Oliguria (<300 mL/day or <30 mL/h) • Hematocrit >0.45 • Hyponatremia (sodium <135 mmol/L) • Hypo-osmolality (osmolality <282 mOsm/kg) • Hyperkalemia (potassium >5 mmol/L) • Hypoproteinemia (serum albumin <35 g/L) • Ovarian size usually >12 cm

(OHSS: ovarian hyperstimulation syndrome; RCOG: Royal College of Obstetricians and Gynaecologists)

CHAPTER 26: Ovarian Hyperstimulation Syndrome: Prevention and Cure

- *Late OHSS:* It occurs 10 days after hCG trigger. It is mostly due to increased endogenous hCG (pregnancy) mainly related to the secretion of placental hCG.

Most cases of OHSS are self-limiting requiring only supportive management.

PATHOPHYSIOLOGY[3-6]

- As of today, the exact cause of OHSS is still not clearly understood.
- Human chorionic gonadotropin is one of the most important triggers for OHSS.
- This causes increase in vascular endothelial growth factor-A (VEGF-A).
- VEGF-A further with its effect on receptor-2 (VEGFR-2) activates and increases angiogenesis and increases permeability of blood vessels.
- This releases intraovarian renin angiotensin system (RAS), which regulates permeability, angiogenesis, and proliferation of endothelial tissue.
- This drastic increase in RAS due to hCG exacerbates OHSS. It is corroborated by the high renin activity seen in the follicular fluid of women with OHSS.
- The underlying feature of OHSS is increased capillary permeability leading to a fluid shift from the intravascular space to third space compartments.
- Lightman et al. identified elevated FF levels of renin, angiotensin II, and angiotensin III from stimulated compared to unstimulated controls.[3]
- *Vascular endothelial growth factor (VEGF), interleukin 8 (IL-8), and hCG:* VEGF is a vasoactive glycoprotein (cytokine) which stimulates endothelial cell proliferation, cell permeability, and angiogenesis.
- Other possible mechanisms for the development of OHSS have been suggested, including FSH receptor variability **(Fig. 1)**.

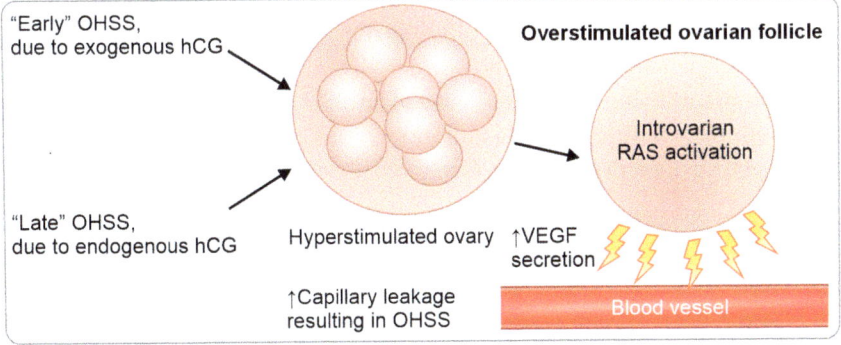

Fig. 1: Pathophysiology of OHSS. (hCG: human chorionic gonadotropin; OHSS: ovarian hyperstimulation syndrome; RAS: renin angiotensin system; VEGF: vascular endothelial growth factor)

RISK STRATIFICATION[7-9]

- *Primary prevention:* In this, the women is graded based on her risk factors into high, normal, or low risk for OHSS. The induction is individualized as per the risk.
- *Secondary prevention:* Herein the patient already has an excessive response to COS. Hence, it uses measures to reduce the symptoms of OHSS.

WHAT ARE THE MEASURES FOR OHSS PREVENTION?

- Recognize preexisting risk factors and individualize ovarian stimulation protocol
- *Secondary prevention:* Prevent progression, e.g., cryopreservation
- However, early OHSS cannot be avoided completely.

Identifying "at-risk" woman:[10]
- Young women <26 years
- Low body mass index (BMI)
- Polycystic ovarian disease (PCOD)
- Women with previous history of OHSS
- *Anti-Müllerian hormone (AMH):* High pretreatment basal AMH concentration (AMH >3.36 ng/mL—sensitivity 90.5%, specificity 81.3%)
- Absolute serum estradiol (E2) concentrations
- Ultrasonographic markers—antral follicular count (AFC). Women with a high AFC (≥24) have high risk of moderate-to-severe OHSS as compared with women with AFC <24 (8.6% vs. 2.2%)
- When the number of follicles of size 2–8 mm is >12

Secondary risk factors:
- During controlled ovarian stimulation (COS), ultrasound and serum E2 monitoring
- Number of developing follicles on the day of hCG administration (>14 follicles with a diameter of 11 mm)
- Number of oocytes retrieved
- None are independently predictive of OHSS
- Combination of ≥18 follicles on ultrasound (diameter ≥11 mm) and E2 ≥ 5,000 ng/L on the day of hCG trigger (sensitivity 83%, specificity 84%)

Primary prevention—keeping the intent right:
- Selection of patients
- Weight loss
- Insulin sensitizers
- Investigations
- AMH/AFC correlation
- Previous history

CHAPTER 26: Ovarian Hyperstimulation Syndrome: Prevention and Cure

Prevention—cautious treatment:
- Individualized protocols iCOS (individualized controlled ovarian stimulation)
- Utilizing adjuvant insulin sensitizer (metformin) therapy
- Reducing the gonadotropin dose and duration
- Battle between the recombinant follicle-stimulating hormone (rFSH), human menopausal gonadotropin (hMG), luteinizing hormone (LH), and hCG
- Antagonist protocol
- Step up if required after 5–7 days
- Use STEP-UP protocol for stimulation rather than STEP-DOWN protocol in these high-risk women
- Plan an agonist trigger
- Close monitoring

■ TRIGGERING OVULATION[10-12]

- *Exogenous hCG:* Long half-life (2–3 days), however, causes prolonged luteotrophic effects, multiple corpus luteum, and higher P4 and E2.
- Lowest dose can be used (i.e., 2,000–5,000 IU) or must not be used at all.
- GnRH agonists (GnRHa) produce a shorter midcycle gonadotropin surge (24–36 hours).
- This LH surge induces ovulation without being sustained for a long time and hence avoids OHSS.
- "Freeze all" approach
- *Dual trigger:* Add 2,000 IU of hCG to GnRHa trigger
- *Improved pregnancy, implantation and live birth rates, the propensity for OHSS remains very possible*
- Longer half-life of hCG compared to LH, >24 h versus 60 minutes facilitating (OHSS) due to the sustained luteotropic activity and the production of vascular permeability mediators.
- The utilization of GnRH agonist for triggering ovulation in antagonist cycles has been a breakthrough in the elimination of OHSS **(Fig. 2)**.

■ GnRH ANTAGONIST IN OHSS PREVENTION[11,12]

- Ovary has been shown to be primary source of VEGF secretion
- *VEGF:* Key role in increase of vascular permeability
- Ovary—GnRH receptors
- Shown to inhibit expression of VEGF in human granulosa luteal cell cultures
- *Hypothesis:* Direct action of GnRH antagonist on ovary
- *Luteal administration:* Associated with a significant and rapid ↓ serum VEGF levels starting as early as 2 days after GnRH antagonist

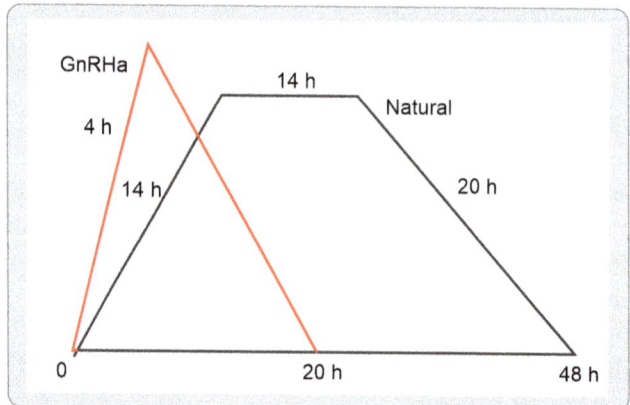

Fig. 2: LH surge after GnRH agonist trigger versus natural cycle. (LH: luteinizing hormone; GnRHa: gonadotropin-releasing hormone agonist)

- Luteolytic effect
- When to start, dose, and how long
- Start postoocyte retrieval immediately and to be continued daily for 8 days, e.g., cetrorelix acetate or ganirelix acetate 0.25 mg subcutaneously

■ SECONDARY PREVENTION

Coasting[13]

- The stimulation dose is either reduced drastically or stopped completely when the serum estradiol levels are rising to a particular value and/or a critical number of follicles are seen on folliculometry.
- The trigger is also delayed till the estradiol value significantly reduces.
- The hCG trigger is given only after that and transvaginal oocyte retrieval (TVOR) is done followed by embryo transfer or freezing depending upon the E2.
- Generally employed for <3 days.
- Coasting by withholding gonadotropins
- Initiated between 2,500 and 3,500 pg/mL of E2 or >30 small developing follicles
- Ulug et al. found reduced implantation and pregnancy rates in cycles coasted for >4 days.
- A longer duration of coasting seemed to affect the endometrial receptivity or its synchronization with embryonic age.
- A reduction in the number and quality of oocytes retrieved in a coasted cycle has been reported.[14,15]
- Cochrane review 2002 identified 13 studies examining the effects of coasting, but only one met their inclusion criteria. The authors concluded that there was insufficient evidence to determine whether coasting was an effective strategy for preventing OHSS.

Cryopreservation of Embryos[16-20]
- After COS and TVOR, all embryos are cryopreserved.[16-20]
- The embryos are then transferred in the next cycle.
- With advancement in cryopreservation techniques, the success rate for frozen embryo transfer (FET) pregnancies is much better than fresh ET.

Cycle Cancellation
- The most successful method which can prevent OHSS is not giving the trigger and cancelling the cycle.
- In spite of cancelling the cycle, sometimes endogenous LH surge can happen and still lead to OHSS.
- Financial impact.
- Psychological distress.

Alternative Methods of Prevention
Colloid Infusion
Colloids can be given during oocyte retrieval as they bind to and deactivate vasoactive mediators responsible for OHSS as seen in **Table 2**.

Intravenous colloids:[21,22]
Albumin:
- May bind to the vasoactive agents responsible for the development of OHSS and facilitate their removal from the circulation.
- Albumin administration could increase plasma osmotic pressure, helping to maintain the intravascular volume.
- Attenuate the effects of hypovolemia, hemoconcentration, and ascites.
- Human albumin solution 25% may be used as a plasma volume expander.
- *Dose:* 50–100 g, infused over 4 hours and repeated 4- to 12-hourly.[22]
- Strict fluid balance recording should be followed for these patients.
- However, the evidence supporting the use of IV albumin for the reduction of OHSS is not strong.

Hydroxyethyl starch 6%:
- Colloid helps in expansion of the intravascular compartment.[21,22]
- Shift of fluid from the third spaces
- No major side effects unlike albumin
- Caution in cardiopulmonary compromised patients as may lead to pulmonary edema

Cabergolin[23,24]
- Dopamine-r2 agonist
- Reversed VEGFR-2-dependent vascular permeability (VP) without affecting luteal angiogenesis through partial inhibition of ovarian VEGFR-2 phosphorylation levels.

TABLE 2: Summary of recommendations for strategies to prevent OHSS.

Sr. No.	Intervention	Recommendation	Effect of intervention	Level of evidence
1.	Reducing gonadotropin dose	Recommended	"Step-up regimen" has a lower risk of OHSS, cycle cancellation from hyperstimulation, and higher rate of monofollicular ovulation in contrast to other protocols	1b, 4
2.	Reducing gonadotropin duration	Utilized as clinically appropriate	• "Mild" stimulation protocol with GnRH antagonist for late suppression has a lower risk of OHSS and multiple pregnancies and is cost-effective	1b
			• It also is less effective in terms of pregnancy rates than "long" protocols	1a
3.	Individualized COS (iCOS)	Further research required	iCOS can reduce OHSS rates and associated cycle cancellations. It also produces a significant oocyte yield and good pregnancy rates	1b, 2a
4.	GnRHa as an ovulation trigger	Recommended	GnRHa use virtually eliminates OHSS rates	1b
5.	hCG as an ovulation trigger	Further research required	Lowest dose of hCG does not seem to reduce OHSS rates	2a, 2b, 4
6.	Adjuvant metformin therapy	Recommended	Metformin is associated with a lower risk of OHSS and increased clinical pregnancy rate	1a, 4
7.	Cabergoline	Recommended	Cabergoline reduces the incidence of OHSS without an effect on pregnancy rates	1a
8.	Hydroxyethyl starch	Utilized as clinically appropriate	HES causes a decrease in OHSS without an effect on pregnancy rates	1a
9.	Coasting	Further research required	Coasting does not completely prevent OHSS, is associated with a lower oocyte yield, and has no benefit in contrast to other interventions. The protocols are also very diverse	1a, 4

Contd...

CHAPTER 26: Ovarian Hyperstimulation Syndrome: Prevention and Cure

Contd...

Sr. No.	Intervention	Recommendation	Effect of intervention	Level of evidence
10.	Cryopreservation	Utilized as clinically appropriate	• Cryopreservation alone does not reduce rates of OHSS	1a
			• GnRHa followed by cryopreservation virtually eliminates OHSS	1b
11.	Cycle cancellation	Utilized as clinically appropriate	Cancellation completely eliminates risk of OHSS but has a high financial and emotional burden	4
12.	Adjunct GnRHa use	Not recommended	GnRHa use increases the associated costs and rate of OHSS while lowering the pregnancy rates	1a
13.	Aromatase inhibitors for OI	Not recommended	AIs have shown no reduction in rates of OHSS in contrast to other methods of OI	1a
14.	rhLH	Not recommended	rhLH use does not reduce the risk of OHSS and has higher costs and lower pregnancy rates	1a, 1b
15.	hCG for luteal phase support	Not recommended	Progesterone significantly reduces the risk of OHSS with improved clinical pregnancy rates and live birth rates in comparison to hCG for LPS	1a
16.	Albumin infusion	Not recommended	Albumin does not reduce OHSS rates and may cause lower pregnancy rates. There are also associated risks with anaphylaxis and disease transmission	1a
17.	Vasopressin V1a receptor antagonist	Further research required	It appears to reduce the ovarian weight gain and multiple corpus luteum development in OHSS	2b

(GnRH: gonadotropin-releasing hormone; hCG: human chorionic gonadotropin; OHSS: ovarian hyperstimulation syndrome; OI: ovulation induction; rhLH: recombinant human luteinizing hormone)
Source: RCOG guidelines.

- No luteolytic effects (serum progesterone levels and luteal apoptosis unaffected) were observed.
- Administration of cabergoline (5–10 µg/kg/d) decreased the occurrence of OHSS from 65% (controls) to 25% (treatment).
- Cabergoline needs to be started from the day of trigger for the next 7–14 days.
- No effect on luteal angiogenesis/luteal phase.
- Commenced on day of hCG trigger at a dose of 0.5 mg for 8 days.

Letrozole (Fig. 3)

- Nonsteroidal aromatase inhibitor
- Inhibits conversion of androgens into estrogens (E)
- Drastically reduces estradiol levels
- Ideal option—freeze oocytes/embryos, high responders, and cancer patients
- 1–5 mg/day, inhibits aromatase activity (97–99%)

Discussion:
- Letrozole during luteal phase
- Significant ↓ Sr E2, from day 5 after hCG administration
- On day 7 post-hCG administration, E2 levels reached basal values in many participants
- ↓ Moderate and severe early onset OHSS

Letrozole in OHSS Prevention[25,26]

- *Letrozole during luteal phase:* May be a new approach to reduce risk for thrombosis associated with OHSS (patients who will freeze or donate their eggs)—by suppressing circulating E2 levels and diminishing insult to coagulation/fibrinolytic system.
- Duration of luteal phase was significantly shorter in the letrozole group.

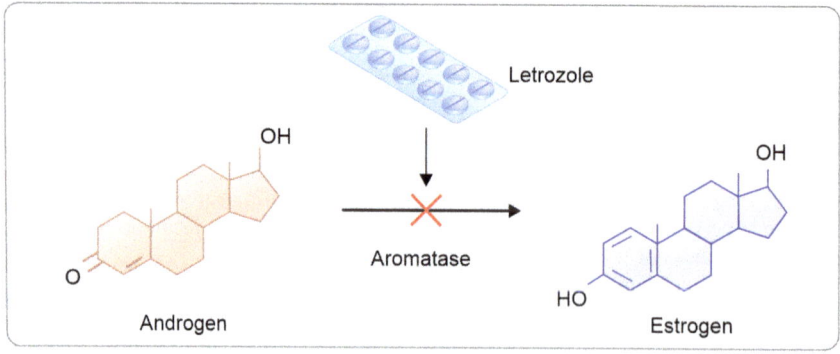

Fig. 3: Mechanism of action of letrozole.

- Our results verified the concept of luteolytic effect and corpus luteum dysfunction after letrozole.

Literature Review—Letrozole
- Can reduce endometriosis like lesions that parallel a decrease of VEGF[27]
- Significantly decrease level of VEGF in residual tissue in patients with breast cancer[27]
- *Two cells and two hormones theory:* Reduction in E2 can relieve E2-induced hypothalamic-pituitary negative feedback, ↑ LH[26]
- ↑ LH is conducive to P synthesis, thus increasing its level
- VEGF is blocked, corpus luteum formation is affected and ↓ P[26,27]

Glossary for levels of evidence:
- *1a:* Systematic review and/or meta-analysis
- *1b:* ≥1 RCT
- *2a:* ≥1 well-designed controlled study without randomization
- *2b:* ≥1 well-designed quasi experimental study
- *3:* ≥1 well-designed descriptive study
- *4:* Committee or expert opinions

DANGER SIGNS OF OHSS
- Decreased urine output
- Tense ascites
- Dyspnea at rest
- Thromboembolism
- Ovarian torsion rarely

MANAGEMENT OF OHSS

Outpatient Management (Level of Evidence D)[24]
- Can be done if the women are counseled adequately and have understood fluid intake and output monitoring.
- Their renal function may be compromised and hence nonsteroidal anti-inflammatory agents should not be used.
- These women should also be given thromboprophylaxis [low molecular weight heparin (LMWH)]. Duration of LMWH should be individualized.
- Paracentesis of ascitic fluid can be carried out on an outpatient basis under ultrasound guidance.
- Currently, there is lack of evidence to support use of dopamine agonists or gonadotropin-releasing hormone antagonists in established cases of OHSS.
- Her laboratory investigations such as complete blood count (CBC), liver function test (LFT), renal function test (RFT), and coagulation profile

should be repeated if the severity of OHSS is worsening. Hematocrit is an excellent indicator of the degree of intravascular volume depletion.

When do these women require hospital admission?[28]
- Unable to achieve satisfactory pain relief
- Not able to maintain adequate fluid intake
- Excessive nausea and vomiting
- Show signs of worsening of symptoms in spite of outpatient management
- Not able to go for regular outpatient follow-up
- Women with critical OHSS

Management of OHSS:[28,29]
- Analgesia and antiemetics
- Fluid replacement by increasing oral fluid intake guided by thirst
- If there is hemoconcentration despite volume replacement with intravenous fluids, she may need invasive monitoring.
- Diuretics deplete intravascular volume and hence should be avoided.
- A multidisciplinary approach is necessary especially if there is persistent oliguria in spite of fluid replacement and drainage of ascites.

When to do paracentesis?[28,29]
- If there is severe abdominal pain and distension due to ascites.
- Breathlessness or respiratory compromise due to increased intra-abdominal pressure or ascites.
- Persistent low urine output in spite of adequate volume replacement due to increased abdominal pressure with reduced renal perfusion.
- Paracentesis should be carried out under ultrasound guidance and can be performed abdominally or vaginally.

Anticoagulant therapy:[28]
- The duration of LMWH prophylaxis should be individualized according to patient risk factors.
- Those with moderate OHSS should be further evaluated for predisposing risk factors related to increased risk for thrombosis. Further, they should be prescribed LMWH or antiembolism stockings.

Specific Treatment for Late OHSS
- Do not give hCG in the luteal phase.
- Give progesterone as luteal phase support.
- Supportive management as discussed earlier.
- Cabergoline may be tried although studies are currently not supporting this therapy.
- Avoid isotonic solutions such as RL, NS, as they will increase the fluid in the third space.

CHAPTER 26: Ovarian Hyperstimulation Syndrome: Prevention and Cure

- Give colloids to maintain the intravascular compartment.
- In extreme cases, medical termination of pregnancy (MTP) may remain as the only option.

CONCLUSION

To conclude OHSS cannot be prevented completely but the incidence can be reduced by predetecting women who are at high risk. Also certain steps can be followed in these high risk women to avoid OHSS. Individualization is the key to prevent OHSS.

KEY POINTS

- Incidence of OHSS can be markedly reduced.
- Antagonist protocol for COS and freeze all policy may help prevent primary OHSS.
- Various medical therapy like Cabergoline, Letrozole and GnRH antagonist can be given in selected cases.
- Early diagnosis and prompt management is the key to management of OHSS before it progress in severity.
- Risk of secondary OHSS has markedly reduced due to "Freeze all protocol".

REFERENCES

1. Delvinge A, Rozenberg S. Epidemiology and prevention of ovarian hyperstimulation syndrome (OHSS): a review. Hum Reprod Update. 2002;8(6):559-77.
2. Nastri CO, Teixeira DM, Moroni RM, Leitao VM, Martins WP. Ovarian hyperstimulation syndrome: pathophysiology, staging, prediction and prevention. Ultrasound Obstet Gynecol. 2015;45(4):377-93.
3. Goldsman MP, Pedram A, Dominguez CE, Ciuffardi I, Levin E, Asch RH. Increased capillary permeability induced by human follicular fluid: a hypothesis for an ovarian origin of the hyperstimulation syndrome. Fertil Steril. 1995;63(2):268-72.
4. Tollan A, Holst N, Forsdahl F, Fadnes HO, Oian P, Maltau JM. Transcapillary fluid dynamics during ovarian stimulation for in vitro fertilization. Am J Obstet Gynecol. 1990;162(2):554-8.
5. Aboulghar MA, Mansour RT. Ovarian hyperstimulation syndrome: classifications and critical analysis of preventive measures. Hum Reprod Update. 2003;9(3):275-89.
6. Mathur RS, Akande AV, Keay SD, Hunt LP, Jenkins JM. Distinction between early and late ovarian hyperstimulation syndrome. Fertil Steril. 2000;73(5):901-7.
7. Christin-Maitre S, Hugues JN, Recombinant FSH Study Group. A comparative randomized multicentric study comparing the step-up versus step-down protocol in polycystic ovary syndrome. Hum Reprod. 2003;18(8):1626-31.
8. Homburg R, Levy T, Ben-Rafael Z. A comparative prospective study of conventional regimen with chronic low-dose administration of follicle-stimulating hormone for anovulation associated with polycystic ovary syndrome. Fertil Steril. 1995;63(4):729-33.

9. Nugent D, Vandekerckhove P, Hughes E, Arnot M, Lilford R. Gonadotrophin therapy for ovulation induction in subfertility associated with polycystic ovary syndrome. Cochrane Database Syst Rev. 2000;(4):CD000410.
10. Joint SOGC-CFAS Clinical Practice Guideline. The diagnosis and management of ovarian hyperstimulation syndrome. J Obstet Gynaecol Canada. 2011; 2068:1156-62.
11. Kolibianakis EM, Papanikolaou EG, Tournaye H, Camus M, van Steirteghem AC, Devroey P. Triggering final oocyte maturation using different doses of human chorionic gonadotropin: a randomized pilot study in patients with polycystic ovary syndrome treated with gonadotropin-releasing hormone antagonists and recombinant follicle-stimulating hormone. Fertil Steril. 2007;88(5):1382-8.
12. Kashyap S, Parker K, Cedars MI, Rosenwaks Z. Ovarian hyperstimulation syndrome prevention strategies: reducing the human chorionic gonadotropin trigger dose. Semin Reprod Med. 2010;28(6):475-85.
13. Delvigne A, Rozenberg S. A qualitative systematic review of coasting, a procedure to avoid ovarian hyperstimulation syndrome in IVF patients. Hum Reprod Update. 2002;8(3):291-6.
14. Ulug U, Bahceci M, Erden HF, Shalev E, Ben-Shlomo I. The significance of coasting duration during ovarian stimulation for conception in assisted fertilization cycles. Hum Reprod. 2002;17(2):310-3. doi: 10.1093/humrep/17.2.310.
15. Delvigne A, Rozenberg S. Review of clinical course and treatment of ovarian hyperstimulation syndrome (OHSS). Hum Reprod Update. 2003;9:77-96
16. D'Angelo A. "Ovarian hyperstimulation syndrome prevention strategies: cryopreservation of all embryos. Semin Reprod Med. 2010;28(6):513-8.
17. D'Angelo A, Amso N. Embryo freezing for preventing ovarian hyperstimulation syndrome. Cochrane Database Syst Rev. 2007;(3):CD002806.
18. Herrero L, Mart´ınez M, Garcia-Velasco JA. Current status of human oocyte and embryo cryopreservation. Curr Opin Obstet Gynecol. 2011;23(4):245-50.
19. Dolmans M, Marotta M, Pirard C, Donnez J, Donnez O. Ovarian tissue cryopreservation followed by controlled ovarian stimulation and pick-up of mature oocytes does not impair the number or quality of retrieved oocytes. J Ovarian Res. 2014;7:80.
20. Roque M. Freeze-all policy: is it time for that? J Assist Reprod Genet. 2015 Feb;32(2):171-6. doi: 10.1007/s10815-014-0391-0. Epub 2014 Nov 27.
21. Youssef MA, Al-Inany HG, Evers JL, Aboulghar M. Intra-venous fluids for the prevention of severe ovarian hyperstimulation syndrome. Cochrane Database Syst Rev. 2011;(2):CD001302.
22. Practice Committee of the American Society for Reproductive Medicine. Ovarian hyperstimulation syndrome. Fertil Steril. 2008;90 Suppl 5:S188-93.
23. Tang H, Hunter T, Hu Y, Zhai SD, Sheng X, Hart RJ. Cabergoline for preventing ovarian hyperstimulation syndrome. Cochrane Database Syst Rev. 2012;(2):CD008605.
24. Leitao VMS, Moroni RM, Seko LMD, Nastri CO, Martins WP. Cabergoline for the prevention of ovarian hyperstimulation syndrome: systematic review and meta-analysis of randomized controlled trials. Fertil Steril. 2014;101(3):664-75.e7.
25. He Q, Liang L, Zhang C, Li H, Ge Z, Wang L, et al. Effects of different doses of letrozole on the incidence of early-onset ovarian hyperstimulation syndrome after oocyte retrieval. Syst Biol Reprod Med. 2014;60(6):355-60.

CHAPTER 26: Ovarian Hyperstimulation Syndrome: Prevention and Cure

26. Choudhary RA, Vora PH, Darade KK, Pandey S, Ganla KN. A Prospective Comparative Study of Luteal Phase Letrozole Versus Ganirelix Acetate Administration to Prevent Severity of Early Onset OHSS in ARTs. Int J Fertil Steril. 2021;15(4):263-8.
27. Linderholm BK, Hellborg H, Johansson U, Elmberger G, Skoog L, Lehtiö J, et al. Significantly higher levels of vascular endothelial growth factor (VEGF) and shorter survival times for patients with primary operable triple-negative breast cancer. Ann Oncol. 2009;20(10):1639-46.
28. Royal College of Obstetricians and Gynaecologists. (2016). The Management of Ovarian Hyperstimulation Syndrome, Green-top Guideline No. 5. Available from: https://www.rcog.org.uk/guidance/browse-all-guidance/green-top-guidelines/the-management-of-ovarian-hyperstimulation-syndrome-green-top-guideline-no-5/. [Last accessed April, 2024]
29. Smith V, Osianlis T, Vollenhoven B. Prevention of Ovarian Hyperstimulation Syndrome: A Review. Obstet Gynecol Int. 2015;2015:514159.

Section 12

Mixed Bag

- **Mild and Minimal Stimulation**
  Bushra Khan, Sunita Tandulwadkar
- **Dual Stimulation**
  Hrishikesh D Pai, Sheetal Sawankar
- **Low-cost In Vitro Fertilization**
  Priya Bhave, Ashita Punjabi Hakhoo
- **Immunotherapy in Assisted Reproduction Treatment**
  Sapna Ahuja
- **Fertility Toolbox**
  Mrinmayi Dharmadhikari, Ameet S Patki

Chapter 27

Mild and Minimal Stimulation

Bushra Khan, Sunita Tandulwadkar

■ INTRODUCTION

Worldwide various ovarian stimulation protocols are being used to achieve an optimal ovarian response. Depending on the patient factors and cause of infertility, stimulation protocols can be customized to their needs. Oocytes can be collected from natural or stimulated cycles for in vitro fertilization (IVF). Many concerns surrounding conventional stimulation protocols such as hyperstimulation and multiple births can be overcome by milder more physiological approach to ovarian stimulation in IVF.[1] Despite the mentioned benefits of milder protocols like fewer complications, better tolerability, and lesser drugs at a lower cost, this protocol has not received much popularity. Nevertheless, mild stimulation was adopted greatly few years back when evidence proved that avoiding ovarian hyperstimulation syndrome (OHSS) was critical for every cycle although if we use "freeze-all" technique in conventional IVF, much of OHSS risk is eliminated.

Mild stimulation IVF uses lower doses of drugs aimed at achieving a mild response and is perfect for women wishing to minimize medication, reduce the risk of OHSS, and reduce the physical and emotional impact of treatment on their lives.

■ OVULATION INDUCTION

Ovarian stimulation refers to administration of various gonadotropic drugs to stimulate ovaries to produce many follicles. Concept remains to overexaggerate the normal physiological single dominant follicle selection, development, and ovulation.[2]

Controlled Ovarian Hyperstimulation

Controlled ovarian stimulation aims at producing more than 3 follicles in a single stimulated cycle so that enough number of eggs can be retrieved to maintain the good chances of pregnancy. Although the debate is still going on regarding the number of oocytes retrieved, whether "less is more" or "more is better" (Macklon et al., 2006), there are a number of benefits connected with milder stimulation protocols. Factors to consider before choosing a particular protocol are patient age, ovarian reserve testing, related frequent clinic visits, risk of OHSS, cost, and intensive monitoring of patient.[3]

CONCEPTS OF FOLLICLE DEVELOPMENT REGULATION RELEVANT TO OVARIAN STIMULATION

There is continuous process of recruitment of follicles from the basic residual pool of primordial follicles to antral follicles. This process is random and takes several months.[4] During initial phase of recruitment, few follicles enter the stage of growth, and others remain dormant or in latent phase. From the recruited primordial follicles, majority become atretic **(Fig. 1)**. The transition from the preantral to the antral stage and onwards is promoted by follicle-stimulating hormone (FSH). Second process is called cyclical recruitment of developing follicles where antral follicles develop under the action of various hormones to a more advanced follicular stage.[5] Depending upon FSH levels in the cycle, a cohort of antral follicles escape apoptosis and become gonadotropin dependent and continue to grow whereas others get

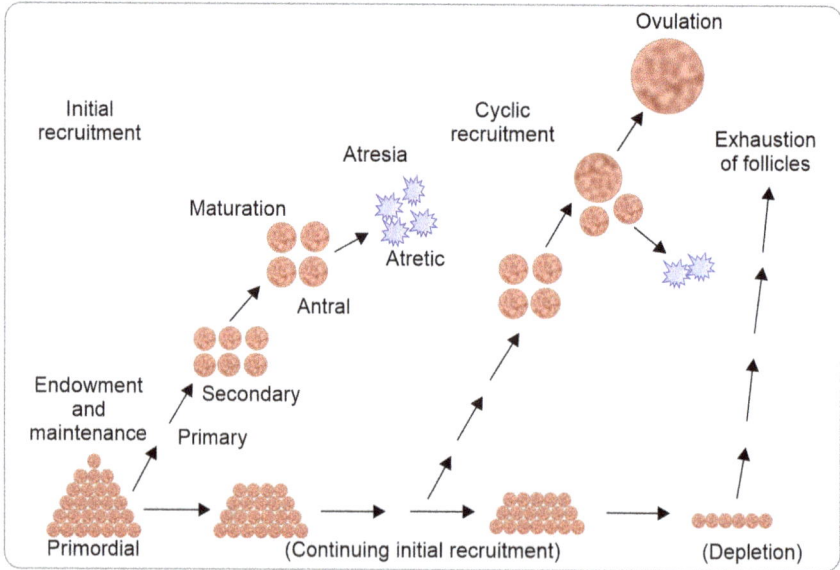

Fig. 1: Developmental stages of ovarian follicles: endowment and maintenance, initial recruitment, maturation, atresia or cyclic recruitment, ovulation, and exhaustion. There are a fixed number of primordial follicles in each lady at early intrauterine life which are at resting phase. At puberty, a defined number of follicles remain as others get atretic. Growth of dominant follicle initiates at puberty or sometimes before reproductive life. This is called initial recruitment. Throughout reproductive life follicles are in a dynamic state, they develop from primordial–primary–secondary stages–antral follicle. This follows cyclical recruitment where a preovulatory stage is achieved. Eventually, depletion of the pool of resting follicles leads to ovarian follicle exhaustion and senescence.
Source: From McGee EA, Hsueh AJ. Initial and cyclic recruitment of ovarian follicles. Endocr Rev. 2000;21:200-14.

apoptotic. In dominant follicles, FSH induces steroidogenesis by increasing aromatase activity in granulosa cell, and luteinizing hormone (LH) receptor sensitivity, therefore intraovarian conversion of androgens to estradiol (E2) increases in follicular compartment.

FSH Threshold and FSH Window

During luteofollicular transition, corpus luteum starts to vanish and FSH levels start to rise under the influence of pulsatile secretion of gonadotropin-releasing hormone (GnRH). There is declining levels of E2, inhibin A, and progesterone. Followed by decline in FSH levels due to negative feedback of inhibin B and E2,[6,7] naturally only one or two follicles escape through the FSH window, whereas in a stimulated cycle prolonged doses of FSH are administered to keep the FSH window open, facilitating a greater number of follicles to become dominant in a single cycle. FSH threshold is the minimum level of FSH hormone required by the follicle to become dominant, hence each dominant follicle needs to be crossing the FSH threshold to be able to release an oocyte[8] **(Fig. 2)**.

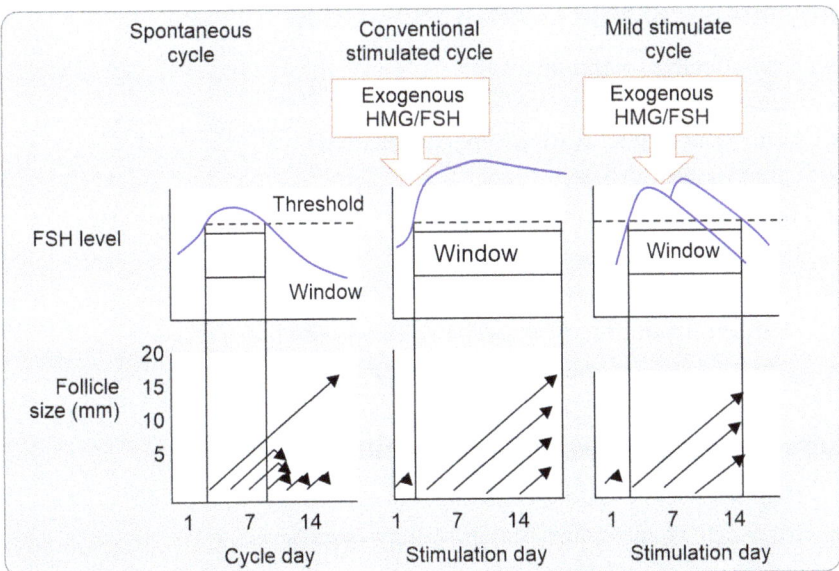

Fig. 2: The FSH threshold and FSH window concept for monofollicular development (left), conventional stimulation protocol strategy to achieve multifollicular development (middle). Each arrow represents a developing follicle. Last panel shows the concept of multifollicular development in a mild stimulation cycle, where a lesser amount of FSH is administered to patient. (FSH: follicle-stimulating hormone; HMG: human menopausal gonadotropin)
Source: From Macklon NS, Stouffer RL, Giudice LC, Fauser BC. The science behind 25 years of ovarian stimulation for in vitro fertilization. Endocr Rev. 2006;27:170-207.

NEW APPROACHES TO MILD OVARIAN STIMULATION FOR IVF

The terms "natural", "patient friendly", "mild", "minimal", and "minimally stimulating" IVF are commonly used to describe low-dose protocols for patients and such protocols have gained immense popularity. Whereas, for clinical relevance, "natural cycle IVF", "modified natural cycle", and "mild ovarian stimulation for IVF" are terms commonly used.[9]

Unlike conventional ovarian stimulation where high doses of gonadotropins are used, in mild ovarian stimulation, oral agents like clomiphene citrate (CC) and aromatase inhibitors are used.[10] If need be then low doses of gonadotropins, GnRH antagonists, and recombinant human chorionic gonadotropin (rhCG) can be used too. As mentioned before, aim is to achieve a milder and patient friendly response of ovarian stimulation especially in patients who have low ovarian reserve.

To avoid or overcome early follicular luteinization, add-back therapy with GnRH antagonist in the late follicular phase is proposed specifically in modified natural cycle ovarian stimulation.[11]

Advantages of Mild Ovarian Stimulation

- Cost-effective treatment cycle
- Minimal risk of multiple pregnancy
- Low risk of OHSS (ovarian hyperstimulation)
- Good-quality oocytes
- Total gonadotropin dose less
- Better endometrium for fresh transfer
- Less stressful for patient
- Oral administration of drugs and wider availability of drugs
- Extensive cycle monitoring is not required.

Disadvantages of Mild Ovarian Stimulation

- High chances of cycle cancellation
- No oocyte recovered or immature oocytes retrieved
- May be lower success rates
- Premature ovulation

CLASSIFICATION AND TERMINOLOGY

International Society for Mild Approaches in Assisted Reproduction (ISMAAR) classified mild stimulation protocols according to the drugs used in each protocol **(Table 1)**.[12]

TABLE 1: Different protocols of minimal stimulation IVF.

Protocol	Ovarian stimulation	Prevention of premature LH surge	Ovulation trigger	Luteal phase support
Natural cycle IVF	None	None	None	None
Modified natural cycle IVF	None/gonadotropins add-back	None/GnRH antagonist	hCG	Yes
Mild IVF	Clomiphene, letrozole, early or late low-dose gonadotropins	GnRH antagonist	hCG	Yes
Conventional IVF	High-dose gonadotropins	GnRH agonist or antagonist	hCG or GnRH agonist	Yes

(GnRH: gonadotropin-releasing hormone; hCG: human chorionic gonadotropin; IVF: in vitro fertilization; LH: luteinizing hormone)

■ MILD STIMULATION

Ovary is expected to be mildly stimulated during such protocols, hence the protocol itself is called mild ovarian stimulation where to achieve multifollicular growth antiestrogens can be used such as CC or letrozole or low-dose gonadotropins. Along with the above drugs, GnRH antagonist is used to suppress endogenous LH.[13] CC is given from day 3 to day 7 of the stimulation cycle at 100 mg dose or letrozole 2.5–5 mg from day 3 to day 7 of the cycle (Grabia et al.). Gonadotropins (HMG or rFSH) are given at dose of 150 IU from day 9 of the stimulation cycle. Ultrasound monitoring starts from day 9 and GnRH antagonist is started when follicle reaches 14 mm size, and it is continued till trigger. Ovum pickup takes place 35–36 hours after trigger. Luteal phase is supported with progesterone.[14]

Indications:
- Young patients[11]
- Good ovarian reserve
- Low socioeconomic patients
- Women with low-ovarian reserve (poor responders)
- Women with previous multiple IVF failures
- Women above the age of 40 years
- Women with previous OHSS and polycystic ovary syndrome (PCOS) patients (hyper-responders)

A retrospective trial when compared conventional IVF to mild IVF using clomiphene (with or without the GnRH antagonist) showed similar clinical pregnancy rate (37% for minimal stimulation and 41% for conventional IVF).[14] Weigert et al. compared the success of mild IVF using clomiphene and gonadotropins to conventional IVF in a randomized controlled study. The pregnancy rate per initiated cycle in the mild stimulation cycle (35.1%) was not statistically different from that in the conventional IVF group (29.3%).[15] CC is a leading competitive inhibitor of estrogen at hypothalamus. It acts through inhibiting positive feedback and increasing GnRH.

Aromatase inhibitors or letrozole is used in some cases of mild stimulation to reduce the total gonadotropin dosage and to allow multifollicular growth during mild ovarian stimulation cycles.[16] Letrozole is used as an alternative to clomiphene and it has shown good prognosis in IVF patients. A clinical pregnancy rate of 27% was reported in letrozole group.[17] Letrozole has a short half-life of 45 hours and estrogen receptors are not downregulated, hence lesser side effects on endometrium and cervix.

Another component of mild stimulation is only gonadotropin cycle, which means no oral ovulogens are used prior to gonadotropins in a stimulated cycle but, however, the total dose of gonadotropins is minimal with intension of total cycle cost reduction. Hence, there is reduction of incidence of complications which are common with conventional protocols, specially one can have an OHSS-free clinic while practicing mild ovarian stimulation protocols.

Gonadotropins can be initiated from day 2 or day 3 of stimulation cycle or may be later in the follicular phase; however, early start of gonadotropin results in multifollicular growth.[18] Fernandez-Shaw et al. reported the efficacy of the low gonadotropins IVF protocol in 79 young women with a good prognosis. Patients with PCOS, severe endometriosis, ovarian failure, or elevated early follicular FSH or estradiol were excluded. When compared results of mild stimulation with conventional stimulation protocols, mild stimulation resulted in lower number of embryo when compared to conventional dose gonadotropins (150 IU); however, the pregnancy rates were not different (51.8 vs. 50.7%) **(Fig. 3)**.[13]

Follicular Aspiration in Mild Stimulation

To achieve highest numbers of oocytes, procedure is done meticulously and follicular flushing is done during oocyte pickup procedure. The needle used is a special type double lumen measuring 17 G/19 G needle.

There are few centers across the world who practice doing IVM for small size follicles/oocytes.

Minimal Stimulation IVF and Single Embryo Transfer

As a well-known fact, mild stimulation significantly reduces chances and complications of multiple pregnancies, henceforth total embryos made and transferred in mild IVF are less. This concept theoretically reduces the concerned complications as compared to conventional protocols.[19] A randomized controlled trial took place where four cycles of mild stimulation with single embryo transfer were compared with three cycles

CHAPTER 27: Mild and Minimal Stimulation

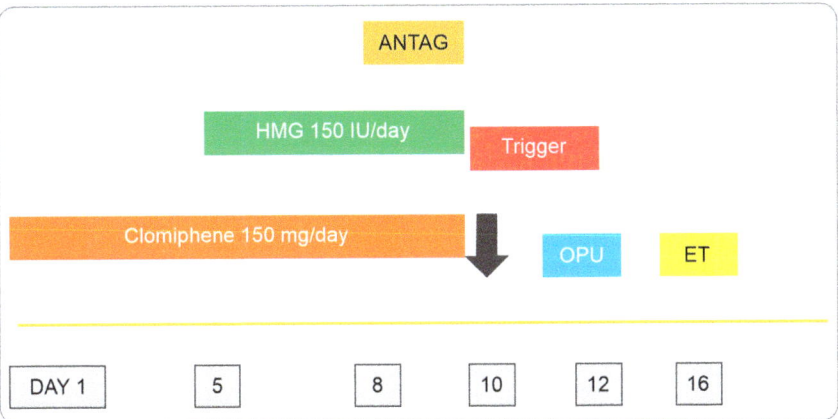

Fig. 3: *Mild stimulation protocol.* Diagrammatic representation of mild stimulation protocol where clomiphene is continued till day of trigger, from day 5 of stimulation HMG is added till day of trigger. GnRH antagonist is added once the follicles reach 14 mm and trigger with recombinant hCG is given when follicles reach 18 mm. 35–36 hours later OPU is done. Fresh transfer can be performed in the same cycle. (GnRH: gonadotropin-releasing hormone; hCG: human chorionic gonadotropin; HMG: human menopausal gonadotropin; OPU: ovum pick-up)

of conventional IVF with three embryos transferred. Heijnen et al. selected patients younger than 38 years of age with regular cycles and normal BMI. When compared, total duration of stimulation, gonadotropin dose, number of oocytes retrieved, and embryos transferred were lower in mild stimulation. The 1-year cumulative term live birth rate per couple (43.4%) in the mild IVF group was not inferior to that of the conventional IVF group (44.7%). The proportion of multiple pregnancy rates per couple in 1 year in the mild IVF group (0.5%) was significantly lower than that in the conventional IVF group (13.1%).[20,21]

It is well established that better quality embryos are made in mild stimulation cycles as compared to conventional cycles[22] of ovarian stimulation, probably because of fewer stimulation strategy. When reviewed various articles comparing mild stimulation and conventional stimulation in poor and normal responders, no difference was found in good-quality embryos.[23]

A relationship between ovarian stimulation and aneuploidy rates of embryos has also been proposed based on a large sample size, multicenter, and cross-sectional data set.[24]

Luteal Phase Support

As stimulated cycles have homes at a supraphysiological level, luteal phase has to be supported extensively in IVF cases. However, there is insufficient evidence supporting need of luteal support in natural or minimal stimulated cycles. Especially in clomiphene mild stimulation cycles, endometrium is negatively affected hence luteal support is mandatory in these cycles.[22]

Vitrification

Minimal stimulation IVF has many benefits like being low cost, fewer medications, and better quality embryos. In especially clomiphene cycles, two-step sequential frozen embryo transfers are preferred. To achieve this vitrification plays a very important role. Cryopreserved embryo transfers with mild stimulation protocols yield much higher pregnancy rates. Vitrification strategy is the best method to achieve embryo–endometrium synchrony and better results.

■ CONCLUSION

It has become a myth that higher stimulation dose improves pregnancy outcomes in poor responders because of much recent data challenging this theory. The American Society for Reproductive Medicine recommended that in patients who are considered to be poor responders, "strong consideration" should be given to a mild ovarian stimulation protocol (≤150 IU FSH) due to lower costs and comparable pregnancy rates.[25]

Developing cost-effective and affordable IVF will increase access to treatment in many parts of the world where patients have to self-fund their care and may also convince more health insurance companies to cover IVF expenses. The true real-world cost of IVF should take into account not only the actual cost of treatment but also resources required for the management of complications such as OHSS, and added costs related to pregnancy complications and additional perinatal care, including any long-term healthcare costs for the mother and her offspring.

■ KEY POINTS

- Minimal or mild stimulation is an art of ART where we use the minimal or fixed quantity of gonadotropins to stimulate a patient.
- Drugs commonly used along with gonadotropins in minimal stimulation are clomiphene citrate, letrozole, and camoxiphen.
- The maximum allowed gonadotropins dose is 150 IU of either FSF or HMG.
- Minimal stimulation is supposed to be the best protocol for extreme responders like poor ovarian reserve and PCOS if we want to do a fresh embryo transfer cycle.
- The aneuploidy rates cost of the cycle and other side effects related to supraphysiological levels of steroids are avoided here.

REFERENCES

1. Geeta N, Adrija D, Bart F. Mild Stimulation for In Vitro Fertilization. Fertil Steril. 2017;108:558-67.
2. Fauser BC, Devroey P, Macklon NS. Multiple birth resulting from ovarian stimulation for subfertility treatment. Lancet. 2005;365:1807-16.
3. Macklon NS, Stouffer RL, Giudice LC, Fauser BC. The science behind 25 years of ovarian stimulation for in vitro fertilization. Endocr Rev. 2006;27:170-207.
4. McGee EA, Hsueh AJ. Initial and cyclic recruitment of ovarian follicles. Endocr Rev. 2000;21:200-14.
5. Fauser BC, Van Heusden AM. Manipulation of human ovarian function: Physiological concepts and clinical consequences. Endocr Rev. 1997;18:71-106.
6. Baird DT. A model for follicular selection and ovulation: Lessons from superovulation. J Steroid Biochem. 1987;27:15-23.
7. Fluker MR, Marshall LA, Monroe SE, Jaffe RB. Variable ovarian response to gonadotropin-releasing hormone antagonist-induced gonadotropin deprivation during different phases of the menstrual cycle. J Clin Endocrinol Metab. 1991;72:912-9.
8. The Thessaloniki ESHRE/ASRM Sponsored PCOS Consensus Workshop Group. Consensus on infertility treatment related to polycystic ovary syndrome. Human Reprod. 2008;23(3):462-77.
9. Zegers-Hochschild F, Adamson GD, Dyer S, Racowsky C, de Mouzon J, Sokol R, et al. The International Glossary on Infertility and Fertility Care, 2017. Fertil Steril. 2017;108:393-406.
10. Pelinck MJ, Hoek A, Simons AH, Heineman MJ. Efficacy of natural cycle IVF: a review of the literature. Hum Reprod Update. 2002;8:129-39.
11. Verberg MF, Macklon NS, Nargund G, Frydman R, Devroey P, Broekmans FJ, et al. Mild ovarian stimulation for IVF. Hum Reprod Update. 2009;15:13-29.
12. Nargund G, Fauser BC, Macklon NS, Ombelet W, Nygren K, Frydman R. The ISMAAR proposal on terminology for ovarian stimulation for IVF. Hum Reprod. 2007;22:2801-4.
13. Fernandez-Shaw S, Perez Esturo N, Cercas Duque R, Pons Mallol I. Mild IVF using GnRH agonist long protocol is possible: comparing stimulations with 100 IU vs. 150 IU recombinant FSH as starting dose. J Assist Reprod Genet. 2009;26:75-82.
14. Williams SC, Gibbons WE, Muasher SJ, Oehninger S. Minimal ovarian hyperstimulation for in vitro fertilization using sequential clomiphene citrate and gonadotropin with or without the addition of a gonadotropin-releasing hormone antagonist. Fertil Steril. 2002;78:1068-72.
15. Weigert M, Krischker U, Pohl M, Poschalko G, Kindermann C, Feichtinger W. Comparison of stimulation with clomiphene citrate in combination with recombinant follicle-stimulating hormone and recombinant luteinizing hormone to stimulation with a gonadotropin-releasing hormone agonist protocol: a prospective, randomized study. Fertil Steril. 2002;78:34-9.
16. Mitwally MF, Casper RF. Aromatase inhibition reduces gonadotrophin dose required for controlled ovarian stimulation in women with unexplained infertility. Hum Reprod. 2003;18:1588-97.

17. Grabia A, Papier S, Pesce R, Mlayes L, Kopelman S, Sueldo C. Preliminary experience with a low-cost stimulation protocol that includes letrozole and human menopausal gonadotropins in normal responders for assisted reproductive technologies. Fertil Steril. 2006;86:1026-8.
18. de Jong D, Macklon NS, Fauser BC. A pilot study involving minimal ovarian stimulation for in vitro fertilization: extending the "follicle-stimulating hormone window" combined with the gonadotropin-releasing hormone antagonist cetrorelix. Fertil Steril. 2000;73:1051-4.
19. Ledger WL. Favourable outcomes from "mild" in-vitro fertilisation. Lancet. 2007;369:717-8.
20. Heijnen EM, Eijkemans MJ, De Klerk C, Polinder S, Beckers NG, Klinkert ER, et al. A mild treatment strategy for in-vitro fertilisation: a randomised non-inferiority trial. Lancet. 2007;369:743-9.
21. Roque M, Haahr T, Geber S, Esteves SC, Humaidan P. Fresh versus elective frozen embryo transfer in IVF/ICSI cycles: a systematic review and meta-analysis of reproductive outcomes. Hum Reprod Update. 2019;25:2-14.
22. Baart EB, Martini E, Eijkemans MJ, Van Opstal D, Beckers NG, Verhoeff A, et al. Milder ovarian stimulation for in-vitro fertilization reduces aneuploidy in the human preimplantation embryo: a randomized controlled trial. Hum Reprod. 2007;22:980-8.
23. Nargund G, Datta AK, Fauser B. Mild stimulation for in vitro fertilization. Fertil Steril. 2017;108:558-67.
24. McCulloh DH, Alikani M, Norian J, Kolb B, Arbones JM, Munne S. Controlled ovarian hyperstimulation (COH) parameters associated with euploidy rates in donor oocytes. Eur J Med Genet. 2019;62(8):103707.
25. ASRM. Comparison of pregnancy rates for poor responders using IVF with mild ovarian stimulation versus conventional IVF: a guideline. Fertil Steril. 2018;109:993-9.

Dual Stimulation

Hrishikesh D Pai, Sheetal Sawankar

■ INTRODUCTION

Management of poor ovarian responders (POR) remains a challenge despite the remarkable progress in assisted reproductive technologies, simply because they do not respond to treatment. It is a frustrating condition for patients as well as clinicians. Based on the differences in the definition of poor response, the prevalence of POR varies from 5.6 to 35.1%.[1-5] Such a wide range is indeed indicative of a heterogeneous population of patients. Hence, several definitions have been proposed to classify "poor responders," namely up to 41 according to the systematic review by Polyzos and Devroey,[6] and numerous protocols and strategies have been proposed to treat such poor prognosis patients. There is still no clear superiority of one treatment versus another to improve the reproductive outcome. The Bologna consensus criteria were first described in 2011 under the auspices of the European Society of Human Reproduction and Embryology (ESHRE) and have been a great achievement for classifying such patients.[7] According to this criteria, at least two of the following characteristics must be present to define "a poor responder patient": advanced maternal age (>40 years) and/or scarce response to a previous conventional stimulation (≤3 oocytes) and/or reduced ovarian reserve (antral follicle count—AFC <5-7 follicles, and/or anti-Müllerian hormone—AMH <1.1 ng/mL).

Since the oocyte competence can be severely affected by numerous factors, maternal age being the most important factor,[8,9] there was a lot of criticism and hence the classification should be more patient oriented. A new classification by a panel of experts, known as the POSEIDON (Patient-Oriented Strategies Encompassing IndividualizeD Oocyte Number) group,[10] has been introduced to better categorize the spectrum of poor responder patients. The POSEIDON group focused on tailoring the stimulation protocol so as to increase the chances of obtaining an euploid blastocyst, which was proposed as main goal of controlled ovarian stimulation (COS). This group then introduced the concept of "suboptimal response." In this group of patients collecting 4-9 oocytes, 4 subclusters were outlined according to both the ovarian reserve and the maternal age. In the POSEIDON criteria, the patients are divided in four subgroups based on the number of oocytes collected and the maternal age and ovarian reserve. Especially, groups 3 and 4 are represented from women younger than 35 or older than 35, respectively, with a compromised ovarian reserve (AFC <5 and AMH <1.2 ng/mL), an issue, which cannot be resolved pharmacologically, as already reported in several studies.[11-18]

Overall, the pregnancy rates attained with in vitro fertilization (IVF) in POR patients are low being less than 8%.[19-22] Polyzos and colleagues[21] in a cohort of 485 PORs reported a live birth rate (LBR) per cycle of 7.1% in patients <40 years and 5.2% in women ≥40 years old; in this study, the only independent variable related to the LBR was the number of oocytes. Indeed, the number of eggs is a robust surrogate outcome for LBR in IVF across all female age groups;[23] in women aged 35–37, the estimated effect of collecting three oocytes compared with two oocytes was a relative increase in the observed LBR by about 28%.[23] Thus, retrieving even one extra oocyte in this patient population makes a big difference in prognosis and any treatment modality that would increase the number of oocytes would be a very important step to improve reproductive outcome.

Establishment of excellent cryopreservation techniques along with our enhanced understanding of the physiologic, biochemical, and molecular mechanisms underlying antral follicular wave dynamics[24-26] has permitted the first description of double stimulation (DS) in 2013.[27] It initially started with random start and luteal phase stimulation (LPS) protocols for cancer patients and, more recently, the DuoStim protocol (follicular and LPS during the same menstrual cycle).

This chapter aims to tell the efficacy of dual stimulation protocol especially in poor ovarian reserve patients.

PATHOPHYSIOLOGY OF DUAL STIMULATION: THEORIES OF FOLLICULAR DEVELOPMENT

The physiologic mechanisms underlying selection and recruitment of antral follicles in women are not fully understood. Follicular development is an extremely dynamic process. It was initially thought, as per the classic theory (single recruitment episode theory), that a single cohort of antral follicles grows during the follicular phase of the ovarian cycle after luteal regression. However, this theory has been overtaken by the evidence of multiple waves arising during an ovarian cycle in many mammals. Such evidence, at first reported in large animal models,[28-33] was confirmed also in humans leading to the definition of two further theories of follicle recruitment:[27] the continuous recruitment theory, according to which the follicles start growing and regress continuously during the ovarian cycle; and the waves theory, according to which multiple cohorts (also referred to as "waves") of antral follicles are recruited per ovarian cycle.

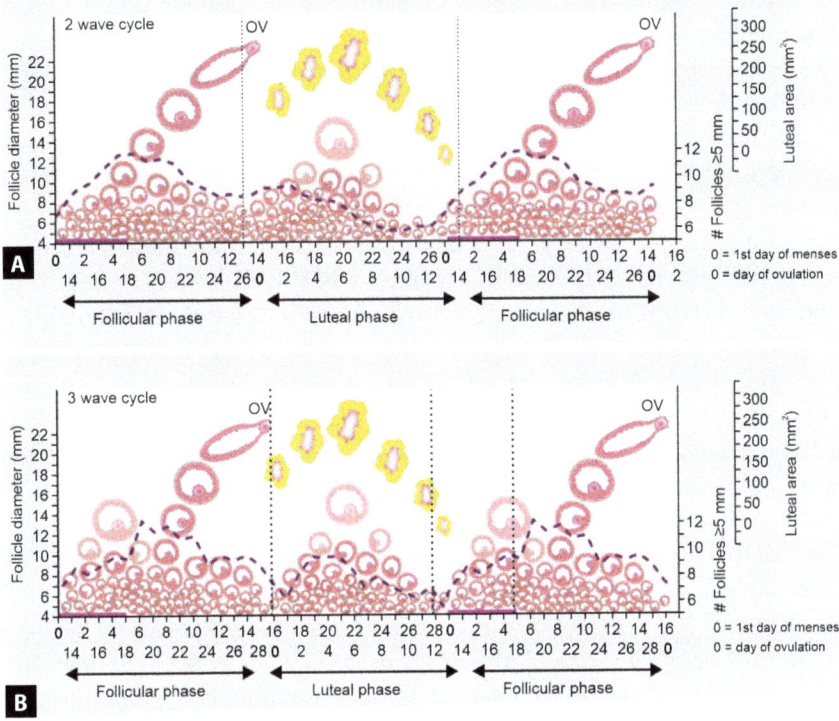

Figs. 1A and B: Ovarian follicular waves during menstrual cycle—multifollicular wave pattern.

Several intraovarian regulators, follicle-stimulating hormone (FSH) and progesterone levels, and inflammatory markers (e.g., serum C-reactive protein) were all proposed as modulators of the dynamics behind the origin of follicular waves.[26,27,34] From a clinical perspective, the growing knowledge of human ovarian follicular waves opened new options for COS to improve the efficiency and possibly the efficacy of IVF.

The multifollicular wave theory challenges the classical concept of folliculogenesis and is the basis for dual stimulation **(Figs. 1A and B)**.

■ STEPS TO PERFORM A DUAL STIMULATION CYCLE

The DS/DuoStimulation protocol is performed in a single menstrual cycle and it consists of the follicular phase stimulation (FPS) and the LPS. This protocol is done with an intent to have more number of retrieved oocytes in the same cycle. It is primarily done for POR patients, even fertility preservation cases or cancer patients benefit from this approach where time is of essence.

As per the current evidence, in POR patients, we can either use mild ovarian stimulation protocols (low-dose gonadotropins with or without oral ovulogens) or we can use the standard dose conventional ovarian stimulation protocols but mild OS protocols offer comparable reproductive outcome albeit lower cost.[35,36]

For dual stimulation, various OS protocols and regimens have been described for FPS and LPS. To all patients undergoing DuoStim, before the FPS, luteal estradiol priming may be started to promote synchronization and coordination of follicular growth.[37,38]

As discussed earlier, we can either use mild OS or the conventional regimens for FPS and LPS. For mild OS, oral ovulogens such as clomiphene citrate (CC) and letrozole (LE) with/without low-dose exogenous gonadotropins can be used. The other protocol is the conventional protocol where 225–450 IU daily dose of exogenous FSH with/without luteinizing hormone (LH)/LH-like activity can also be used for FPS and LPS **(Fig. 2)**.

Different treatment modalities have been used to prevent premature LH surge during FPS and LPS including gonadotropin-releasing hormone antagonist (GnRH-ant) use, exogenous progestins, and/or ibuprofen. A flexible GnRH-ant protocol is most commonly used where the antagonist is started when the leading follicle attains a mean diameter of 12–14 mm and is continued until the day of trigger. Exogenous progestins may also be used for this purpose, especially during LPS, not only to avoid premature LH surge but also to avoid menses during oocyte retrieval[39] to decrease the risk of infection.[40,41]

In the Shanghai protocol, the drugs used for COS were CC 25 mg/day, LE 2.5 mg/day, and mild dose of human menopausal gonadotropin 150–225 IU/day. The final trigger was induced by triptorelin followed by ibuprofen 0.6 g the day of trigger and the day after, in both FPS and LPS. Although ibuprofen was used in some studies, the precise role to avoid premature ovulation in this patient population needs to be proven in further studies.[42,43]

Gonadotropin-releasing hormone agonist (GnRHa) is most commonly used to trigger final oocyte maturation for both FPS and LPS.

In 2016, the authors published a proof-of-concept study where a DuoStim protocol was adopted together with a preimplantation genetic testing (PGT-A)

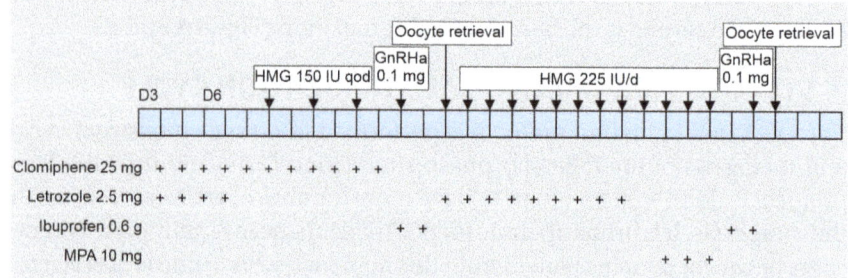

Fig. 2: The protocol of double stimulation during the follicular and luteal phases in patients with poor ovarian response. (GnRHa: gonadotropin-releasing hormone agonist; HMG: human menopausal gonadotropin; MPA: medroxyprogesterone acetate; qod: every other day)
Source: Shanghai protocol

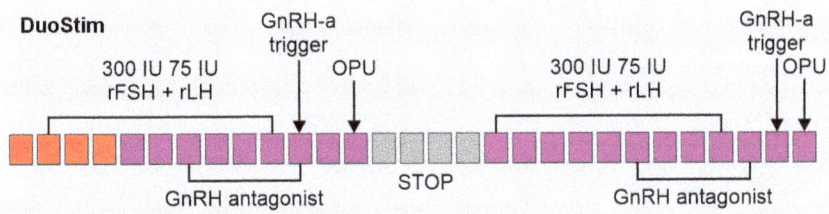

Fig. 3: DuoStim protocol. (GnRH: gonadotropin-releasing hormone; OPU: oocyte pick-up; rFSH: recombinant follicle-stimulating hormone; rLH: recombinant luteinizing hormone)

program in poor prognosis patients.[44] They found out that the application of DuoStim in this thorny patient population improved the chances of obtaining at least one euploid blastocyst from 40–70% in the same menstrual cycle **(Fig. 3)**.

CURRENT AVAILABLE EVIDENCE COMPARING FPS AND LPS IN POR PATIENTS

Concomitant FPS and LPS were first reported in a 41-year-old POR woman by Xu and Li in 2013.[27] In that case, they used a combination of 50–100 mg CC coupled with a daily dose of 150 IU FSH, for both FPS and LPS. She was triggered by GnRHa in the FPS and 10,000 IU urinary human chorionic gonadotropin (uhCG) for LPS. The oocyte retrieval was done 21 and 25 hours after triggering in FPS and LPS, respectively. Unfortunately, the patient did not conceive with frozen embryo transfer (FET) of the available embryo. Since this initial case report, several studies with different design, different OS regimens during FPS and LPS, and number of patients have been reported in PORs.[40,41,44,45-53]

In 2016, Wei and colleagues[47] confirmed the initial results of Kuang and colleagues, with the same protocol adopted in 23 POR patients fulfilling Bologna criteria; and they found out that the number of oocytes was significantly higher with LPS when compared with FPS (3.5 ± 3.4 vs. 1.6 ± 1.1, $p = 0.01$).

Many randomized controlled trials (RCTs) also showed that the number of oocytes retrieved, normal fertilized oocytes, cleaved embryos, cryopreserved embryos, and good-quality embryos and the blastocyst formation rate of the LPS stage were significantly higher than those of the FPS stage.

Many factors could be involved in increasing the oocyte number when performing LPS stimulation. Indeed high level of estradiol and progesterone reached after FPS may:
- Synchronize the cohort of antral follicles in anovulatory waves
- Stimulate the proliferation of FSH receptors in granulosa cells resulting overall in a better response to the stimulation

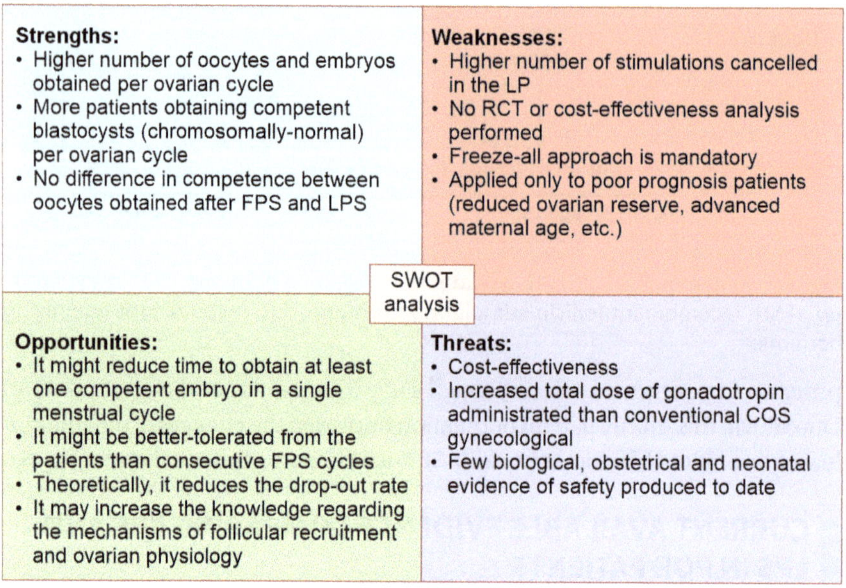

Strengths:	Weaknesses:
• Higher number of oocytes and embryos obtained per ovarian cycle • More patients obtaining competent blastocysts (chromosomally-normal) per ovarian cycle • No difference in competence between oocytes obtained after FPS and LPS	• Higher number of stimulations cancelled in the LP • No RCT or cost-effectiveness analysis performed • Freeze-all approach is mandatory • Applied only to poor prognosis patients (reduced ovarian reserve, advanced maternal age, etc.)
Opportunities:	Threats:
• It might reduce time to obtain at least one competent embryo in a single menstrual cycle • It might be better-tolerated from the patients than consecutive FPS cycles • Theoretically, it reduces the drop-out rate • It may increase the knowledge regarding the mechanisms of follicular recruitment and ovarian physiology	• Cost-effectiveness • Increased total dose of gonadotropin administrated than conventional COS gynecological • Few biological, obstetrical and neonatal evidence of safety produced to date

Fig. 4: DuoStim SWOT analysis. (FPS: follicular phase stimulation; LPS: luteal phase stimulation; RCT: randomized controlled trial; COS: controlled ovarian stimulation)

- Increase the angiogenic factors
- Enhance the sensitivity of the granulosa cells to FSH
- Possible flare-up effect derived from GnRH agonist trigger which might induce a downregulation in the expression of AMH in the follicles from the anovulatory wave

SWOT ANALYSIS OF DuoStim

To outline the advantages and disadvantages of DuoStim, a SWOT analysis was conducted **(Fig. 4)**, which was an efficient analytical framework useful to summarize the strengths, weaknesses, opportunities, and threats of a technology.

The strengths of this approach make it very promising. However, many more studies are needed in the future to restrict its weaknesses, shed light on its possible threats, and realize its opportunities.

CONCLUSION

The concept of multifollicular wave recruitment in a single ovarian cycle in women has opened important clinical implications for the treatment of poor prognosis patients. And time is very crucial for obtaining higher number and better quality oocytes in a shorter duration for these POR patients and even in cancer patients. The number of oocytes obtained in the LPS stage is greater than that in FPS stage. GnRHa or recombinant hCG as the trigger medicine may be better than uhCG during both the FPS and LPS stages for POR undergoing the DuoStim protocol.

Patients of dual stimulation require a mandatory freeze-all cycle and hence there is lack of cost-effectiveness. Since dual stimulation exploits the anovulatory waves of follicular recruitment, there should be a thorough biological and clinical investigation before it can be generally implemented. Before we use dual stimulation widely, we should do (1) an RCT comparing double-FPS versus DuoStim, (2) the application of DuoStim in cancer patients for fertility preservation, (3) as well as in prospective analyses focused on patients clustered according to either the Bologna criteria or the POSEIDON stratification. Until the results would be produced, DuoStim should be clinically applied only to poor prognosis patients and/or to whom time represents a critical issue like cancer patients.

■ KEY POINTS

- *Concept:* Dual stimulation involves two rounds of ovarian stimulation within a single menstrual cycle, typically one during the follicular phase and one during the luteal phase.
- *Purpose:* It aims to maximize the number of eggs retrieved in a shorter period, which is particularly beneficial for women with low ovarian reserve or poor responders.
- *Protocol:* The first stimulation begins at the start of the menstrual cycle, and after egg retrieval, a second stimulation starts a few days later.
- *Benefits:* Increases the total number of eggs retrieved and potentially improves cumulative pregnancy rates.
- *Timing:* It reduces the overall time required for egg retrieval compared to conventional IVF cycles spaced months apart.
- *Candidates:* Often recommended for patients with diminished ovarian reserve, older women, or those needing fertility preservation (e.g., cancer patients).
- *Hormonal considerations:* Involves careful monitoring of hormone levels to optimize the timing of stimulation and egg retrievals.
- *Research and evidence:* Ongoing studies suggest it can be an effective strategy, but it may not be suitable for all patients, and further research is needed to refine protocols and determine long-term outcomes.
- *Potential challenges:* Requires close monitoring, may increase the risk of ovarian hyperstimulation syndrome (OHSS), and can be more physically and emotionally demanding for patients.
- *Clinical practice:* Still an emerging approach, and not all fertility clinics may offer dual stimulation protocols.

REFERENCES

1. Biljan MM, Buckett WM, Dean N, Phillips SJ, Tan SL. The outcome of IVF-embryo transfer treatment in patients who develop three follicles or less. Hum Reprod. 2000;15:2140-4.
2. Inge GB, Brinsden PR, Elder KT. Oocyte number per live birth in IVF: were Steptoe and Edwards less wasteful? Hum Reprod. 2005;20:588-92.
3. Veleva Z, Järvelä IY, Nuojua-Huttunen S, Martikainen H, Tapanainen JS. An initial low response predicts poor outcome in in vitro fertilization/intracytoplasmic sperm injection despite improved ovarian response in consecutive cycles. Fertil Steril. 2005;83:1384-90.
4. Hendriks DJ, te Velde ER, Looman CW, Bancsi LF, Broekmans FJ. Expected poor ovarian response in predicting cumulative pregnancy rates: a powerful tool. Reprod Biomed Online. 2008;17:727-36.
5. Orvieto R, Meltcer S, Nahum R, Rabinson J, Anteby EY, Ashkenazi J. The influence of body mass index on in vitro fertilization outcome. Int J Gynaecol Obstet. 2009;104:53-5.
6. Polyzos NP, Devroey P. A systematic review of randomized trials for the treatment of poor ovarian responders: is there any light at the end of the tunnel? Fertil Steril. 2011;96:1058-61.e7.
7. Ferraretti AP, La Marca A, Fauser BC, Tarlatzis B, Nargund G, Gianaroli L; ESHRE working group on Poor Ovarian Response Definition. ESHRE consensus on the definition of 'poor response' to ovarian stimulation for in vitro fertilization: the Bologna criteria. Hum Reprod. 2011;26:1616-24.
8. Ferraretti AP, Gianaroli L. The Bologna criteria for the definition of poor ovarian responders: is there a need for revision? Hum Reprod. 2014;29:1842-5.
9. Younis JS, Ben-Ami M, Ben-Shlomo I. The Bologna criteria for poor ovarian response: a contemporary critical appraisal. J Ovarian Res. 2015;8:76.
10. Poseidon Group (Patient-Oriented Strategies Encompassing IndividualizeD Oocyte Number), Alviggi C, Andersen CY, Buehler K, Conforti A, De Placido G, et al. A new more detailed stratification of low responders to ovarian stimulation: from a poor ovarian response to a low prognosis concept. Fertil Steril. 2016;105:1452-3.
11. Duffy JM, Ahmad G, Mohiyiddeen L, Nardo LG, Watson A. Growth hormone for in vitro fertilization. Cochrane Database Syst Rev. 2010;(1):CD000099.
12. Yeung T, Chai J, Li R, Lee V, Ho PC, Ng E. A double-blind randomised controlled trial on the effect of dehydroepiandrosterone on ovarian reserve markers, ovarian response and number of oocytes in anticipated normal ovarian responders. BJOG. 2016;123:1097-105.
13. Yeung TW, Chai J, Li RH, Lee VC, Ho PC, Ng EH. A randomized, controlled, pilot trial on the effect of dehydroepiandrosterone on ovarian response markers, ovarian response, and in vitro fertilization outcomes in poor responders. Fertil Steril. 2014;102:108-115.e1.
14. Yeung TW, Li RH, Lee VC, Ho PC, Ng EH. A randomized double-blinded placebo-controlled trial on the effect of dehydroepiandrosterone for 16 weeks on ovarian response markers in women with primary ovarian insufficiency. J Clin Endocrinol Metab. 2013;98:380-8.
15. Balasch J, Fabregues F, Penarrubia J, Carmona F, Casamitjana R, Creus M, et al. Pretreatment with transdermal testosterone may improve ovarian

response to gonadotrophins in poor-responder IVF patients with normal basal concentrations of FSH. Hum Reprod. 2006;21:1884-93.
16. Fabregues F, Penarrubia J, Creus M, Manau D, Casals G, Carmona F, et al. Transdermal testosterone may improve ovarian response to gonadotrophins in low-responder IVF patients: a randomized, clinical trial. Hum Reprod. 2009;24:349-59.
17. Bosdou JK, Venetis CA, Dafopoulos K, Zepiridis L, Chatzimeletiou K, Anifandis G, et al. Transdermal testosterone pretreatment in poor responders undergoing ICSI: a randomized clinical trial. Hum Reprod. 2016;31:977-85.
18. Polyzos NP, Davis SR, Drakopoulos P, Humaidan P, De Geyter C, Vega AG, et al. Testosterone for poor ovarian responders: lessons from ovarian physiology. Reprod Sci. 2018;25(7):980-2.
19. Busnelli A, Papaleo E, Del Prato D, La Vecchia I, Iachini E, Paffoni A, et al. A retrospective evaluation of prognosis and cost-effectiveness of IVF in poor responders according to the Bologna criteria. Hum Reprod. 2015;30:315-22.
20. La Marca A, Grisendi V, Giulini S, Sighinolfi G, Tirelli A, Argento C, et al. Live birth rates in the different combinations of the Bologna criteria poor ovarian responders: a validation study. J Assist Reprod Genet. 2015;32:931-7.
21. Polyzos NP, Nwoye M, Corona R, Blockeel C, Stoop D, Haentjens P, et al. Live birth rates in Bologna poor responders treated with ovarian stimulation for IVF/ICSI. Reprod Biomed Online. 2014;28:469-74.
22. Sfontouris IA, Kolibianakis EM, Lainas GT, Navaratnarajah R, Tarlatzis BC, Lainas TG. Live birth rates using conventional in vitro fertilization compared to intracytoplasmic sperm injection in Bologna poor responders with a single oocyte retrieved. J Assist Reprod Genet. 2015;32:691-7.
23. Sunkara SK, Rittenberg V, Raine-Fenning N, Bhattacharya S, Zamora J, Coomarasamy A. Association between the number of eggs and live birth in IVF treatment: an analysis of 400 135 treatment cycles. Hum Reprod. 2011;26:1768-74.
24. Baerwald AR, Adams GP, Pierson RA. A new model for ovarian follicular development during the human menstrual cycle. Fertil Steril. 2003;80:116-22.
25. Baerwald AR, Adams GP, Pierson RA. Ovarian antral folliculogenesis during the human menstrual cycle: a review. Hum Reprod Update. 2012;18:73-91.
26. Baerwald AR, Adams GP, Pierson RA. Characterization of ovarian follicular wave dynamics in women. Biol Reprod. 2003;69:1023-31.
27. Xu B, Li Y. Flexible ovarian stimulation in a poor responder: a case report and literature review. Reprod Biomed Online. 2013;26:378-83.
28. Adams GP, Singh J, Baerwald AR. Large animal models for the study of ovarian follicular dynamics in women. Theriogenology. 2012;78:1733-48.
29. Jacob JC, Gastal EL, Gastal MO, Carvalho GR, Beg MA, Ginther OJ. Follicle deviation in ovulatory follicular waves with one or two dominant follicles in mares. Reprod Domest Anim. 2009;44:248-54.
30. Jacob JC, Gastal EL, Gastal MO, Carvalho GR, Beg MA, Ginther OJ. Temporal relationships and repeatability of follicle diameters and hormone concentrations within individuals in mares. Reprod Domest Anim. 2009;44:92-9.
31. Ginther OJ, Knopf L, Kastelic JP. Temporal associations among ovarian events in cattle during oestrous cycles with two and three follicular waves. J Reprod Fertil. 1989;87:223-30.

32. Ginther OJ, Jacob JC, Gastal MO, Gastal EL, Beg MA. Development of one vs multiple ovulatory follicles and associated systemic hormone concentrations in mares. Reprod Domest Anim. 2009;44:441-9.
33. Ginther OJ. The mare: a 1000-pound guinea pig for study of the ovulatory follicular wave in women. Theriogenology. 2012;77:818-28.
34. Clancy KB, Baerwald AR, Pierson RA. Systemic inflammation is associated with ovarian follicular dynamics during the human menstrual cycle. PLoS One. 2013;8:e64807.
35. Practice Committee of the American Society for Reproductive Medicine. Comparison of pregnancy rates for poor responders using IVF with mild ovarian stimulation versus conventional IVF: a guideline. Fertil Steril. 2018;109:993-9.
36. Youssef MAF, van Wely M, Mochtar M, Fouda UM, Eldaly A, El Abidin EZ, et al. Low dosing of gonadotropins in in vitro fertilization cycles for women with poor ovarian reserve: systematic review and meta-analysis. Fertil Steril. 2018;109:289-301.
37. Reynolds KA, Outrage KR, Jimenez PT, Rhee JS, Tuuli MG, Jungheim ES. Cycle cancellation and pregnancy after luteal estradiol priming in women defined as poor responders: a systematic review and meta-analysis. Hum Reprod. 2013;28:2981-89.
38. Chang X, Wu J. Effects of luteal estradiol pre-treatment on the outcome of IVF in poor ovarian responders. Gynecol Endocrinol. 2013;29:196-200.
39. Ata B, Capuzzo M, Turkgeldi E, Yildiz S, La Marca A. Progestins for pituitary suppression during ovarian stimulation for ART: a comprehensive and systematic review including meta-analyses. Hum Reprod Update. 2021;27:48-66.
40. Kuang Y, Chen Q, Hong Q, Lyu Q, Ai A, Fu Y, et al. Double stimulations during the follicular and luteal phases of poor responders in IVF/ICSI programmes (Shanghai protocol). Reprod Biomed Online. 2014;29:684-91.
41. Zhang W, Wang M, Wang S, Bao H, Qu Q, Zhang N, et al. Luteal phase ovarian stimulation for poor ovarian responders. JBRA Assist Reprod. 2018;22:193-8.
42. Kawachiya S, Matsumoto T, Bodri D, Kato K, Takehara Y, Kato O. Short-term, low-dose, non-steroidal anti-inflammatory drug application diminishes premature ovulation in natural-cycle IVF. Reprod Biomed Online. 2012;24:308-13.
43. Kadoch IJ, Al-Khaduri M, Phillips SJ, Lapensée L, Couturier B, Hemmings R, et al. Spontaneous ovulation rate before oocyte retrieval in modified natural cycle IVF with and without indomethacin. Reprod Biomed Online. 2008;16:245-9.
44. Ubaldi FM, Capalbo A, Vaiarelli A, Cimadomo D, Colamaria S, Alviggi C, et al. Follicular versus luteal phase ovarian stimulation during the same menstrual cycle (DuoStim) in a reduced ovarian reserve population results in a similar euploid blastocyst formation rate: new insight in ovarian reserve exploitation. Fertil Steril. 2016;105:1488-95.e1.
45. Zhang Q, Guo XM, Li Y. Implantation rates subsequent to the transfer of embryos produced at different phases during double stimulation of poor ovarian responders. Reprod Fertil Dev. 2017;29:1178-83.
46. Rashtian J, Zhang J. Luteal-phase ovarian stimulation increases the number of mature oocytes in older women with severe diminished ovarian reserve. Syst Biol Reprod Med. 2018;64:216-9.

47. Wei LH, Ma WH, Tang N, Wei JH. Luteal-phase ovarian stimulation is a feasible method for poor ovarian responders undergoing in vitro fertilization/intracytoplasmic sperm injection—embryo transfer treatment compared to a GnRH antagonist protocol: a retrospective study. Taiwan J Obstet Gynecol. 2016;55:50-4.
48. Jin B, Niu Z, Xu B, Chen Q, Zhang A. Comparison of clinical outcomes among dual ovarian stimulation, mild stimulation and luteal phase stimulation protocols in women with poor ovarian response. Gynecol Endocrinol. 2018;34:694-7.
49. Madani T, Hemat M, Arabipoor A, Khodabakhshi SH, Zolfaghari Z. Double mild stimulation and egg collection in the same cycle for management of poor ovarian responders. J Gynecol Obstet Hum Reprod. 2019;48:329-33.
50. Alsbjerg B, Haahr T, Elbaek HO, Laursen R, Povlsen BB, Humaidan P. Dual stimulation using corifollitropin alfa in 54 Bologna criteria poor ovarian responders—a case series. Reprod Biomed Online. 2019;38:677-82.
51. Luo Y, Sun L, Dong M, Zhang X, Huang L, Zhu X, et al. The best execution of the DuoStim strategy (double stimulation in the follicular and luteal phase of the same ovarian cycle) in patients who are poor ovarian responders. Reprod Biol Endocrinol. 2020;18:102.
52. Bourdon M, Santulli P, Maignien C, Pocate-Cheriet K, Marcellin L, Chen Y, et al. The ovarian response after follicular versus luteal phase stimulation with a double stimulation strategy. Reprod Sci. 2020;27:204-10.
53. Vaiarelli A, Cimadomo D, Alviggi E, Sansone A, Trabucco E, Dusi L, et al. The euploid blastocysts obtained after luteal phase stimulation show the same clinical, obstetric and perinatal outcomes as follicular phase stimulation-derived ones: a multicenter study. Hum Reprod. 2020;35:2598-608.

Chapter 29: Low-cost In Vitro Fertilization

Priya Bhave, Ashita Punjabi Hakhoo

■ INTRODUCTION

Around 80 million couples are impacted by infertility worldwide causing a significant psychological burden.[1] In India, having a child is considered important to promote family lineage and also to ensure economic security in older ages. Often the infertile couples are subjected to scrutiny and sometimes ostracized at the hands of society for the childlessness. It is important that infertility should be considered as a social and public health issue impacting detrimentally a significant proportion of population.[2] The advent of assisted reproductive technology (ART) has made it possible for couples with tubal factor, severe male infertility, decreased ovarian reserve, and those not responding to conventional treatments to bear offsprings. But the cost of in vitro fertilization (IVF) and intracytoplasmic sperm injection (ICSI) still remains nonaffordable to many couples and, therefore, there is wide variation in utilization of ART services even in developed countries. In 2001, the World Health Organization (WHO) recommended that infertility be considered a global health problem and stressed on measures to develop low-budget ART.[3] However, devising a low-cost IVF model should not only include direct but also indirect costs associated with IVF.

■ DIRECT COSTS

Direct costs include those directly incurred in treatment like expenditures on medical consultations, ultrasonography, hormones and medications, procedures, laboratory and embryology services, and hospital charges. The affordability of IVF treatment to a consumer is determined by the underlying cost of treatment, the level of public or third-party insurance to subsidize this cost, and the income of consumers.[4] For example, with the condition of transferring the restricted number of embryos according to female's age, Belgian Government reimburses the laboratory expenses for up to six IVF cycles up to the age of 42 years.[5] In Australia, there are no limitations and treatment is publicly funded.[6] In contrast, in the USA, the brunt of ART expenditure is on the consumer's pocket. Despite its high prevalence, infertility treatment still remains an area of low priority. Health authorities need to devise an appropriate funding framework to make ART services affordable and accessible to all.

INDIRECT COSTS

Indirect costs include the cost incurred on travelling to clinic, the loss of wages, treatment complications [e.g., ovarian hyperstimulation syndrome (OHSS)], and extra expenditures involved in caring of multiple births.[4] Cost analyses have shown that expenditure on twin pregnancy during the perinatal period is almost triple of a singleton pregnancy.[7,8]

STRATEGIES TO REDUCE IVF COST

High costs of IVF are largely due to expenditures for investigations, medications, and laboratory equipment. Adverse effects from IVF also contribute to strain on healthcare resources **(Table 1)**.

Relevant Investigations

Basic investigations should include semen analysis, transvaginal sonography, and serum anti-Müllerian hormone (AMH) in selected cases. Sometimes, hysteroscopy may be necessary to investigate and treat intrauterine abnormalities such as submucosal fibroids, septa, polyps, and intrauterine adhesions. With advent of office endoscopy, these can be done using an ambulatory approach in "one-stop subfertility clinics". Using transvaginal hydrolaparoscopy, reproductive organs can be directly visualized and tubal patency can be assessed in an outpatient setting.[9-11] Avoid duplicate and unnecessary investigations.

Ovarian Stimulation

Mild Stimulation Protocols

In a study by Polinder et al., patients randomized to mild-IVF had an increase in total number of cycles completed throughout the year, and

TABLE 1: The expenditure and strategies to reduce cost in IVF.

Expenditure in IVF	Strategies to reduce cost
Offering unnecessary IVF	Careful patient selection
Investigations	Simplifying investigative methods
Medications	Reducing the cost of ovarian stimulation
Laboratorial equipment	Simplifying the procedures and equipment in the laboratory
Treating adverse effects	Minimizing the complications of IVF

(IVF: in vitro fertilization)
Source: Teoh PJ, Maheshwari A. Low-cost in vitro fertilization: current insights. Int J Womens Health. 2014;6:817-27.

mild-IVF (MD-IVF) was determined to be a cost-effective alternative to conventional IVF (conv-IVF).[12] Higher costs involved in conventional IVF were attributed to increased obstetrics and neonatal costs in multiple pregnancies.

Mild ovarian stimulation saves the direct costs by reducing the costs associated with higher gonadotropin doses and also the indirect costs associated with complications such as OHSS and multiple gestations.[13]

A recent meta-analysis found no difference in pregnancy outcomes between mild and conventional stimulation in poor, normal, or high responders of IVF. Cycle cancellation rates were higher in poor responders only undergoing MD-IVF. Even though fewer oocytes were retrieved or fewer embryos created in MD-IVF group, the chance of obtaining high-grade embryos was found to be no different in poor, normal, as well as hyper-responders.[14]

Choice of Gonadotropins

A Cochrane review comprising 42 trials comparing recombinant follicle-stimulating hormone (rFSH) to any of the other gonadotropins [human menopausal gonadotropin (HMG), FSH-P, and FSH-HP] found no statistically significant difference in live birth rates. It concluded that clinical choice of gonadotropin should depend on convenience, availability, and cost of gonadotropin.[15] Using urinary preparations can decrease the cost of the stimulation protocol.

Prevention of Luteinizing Hormone Surge

Clomiphene citrate (CC), owing to its property to cause central inhibition, has been shown in many studies to prevent premature luteinizing hormone (LH) surge. It is a cheaper drug as compared to gonadotropin-releasing hormone (GnRH) agonists and antagonists.[16,17] Along with other cost-cutting measures, Aleyamma et al. achieved an acceptable live birth rate per transfer of 19% with one cycle IVF costing around US$ 675 and US$ 725 for an ICSI treatment.[18] In a prospective study, MPA was shown as an effective oral drug to prevent LH surge in women undergoing controlled ovarian hyperstimulation (COH). The incidence of LH in the study was 0.7% with no statistically significant difference in pregnancy outcomes.[19]

Monitoring of IVF Cycle

Using only ultrasonography, follicular monitoring can be done during IVF stimulation without the need for expensive endocrine investigations.[2] Cochrane review found no increase in clinical pregnancy rates while comparing combined monitoring by transvaginal ultrasound (TVUS) and serum estradiol with monitoring by TVUS alone, although the evidence was of low quality.[20]

Laboratory Considerations
INVO: Simple, Cost-effective ART
Intravaginal culture of oocytes (INVO) procedure is a simple and effective infertility treatment that uses a new device, the INVO cell. The INVO procedure consists of fertilization of oocyte(s) and development of embryo in early stages in the INVO cell placed into the maternal vaginal cavity for incubation. In this technique, vaginal cavity acts as surrogate for expensive IVF laboratory.

Over 800 cycles have been published worldwide which showed a clinical pregnancy rate of 19.6%. The INVO technology can be performed in an office setting with minor capital equipment.[21] This technology can help in providing low-cost, accessible IVF treatment to developing countries.

The Walking Egg Project
The Walking Egg nonprofit organization aims to raise awareness regarding infertility in resource-poor countries and make infertility treatments including ART available and accessible to the population. By simplifying the diagnostic and IVF laboratory procedures and by modifying the ovarian stimulation protocols for IVF-assisted reproductive techniques can be offered at affordable prices.[2] As part of the project, a new simplified method of IVF culturing called the "tWE lab method" has been devised **(Figs. 1A to E)**.

It is a closed system that enables fertilization and embryo development to occur undisturbed in the same tube until day 3 following which the embryo transfers are done. The method employs a simple chemical reaction to produce CO_2 de novo, namely a combination of a weak base (sodium bicarbonate), a weak acid (citric acid), and water. Fertilization and embryo development and selection of embryos for transfer can be done without opening vacutainers.[22] This method can save exuberant costs associated with conventional culture in complex IVF laboratories.[2]

Media
Use of monophasic media over sequential media has the advantage of continuous embryo development without the need for media renewal on day 3. It could prevent exposure of an embryo to fluctuating environmental changes (pH, temperature) besides requiring fewer resources, and less media, thus reducing the cost of IVF.

Reducing Complications of IVF
Ovarian Hyperstimulation Syndrome
In a recent meta-analysis, use of mild dose IVF was associated with reduced incidence of OHSS both in normal and high responders at a moderate quality of evidence[14] **(Box 1)**.

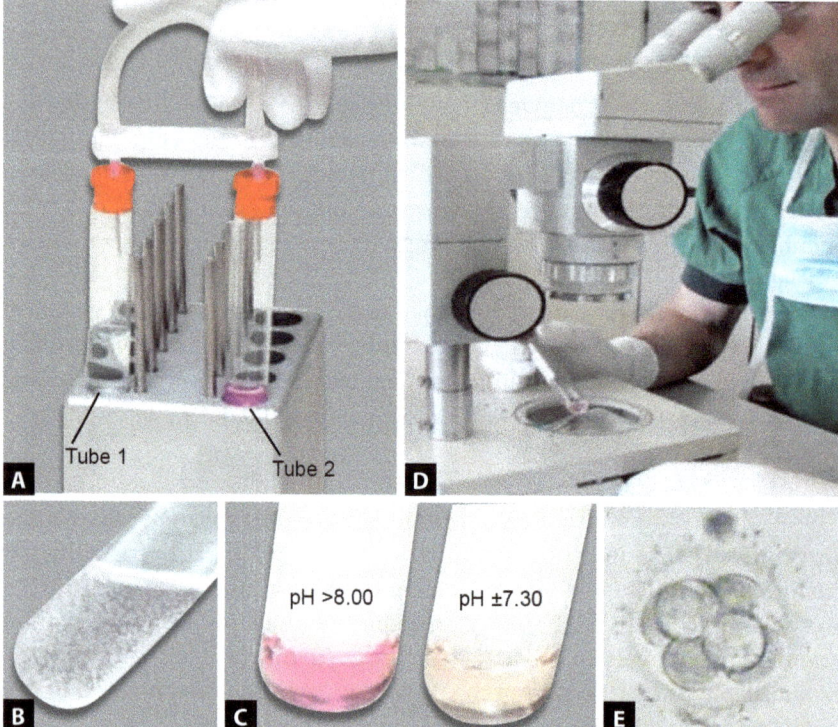

Figs. 1A to E: tWE lab method: (A) Connection between tube 1 with citric acid and sodium bicarbonate in water and tube 2 with IVF culture medium transfers enough CO_2 gas; (B) produced by the chemical reaction between the acid and the base to equilibrate the pH of the medium to ± 7:30; (C) Fertilization and embryo scoring by looking through the glass tube (D and E).

BOX 1: Practical guide to low-cost IVF.

- *Relevant investigations avoiding duplicate/unnecessary investigations:* Semen analysis, TVS baseline, AMH in selected cases, and office hysteroscopy when required
- *Ovarian stimulation:* Mild stimulation, urinary gonadotropins, CC to prevent LH surge, and USG monitoring of IVF cycle
- *Laboratory considerations: Monophasic media:* Less use of disposables, culture media, and less embryo manipulation
- *Reducing IVF complications:* OHSS—mild stimulation and multiple pregnancy—single embryo transfer

(AMH: anti-Müllerian hormone; CC: clomiphene citrate; IVF: in vitro fertilization; LH: luteinizing hormone; TVS: transvaginal sonography; USG: ultrasonography)

Multiple Pregnancy

Mild stimulation with practice of elective single embryo transfer can significantly reduce the incidence of IVF multiple pregnancies and the associated costs and complications.[23]

■ CONCLUSION

Infertility has been ranked the fifth-highest generator of disability among the global population of all people under the age of 60 years by WHO.[24] Public funding for IVF has been dismally low leading to dearth of utilization even in developed countries.[4] Infertility treatment has always been an area of low priority for health sector authorities. It is high time to realize the social and mental impact of infertility and make ART services affordable for all. Evaluation of expenditure should consider direct as well as indirect costs. While developing cost-effective strategies, it should be borne in mind that low-cost IVF should not lead to low-quality IVF.

■ KEY POINTS

- For the countries like India where ART cycles are neither government supported nor by insurance low budget IVF can make IVF affordable to masses.
- Minimal stimulation prevents unwanted side effects of ART and gives parallel success in selected group of patients.
- Low budget IVF should be a priority for all the ART units to make it more acceptable and smooth.
- Infertility impacts millions of couples worldwide. IVF/ICSI has evolved to cater to various causes of infertility but its high cost is an important deterrent to its accessibility.
- In countries like India, where IVF is neither government sponsored nor covered in insurance, its imperative to devise strategies to reduce IVF cost.
- Strategies to reduce cost of IVF include scrupulous selection of patients requiring IVF, performing relevant investigations, reducing cost of ovarian stimulation including minimal stimulation, simplifying laboratory procedures and equipment and reducing complications.

■ REFERENCES

1. James KS, Skirbekk V, Van Bavel J. Education and the global fertility transition. Vienna Yearbook Popul Res. 2012;10:1-8.
2. Ombelet W. The Walking Egg Project: Universal access to infertility care—from dream to reality. Facts Views Vis Obgyn. 2013;5(2):161-75.
3. Vayena E, Rowe P, Griffin PD. Current practices and controversies in assisted reproduction: report of a World Health Organization meeting. Geneva: World Health Organization; 2002.

4. Chambers GM, Adamson GD, Eijkemans MJ. Acceptable cost for the patient and society. Fertil Steril. 2013;100:319-27.
5. Gordts S. Belgian legislation and the effect of elective single embryo transfer on IVF outcome. Reprod Biomed Online. 2005;10:436-41.
6. Chambers GM, Sullivan EA, Ishihara O, Chapman MG, Adamson GD. The economic impact of assisted reproductive technology: a review of selected developed countries. Fertil Steril. 2009;91:2281-94.
7. Chambers GM, Chapman MG, Grayson N, Shanahan M, Sullivan EA. Babies born after ART treatment cost more than non-ART babies: a cost analysis of inpatient birth-admission costs of singleton and multiple gestation pregnancies. Hum Reprod. 2007;22:3108-15.
8. Lukassen HG, Schonbeck Y, Adang EM, Braat DD, Zielhuis GA, Kremer JA. Cost analysis of singleton versus twin pregnancies after in vitro fertilization. Fertil Steril. 2004;81:1240-6.
9. Teoh PJ, Maheshwari A. Low-cost in vitro fertilization: current insights. Int J Womens Health. 2014;6:817-27.
10. Cicinelli E, Matteo M, Causio F, Schonauer LM, Pinto V, Galantino P. Tolerability of the mini-pan-endoscopic approach (transvaginal hydrolaparoscopy and minihysteroscopy) versus hysterosalpingography in an outpatient infertility investigation. Fertil Steril. 2001;76(5):1048-51.
11. Watrelot A, Nisolle M, Chelli H, Hocke C, Rongières C, Racinet C, International Group for Fertiloscopy Evaluation. Is laparoscopy still the gold standard in infertility assessment? A comparison of fertiloscopy versus laparoscopy in infertility. Results of an international multicentre prospective trial: the 'FLY' (Fertiloscopy-LaparoscopY) study. Hum Reprod. 2003;18(4):834-9.
12. Polinder S, Heijnen EM, Macklon NS, Habbema JD, Fauser BJ, Eijkemans MJ. Cost-effectiveness of a mild compared with a standard strategy for IVF: A randomized comparison using cumulative term live birth as the primary endpoint. Hum Reprod. 2008;23:316-23.
13. Crawford NM, Sahay KM, Mersereau JE. Mild Stimulation versus Conventional IVF: A Cost-Effectiveness Evaluation. Open J Obstet Gynecol. 2016;6:180-8.
14. Datta AK, Maheshwari A, Felix N, Campbell S, Nargund G. Mild versus conventional ovarian stimulation for IVF in poor, normal and hyper-responders: a systematic review and meta-analysis. Hum Reprod Update. 2021;27(2):229-53.
15. van Wely M, Kwan I, Burt AL, Thomas J, Vail A, Van der Veen F, et al. Recombinant versus urinary gonadotrophin for ovarian stimulation in assisted reproductive technology cycles. Cochrane Database Syst Rev. 2011;2011(2):CD005354.
16. Verberg MF, Macklon NS, Nargund G, Frydman R, Devroey P, Broekmans FJ, et al. Mild ovarian stimulation for IVF. Hum Reprod Update. 2009;15:13-29.
17. Teramoto S, Kato O. Minimal ovarian stimulation with clomiphene citrate: A large-scale retrospective study. Reprod Biomed Online. 2007;15(2):134-48.
18. Aleyamma TK, Kamath MS, Muthukumar K, Mangalaraj AM, George K. Affordable ART: a different perspective. Hum Reprod. 2011;26(12):3312-331.
19. Kuang Y, Chen Q, Fu Y, Wang Y, Hong Q, Lyu Q, et al. Medroxyprogesterone acetate is an effective oral alternative for preventing premature luteinizing hormone surges in women undergoing controlled ovarian hyperstimulation for in vitro fertilization. Fertil Steril. 2015;104:62-70.

20. Kwan I, Bhattacharya S, Kang A, Woolner A. Monitoring of stimulated cycles in assisted reproduction (IVF and ICSI). Cochrane Database Syst Rev. 2014;(8):CD005289.
21. Frydman R, Ranoux C. INVO: a simple, low cost effective assisted reproductive technology. ESHRE Monographs. 2008;1:85-9.
22. Ombelet W, Van Blerkom J, Klerkx E, Janssen M, Dhont N, Mestdagh G, et al. The tWe LAB Simplified IVF Procedure: First Birth after freezing/thawing. Facts Views Vis Obgyn. 2014;6(1):45-9.
23. McLernon DJ, Harrild K, Bergh C, Davies MJ, de Neubourg D, Dumoulin JC, et al. Clinical effectiveness of elective single versus double embryo transfer: meta-analysis of individual patient data from randomised trials. BMJ. 2010;341:c6945.
24. World Health Organization. (2011). World Report on Disability. Available from: https://www.who.int/publications/i/item/9789241564182. [Last accessed May, 2024].

Chapter 30

Immunotherapy in Assisted Reproduction Treatment

Sapna Ahuja

■ INTRODUCTION

In vitro fertilization (IVF) has come a long way, since the birth of the first IVF baby Louise Brown in 1978. Though there have been improvements in the success rates of both fresh and frozen cycles, there is a group of patients who will fail to implant good-quality embryos, even genetically tested euploid embryos, repeatedly. The most common cause of implantation failure and miscarriage relates to chromosomal abnormalities of the embryo.[1] While future research may show that some of these cases are still due to embryonic problems, an immunological imbalance leading to a failure of implantation offers a plausible explanation.

The global reproductive scientific community agrees around the role of the immunological factor in implantation, however, the controversy is due to the lack of good-quality evidence, the lack of standardized and validated immunological tests, the cost, and the short- and long-term risks of immunomodulatory drugs for both mother and fetus. Robust data, i.e., randomized controlled trials (RCTs) around the subject are sparse, with the studies being poorly designed, heterogenous, reporting on small numbers of patients and only few reporting on live births. Some of these studies use multiple agents in treatment, to optimize the outcome, making it difficult to attribute any change to a particular drug.

In UK, the regulatory body, Human Fertilisation Embryology Authority (HFEA), classifies reproductive immunology testing and treatments as a "treatment add-on" (an optional additional treatment that may be offered to patients in addition to IVF) with a "red rating". They give a red rating for an add-on where there is no good-quality evidence in the form of RCTs to show improved live birth rates (LBRs), or where there are concerns about safety.

▌ IMMUNOLOGICAL TESTING AND THE RATIONALE FOR IMMUNOTHERAPY

Recurrent implantation failure (RIF) is commonly defined as the inability to achieve a clinical pregnancy after transfer of at least four embryos, over three fresh or frozen cycles, in a woman under the age of 40.[2,3] While the

CHAPTER 30: Immunotherapy in Assisted Reproduction Treatment

cause of RIF is considered idiopathic in about 50% of cases, one of the factors implicated is that—the maternal immune system fails to adapt and accept the semi-allograft fetus.[4,5]

Peter Medawar, in 1953, introduced the concepts of the fetal transplant and maternal immunosuppression.[6] According to this theory, the fetal antigens were not presented to the maternal lymphocytes or the lymphocytes were functionally suppressed. Wegmann,[7] in 1993, hypothesized that the maternal antigens were presented, but the maternal immune response shifted to the anti-inflammatory TH2 response to allow implantation to continue. Sacks[8] subsequently hypothesized that pregnancy is a state of immune activation, where there is an altered balance between the innate and adaptive immune systems.

Due to the lack of consensus and standardization of tests, clinicians use different tests and ranges to advocate treatments, as shown in **Figure 1**. Here we briefly discuss the commonly used tests, the T Helper cells, also called the CD4+ cells, are the key mediators of immune system. Cytokines are signalling proteins produced by cells and act as messengers. Interleukin 2 (IL2), interferon-γ (IFN-γ), and tumor necrosis factor-α (TNFα) are produced by TH1 cells, whereas IL4, IL5, IL6, IL10, and IL13 are secreted by Th2 cells.[9] Lower transforming growth factor-$\beta 1$ (TGF$\beta 1$), an anti-inflammatory cytokine, and raised IL-1β (IL1β), a pro-inflammatory cytokine, have been reported in patients with RIF.[10] Th2 predominance has been linked to positive pregnancy outcomes in those undergoing assisted reproduction,[10,11] and Th1 predominance may result in pregnancy loss.[12,13]

The right cytokine milieu is essential for angiogenesis, trophoblast invasion, and embryo implantation.[14] Though Treg cells and Th17 cells play an important role in implantation, these cytokines are not as commonly measured.[9]

Winger et al.[15] described that the normal range of TNFα/IL10 ratio was 13.2–30.6 and the levels of >30.6 and >20.5 for TNFα/IL10 and IFNχ/IL10,

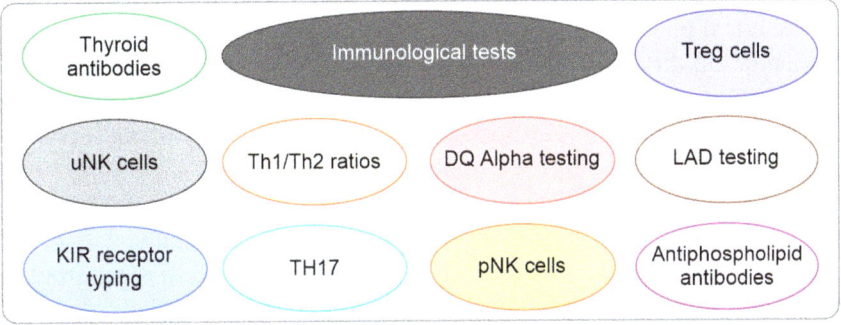

Fig. 1: Some of the immunological tests carried out to investigate an immunological factor in recurrent implantation failure.

respectively were being elevated. Liang et al.,[10] more recently, reported that the cytokine ratios TNFα/TGFβ1, IFNχ/IL4, IFNχ/TGFβ1, IFN/χIL10, IL6/TGFβ1, IL6/IL10, and IL1χ/TGFβ1 in peripheral blood have been shown to be significantly higher in patients with RIF when compared to control groups, supporting the hypothesis that cytokine ratios may impact clinical outcomes in assisted reproduction.

Natural killer (NK) cells were first described in 1975. They are types of lymphocytes in peripheral blood named due to their effector functions in killing target cells. The peripheral blood NK (pNK) cells account for ~15% of total lymphocytes.[16] 90% of pNK cells have a CD56dim CD16+ phenotype and are potently cytotoxic; whereas, 10% are CD56bright CD16+ which produce cytokines including IFNγ that have poor cytotoxic ability.[17-19] CD56bright and CD56dim share some phenotypic traits with uterine NK (uNK) cells,[19] including the expression of high levels of killer cell immunoglobulin-like receptors (KIR) that are responsible for self-tolerance.[20]

Ramos-Medina et al.[21] showed that in the RIF population, significantly higher levels of activated CD56dimCD16+CD69+ pNK cells were present in those who failed to achieve a pregnancy ($n = 75$) compared to those who were pregnant.

Uterine natural killer cells (uNK) are lymphocytes found in abundance in the decidua during implantation and in early pregnancy. Their presence is important for trophoblast invasion, transformation of the spiral arteries and placental development. There is a lack of consensus and standardization on the number/percentage of stromal uNK cells in a normal pregnancy, in early miscarriage and RIF.

The uNK cells vary depending on the stage of the menstrual cycle. Due to the invasive nature of an endometrial biopsy required to measure uNK cells, and, the lack of consensus on the number/percentage of stromal uNK cells in a normal pregnancy compared to a healthy control group, there remains controversy with regard to the significance of uNK cells and reproductive outcomes.

Progesterone and IL15 lead to an increase in uNK cell proliferation in the luteal phase leading to embryo implantation.[19,22] These cells lead to implantation through endothelial cell-modulating factors such as vascular endothelial growth factor (VEGF), which results in angiogenesis and vascularization, control of trophoblast remodeling, and cytokine secretion in the uterus.[23-25]

A meta-analysis by Seshadri et al.[18] reported no significant difference in the percentage of pNK or uNK cells in infertile women compared with fertile controls. Pooled studies demonstrated that when pNK cells were reported as absolute numbers, there was a significantly higher NK cell number in infertile women in comparison with a fertile group. There is a large variation in the numbers of pNK cells in healthy individuals.[26]

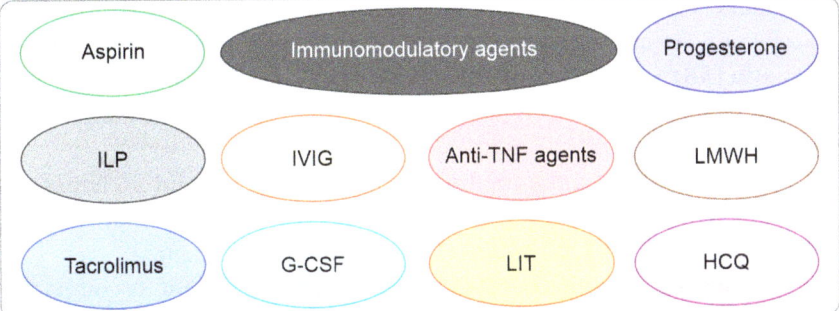

Fig. 2: Some of the immunomodulant treatments carried out to treat an immunological factor in recurrent implantation failure. (G-CSF: granulocyte colony-stimulating factor; HCQ: hydroxychloroquine; ILP: intralipid; IVIG: intravenous immunoglobulin; LMWH: low-molecular-weight heparin; TNF: tumor necrosis factor)

Despite intensive research, the role of uNK cells in pregnancy remains uncertain.[27]

There are no standardized and validated tests for pNK or uNK cells. Further research is needed to clarify the role of THI/TH2 ratios, pNK, and uNK cell testing in women with reproductive failure. Despite the lack of consensus and the value of these measurements being controversial, a number of couples request and are offered pNK and/or uNK cell testing.[22,28] The RCOG[29] in their scientific impact paper—"The Role of Natural Killer Cells in Human Fertility" concluded that women undergoing uNK cell testing should be advised that there are no proven effective treatments for those with "abnormal results".

Clinicians and institutions have been using different combinations of the tests discussed here, see **Figure 1**, to identify immunological dysfunction and consider immunomodulant treatments, see **Figure 2**. There are no national or international guidelines or any consensus.

■ IMMUNOMODULATORY AGENTS

Low Dose Aspirin (LDA)

Action: Aspirin inhibits the enzyme cyclooxygenase and decreases the production of prostaglandins. In platelets, this action effectively stops the production of thromboxane, which is a vasoconstrictor, leading to vasodilatation.

The proposed beneficial effects of aspirin in assisted reproduction are:
- Reduction of inflammation in the uterine cavity
- Improvement of uterine and ovarian perfusion, which might improve endometrial receptivity and ovarian responsiveness[30,31]
- It can also lead to cytokine production, placental cell apoptosis, and impacts trophoblast implantation.[32]

A meta-analysis of six RCTs by Gelbaya et al.[33] comparing aspirin to placebo or no treatment during ART found no beneficial effect on pregnancy [risk ratio (RR) 1.09; 95% confidence interval (CI) 0.92–1.29], LBR per cycle (RR 0.87; 95% CI 0.57–1.34), or LBR per embryo transfer (RR 1.08; 95% CI 0.83–1.40).

Similarly, another meta-analysis by Khairy et al.[34] found no benefit of aspirin compared to placebo or no treatment for clinical pregnancy rate (PR) (RR 1.11; 95% CI 0.95–1.31) or LBR (RR 0.94; 95% CI 0.64–1.39).

Dentali et al.,[35] in 2012, published a meta-analysis of 17 RCTs comparing aspirin with no aspirin or placebo in IVF/intracytoplasmic sperm injection (ICSI) couples showed a higher PR (OR 1.19; 95% CI 1.01–1.39) but did not show a benefit for LBR (OR 1.08; 95% CI 0.90–1.29).

A Cochrane review published in 2016[36] along with many other published RCTs concluded that treatment with low-dose aspirin does not improve pregnancy outcomes in terms of implantation, clinical pregnancy, ongoing pregnancy, or LBRs in an unselected population of women undergoing IVF or ICSI.

Adverse effects: Maternal gastrointestinal side effects can occur, though at doses of 75–81 mg/day, side effects are unlikely.

Due to the easy availability, low cost, and low risk of side effects, LDA tends to be used frequently during IVF treatment despite the lack of evidence of benefit.

Low-molecular-weight Heparin

While low-molecular-weight heparin (LMWH) was initially used in ART due to its antithrombotic action, other early implantation and immunomodulatory effects were identified which has led to it being used frequently in the ART setting.[37]

The LMWH actions include the following:
- Prevention of complement activation in pregnant patients with antiphospholipid antibodies[38]
- The complex heparin binding epidermal growth factor appears to facilitate an invasive phenotype of the trophoblast and inhibits apoptosis.[38]
- It increases the free levels of insulin-like growth factor-I (IGF-I) and IGF II, which increase trophoblast invasion.[39]
- It has been shown to induce transcription of matrix metalloproteinases, which regulate cell–cell interactions facilitating trophoblast invasion.

Qublan et al.[40] reported the effect of heparin in women with failed IVF attempts and at least one thrombophilia disorder. They reported a significantly higher implantation rate (IR) (19.8% vs. 6.1%), PR (31% vs. 9.6%), and LBR (23.4% vs. 2.4%) and a reduced miscarriage rate in the heparin intervention group.

Urman et al.[41] and Noci et al.[42] did randomized studies of 150 and 172 women with RIF respectively, with LMWH in the luteal phase in the intervention group. Both studies failed to show any significant increase in clinical pregnancy, ongoing pregnancy, live birth, or IRs.

Potdar et al.[39] carried out a systematic review and meta-analysis to evaluate the effect of LMWH on LBRs and IRs in women with RIF. Approximately eight women required treatment to achieve one extra live birth. They concluded that the use of LMWH significantly improved LBR by 79% compared with the control group.

Adverse effects—include injection site bruising/bleeding, erythema, discoloration, delayed hypersensitivity, thrombocytopenia, alopecia, osteoporosis, and transient transaminase elevation.

Similar to aspirin, due to the relative safety, low cost, and simple administration, LMWH is frequently used by clinicians in the setting of RIF.

Glucocorticoids

It has been proposed that glucocorticoids may improve the intrauterine environment by:
- Suppressing endometrial inflammation
- Acting as immunomodulators to reduce the uterine NK cell count and normalize the cytokine expression profile in the endometrium

The suppression of Th1 and promotion of Th2 and Treg cells have been demonstrated in the murine model, using corticosteroids.[43-45]

Retrospective analysis by Taniguchi[46] and Geva[47] reported beneficial effects of glucocorticoid treatment in autoantibody seropositive women with implantation failure and in women with antinuclear antibodies, respectively.

Fawzy et al.[48] published a prospective, randomized, placebo-controlled trial of 160 women with idiopathic RIF. They reported that the combination of 20 mg of prednisolone with progesterone and enoxaparin (and also enoxaparin alone) significantly increased the LBR when compared to no treatment: combination group—45/53 (85%); enoxaparin group—46/57 (80.7%); and no treatment group—24/50 (48%).

The Cochrane review by Boomsma et al.[49] investigated peri-implantation glucocorticoids to improve clinical outcomes in subfertile women undergoing IVF or ICSI. The review included fourteen studies (involving 1,879 couples) and concluded that there was no evidence that glucocorticoids improved the PRs and clinical outcomes (13 RCTs; OR 1.16, 95% CI 0.94-1.44). A subgroup analysis of 650 women undergoing IVF (6 RCTs) showed a significantly higher PR in favor of glucocorticoids (OR 1.50, 95% CI 1.05-2.13).

Adverse effects—include high blood pressure, diabetes, premature birth, gastric ulceration, Cushing's syndrome, hypocalcemia, osteoporosis, skin thinning, and dry skin (BNF, 2015). A meta-analysis of corticosteroid safety concluded that they do not present a major teratogenic risk, but lead to a 3–4-fold increased risk of a fetal oral cleft.[50]

Tumor Necrosis Factor-Alpha Blockers

Tumor necrosis factor-α is a naturally occurring cytokine involved in cell-mediated immunity. Humira (adalimumab/anti-TNF-α) is recombinant human IgG1 monoclonal antibody, specific for human TNF. It decreases the cell-mediated immune response from Th1 lymphocytes by neutralizing TNF-α.

Humira (adalimumab) actions include the following:[27,51]
- Humira binds specifically to TNF-α, hence blocking its interaction with the p55 and p75 cell surface TNF receptors.
- It lyses cells, that express TNF surface receptors in vitro, in the presence of complement.
- It modulates the inflammatory responses that are induced by TNF, including changes in the adhesion molecules responsible for leukocyte migration.
- Humira reduces the inflammatory response by inhibiting TNFα. This action occurs via the blockade of fibrinogen-like protein 2 (FGL2), possibly leading to a shift in the Th1/Th2 imbalance in RIF and recurrent pregnancy loss (RPL).

An observational study of 75 idiopathic RIF patients was published by Winger et al.[52] Women were given LMWH and aspirin either with intravenous immunoglobulin (IVIG) or Humira or both. This small study reported a significant improvement in the PR in the combined treatment group (80% in 41 individuals), and concluded that Humira and IVIG significantly improves IVF outcomes in infertile women with Th1/Th2 cytokine elevation.

The same group published another retrospective observational study,[53] in 76 women with RIF. They looked at the Th1/Th2 cytokine ratio (TNFα/IL10) before and after treatment with Humira and IVIG, administered 90–120 days before embryo transfer. The cohort was separated into two groups depending on the TNFα/IL10 ratios (30.6–39 for group 1 and >39 for group two). While there was a statistically significant reduction in TNFα/IL10 ratios following immunomodulation, there was a nonsignificant increase in IR, clinical PR, LBR, and delivery rate per embryo transferred, when comparing the two groups.

Adverse effects: These include infection—chronic infections such as tuberculosis and septicemia, lymphoma, demyelinating disease, autoantibody induction, congestive heart failure, injection site reactions, lupus-like syndrome, severe allergic reactions to the drug, etc.[54]

The TNF-α inhibitors such as Humira are classified as FDA Category B. This is to reflect limited evidence in a small number of pregnant women and women of childbearing age, where these drugs have not shown any increase in the frequency of malformation, or other direct or indirect harmful effects on the human fetus.

The risks of short-term use (2-4 injections over a period of 8-14 weeks) of Humira in appropriately screened women are minimal. The published studies are few with a small number of patients and with no randomized studies. When considering the use of TNF-α blockers in this setting, careful case selection, appropriate counseling, informed consent involving the couple, and strict protocols and supervision under an experienced team are essential.

Intravenous Immunoglobulin

Intravenous immunoglobulin is a protein concentrate of human immunoglobulin G (IgG) from pooled human plasma, for intravenous administration.

The IVIG actions include the following:
- Modulation of T cells, B cells, and macrophages—leading to interference with antibody production and degradation
- Modulation of complement and cytokines
- Cell growth regulation
- Reduction in peripheral cytotoxic NK cells
- Enhancement of Treg cells
- Downregulation of B cells that are responsible for antibody production

Those who believe in immunomodulation treatments argue that these effects lead to a decrease in the Th1 cytotoxic response with the Th2 response predominating and, therefore, improved implantation mechanisms.

A retrospective observational study[21] of women with RIF/recurrent miscarriage, given 0.4 g/kg IVIG, in the ET cycle/three weekly during the first trimester and then 0.2 g/kg, four weekly up to 35-36 weeks pregnancy, led to a significant increase in the LBRs (from 17.9 to 80% in the RIF group and from 30.8 to 96.3% in the recurrent miscarriage group).

A meta-analysis[55] of nine randomized studies including 2,415 women evaluated the role of IVIG in RIF. The authors concluded that there was a statistically significant increase in live birth—406 of 816 (49.8%) in the IVIG treatment group compared to 506 of 1,599 (31.6%) in the non-IVIG group.

Stephenson et al.[56] carried out a randomized trial reporting on 39 fresh IVF cycles. The LBRs were 4/26 (15%) for the IVIG group and 3/25 (12%) for the placebo group (P = 0.52). They concluded that IVIG did not improve the LBR in couples with repeated unexplained IVF failure.

Placido et al.[57] reported on eighteen patients randomized to the IVIG treatment group and 21 in the placebo arm. Though the increase in PR was not statistically significant (33.3 vs. 19.1), the IR in the IVIG group was remarkably higher as compared to the placebo group (17.7% vs. 6.5%).

Adverse effects: These include headache, muscle pain, fever, chills, low back pain, rarely thromboembolism, renal failure, aseptic meningitis, hemolytic reactions, anaphylactic reactions, lung disease, enteritis, dermatologic disorders, and infectious diseases.[58] Christiansen[59] demonstrated no congenital malformation with an adverse effects profile consisting of headache and skin rash.

The conflicting results lead to a strong need for further RCTs to support the clinical benefits of IVIG in RIF patients. Serious side effects of IVIG are rare. However, the cost is prohibitive and long-term safety data are lacking. Again, appropriate counseling, informed consent involving the couple, and strict protocols and supervision under an experienced team are essential.

Intralipids

Intralipid® 20% (A 20% IV fat emulsion) is a sterile, nonpyrogenic fat emulsion, made up of 20% soybean oil, 1.2% egg yolk phospholipids, 2.25% glycerin, and water for injection.

Possible actions of ILP include:
- Modulating certain immune cellular mechanisms, by downregulating cytotoxic/activated NK cells
- They may suppress proinflammatory cellular (type-1) cytokines such as IFN-γ and TNF-α.
- Corticosteroids such as dexamethasone and prednisolone can enhance the above effect by suppressing cytotoxic/activated T-lymphocytes.

It has been suggested that ILPs reduce the pNK cell count and suppress pNK cell cytotoxicity in patients with RIF and RPL.[60,61]

In a small, observational study of women with RIF/RPL and elevated pNK cells, the women were given either IVIG ($n = 242$) or ILP therapy ($n = 200$) resulting in LBRs of 61% and 56%, respectively. The pregnancy outcomes were similar in these two groups.[60]

One RCT[62] evaluated ILP in 296 women ($n = 144$ in the treatment group, $n = 152$ controls) with unexplained secondary infertility, recurrent spontaneous abortion, and elevated NK cell activity (>12%). This study reported ILP given on the day of oocyte retrieval was associated with a statistically significant increase in ongoing PR and LBR (treatment group 37.5% vs. controls 22.4%), a nonsignificant increase in chemical PR, and a nonsignificant reduction in spontaneous abortion rate.

Singh et al.[63] carried out a single blinded RCT of 105 subjects with previous failed IVF. There was a significant difference in the biochemical PR in the ILP group [(40.38% vs. control 16%), RR = 2.5 (1.23–5.16 CI)], clinical PR [(34.62% vs. 14%), RR = 2.5 (1.13–5.40 CI)], IR [(16.6% vs. 6.6%), RR = 2.5 (1.18–5.41 CI)], and take home baby rate [28.8% vs. 10%, $p = 0.024$, RR = 2.8 (1.1–7.3)]. The adjusted odds ratio for clinical pregnancy in women who received ILP versus placebo was 3.1.

Adverse effects: These include headache, dizziness, flushing, nausea, clotting, infection, hypersensitivity, thrombocytopenia, iatrogenic infections, hepatomegaly, jaundice, cholestasis, splenomegaly, leukopenia, and fat overload syndrome.[60]

The relatively easy availability and administration, rarity of side effects, and acceptable cost have led to ILPs being used more frequently by many clinics, in women with previous IVF failures, even without any laboratory testing. Short and long-term data to show the impact of ILPs on the fetus are lacking.

Granulocyte Colony-Stimulating Factor

Granulocyte colony-stimulating factor (G-CSF) belongs to the family of colony-stimulating factors (CSFs) synthesized by multiple cell types (e.g., endothelial cells, fibroblasts, macrophages, and lymphocytes).[65,66]

It has been investigated to improve embryo euploidy rates, thin endometrium, and to increase implantation.

A recent meta-analysis[67] of 10 RCTs, involving 1,016 IVF-ET cycles, reported that G-CSF administration could significantly improve clinical pregnancy rate (CPR, RR 1.89, 95% CI 1.53-2.33), while it had no beneficial effect on embryo IR (RR 1.84, 95% CI 0.84-4.03). A subgroup analysis showed that both uterine infusion and subcutaneous injection can produce an increase in CPR, with the pooled RRs (95% CI) being 1.46 (1.04-2.05) and 2.23 (1.68-2.95), respectively. Pooled data in the RIF group showed a higher PR and IR in G-CSF group as compared to that in the control, with the RRs (95% CI) 2.07 (1.64-2.61) and 1.52 (1.08-2.14), respectively.

Jain et al.[68] published a randomized double-blinded placebo-controlled trial including 150 women undergoing fresh embryo transfer. Patients in the intervention group received intrauterine perfusion of 300 µg (0.5 mL) of G-CSF and patients in placebo group received intrauterine perfusion of 0.5 mL normal saline. Clinical PR was 27.6% in the intervention group compared to 18.9% in the placebo group and the difference was not statistically significant. There was no statistically significant difference between biochemical PR, IR, ongoing PR, LBR, and endometrial parameters between the two groups.

Adverse effects: These include mucositis, splenic enlargement, hepatomegaly, transient hypotension, epistaxis, urinary abnormalities, osteoporosis, exacerbation of rheumatoid arthritis, anemia, and pseudogout (BNF, 2015). When used as an intrauterine infusion or as a single subcutaneous dose before transfer, it is very rare to get any adverse effects.

Tacrolimus

Tacrolimus is an immunosuppressive drug, used to prevent rejection in patients undergoing a transplant.

Actions include:
- It inhibits antigen-induced lymphocytic proliferation, cytotoxic T-cell formation, IL-2 receptor expression, and the production of IL-2 and IFN-γ
- A reduction of inflammatory cytokines TNFα, IL1β, and IL6 mediated through inhibition of calcineurin leads to its immunosuppressive activity.[69]

A prospective cohort study of 42 patients with RIF was published by Nakagawa et al.[70] 25 patients received tacrolimus from 2 days prior to the embryo transfer, until a positive pregnancy test. The clinical PR and LBR in the treatment group were 64% versus 0% and 60% versus 0%, respectively.

The same group published a larger prospective cohort study[71] of 124 women with RIF and elevated Th1/Th2 cell (CD4+ IFN-γ+ /CD4+ IL-4+) ratios (≥10.3) treated with tacrolimus. 52/124 women achieved a clinical pregnancy (41.9%). Pregnancy beyond 12 weeks was statistically higher in the low Th1/Th2 group (46.3%) in comparison with the high Th1/Th2 group (23.8%).

Another group[72] reported on 10 RIF patients with elevated Th1/Th2 cell ratios. Tacrolimus significantly increased the expression of LIF, IL-10, and IL-17 and decreased the expression of IL-4, IFN-γ, and the IFN-γ/IL-10 ratio. The IR was 40%, clinical PR 50%, and the LBR was 35%, in RIF patients with elevated Th1/Th2 ratios.

Tacrolimus has demonstrated safety for both the mother and fetus.[73] However, with only few small studies published, good quality data and great caution is required before recommending tacrolimus to improve outcomes in assisted reproduction treatment.

Hydroxychloroquine

Hydroxychloroquine (HCQ) is an anti-inflammatory drug and widely used as an antimalarial and an immunomodulant.

In one study[74] of 17 women with RIF and elevated TNF-α/IL-10 ratios, HCQ administration (400 mg/orally per day) reported a reduction in the TNF-α/IL-10 ratio.

While there is no evidence of benefit in RIF, the overall safety of HCQ use is well established.[75]

■ CONCLUSION

The role of the immune system in implantation and pregnancy is well recognized. However, there is no consensus among the scientific community with regard to the role of immunological testing and immunomodulation treatments in women with RIF.

While embryonic causes may offer a likely explanation for this in many cases, the role of the maternal immune system offers a plausible explanation in selected patients. Good-quality RCTs are required to add to the existing

CHAPTER 30: Immunotherapy in Assisted Reproduction Treatment

scientific literature to substantiate the role of immunomodulation in selected subgroups of women.

International professional bodies should come together and review the upcoming evidence to advise the reproductive medicine community, regarding the best available tests and treatments. National and international databases should be set up to report treatment outcomes and short- and long-term adverse effects of these treatments to inform both clinicians and patients.

The Food and Drug Administration (FDA) pregnancy safety categories for majority and outcomes of these immunomodulant therapies such as IVIG, corticosteroids, tacrolimus, ILP therapy are category C medications, requiring careful "benefit to risk" evaluation. While all immunomodulant medications have side effects, some of which can be serious, these treatments are used in many medical immunological conditions with good maternal and fetal outcomes.

Albert Einstein said—"If you want different results, do not do the same things". As clinicians, when faced with a couple with RIF and no obvious explanation, we must consider all the possible factors including immunological dysfunction. Couples with RIF go through multiple cycles with significant physical, emotional, and financial implications which could be avoided with such treatments in selected cases. While indeed, we must first "do no harm", couples should be counseled appropriately and given the information, the time, the choice, and be involved in making informed decisions about their care.

■ KEY POINTS

- An immunological imbalance offers a plausible explanation for lack of implantation.
- There is no consensus or standardization regarding the immunological tests and treatments.
- Low dose aspirin, and low molecular heparin are commonly used in recurrent implantation failure, for their anticoagulant properties and other effects on implantation despite a lack of evidence of benefit.
- Glucocorticoids may be of benefit in a subgroup of patients, but more data is required.
- There are many studies evaluating the use of intralipids, and intravenous immunoglobulin in assisted reproduction, with many showing positive outcomes, but there is a lack of good quality data. Long-term data is lacking.
- There are very few, small studies evaluating the use of TNF alpha blockers-Humira, Hydroxychloroquine and Tacrolimus, in implantation failure, and they should be used with great caution.

- Granulocyte colony-stimulating factor may be used for a thin endometrium and to improve implantation but the evidence is limited.
- Any immunological testing and treatments should be carried out only with careful counseling regarding the evidence, well-selected patients, informed consent, and involving the couple in all decisions.
- Any immunological testing and treatments should be carried out only with experienced teams, using strict protocols.
- The risks from some immunomodulatory agents used carefully, in well-selected and counseled patients, are low, though can come at a significant cost.

REFERENCES

1. Hart R. Physiological aspects of female fertility: role of the environment, modern lifestyle, and genetics. Physiol Rev. 2016;96:873-909.
2. Coughlan C, Ledger W, Wang Q, Liu F, Demirol A, Gurgan T, et al. Recurrent implantation failure: definition and management. Reprod Biomed Online. 2014;28:14-38.
3. Polanski LT, Baumgarten MN, Quenby S, Brosens J, Campbell BK, Raine-Fenning NJ. What exactly do we mean by 'recurrent implantation failure'? A systemic review and opinion. Reprod Biomed Online. 2014;28:409-23.
4. Alijotas-Reig J, Llurba E, Gris J. Potentiating maternal immune tolerance in pregnancy: a new challenging role for regulatory T cells. Placenta. 2014;35:241-8.
5. Laird S, Tuckerman E, Cork B, Linjawi S, Blakemore A, Li T. A review of immune cells and molecules in women with recurrent miscarriage. Hum Reprod Update. 2003;9:163-74.
6. Medawar PB. Some immunological and endocrinological problems raised by the evolution of viviparity in vertebrates: Prevention of allogeneic fetal rejection by tryptophan catabolism. Symp Soc Exp Biol. 1953;7:320-38.
7. Wegmann TG, Lin H, Guilbert L, Mosmann TR. Bidirectional cytokine interactions in the maternal-fetal relationship: is successful pregnancy a TH2 phenomenon? Immunol Today. 1993;14(7):353-6.
8. Sacks G, Sargent I, Redman C. An innate view of human pregnancy. Immunol Today. 1999;20(3):114-8.
9. Saito S, Nakashima A, Shima T, Ito M. Th1/Th2/Th17 and regulatory T-cell paradigm in pregnancy. Am J Reprod Immunol. 2010;63:601-10.
10. Liang P, Diao L, Huang C, Lian RC, Chen X, Li GG, et al. The pro-inflammatory and anti-inflammatory cytokine profile in peripheral blood of women with recurrent implantation failure. Reprod Biomed Online. 2015;31:823-6.
11. Kalu E, Bhaskaran S, Thum M, Vishwanatha R, Croucher C, Sherriff E, et al. Serial estimation of Th1:Th2 cytokines profile in women undergoing in-vitro fertilisation embryo transfer. Am J Reprod Immunol. 2008;59:206-11.
12. Comba C, Bastu E, Dural O, Yasa C, Keskin G, Ozsurmeli M, et al. Role of inflammatory mediators in patients with recurrent pregnancy loss. Fertil Steril. 2015;104:1467-74.

13. Bates M, Quenby S, Takakuwa K, Johnson P, Vince G. Aberrant cytokine production by peripheral blood mononuclear cells in recurrent pregnancy loss? Hum Reprod. 2002;17:2439-44.
14. Mor G, Cardenas I, Abrahams V, Guller S. Inflammation and pregnancy: the role of the immune system at the implantation site. Ann N Y Acad Sci. 2011;1221:80-7.
15. Winger E, Reed J, Ashoush S, El-Toukhy T, Ahuja S, Taranissi M. Elevated preconception CD56 + 16 + and/or Th1:Th2 levels predict benefit from IVIG therapy in subfertile women undergoing IVF. Am J Reprod Immunol. 2011;66:394-403.
16. Robertson M, Ritz J. Biology and clinical relevance of human natural killer cells. Blood. 1990;76:2421-38.
17. Kwak-Kim J, Gilman-Sachs A, Kim C. T helper 1 and 2 immune responses in relationship to pregnancy, nonpregnancy, recurrent spontaneous abortions and infertility of repeated implantation failure. Chem Immunol Allergy. 2005;88:64-79.
18. Seshadri S, Sunkara S. Natural killer cells in female infertility and recurrent miscarriage: a systematic review and meta-analysis. Hum Reprod Update. 2014;20:429-38.
19. Björkström N, Ljunggren H, Michaëlsson J. Emerging insights into natural killer cells in human peripheral tissues. Nat Rev Immunol. 2016;16:311-20.
20. Kim S, Poursine-Laurent J, Truscott S, Lybarger L, Song YJ, Yang L, et al. Licensing of natural killer cells by host major histocompatibility complex class I molecules. Nature. 2005;436:709-13.
21. Ramos-Medina R, García-Segovia A, Gil J, Carbone J, Aguarón de la Cruz A, Seyfferth A, et al. Experience in IVIG therapy for selected women with recurrent reproductive failure and NK cell expansion. Am J Reprod Immunol. 2014;71:458-66.
22. Moffett A, Shreeve N. First do no harm: uterine natural killer (NK) cells in assisted reproduction. Hum Reprod. 2015;30:1519-25.
23. Kalkunte S, Mselle T, Norris W, Wira C, Sentman C, Sharma S. Vascular endothelial growth factor C facilitates immune tolerance and endovascular activity of human uterine NK cells at the maternal-fetal interface. J Immunol. 2009;182:4085-92.
24. Moffett-King A. Natural killer cells and pregnancy. Nat Rev Immunol. 2002;2:656-63.
25. Faas M, de Vos P. Uterine NK cells and macrophages in pregnancy. Placenta. 2017;56:44-52.
26. Angelo L, Banerjee P, Monaco-Shawver L, Rosen JB, Makedonas G, Forbes LR, et al. Practical NK cell phenotyping and variability in healthy adults. Immunol Res. 2015;62:341-56.
27. Lee SK, Na BJ, Kim JY, Hur SE, Lee M, Gilman-Sachs A, et al. Determination of clinical cellular immune markers in women with recurrent pregnancy loss. Am J Reprod Immunol. 2013;70:398-411.
28. Sacks G. Enough! Stop the arguments and get on with the science of natural killer cell testing. Hum Reprod. 2015;30:1526-31.
29. Royal College of Obstetricians and Gynaecologists. (2016). The Role of Natural Killer Cells in Human Fertility (Scientific Impact Paper No. 53). [online] Available from https://www.rcog.org.uk/media/uhzggdwb/sip_53.pdf. [Last accessed May, 2024]

30. Hanevik HI, Friberg M, Bergh A, Haraldsen C, Kahn JA. Do acetyl salicylic acid and terbutaline in combination increase the probability of a clinical pregnancy in patients undergoing IVF/ICSI? J Obstet Gynaecol (Lahore). 2012;32:786-9.
31. Dirckx K, Cabri P, Merien A, Galajdova L, Gerris J, Dhont M, et al. Does low-dose aspirin improve pregnancy rate in IVF/ICSI? A randomized double-blind placebo controlled trial. Hum Reprod. 2009;24:856-60.
32. Panagodage S, Yong HE, Da Silva Costa F, Borg AJ, Kalionis B, Brennecke SP, et al. Low-Dose Acetylsalicylic Acid Treatment Modulates the Production of Cytokines and Improves Trophoblast Function in an in Vitro Model of Early-Onset Preeclampsia. Am J Pathol. 2016;186(12):3217-24.
33. Gelbaya TA, Kyrgiou M, Li TC, Stern C, Nardo LG. Low-dose aspirin for in vitro fertilization: a systematic review and meta-analysis. Hum Reprod Update. 2007;13:357-64.
34. Khairy M, Banerjee K, El-Toukhy T, Coomarasamy A, Khalaf Y. Aspirin in women undergoing in vitro fertilization treatment: a systematic review and meta-analysis. Fertil Steril. 2007;88:822-31.
35. Dentali F, Ageno W, Rezoagli E, Rancan E, Squizzato A, Middeldorp S, et al. Low-dose aspirin for in vitro fertilization or intracytoplasmic sperm injection: a systematic review and a meta-analysis of the literature. J Thromb Haemost. 2012;10:2075-85.
36. Siristatidis CS, Basios G, Pergialiotis V, Vogiatzi P. Aspirin for in vitro fertilisation. Cochrane Database Syst Rev. 2016;11(11):CD004832.
37. Nelson SM, Greer IA. The potential role of heparin in assisted conception. Hum Reprod Update. 2008;14:623-45.
38. Berker B, Taşkin S, Kahraman K, Taşkin EA, Atabekoglu C, Sönmezer M. The role of low-molecular-weight heparin in recurrent implantation failure: a prospective, quasi-randomized, controlled study. Fertil Steril. 2011;95:2499-502.
39. Potdar N, Gelbaya TA, Konje JC, Nardo LG. Adjunct low-molecular-weight heparin to improve live birth rate after recurrent implantation failure: a systematic review and meta-analysis. Hum Reprod Update. 201;19(6):674-84.
40. Qublan H, Amarin Z, Dabbas M, Farraj A-E, Beni-Merei Z, Al-Akash H, et al. Low-molecular-weight heparin in the treatment of recurrent IVF-ET failure and thrombophilia: a prospective randomized placebo-controlled trial. Hum Fertil (Camb). 2008;11:246-53.
41. Urman B, Ata B, Yakin K, Alatas C, Aksoy S, Mercan R, et al. Luteal phase empirical low molecular weight heparin administration in patients with failed ICSI embryo transfer cycles: a randomized open-labeled pilot trial. Hum Reprod. 2009;24:1640-7.
42. Noci I, Milanini MN, Ruggiero M, Papini F, Fuzzi B, Artini PG. Effect of dalteparin sodium administration on IVF outcome in non-thrombophilic young women: a pilot study. Reprod Biomed Online. 2011;22:615-20.
43. Franchimont D. Overview of the actions of glucocorticoids on the immune response: a good model to characterize new pathways of immunosuppression for new treatment strategies. Ann New York Acad Sci. 2004;1024:124-37.
44. Chen X, Oppenheim J, Winkler-Pickett R, Ortaldo J, Om H. Glucocorticoid amplifies IL-2- dependent expansion of functional FoxP3(+) CD4(+)CD25(+) T regulatory cells in vivo and enhances their capacity to suppress EAE. Eur J Immunol. 2006;36:2139-49.

45. Robertson S, Jin M, Yu D, Moldenhauer LM, Davies MJ, Hull ML, et al. Corticosteroid therapy in assisted reproduction—immune suppression is a faulty premise. Hum Reprod. 2016;10:2164-73.
46. Taniguchi F. Results of prednisolone given to improve the outcome of in vitro fertilization-embryo transfer in women with antinuclear antibodies. J Reprod Med. 2005;50:383-8.
47. Geva E, Amit A, Lerner-Geva L, Yaron Y, Daniel Y, Schwartz T, et al. Prednisone and aspirin improve pregnancy rate in patients with reproductive failure and autoimmune antibodies: a prospective study. Am J Reprod Immunol. 2000;43:36-40.
48. Fawzy M, Shokeir T, El-Tatongy M, Warda O, El-Refaiey A, Mosbah A. Treatment options and pregnancy outcome in women with idiopathic recurrent miscarriage: a randomized placebo-controlled study. Arc Gyn Obstetrics. 2008;278:33-8.
49. Boomsma CM, Keay SD, Macklon NS. Peri-implantation glucocorticoid administration for assisted reproductive technology cycles. Cochrane Database Syst Rev. 2012;(6):CD005996.
50. Park-Wyllie L, Mazzotta P, Pastuszak A, Moretti ME, Beique L, Hunnisett L, et al. Birth defects after maternal exposure to corticosteroids: prospective cohort study and meta-analysis of epidemiological studies. Teratology. 2000;62:385-92.
51. Heinz H, Loos M. Activation of the first component of complement, C1: comparison of the effect of sixteen different enzymes on serum C1. Immunobiology. 1983;165:175-85.
52. Winger E, Reed J, Ashoush S, Ahuja S, El-Toukhy T, Taranissi M. Treatment with adalimumab (Humira) and intravenous immunoglobulin improves pregnancy rates in women undergoing IVF. Am J Reprod Immunol. 2009;61:113-20.
53. Winger E, Reed J, Ashoush S, El-Toukhy T, Ahuja S, Taranissi M. Degree of TNFa/IL10 cytokine elevation correlates with IVF success rates in women undergoing treatment with Adalimumab (Humira) and IVIG. Am J Reprod Immunol. 2011;65:610-18.
54. Scheinfeld N. A comprehensive review and evaluation of the side effects of the tumor necrosis factor alpha blockers etanercept, infliximab and adalimumab. J Dermatolog Treat. 2004;15:280-94.
55. Li J, Chen Y, Liu C, Hu Y, Li L. Intravenous immunoglobulin treatment for repeated IVF/ICSI failure and unexplained infertility: a systematic review and a meta-analysis. Am J Reprod Immunol. 2013;70:434-47.
56. Stephenson MD, Fluker MR. Treatment of repeated unexplained in vitro fertilization failure with intravenous immunoglobulin: a randomized, placebo-controlled Canadian trial. Fertil Steril. 2000;74:1108-13.
57. De Placido G, Zullo F, Mollo A, Cappiello F, Nazzaro A, Colacurci N, et al. Intravenous immunoglobulin (IVIG) in the prevention of implantation failures. Ann N Y Acad Sci. 1994;734:232-4.
58. Stiehm ER. Adverse effects of human immunoglobulin therapy. Transfus Med Rev. 2013;27:171-8.
59. Christiansen O, Larsen E, Egerup P, Lunoee L, Egestad L, Nielsen H. Intravenous immunoglobulin treatment for secondary recurrent miscarriage: a randomized, double-blind, placebo-controlled trial. Br J Obs Gyn. 2015;122:500-8.
60. https://www.accessdata.fda.gov/drugsatfda_docs/label/2022/020248s026lbl.pdf

61. Coulam C, Acacio B. Does immunotherapy for treatment of reproductive failure enhance live births? Am J Reprod Immunol. 2012;67:296-304.
62. Roussev R, Ng S, Coulam C. Natural killer cell functional activity suppression by intravenous immunoglobulin, intralipid and soluble human leukocyte antigen-G. Am J Reprod Immunol. 2007;57:262-9.
63. Dakhly DM, Bayoumi YA, Sharkawy M, Gad Allah SH, Hassan MA, Gouda HM, et al. Intralipid supplementation in women with recurrent spontaneous abortion and elevated levels of natural killer cells. Int J Gynaecol Obstet. 2016;135:324-7.
64. Singh N, Davis AA, Kumar S, Kriplani A. The effect of administration of intravenous intralipid on pregnancy outcomes in women with implantation failure after IVF/ICSI with non-donor oocytes: A randomised controlled trial. Eur J Obstet Gynecol Reprod Biol. 2019;240:45-51.
65. Metcalf D. The granulocyte–macrophage colony stimulating factors. Cell. 1985;43:5-6.
66. Würfel W. Treatment with granulocyte colony-stimulating factor in patients with repetitive implantation failures and/or recurrent spontaneous abortions. J Reprod Immunol. 2015;108:123-35.
67. Zhang L, Xu WH, Fu XH, Huang QX, Guo XY, Zhang L, et al. Therapeutic role of granulocyte colony-stimulating factor (G-CSF) for infertile women under in vitro fertilization and embryo transfer (IVF-ET) treatment: a meta-analysis. Arch Gynecol Obstet. 2018;298(5):861-71.
68. Jain S, Mahey R, Malhotra N, Kalaivani M, Sangeeta P, Bhatt A, et al. Effect of Intrauterine Perfusion of Granulocyte Colony-stimulating Factor on Endometrial parameters and In Vitro Fertilization Outcome in Women Undergoing In Vitro Fertilization/Intracytoplasmic Sperm Injection Cycles: A Randomized Controlled Trial. J Hum Reprod Sci. 2018;11(3):254-60.
69. Thomson A, Bonham C, Zeevi A. Mode of action of tacrolimus (FK506): molecular and cellular mechanisms. Ther Drug Monit. 1995;17:584-91.
70. Nakagawa K, Kwak-Kim J, Ota K, Kuroda K, Hisano M, Sugiyama R, et al. Immunosuppression with tacrolimus improved reproductive outcome of women with repeated implantation failure and elevated peripheral blood Th1/Th2 cell ratios. Am J Reprod Immunol. 2015;73:353-61.
71. Nakagawa K, Kwak-Kim J, Kuroda K, Sugiyama R, Yamaguchi K. Immunosuppressive treatment using tacrolimus promotes pregnancy outcome in infertile women with repeated implantation failures. Am J Reprod Immunol. 2017;78.
72. Bahrami-Asl Z, Farzadi L, Fattahi A, Yousefi M, Quinonero A, Hakimi P, et al. Tacrolimus Improves the Implantation Rate in Patients with Elevated Th1/2 Helper Cell Ratio and Repeated Implantation Failure (RIF). Geburtshilfe Frauenheilkd. 2020;80(8):851-62.
73. Nevers W, Pupco A, Koren G, Bozzo P. Safety of tacrolimus in pregnancy. Can Fam Phys. 2014;60:905-6.
74. Ghasemnejad-Berenji H, Ghaffari Novin M, Hajshafiha M, Nazarian H, Hashemi SM, Ilkhanizadeh B, et al. Immunomodulatory effects of hydroxychloroquine on Th1/Th2 balance in women with repeated implantation failure. Biomed Pharmacother. 2018;107:1277-85.
75. Sciascia S, Hunt B, Talavera-Garcia E, Lliso G, Khamashta M, Cuadrado M. The impact of hydroxychloroquine treatment on pregnancy outcome in women with antiphospholipid antibodies. Am J Obstet Gynecol. 2016;214(2):273.e1-273.e8.

Fertility Toolbox

Mrinmayi Dharmadhikari, Ameet S Patki

■ INTRODUCTION

Infertility forms a major health concern affecting all parts of the world. The societal, emotional, community, as well as cultural pressures and distress associated with it make this an important health problem. However, with adequate counseling, appropriate guidance, and proper treatment, many of the infertile patients can receive optimal management. Education, counseling, and appropriate guidance of these couples form key aspects of managing infertility and this can be done at all levels of care.

■ THE FIGO FERTILITY TOOLBOX

The International Federation of Gynecology and Obstetrics (FIGO) fertility toolbox was designed initially for healthcare workers in order to guide them in the management of infertile couples. But now, this toolbox has found a place in guiding anybody who wants to make a difference in the lives of people with infertility. The beauty of this Toolbox lies in the fact that it is applicable in any situation and resource setting. The FIGO fertility toolbox is directed toward empowering people to take action in their setting.[1] The Toolbox is available as a hard copy, electronic version for computers as well as for cell phones **(Fig. 1)**.

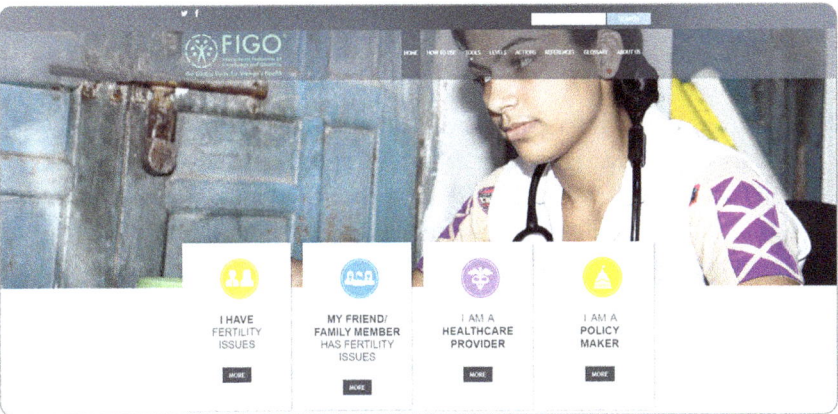

Fig. 1: FIGO fertility toolbox.

Major principles of the toolbox are:
- It focuses on low-resource settings.
- It is flexible and is applicable in almost any country of the world.
- It is aimed primarily at midlevel practitioners such as nurses and midwives to equip them at handling infertility issues better.
- It is usable not only by healthcare professionals but also stakeholders, policymakers, and patients.
- It is easily distributed and accessible by electronic and mobile applications.
- It is innovative and interesting.

What does the toolbox consist of?

This wonderfully designed toolbox consists of seven tools which will help in tackling the disease/disability of infertility. Each of these tools provides information on how to manage a particular aspect of infertility and hence it has widespread application.
- *Tool 1:* The FIGO Fertility Daisy—why we should care about infertility
- *Tool 2:* Overcome personal barriers
- *Tool 3:* Overcome societal barriers
- *Tool 4:* Diagnose infertility
- *Tool 5:* Treat infertility
- *Tool 6:* Refer/resolve infertility
- *Tool 7:* Prevent infertility

In order to understand the working of these tools, we must know the levels of the tools. There are three tiers or levels under which this toolbox is divided. These form the basic framework of the toolbox and also simplify approach and its use by all. These are:
- *The Basic Tools™:* These contain information which is brief and concise. This could be just a simple and brief summarization of the Pyramids of Action. This tool helps in spreading general awareness among healthcare providers, patients, and anyone using this tool as to what aspects and issues need to be addressed in order to help infertile couples. The basic tools are colored orange **(Fig. 2)**.
- *The Support Tools™:* These provide more detailed information so that one knows what to do in order to take action. This includes more intrinsic details on clinical care, diagnosis, referral/resolution, treatment, and support. These may be particularly useful for nurses, midwives, and well-educated healthcare providers who are better equipped with basic knowledge and resources to carry out slightly more complex actions described in the support tools. The support tools are colored green.
- *The Reference Tools™:* These are lists of references providing evidence for the information and recommended actions mentioned in the basic and support tools. Evidence from important references, meta-analyses, highly regarded journals, professional organizations, and national or

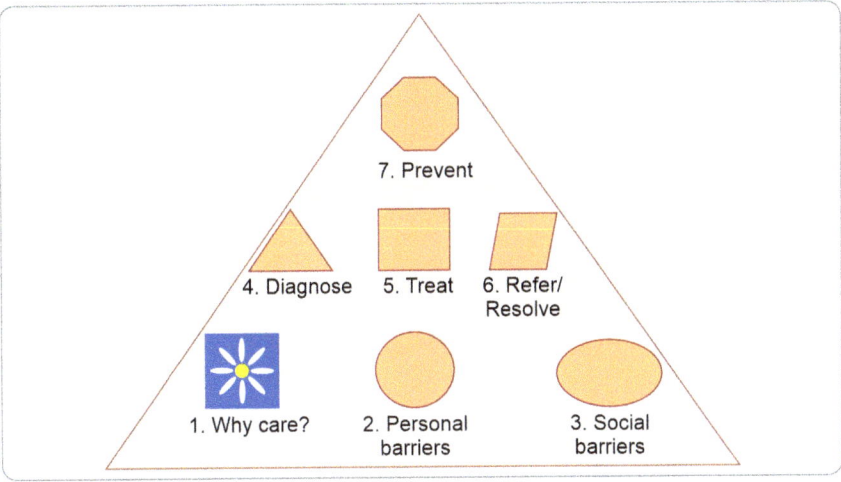

Fig. 2: The tools pyramid.

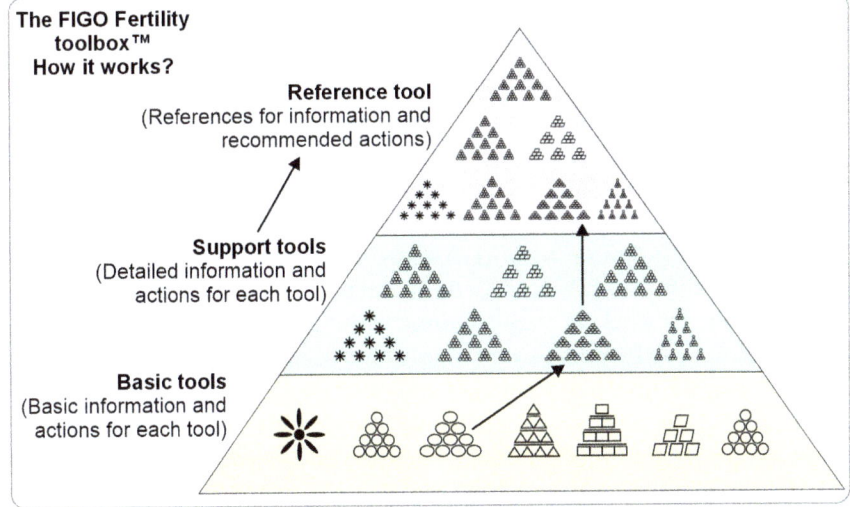

Fig. 3: The Levels Pyramid.

international organizations such as World Health Organization (WHO), American Society for Reproductive Medicine (ASRM), European Society of Human Reproduction and Embryology (ESHRE), International Federation of Fertility Societies (IFFS), and others are used. The reference tools are at the top of the pyramid and colored white.

This color coding keeps one aware of the tool they are working with. You can choose the level you want to work in by simply clicking on it in The Levels Pyramid **(Fig. 3)**.

In order to help healthcare providers as well as those using this toolbox know what action to take, there is The Actions Pyramid **(Fig. 4)**.

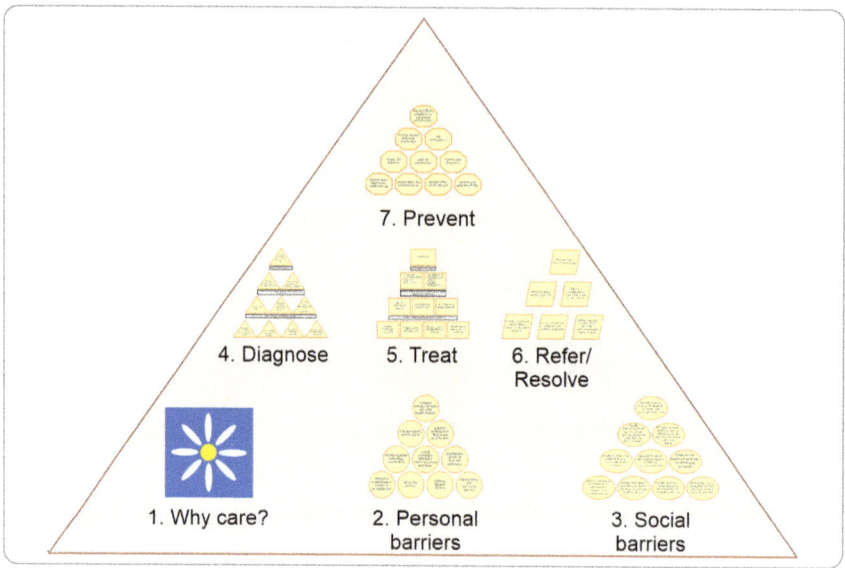

Fig. 4: The Actions Pyramid.

All tools have the shape of a pyramid except Tool 1 that is, The Daisy. The simpler actions which can be undertaken even in low-resource settings are present at the base of the pyramid. These are simple, elementary actions involving fewer people and are often low-cost interventions befitting a low-resource setting. As you move higher up in the pyramid, the actions are more complex requiring more resources. However, this helps the providers to choose whatever action is most befitting their situation including resources and competency. Clicking on the Actions arrow at the top of the page will take you to The Actions Pyramid. Here you can choose the Action you want to work in by clicking the Tool and then the Action in that particular Tool you wish to perform. This can help you in starting with something basic which you think works best for you in your particular situation and slowly you can work your way up the pyramid and build on what you have already achieved. Doing something, no matter how small a huge step in is helping these patients get optimum services and guidance for their problem.

FIGO Fertility Tool 1

Why should you care about infertility?

Basic tool 1: The Daisy—Why should I care? **(Fig. 5)**

- *Quality of life:* Infertility affects the quality of life and can lead to negative psychosocial results including depression and fear. The societal stigma associated with it can cause guilt and regret. This is especially true in the developing countries.
- *Burden of disease:* A review using data from published population surveys on infertility reported that an estimated 9% of women of reproductive age

CHAPTER 31: Fertility Toolbox

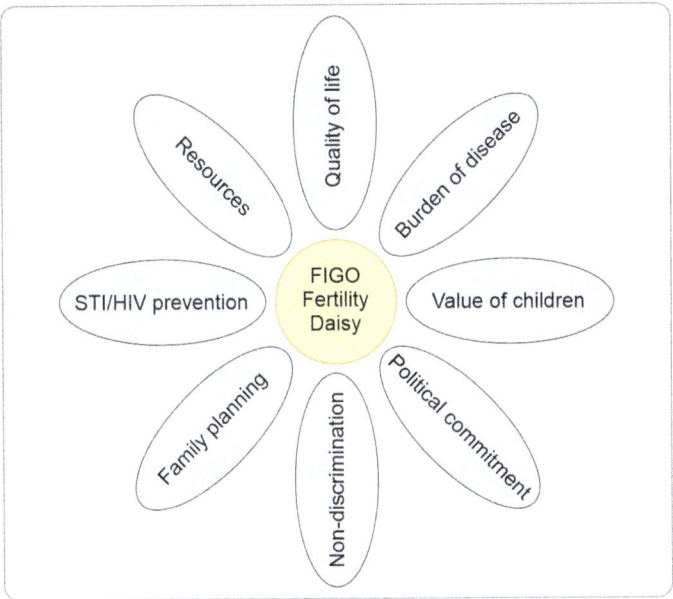

Fig. 5: Basic tool 1—The Daisy. (HIV: human immunodeficiency virus; STI: sexually transmitted infection)

suffered from infertility globally. This amounted to around 72.4 million women worldwide.[2] This will only continue to rise unless couples are educated regarding causes and prevention of infertility.

- *Value of children:* Children have varied importance in different parts of the world. In certain societies, there is so much value attached to children that couples especially women without children are stigmatized. Healthcare providers and policy makers should make an effort to understand their patients better in order to provide better support.
- *Political commitment:* Nations around the world have committed to the Millennium Development Goals (MDGs). The MDGs have been described as a tool that facilitates action, generates discussion, and holds leaders accountable in order to successfully fulfill outlined goals.[3]
- *Nondiscrimination:* There should be no discrimination between rich and poor as both are equally deserving of children.
- *Family planning:* The integration of infertility management into family planning/reproductive health/women's health services helps in efficiently utilizing limited resources and mutually facilitating each service.
- *Sexually transmitted infection (STI)/HIV prevention:* Infertility is a risk factor for STI/HIV acquisition. Both these can be tackled together.
- *Affordability:* This is a major hurdle when it comes to low-resource settings. However, simple yet effective interventions are available in many health settings. The main aim should be to make these accessible to patients who need them the most.

- *Protection of resources:* Inappropriate infertility management chelates precious resources of health systems and households. An optimum use of these resources is important.

Support Tool 1: Provides a more detailed knowledge of the above aspects of The Daisy giving a clearer picture on the burden of disease and importance of infertility treatment and its easy and affordable access even in developing countries for a better mental, physical, and societal health of the people suffering from the same.

Reference Tool 1: Provides references from renowned journals, professional organizations, meta-analyses, and so on for those who want a more thorough knowledge in this aspect.

FIGO Fertility Tool 2

How to overcome personal/patient barriers to fertility care?
Basic tool 2 (Fig. 6):
- *Recognize personal and patient barriers to accessing care:* Personal cultural, religious, and family values that prevent access or limit care need to be recognized and resolved.

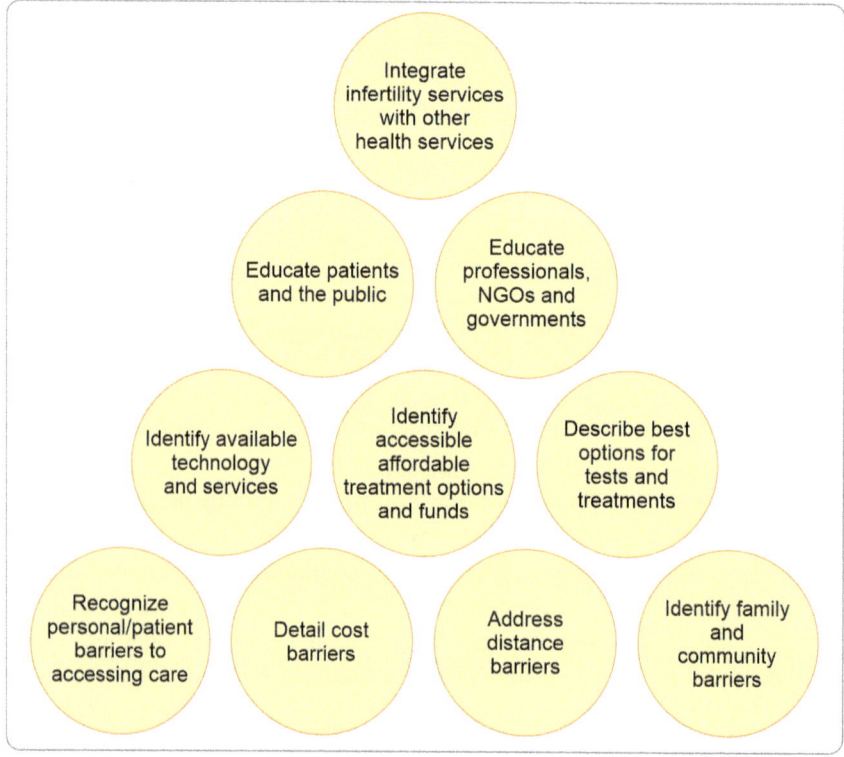

Fig. 6: Basic tool 2.

- *Detail cost barriers:* The cost of infertility is often not covered by available state health services. This can prevent couples from seeking advice or guidance for infertility.
- *Address distance barriers:* Geographical factors modify health-seeking behavior for instance where basic infrastructures in terms of roads and transport are suboptimal.
- *Identify family/community barriers:* Community and family pressures further upset the emotional balance of already stressed infertile couples. The stigmatization associated should be addressed. This can be done with counseling and emotional support.
- *Identify available technology and services:* Basic investigations and treatment for infertility may be available in less resource-rich settings.
- *Identify accessible, affordable treatment options and funds:* Some components of investigation and treatment may be available as part of the general reproductive health programs. Awareness of the cost treatment and possible sources of funds within the family or community can help couples make informed choices.
- *Describe best options for tests and treatment:* Equipping couples with knowledge about cost-effectiveness of tests and treatments can help in decision making.
- *Educate patients and the public:* Fertility awareness and appropriate time for seeking medical help can help overcome personal, cultural, and community hurdles.
- *Educate professionals, NGOs, and governments:* Support from these bodies will substantially improve access to fertility services.
- *Integrate infertility services with other health services:* Use of existing portals of care offers a cost-effective option for fertility services.
- *Recognize personal and patient barriers to accessing care:* These need to be recognized and resolved by the care providers and patients.

*Support tool 2 (**Fig. 7**):* This tool explains how the individual, health care providers, and the infertile can approach personal barriers that prevent access to infertility care. Providing knowledge by education and support groups could be a way forward. Knowledge as to where to seek initial advice will allow couples to access effective medical treatment at the appropriate time and prevent the use of scarce resources on ineffective remedies.[4]

Reference tool 2: This contains a list of references for easy access to gain additional evidence-based information on the recommendations made.

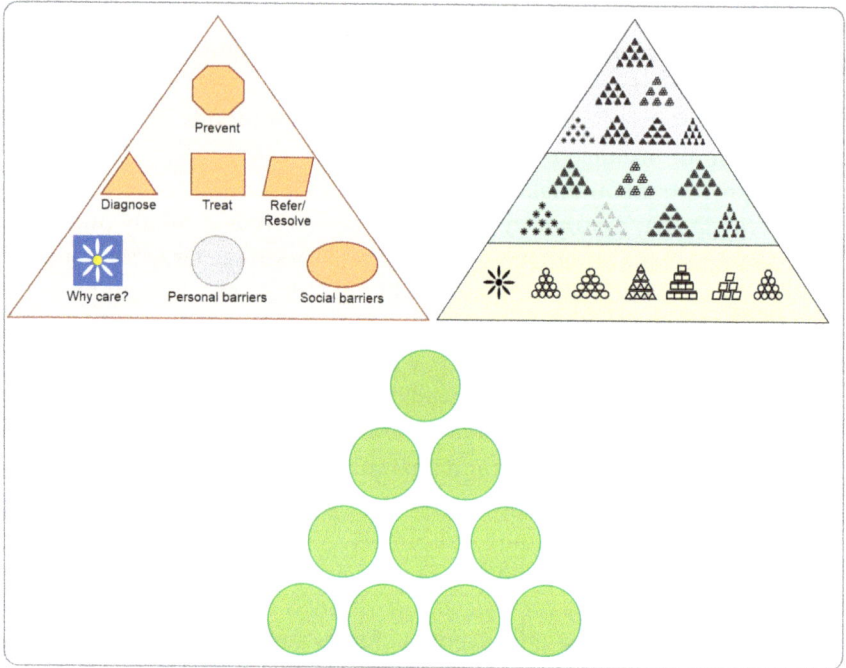

Fig. 7: The support tool 2.

FIGO Fertility Tool 3

How to overcome societal barriers to fertility care?
Basic tool 3 (Fig. 8):

- *Identify and reduce socioeconomic, demographic, religious, and cultural barriers:* In many countries, infertility treatment may be unaffordable and inaccessible. Addressing these barriers and reducing their impact is warranted.
- *Identify and manage competition of infertility with other sexual and reproductive health conditions:* By sharing resources efficiently and by educating the couple.
- *Identify and improve inadequate health care networks and untrained personnel:* Strengthening communication between primary health clinics and referral hospitals is one way of achieving this.
- *Identify and improve inadequate infertility risk factor education and insufficient male partner involvement:* Sex education in schools can reduce STIs and unwanted pregnancies. Involving male partners in infertility treatment can improve the outcomes of fertility treatment.
- *Identify primary care providers (PCPs) and primary healthcare clinics (PHC)* to develop community educational programs for education in reproductive health and prevention and treatment of infertility.

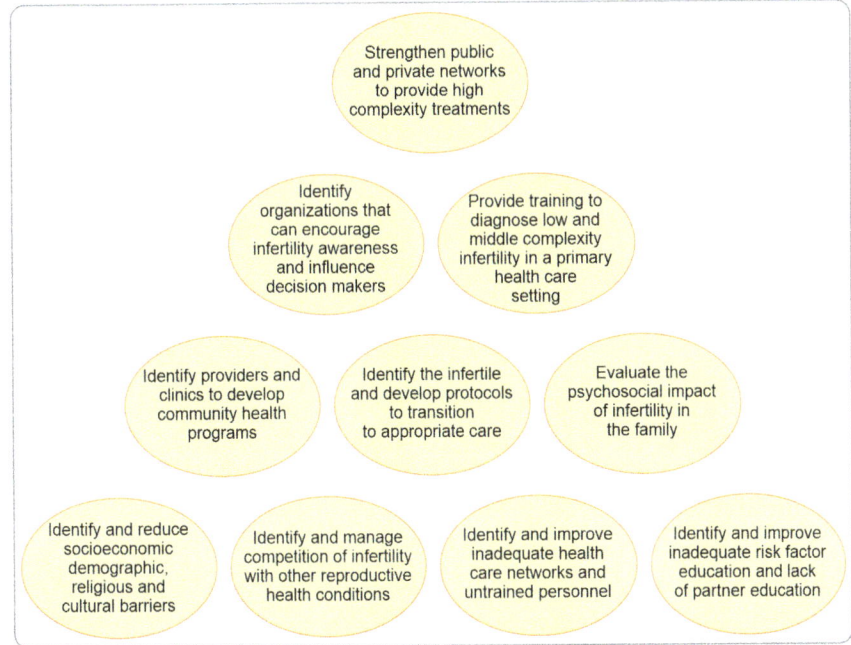

Fig. 8: Basic tool 3.

- *Identify infertile couples and develop protocols to transition to appropriate care in the health network, especially between PHC and upper level of care:* Educate infertile couples on the effect of age, duration of infertility, gynecologic infection, unsafe termination of pregnancies, and other risk factors.
- *Evaluate the psychosocial impact of infertility in the family:* Such patients should be advised and counseled in order to improve their mental status.
- *Identify organizations that can encourage infertility awareness and influence decision makers:* Sensitization of law makers and leaders to infertility issues in order to improve infertility care.
- *Provide training* to diagnose and treat less complicated infertility issues at the PHC setting.
- *Strengthen public and private networks to provide high complexity treatments:* This will reduce the cost of infertility treatment enabling more people to access it.

Support tool 3 *(Fig. 9)*: This tool explains how the individual, health care providers, and the infertile can approach societal barriers that prevent access to infertility diagnosis and treatment in more detail with more complex actions as you go higher up the pyramid.

Reference tool 3: It provides a list of references supporting these recommendations.

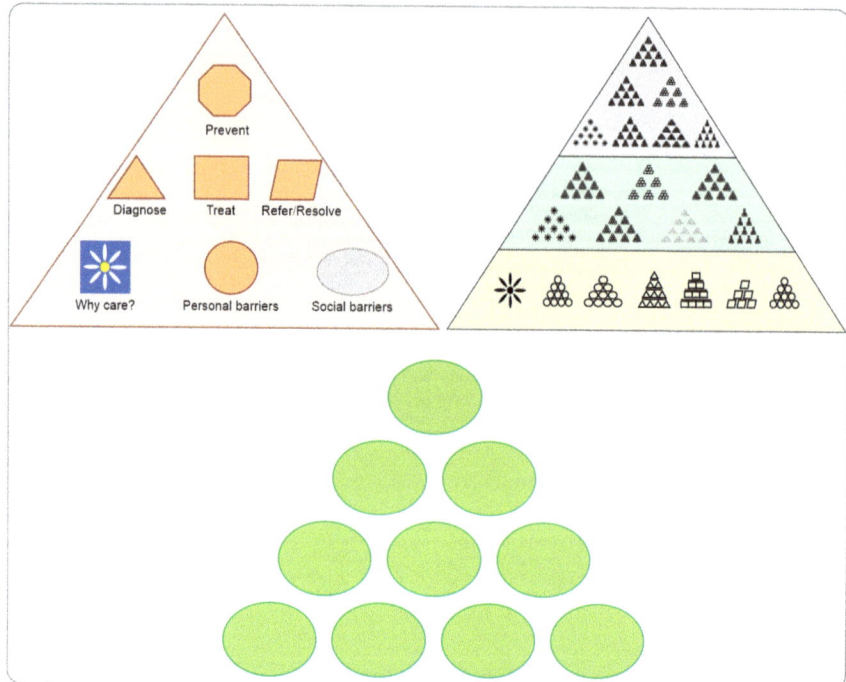

Fig. 9: Support tool 3.

FIGO Fertility Tool 4

How to diagnose infertility?
*Basic tool 4 (**Fig. 10**):*

Level 1 or primary care level services: Advice and counsel—
- *Educate the PCP on history taking:* Teach the PCP to take a simple and appropriate infertility history covering all important aspects.
- *Train the PCP to do a physical examination:* Where possible, teach the PCP to inspect the vagina and cervix and to do a bimanual examination.
- *Determine the patient's fitness for pregnancy:* This should focus on presence of comorbidities.
- *Counsel and manage the patient:* This includes optimizing natural fertility, advising on lifestyle and health, and referring the patient(s) to a higher level of care where appropriate.

Level 2 or intermediate care level services: Perform appropriate and simple tests—
- *Educate and train:* This includes basic education and training in infertility.
- Perform available female and male tests with the aim to exclude tubal pathology and severe male infertility.
- *Counsel and manage the patient:* This includes addressing test results along with counseling of patients as to appropriate treatment.

CHAPTER 31: Fertility Toolbox

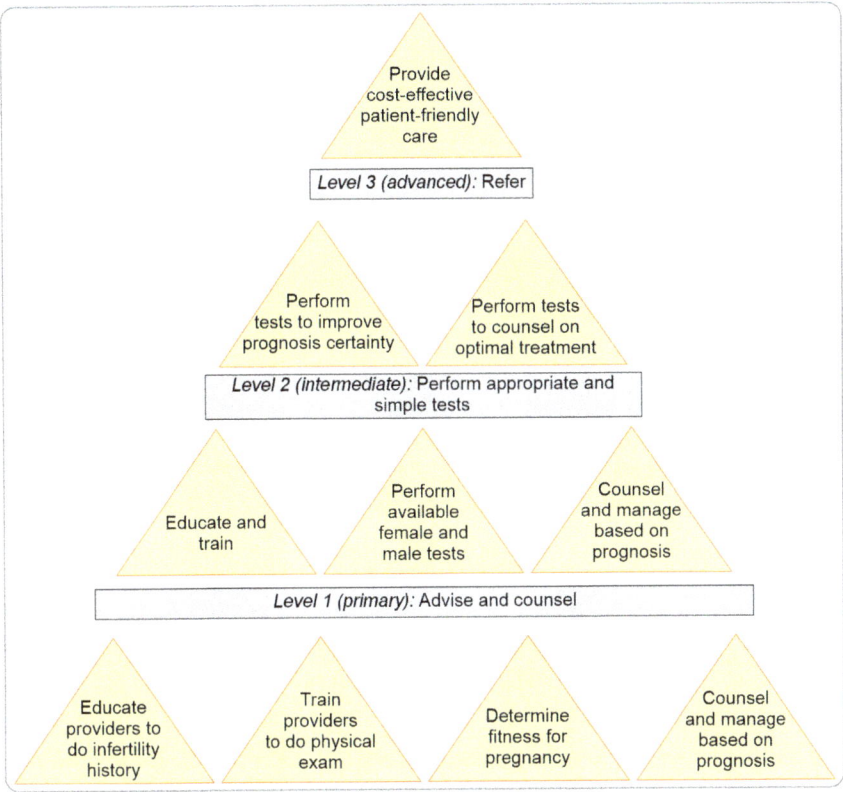

Fig. 10: Basic tool 4.

Level 3 or advanced care level services: Refer—
- *Perform additional tests to improve prognosis:* Appropriate additional tests can be done to confirm diagnosis made at a lower level.
- *Perform female and male tests to decide and counsel on optimal treatment:* Effective and cost-appropriate tests that can improve the diagnosis as well as prognosis should be performed.

Level 4 aspirational goal of diagnostic tests: The ultimate aim is to provide cost-effective and patient-friendly care.

Support tool 4 **(Fig. 11):** This tool further builds up on its basic counterpart and is useful for those working in high-resource settings where more advanced tests are available and can be employed for confirming the cause of infertility. This includes a more detailed and specific history and examination by healthcare providers. Advanced tests such as hysterosalpingography, ultrasonography, semen analysis, sperm function tests, hormonal tests, and hysterolaparoscopy can be performed at this level for a more targeted diagnosis. Once the cause is determined, a better patient counseling and a more sound plan of action for the couple can be charted. This tool moves from the diagnostic to the prognostic approach.

SECTION 12: Mixed Bag

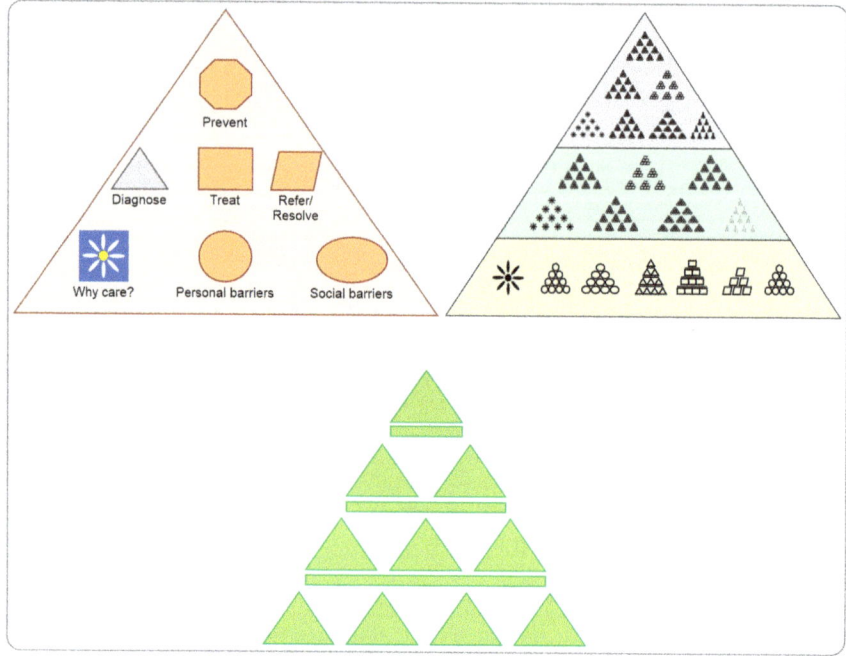

Fig. 11: Support tool 4.

Reference tool 4: This is a list of valuable references supporting the rationale behind the tests and treatments advised and used in the corresponding tool.

FIGO Fertility Tool 5

How to treat infertility?
Basic tool 5 (Fig. 12):

Level 1 or primary care services: Advice and counsel—
The lowest level health care setting includes a primary health center (PHC) with PCP or health provider (HP).

- *Identify treatment resources:* Treatment choices are limited at this level but with appropriate guidance and use of available resources by healthcare providers, infertile couples may be benefited even at this level.
- *Outline causes and outcomes:* Based on the history, physical examination, and diagnostic tests, the cause of infertility should be determined. Available treatment resources should be explained to the patient and used resourcefully in appropriately selected patients.
- *Provide options and get informed consent:* Available treatment options along with their cost, benefit, and risks should be enlisted and explained to the patients and an informed consent obtained after choosing the best option.

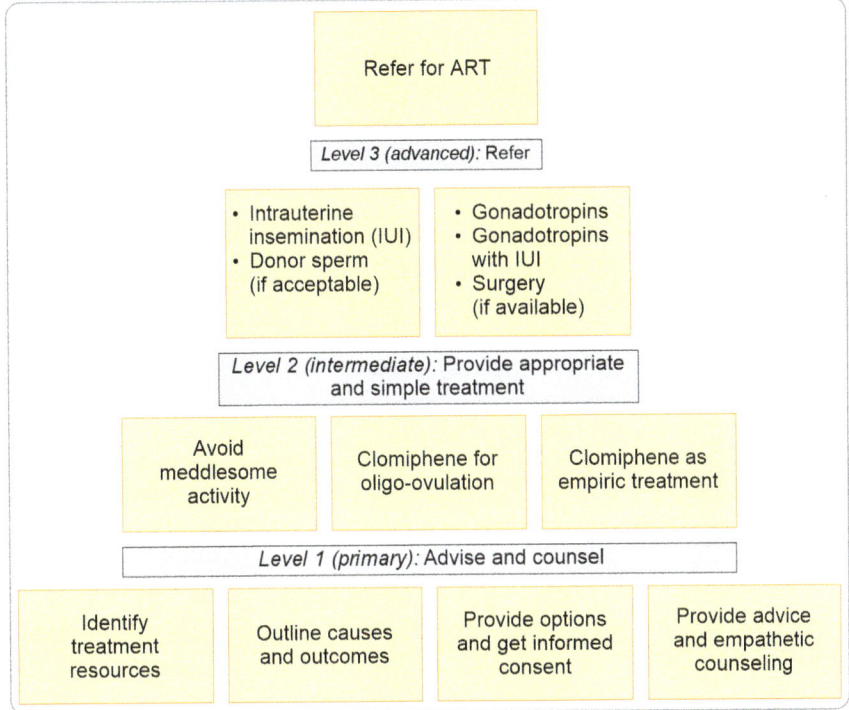

Fig. 12: Basic tool 5.

- *Provide advice and empathetic counseling:* This should continue throughout the course of treatment.

Level 2 or intermediate care level services: Provide appropriate and simple treatment—
- *Avoid meddlesome activity:* These include strict timing of intercourse, use of calendars and basal temperature for monitoring cycles and coitus, extreme diets, unnecessary medications, exercise, or other activities that have not been shown to increase pregnancy rates. These add to the stress and cost of treatment.
- *Clomiphene citrate for oligo-anovulation:* Clomiphene citrate is an effective treatment for oligo- and anovulation. It should be used only in properly selected patients and for the recommended duration.
- *Clomiphene citrate as empiric treatment:* This should be used in properly selected patients and for the recommended amount of time.

Level 3 or advanced care level services: These include tertiary hospitals with more advanced facilities similar to that found in referral hospitals in developed countries.
- (a) *Intrauterine insemination (IUI):* IUI can be used for both male and female infertility as well as erectile dysfunction.

(b) *Donor sperm:* Donor sperm can be used when appropriate with informed couple consents.
- (a) *Gonadotropin stimulation:* This can be used for oligo-anovulation after clomiphene treatment failure.

  (b) *Gonadotropin stimulation with IUI:* This can be used for oligo-anovulation after clomiphene treatment failure and limited empiric follicle-stimulating hormone (FSH)/IUI treatment where IVF is not available.

  (c) *Infertility surgery:* Laparoscopic tubal surgery, myomectomy, adhesiolysis, and endometriosis where indicated. Hysteroscopy may be done for polyps, submucosal myomas, intrauterine adhesions, cornual obstruction, and uterine abnormalities such as septum.

Refer for ART services: The ART services, if accessible, should be used as indicated. Intracytoplasmic sperm injection (ICSI) and preimplantation genetic diagnosis should be used in appropriate patients, where available. The use of donor sperm, donor oocytes, donor embryos, and surrogates/gestational carriers should be used when indicated and available in an ethical manner with appropriate patient consent in accordance with the prevailing laws.

Support tool 5 **(Fig. 13):** This tool comprises advanced level of care and services depending on the available resources, facilities for monitoring the treatment and management of complications in addition to the ones mentioned in the basic tool 5. It involves more widespread knowledge by the caregivers as well as advanced level of care and treatment choices like gonadotrophin stimulation with IUI, donor sperm, and fertility-enhancing surgeries.

Timely referral for patients requiring ART is important to optimize outcome in such couples.

Reference tool 5: This includes important references, meta-analyses, review articles, and other evidence for all the recommendations made in this tool for a better understanding of the topic by healthcare providers.

FIGO Fertility Tool 6

How to refer and/or resolve infertility?
Basic tool 6 **(Fig. 14):**
- *Providers self-learn about referral resources, including adoption:* To facilitate referral, healthcare providers should educate themselves of the available resources and various aspects of the healthcare system.
- *Follow-up treatment outcomes and reassess prognosis:* Follow-up intervals should be fixed for individual patients in order to reassess prognosis.

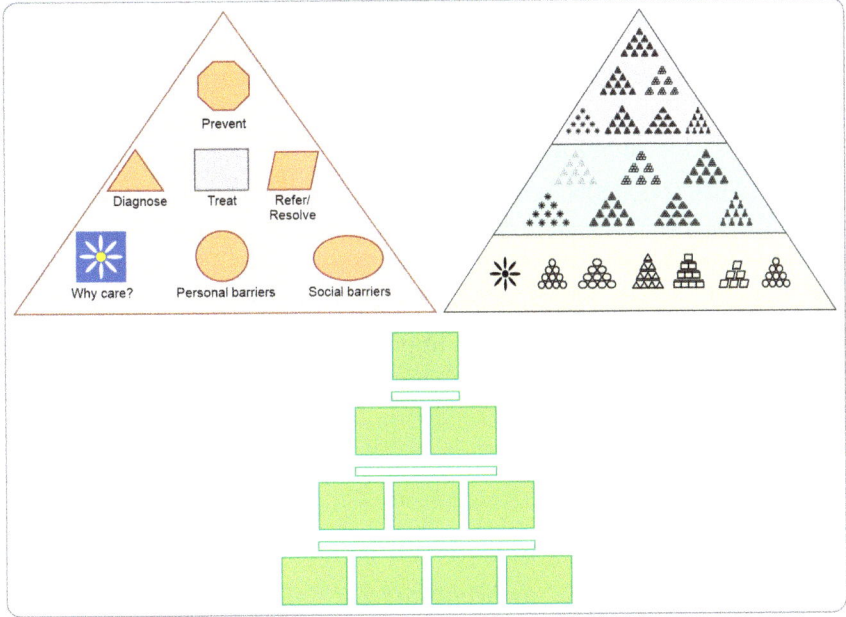

Fig. 13: Support tool 5.

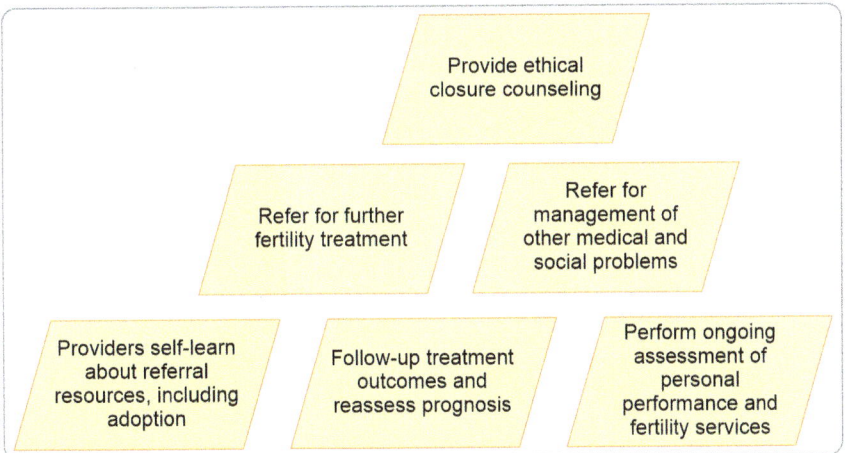

Fig. 14: Basic tool 6.

- *Perform ongoing assessment of self and fertility services:* This is important in order to improve care and should include self-assessment, assessment of quality of care given, and continuous education.
- *Refer for further fertility treatment:* Refer for furthermore specialized fertility treatment in the nearest and most accessible facility for the patient.
- *Refer for management of other medical and social problems.*

- *Provide ethical closure counseling:* It is important to understand the limitations and ethical considerations of infertility treatment. Healthcare providers should recognize when closure is needed and should educate themselves regarding adoption services and offer these to patients when appropriate.

Support tool 6 (Fig. 15): It provides more information with respect to referral services at high-resource settings which are equipped with trained healthcare providers who cannot only provide adequate referral services but also help to resolve fertility issues when the treatment is too complex.

Reference tool 6: This tool provides important references from professional bodies like the World Health Organization for more detailed information with regards to this tool.

FIGO Fertility Tool 7

How to prevent infertility?
Basic tool 7 (Fig. 16):
- *Educate about reproductive health and age*
- *Educate about sex and birth control:* This includes sexual physiology, sex practices, how pregnancy occurs, and methods of birth control.
- *Educate about healthy lifestyle:* Lifestyle factors such as smoking and obesity can substantially reduce fertility. Educational approach should promote healthy living.

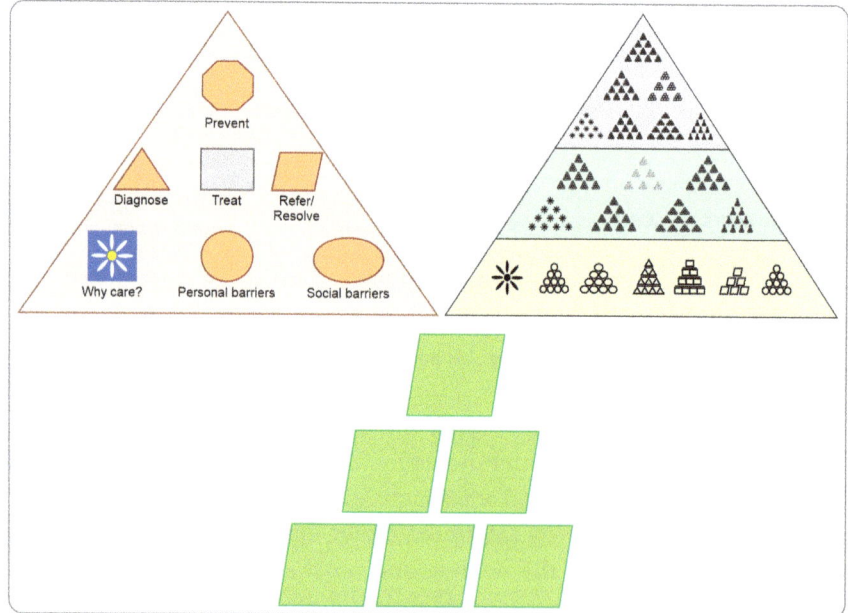

Fig. 15: Support tool 6.

CHAPTER 31: Fertility Toolbox

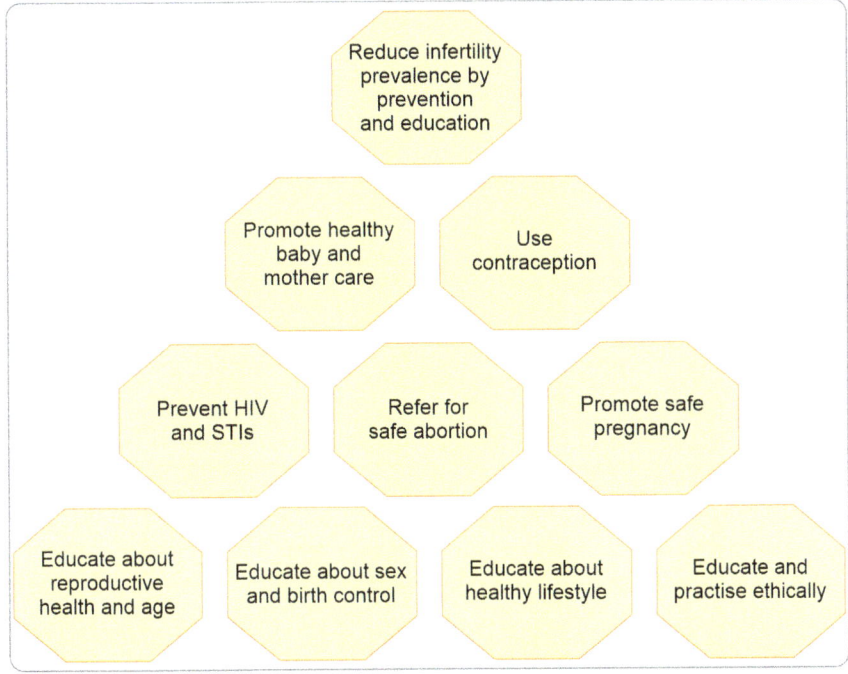

Fig. 16: Basic tool 7. (STI: sexually transmitted infection)

- *Educate and practice ethically:* This is important especially in infertility and all ethical societal and patient aspects need to be considered.
- *Prevent HIV and STIs:* These are preventable causes of infertility. HIV and STI education and prevention therefore forms an important aspect of preventing infertility.
- *Refer for safe abortion:* Unsafe abortion can cause future infertility. Providing education and facilities for safe abortions is important to prevent infertility.
- *Promote safe pregnancy:* Professionals and other providers collaborate with other professionals and organizations to facilitate safe pregnancy.
- *Promote healthy baby and mother care:* Coordination between different institutions for optimal mother and neonatal care is important.
- *Practice family planning:* Preventing unplanned pregnancies and associated risks protects future fertility. Education with respect to contraception, STIs, and safe abortion is of paramount importance and health facilities for these should be accessible to all.
- *Reduce infertility prevalence by prevention and education:* General education and health care prevention strategies can substantially reduce the burden of infertility.

432 SECTION 12: Mixed Bag

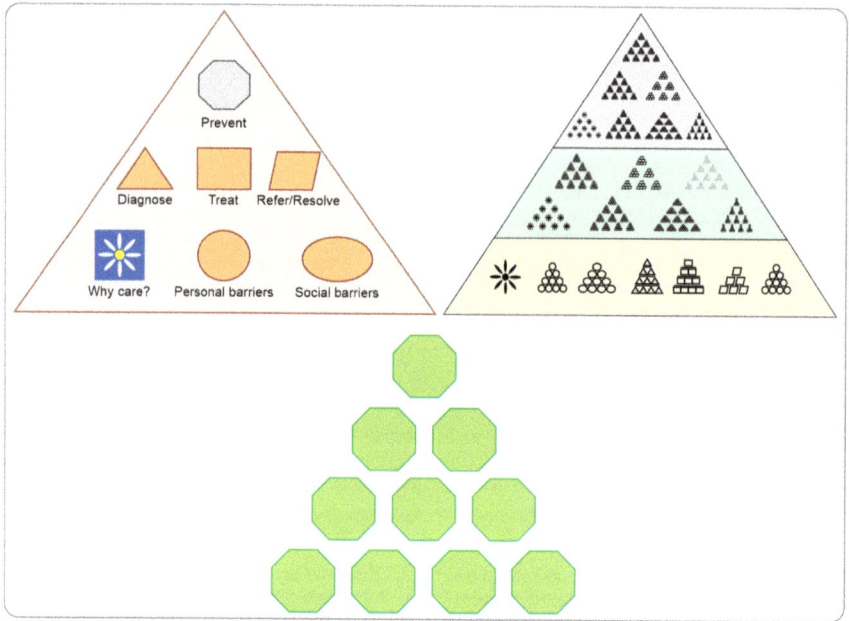

Fig. 17: Support tool 7.

Support tool 7 (Fig. 17): This tool contains detailed knowledge especially for high-resource settings for educating the society on issues concerning fertility, disease prevention, mother and childcare as well as safe delivery. All these have a bearing on fertility and education of the society on these issues will make them better equipped at handling and preventing infertility. Knowledge, after all, is the strongest weapon one can possess.

Reference tool 7: This enlists references on which this particular tool is based for a more thorough understanding of prevention of infertility and related issues.

■ CONCLUSION

In this manner, the fertility toolbox can help infertile couples to get access and guidance to optimum care. The social stigma attached to infertility in many parts of the globe still makes this a pressing issue and, therefore, this toolbox helps in simplifying care of infertile couples which can be provided by absolutely anyone who desires to help these patients. In addition to treatment, it also emphasizes on education not only of patients but also of healthcare providers, sensitization of leader and lawmakers to infertility issues, and also lays importance on the methods of preventing infertility and its knowledge in the society. This is closely related to family planning, safe abortions, safe mother and childcare, and prevention of STIs, and these services can be collaborated with infertility care in order to efficiently use limited resources. The FIGO fertility toolbox provides us a way to make a difference in the field of infertility at individual as well as community level in an efficient and fruitful manner.

■ KEY POINTS

- Infertility is a major health concern affecting couples globally.
- A standardized fertility management is the need of the hour as most couples need adequate counseling as well as support in addition to fertility treatment.
- The FIGO Fertility Toolbox is a ready to use tool which can help all healthcare providers to make a difference in the lives of people with infertility.
- It is applicable in any situation and resource setting.
- It is available as a hard copy as well as in the digital format providing widespread accessibility.
- This Fertility Toolbox has the potential to bring about widespread change in management of fertility.

■ REFERENCES

1. FIGO. The FIGO Fertility Toolbox. [online] Available from http://www.figo.org/news/resources/FIGO_Fertility_Tool_Box.
2. Boivin J, Bunting L, Collins JA, Nygren KG. International estimates of infertility prevalence and treatment-seeking: potential need and demand for infertility medical care. Hum Reprod. 2007;22(6):1506-12.
3. Clemens M, Kenny CJ, Moss TJ. The trouble with the MDGs: Confronting expectations of aid and development success. World Dev. 2007;35(5):735-51.
4. ESHRE Taskforce on Ethics and Law; Pennings G, de Wert G, Shenfield F, Cohen J, Tarlatzis B, et al. Providing infertility treatment in resource poor countries. Hum Reprod. 2009;24(5):1008-11.

Index

Page numbers followed by *b* refer to box, *f* refer to figure, *fc* refer to flowchart, and *t* refer to table.

A

Abdominal distention 234
Actions pyramid 418*f*
Adalimumab 404
Address distance barriers 421
Adenomyomatous polyp 70
Adenomyosis 72
Adenosine
　monophosphate 313*f*
　triphosphate 313*f*
Adhesion 202
Adipose tissue distribution 199
Adjuvant metformin therapy 358
Adjuvant therapy 281, 283, 302
Administration, route of 174
Adolescent polycystic ovarian
　syndrome 315
Adrenal dysfunction, uncontrolled 92
Adrenal zona reticularis 199
Advanced breast cancer,
　treatment of 100
Advanced chemoradiotherapy,
　emergence of 294
Agonist 219, 264*t*, 304
Albumin 357
　infusion 359
Alkylation 147
Allergic reactions, severe 404
Alopecia 103
Alpha-lipoic acid 312, 321
Amino acid 115
　replacement 134
　substitution 147
Aminoglutethimide 100, 102
Anaphylactic reactions 406
Anastrozole 100, 106, 232, 237
Androgens 194, 199
Anechoic myometrial cysts 73
Anemia 407

Angiogenesis 353
Anovulatory infertility 98
Anovulatory polycystic ovary
　syndrome 233
　women, treatment modalities for 311
Antagonist 219, 264*t*, 304
　cycles 113, 151
　protocol 277, 355
　use of 267
Anticoagulant therapy 362
Antiestrogens 237, 239
Anti-Müllerian hormone 3, 26, 27, 29,
　30, 32*f*, 34, 34*f*, 35*f*, 39, 174,
　187*f*, 212, 213*f*, 223*f*, 240, 245,
　246*f*, 259, 275, 276, 289, 302,
　354, 379 391, 394
　actions in ovary, model of 28*f*
　low levels of 29
Antioxidant 194, 197, 198, 221
　intrinsic 321
　pretreatment, effects of 199
　use of 198
Antral follicle 56*f*, 212
　cohort of 370
　count 28, 30, 33*f*, 34, 35*f*, 40, 53, 55,
　119, 174, 187*f*, 212, 223*f*, 245,
　259, 276, 289, 302
　secondary 54*f*
Aplastic anemia 288
Apoptosis 305
Arginine 198
Aromatase enzyme 8
Aromatase inhibitor 100, 102, 104, 105,
　108, 109, 239, 242, 280, 359, 372
　classification of 102, 102*t*
　in ovulation pathway, mechanism of
　action of 101*f*
　role of 100
　selective 330
　use of 106

Arthralgia 103
Artificial cycle 107
Artificial intelligence 350
Artificial reproductive technology 279
Ascites 357
Aseptic meningitis 406
Asherman's syndrome 72
Aspiration needle 345
Aspirin 183, 282, 401
   low dose 401
Assisted fertility journey 26
Assisted reproduction
   effects of aspirin in 401
   technologies 261
   treatment, immunotherapy in 398
Assisted reproductive cycles 149
Assisted reproductive technique 130
   efficacy of 173
   impact of obesity on 216t
   services 428
Assisted reproductive technology 3, 38, 52, 113, 194, 211f, 212, 216, 218, 231, 247, 257, 276, 288, 301, 316, 390
   cycles 339
      luteal phase in 19
   final step of 147
Atypia 70
Autoantibody induction 404
Autoimmune disease 275, 288

B

Basal body temperature 95f
Basal luteinizing hormone 223
Baseline score calculation 55t
Basic tools 416, 419f, 427f, 429f, 431f
Benzopyrans 88, 90
Benzothiophenes 88
Beta follitropin 117
Biochemical pregnancy 76, 152
Birth
   defects 93
   premature 403
Bladder pseudoaneurysm
        hemorrhage 346
Blastocyst
   formation 383
   implantation 329

Blastulation 269
Bleeding 346
   internal 349
Blood
   flow, peripheral 51f
   pressure, high 403
   vessels start 57
Blurred vision 93
Body mass index 43, 55, 108, 119, 130, 213f, 214, 215
   high 108
Bologna criteria 31
Brain's arcuate nucleus 141
Breast 88
   cancer, fertility preservation in 103
   discomfort 234
Breastfeeding 92
Buserelin 147, 161, 174

C

Cabergoline 357, 358
Camoxiphen 376
Cancel cycle 241
Cancer 293
   diagnosis of 288
   patients 385
   therapy regimens, different 293t
Carbohydrate moieties 113
Cell
   growth 319
   malignant 103
   permeability 353
   proliferation 305
Cellular migration 305
Central nervous system 17
Cerebrovascular insufficiency 103
Cervical stenosis 203, 204
Cervix 235
Chemotherapy 215, 275
Chills 406
Chinese hamster ovary cell 117, 251
Cholestasis 407
Chromosomal abnormalities 301
Citric acid 393
Cleaved embryos 383
Clinical pregnancy 151
   rate 103, 106, 197, 303, 315
Clomid babies 87

Clomiphene 87, 90, 91, 94, 95, 231, 240, 270, 304
  contraindications of 93*t*
  indications of 93*t*
  resistant patients 100
  treatment
    extended course 95
    patient selection criteria for 92
Clomiphene citrate 76, 87, 89, 92, 94, 96*f*, 104, 105, 231, 232, 242, 251, 315, 317, 318, 330, 333, 372, 376, 382, 392, 394, 427
  challenge test 26, 28, 30, 39
  dosage schedule of 95*f*
  pharmacokinetics of 90
  side effects of 234
  use of 113
Cochrane 109
Coenzyme Q10 303, 306
Co-existing health issues 224
Cohort of follicles, stimulation of 178
Colloid infusion 357
Colony-stimulating factors, family of 407
Color Doppler
  assessment 50
  perifollicular vascularity on 59*f*
Combination protocols 240
Combined oral contraceptives 260
Common endometrial pathologies, ultrasound diagnosis of 70
Community barriers 421
Complete blood count 361
Conception
  cycles 18, 75
  rates 94
Congestive heart failure 404
Consecutive cycles 294
Controlled ovarian hyperstimulation 49, 52, 67, 186, 196, 212, 231, 267, 303, 369, 392
  cycles 329
Controlled ovarian stimulation 3, 7, 11, 32*f*, 109, 121, 127, 180*f*, 245, 257, 267, 289, 290, 303, 304, 354, 369, 379, 384*f*
Conventional stimulation protocols 374
Corpus luteal cells 329

Corpus luteum 51*f*, 53, 63*f*, 64, 128, 135, 265, 340, 371
  formation of 15
  inadequacy 63*f*
  rescue 18
  role of 15
Cough 103
Cryopreservation 359
Cryopreserved embryo 383
  transfers 376
Cushing's syndrome 403
Cut-back protocol, selective 261
Cycle cancellation 216
Cyclic adenosine monophosphate 114, 148, 161
Cytokines 399
Cytoplasmic maturity 132
Cytoplasmic oocyte maturation 130

D

Dais 419*f*
Decapeptyl 174
Dehydroepiandrostenedione 199
Dehydroepiandrosterone 9*f*, 281, 302, 306
  estradiol conversion from 221*f*
  sulfate 199, 221
Demyelinating disease 404
Deoxyribonucleic acid 117
Depression 103
Dermatologic disorders 406
Deslorelin 147
Detail cost barriers 421
Diabetes 403
Diarrhea 103, 314
Disease, burden of 418
Dizziness 103, 407
Donor sperm 428
Dopamine 357
Double stimulation during follicular and luteal phases, protocol of 382*f*
Double vision 93
Drowsiness 103
Drug, type of 220, 224
Dual stimulation, pathophysiology of 380
DuoStim
  advantages of 384

Index

disadvantages of 384
protocol 383*f*
SWOT analysis of 384, 384*f*
Dydrogesterone 269
Dyspnea 103

E

Ectopic pregnancy, risk of 234
Edema 103
Eggs 288
  mature 294
Embolism 103
Embryo 161, 340
  aneuploidy
    rates of 375
    risk of 276
  cryopreservation of 357
  development 198, 268, 393
  good-quality 219, 383, 398
  implantation 235
    rates 257
  number of 262
  quality 150, 216, 304
    predicting 41
  selection of 393
  transfer 147, 132, 161, 203, 289
    before 404
    difficult 204
Embryo-endometrial crosstalk 128
Embryo-endometrium synchrony 376
Empty follicle syndrome 130, 135, 159
Enclomiphene 90, 98, 232
Endogenous 178
  estrogen 91
  gonadotropins 56
  levels, low 182
  luteinizing hormone 148, 173
    surge 160
Endometrial and embryonic
      development 339
Endometrial cancer 92
Endometrial cavity 68
Endometrial columnar epithelium 76
Endometrial gene 195
  expression 181
Endometrial growth 76, 312
Endometrial hyperplasia 310
Endometrial lips 68

Endometrial maturation 18, 75
Endometrial morphology,
      evaluation of 67
Endometrial peristalsis 75
Endometrial polyp 70
  removal of 202
  ultrasound of 70
Endometrial preparation 11
  protocols for 340
Endometrial ring sign 75
Endometrial thickness,
      measurement of 69*f*
Endometrial-myometrial interface 76
Endometrioma 214
Endometriosis 43, 92, 108, 213, 214,
      223*f*, 275, 348
  causes 213*f*
  diagnosis of 223
  severe 234, 374
Endometriosis-associated pain,
      management of 103, 109
Endometritis 72
  acute 72
  chronic 74*f*
Endometrium 49, 67, 68, 72, 80*f*, 235,
      250, 251, 340
  B-mode features of 76
  inflammation of 75
  monitoring of 75
  morphology of 76
  qualitative assessment of 69
  receptive 78
Endomyometrial junction 67, 69
Endoplasmic reticulum 88
Enteritis 406
Enucleated donor cytoplasm 301
Enzyme 234
  aromatase 100
Epistaxis 407
Erectile dysfunction 427
Escherichia coli 117
Estradiol 28, 119, 303
Estrogen 62, 91, 174, 197, 277
  component 194
  deficient 234
  high 76, 151
  production 11
  receptor 76, 88, 218
    gene 216

modulators, history of selective 87
synthesis in human ovary, regulation of 9*f*
Estrogen-dependent cancers, fertility preservation in 103
Estrogen-sensitive cancers, fertility preservation in 109
Ethical closure counseling 430
Euploid blastocyst 283, 284
Exogenous follicle-stimulating hormone response test 26
Exogenous gonadotropin 56, 96, 175, 231
influence of 27
stimulation 29
Exogenous human chorionic gonadotropin 355
Exogenous progestins 382
Extracellular matrix remodeling 305
Eye irritation 103

F

Family, identify 421
Fat overload syndrome 407
Female reproductive physiology 197
Ferriman–Gallwey score 314
Fertility
decreased 215
preservation 108, 154, 288, 289, 295
stimulation protocols for 288
toolbox 415
treatment 25, 153, 221, 301, 316, 429
Fertilizable ovum 59
Fertilization 198, 216, 268, 393
higher 231
rates 294
Fertilized oocytes, normal 383
Fetal aneuploidy, risk of 41
Fetal implant failure 216
Fever 103, 406
Fibroid 109
uterus 109
Field of infertility, development of triggering options in 133*t*
Final maturation, trigger for 222
Findoles 90
First human clinical test 87
First nonsteroidal antiestrogen 87

Flare-up protocol 175
Flexible start protocol, multiple dose 179*f*
Fluid movement 349
Folic acid 321
Follicle 53, 57, 129
and oocyte targets 290*t*
aspiration of 115
asynchronous development of 179
causing maturation of 101
cumulus, B mode ultrasound image of 61*f*
developing 370, 371*f*
dominant 57*f*
flow correlates 60
mature 53, 175, 233
output rate 43
output ratio 136
reached 280
recruitment of 370
rupture 185
size, measuring 58*f*
to oocyte index 44
Follicle-stimulating hormone 3, 5*f*, 6*f*, 8, 9*f*, 26, 28*f*, 32*f*-34*f*, 34, 49, 91, 93, 101, 101*f*, 114, 116*f*, 127, 134, 160, 174, 176*f*, 179*f*, 180*f*, 187*f*, 194, 213, 223, 223*f*, 238*f*, 239, 245, 246*f*, 247, 258, 277, 291, 302, 311*f*, 318, 370, 371*f*, 381, 428
altered 310
chemical structure of 115*f*
dose protocol, individualization of 261
highly purified 237
levels 231
polymorphisms of 149
receptors 114
threshold 371
treatment 236
window 371
Follicular aspiration in mild stimulation 374
Follicular atresia 38
Follicular blood flow 61
Follicular cohort matures, primary 261
Follicular development 40, 277
stages of 49
theories of 380

Follicular dynamics, abnormal 164, 165
Follicular growth, stages of 127
Follicular maturation 233
    abnormal 139
    stage of 115
Follicular phase 13
    prolongation of 130
    stimulation 281, 381, 384f
Follicular recruitment
    stage of 183
    synchronization of 173
Follicular size 57
Follicular synchronization 194
Follicular volume, ratio of 62
Folliculogenesis 4, 5f, 10, 38
    ovarian hormonal control of 6
Free androgen index 319
Freeze embryos 288
Freeze-all technique 369
Freezing ovarian cortical tissue 288
Fresh embryo transfer 339, 407
Frozen embryo transfer 107, 134, 135, 339, 383
    cycles 107, 339
        luteal phase support in 339
Frozen-thawed embryo transfer 266
Fulfilling pregnancy rates 102

G

Gastric ulceration 403
Gel instillation 68
Gene mutations, effect of various 217t
Genetic disorder 275
Genetic factors 216
Germ layers 4f
Germinal vesicle 137
Gestational diabetes 316
Gestations, multiple 392
Glucagon-like peptide-1 319
    receptor agonists 312
Glucocorticoids 403
Gluconeogenesis, restoration of 313f
Glucose transporter 2 313f
Glycogen synthesis 321
Glycoprotein hormones 113
Glycosylation 117
Glycosylation, sites for 115

Gonadal dysgenesis 4
Gonadotoxicity 293
Gonadotropin 55, 96, 105, 113, 118, 119, 119b, 120, 127, 128, 173, 175, 196, 220, 231, 237, 239-242, 247, 248, 259, 260, 270, 277, 278, 335, 374, 392
    comparative effectiveness of 237
    consumption 56
    dosage 268
    dose of 64, 119, 186, 222, 278, 279, 295, 375
        effect of 220f
        reduced 269
    duration, reducing 358
    formulations 239t
    future of 120
    history of development of 114t
    hormones 113
    in folliculogenesis, role of 8
    in ovulation, role of 8
    injections 240
    low 374
        doses of 250, 304, 372
    of urinary origin 113
    preovulatory natural 137
    preparations 116, 117
        development of 238f
    recombinant 237
    requirement 216, 253
    secretion 173
    starting dose of 159
    step-down protocol 260
    step-up dose protocol, low-dose 260
    stimulation 241, 428
        initiation of 173
    structure of 113
    surge 137
        stimulation, mid-cycle for 265
    types of 237
        protocol with 277
    urinary-derived 237
    uses of 118, 239
    with gonadotropin-releasing hormone
        agonist 239
        antagonist 239

Gonadotropin-releasing hormone 5, 6*f*,
    15, 32*f*, 91, 96*f*, 103, 113, 134,
    142, 175*f*, 176, 176*f*, 179*f*-181*f*,
    182, 187*f*, 194, 219, 232, 248*f*-
    250*f*, 264, 311*f*, 331, 359, 371,
    373, 383*f*, 392
  agonist 98*f*, 138*f*, 142, 160, 173, 174,
    176, 181, 183-185, 246, 248*f*,
    333, 356*f*, 382, 382*f*
    advantages of 177, 265
    as trigger, advantages of 265
    cycle 184, 196
    disadvantages of 177
    drawbacks to 150
    injection 150
    protocols 174
    trigger 265
    trigger, pros of 149
    use of 159, 173
  agonist in in vitro fertilization
    advantages for use of 182*t*
    disadvantages for use of 182*t*
  analogs 185
    efficacy of 183
    role of 7
  antagonist 173, 177-179, 181, 181*f*,
    183, 184, 186, 201, 278, 290,
    355, 372, 375*f*, 382
    advantages of 264
    flexible protocol 249*f*
    role of 7
    salvage protocol 263
  antagonist protocol 178, 263, 265
    advantages of 264
    early 266
  antagonists in in vitro fertilization
    advantages for use of 182*t*
    disadvantages for use of 182*t*
  polymorphisms of 149
  trigger, failure of 150
Gonadotropin-stimulated cycle 57, 277
Goserelin 147, 174
Grade B endometrium 77*f*
Granulocyte colony-stimulating factor
    401*f*, 407, 410
Granulosa cell 3, 27, 115, 138, 163, 371
  apoptosis 215
  luteinization of 13
  proliferation 160

Growth hormone 221, 281, 303, 306
  releasing factor 183
  use of 183
Gynaecological applications 109
Gynecology, indications in 102

H

Hair
  dryness of 234
  loss of 234
Headache 103, 234, 406, 407
Health problem 415
Healthcare providers 417
Healthy baby and mother care,
    promote 431
Healthy lifestyle, educate about 430
Hematopoietic stem cell
    transplantation 293
Hemoconcentration 357
Hemolytic reactions 406
Hepatic disease 92
Hepatic impairment
  history of 92
  severe 104
Hepatomegaly 407
Heterogeneous population 379
Hilar cells produce 42
Hirsutism 315
Histrelin 147
Hormonal considerations 385
Hormonal milieu, natural 339
Hormonal regulation 11
Hormone 29
  control menstrual cycle 6*f*
  replacement therapy 339
  theory 361
Hospital admission 362
Human albumin solution 357
Human chorionic gonadotropin 10, 76,
    96, 96*f*, 115, 116*f*, 118, 127, 129,
    134, 135, 138*f*, 142, 147, 149*f*,
    160, 175*f*, 176*f*, 219, 179*f*-181*f*,
    187*f*, 222, 223*f*, 238*f*, 246, 248*f*-
    250*f*, 253*f*, 258, 260, 265, 329,
    332, 359, 373, 375*f*
  administration 152
  biological functions of 129*t*
  dose as trigger 130

double-edged sword 132
gold standard 128
increased glycosylation of 149*f*
low-dose 304
ovulation trigger 160
support, low-dose 152
trigger 278
  sliding scale protocol for 262
urinary and recombinant
  varieties of 131*t*
Human fertilisation embryology
  authority 398
Human immunodeficiency virus 419*f*
  prevention 419, 431
Human luteinizing hormone 277
Human menopausal gonadotropin 98*f*,
  113, 114, 116, 134, 179*f*-181*f*,
  187*f*, 232, 238*f*, 239, 246, 266,
  269, 277, 304, 333, 355, 371*f*,
  375*f*, 382*f*, 392
  discovery of 232
  highly purified 237
Human ovaries 306
Humira actions 404
Hydrosalpinx 72
Hydroxychloroquine 401*f*, 408, 409
Hydroxyethyl starch 357, 358
Hyperandrogenemia 310
Hyperandrogenism 310, 314
Hypercholesterolemia 103
Hyperechoic vertical shadows 73
Hyperhidrosis 103
Hyperinsulinemia 310
  effect of 311*f*
Hyper-responders, protocols for 260
Hyper-response in hyper-responders,
  control 260*t*
Hypersensitivity 407
Hyperstimulation 369
Hypertension 103
Hypertension, pregnancy-induced 316
Hypertensive disorders 341
Hypertriglyceridemia, risk of 92
Hypocalcemia 403
Hypoechoic vertical shadows 73
Hypogonadotropic hypogonadism 136,
  142, 332
Hypopituitarism 251
Hypothalamic amenorrhea 251, 332

Hypothalamic dysfunction 92
Hypothalamic-pituitary axis 100
Hypothalamic-pituitary-adrenal
  axis 216
Hypothalamic-pituitary-gonadal
  axis 214, 216
Hypothalamic-pituitary-ovarian
  axis 247, 303
  dysfunction 139, 293
Hypothalamo-pituitary suppression 194
Hypovolemia 357
Hysteroscopy 201
  abnormalities 203
  adhesiolysis 72
  screening 194

I

Iatrogenic infections 407
Immune checkpoint inhibitors 43
Immune system 17
  key mediators of 399
  role of 408
Immunological tests 399*f*
Immunomodulant therapies 409
Immunomodulant treatments 401*f*
Immunomodulatory agents 401
Immunotherapy, rationale for 398
Impaired ovarian
  reserve 29
  response 276
Implantation failure 409
Implantation rates 184
In vitro fertilization 25, 32*f*, 38, 55, 78,
  92, 119, 134, 147, 182, 183, 194,
  211, 216, 218, 232, 238*f*, 241,
  245, 249*f*, 257, 260, 270, 275,
  289, 304, 320, 331, 345, 369,
  373, 390, 391, 394, 394*b*, 398
  cost, strategies to reduce 391
  cycle 55*t*, 119*b*
    monitoring of 392
    pretreatment in 194
    segmentation of 266
  implications of hyper-response
    in 258
  low-cost 390
  mild stimulation 96, 369
  minimal stimulation 374

outcome 160, 216
ovarian hyperstimulation for 186
reduce cost in 391*t*
reducing complications of 393
stimulation 247, 249*f*
success rate in 159
treatment 53, 279
Inadequate progesterone production 63
Indoles 88
Infection 347, 407
  severe 347
Infectious diseases 406
Infectious spillage 347
Infertile
  couples, identify 423
  women 400
    inducement of ovulation in 88
Infertility 216, 231, 301, 395, 415, 418
  identify and manage
    competition of 422
  in family, psychosocial impact of 423
  male factor 234, 335
  prevalence by prevention and
    education, reduce 431
  surgery 428
  unexplained 92, 107, 233
Inflated bubble diffused 140
Inhibin B 28, 43
Inhibitory factors, role of 11
Inhibits follicular maturation 310
Injection site reactions 404
Inositol 292, 310, 319
  glycan system 320*f*
Insemination sample 241
Insomnia 103
Insulin 320*f*
  dependent epimerase 321
  resistance 310, 320
  sensitizers 310, 311, 312*b*, 321, 354
  stimulates 310
Insulin-like growth factor 214, 312*f*, 402
  binding protein 129
Intensive luteal phase support 151
Interleukin 8 353
International Federation of Fertility
  Societies 417
Intestinal injury 347
Intra-abdominal bleedings, severe 346
Intracytoplasmic sperm injection 137,
    199, 214, 321, 390, 428

Intraendometrial vascularization 78
Intrafollicular milieu 268
Intralipid 401*f*, 406
Intramuscular injections, painful 102
Intramuscular route 118
Intrauterine
  abnormalities 391
  adhesions 72, 391
Intrauterine insemination 55, 92, 105,
    106, 119, 119*b*, 231, 247, 329,
    333, 334, 427
  cycle 118, 185, 329
    ovarian stimulation protocols
      for 229
  ovarian stimulation protocols in 231
  timing of 241
Intravenous colloids 357
Intravenous immunoglobulin 401*f*,
    404, 405
  actions 405
In-vitro fertilization
  high responders in 107
  poor responders in 107
Irritability 103
Ischemic heart disease 103

J

Jaundice 407
Joint luteinizing hormone 135

K

Kallmann's syndrome 6
Killer cell immunoglobulin 400
Killing target cells 400
Kiss-1 neurons 141
Kisspeptin 120, 140

L

Lactic acidosis 314
Laparoscopic ovarian drilling 318
L-arginine 198
Letrozole 102, 105-107, 231, 232, 234,
    235, 240, 242, 251, 270, 279,
    280, 294, 304, 315, 330, 360,
    361, 376, 382
  alone 315

course of 104
cycles 330
during luteal phase 360
group 236
mechanism of action of 360*f*
treatment, duration of 236
Leukopenia 103, 407
Leuprolide 161, 174
   acetate 247
      injection 278
Leuprorelin 147
Light sensitivity 93
Lipid synthesis 319
Lipoprotein, very low-density 319
Live birth 216
   cumulative 261
      rate 94, 103, 106, 164, 194, 212, 232, 303, 315, 317
Liver
   function test 361
   sialoprotein receptors 115
Long protocol 176*f*
Low back pain 406
Low molecular weight 120, 121
   heparin 361, 401*f*, 402
      actions 402
Low prognosis patients 35*f*
Lower mid-luteal progesterone level 330
Low-resistance perifollicular flow, pulse Doppler image of 59*f*
Lung disease 406
Lupus-like syndrome 404
Luteal phase 13
   defect 18
   deficiency 92, 252, 329
      causes of 330
      concept of 329
      effects of 330
   effect of trigger on 331
   endocrine changes 15
   insufficiency 151
   physiology of 13
   stimulation 280, 384*f*
      efficacy of additional 340
   supplementation 187
   support 134, 241, 327, 333, 333*t*, 339, 375
Luteal supplementation 251
Luteal support, required 339

Luteal-follicular transition phase 266
Luteinized unruptured follicle 62, 64
Luteinizing granulosa cells 132, 160
Luteinizing hormone 4, 5*f*, 6*f*, 9*f*, 13, 14, 26, 42, 49, 75, 91, 113-115, 116*f*, 127, 128*f*, 129, 134, 138*f*, 142, 148, 149*f*, 160, 182, 194, 214, 223*f*, 232, 238*f*, 239, 245, 249*f*, 304, 310, 311*f*, 355, 371, 373, 394
   activity 117
   chemical structure of 116*f*
   during controlled ovarian stimulation, role of 9
   gene 282
   natural 340
   premature 219, 392
   receptor 8, 14
      polymorphisms of 149
   role of 251
   supplementation 181
   surge 11, 62, 356*f*
      prevention of 392
Luteofollicular transition 371
Luteolysis 18, 132, 135, 153
   prevention of 128
   story 141
Lymphoma 404

M

Male infertility, severe 390
Mammals 380
Mammary gland 88
Maternal gastrointestinal side effects 402
Maternal immune system 408
Mature follicle, B mode ultrasound image of 58*f*
Mature oocyte 161
   rate 150
Meddlesome activity, avoid 427
Medical termination of pregnancy 363
Medroxyprogesterone acetate 95, 98*f*, 267, 382*f*
Meiosis, resumption of 132
Melatonin 303
Memory loss 103
Menstrual cycle 10, 13, 180, 233, 245
   till menses 175

Menstrual cyclicity 312
Menstrual frequency 319
Menstruation 278
Mental disorders, risk of 215
Messenger ribonucleic acid 135
Metabolic aberrances 310
Metabolic syndrome, risk of 320
Metaphase oocyte
   mature 249
   number of mature 283
Metastatic breast cancer, treatment of 88
Metformin 105, 194*f*, 200, 204, 292, 310-312, 314-318, 318*b*, 320
   action, role of genetic factor in 313
   for ovulation induction, guidelines for 318
   indications for 314
   inhibition of 313*f*
   mechanism of action of 313*b*
   side effects of 314
   therapy 316
      duration of 314
   transport 313
   use of 317*b*
Methylenetetrahydrofolate reductase 218
Microdose flare protocol 176, 176*f*
Midluteal serum progesterone 330
Midluteal ultrasound parameters 64*t*
Minimal stimulation 369
   in vitro fertilization, different protocols of 373*t*
   protocol 96*f*
Miscarriage 76, 93, 151, 216
   early 152
   late 317
   rate 94, 105, 216, 316
      groups for 105
      higher early 150
Mitochondrial complex, metformin-induced inhibition of 313*f*
Mitochondrial glycerol phosphate dehydrogenase 313*f*
Mixed bag 367
Monacolin 321
Monofollicular development 371*f*
Monofollicular ovulation 235
Mono-ovulation 101
Morphogenesis 319

Mother's genetic fingerprinting 302
Motility 198
Mouth, dry 103
Mucositis 407
Multifollicular growth 374
Multifollicular wave theory 381
Multiple births 369
Multiple dose protocol 178, 179*f*
Multiple follicles
   development of 239
   maturation of 233
Multiple pregnancy 93, 101, 234, 241, 395
   incidence of 185
   lower risk of 261
   rate 104-106, 236
   risk for 237
Muscle pain 406
Mutations, activating 258
Myalgia 103
Myoinositol 198, 319, 321
   plays 320
Myometrial contraction, inhibition of 129
Myometrial vasodilatation 128
Myometrium 129
   isoechoic to 76

N

N-acetyl cysteine 198
Nafarelin 147, 174
Naphthalenes 90
Nasal spray 174
National Health Service 231
Natural cycle 107, 148, 340
   in vitro fertilization 113, 279, 304
   modified 340
Natural killer cells 17, 129, 400
Nausea 234, 314, 407
Neoangiogenesis 129
Neonatal morbidity 317
Neuroendocrine
   abnormalities 139
   control 4
Neurokinin B antagonist 120
   oral preparations 120
Nitric oxide, action of 221
Nondiscrimination 419

Nonpolycystic ovarian syndrome 92
Nonsterile vagina 347
Nonsteroidal antiestrogens 88
Nonsteroidal anti-inflammatory
    drugs 281
Nonsteroidal compounds 90
Nonstimulated and stimulated cycles
    endocrinology of 1, 3
    luteal phase mystery of 13
Norethisterone 196
Normal corpus luteal flow
    on color Doppler 63f
    on pulse Doppler 63f
Normo-ovulatory women 195
Nuclear maturation 160
Nuclear membrane 137
Nutritional status 43

O

Obese infertile women 321
Obesity 349
Oligo-anovulation, clomiphene
    citrate for 427
Oligoasthenoteratospermia 118
One-stop subfertility clinics 391
Oocyte 3, 97, 150, 185, 195, 222, 241,
        289, 371
    and ovulation, maturation of 138
    collection 348
    competence 379
    cryopreservation, cycles of 294
    cumulus complex 137
    decreases, number of 301
    donation cycles 184
    environment and function 321
    intravaginal culture of 393
    maturation 136, 268
        completion of 127
        last stage of 97
        role of triggering in final 10
    maturity 262
    meiosis, resumption of 13
    midcycle 5
    number of 161, 216, 245, 374, 384
        mature 252
    oxidative stress of 321
    quality 25, 31, 153, 211, 216
        improve 304

quantity and quality 35f
reserve, declining 301
retrieval 97, 132, 180, 246f, 275, 345
    technique 348
retrieved
    after in vitro fertilization of 305
    number of 178, 267, 369, 375, 383
    transabdominal-guided 345
yield 294
Oocyte pick-up 134, 147, 259, 345,
        350, 383f
    technique, principles of 345
Optimal ovarian response 369
Oral antioxidants 203
Oral biguanide 200
Oral contraceptive pill 103, 136, 174,
        175f, 179, 184, 185, 194, 195,
        197, 248, 267, 277, 303, 315
    effectiveness of 194
    pretreatment with 185
Oral dehydroepiandrosterone 302
Oral dydrogesterone 336, 340
Oral hypoglycemic agent 311
Oral ovulogens 185
Organic cation transporter 1 313f
Organic intracranial lesions 92
Organogenesis 3
Osteoporosis 403, 407
Outpatient management 361
Ovarian adhesions, prevalence of 348
Ovarian androgen 42
    production, reduces 312
Ovarian angiogenesis dysfunction 42
Ovarian biopsy 29
Ovarian blood flow 29
Ovarian cancer 93
Ovarian condition 212
Ovarian cycle 380
Ovarian cyst 92
Ovarian damage risk 293t
Ovarian development, malfunction in 4
Ovarian drilling 105
Ovarian endometriosis 293
Ovarian enlargement 234
    moderate 93
Ovarian failure 374
Ovarian follicles 114
    developmental stages of 370f
    pool, qualitative decline of 27f

Ovarian follicular waves during
		menstrual cycle 381*f*
Ovarian function 38, 293
Ovarian germline stem cells 306
Ovarian hyperstimulation 263, 372
	risk of 118, 121, 252
Ovarian hyperstimulation syndrome
		10, 32*f*, 55, 93, 101, 106, 119,
		128, 129, 131, 134, 135, 142,
		147, 173, 182, 183, 187*f*, 200,
		216, 234, 241, 258, 264, 270,
		289, 352, 353*f*, 359, 369, 385,
		391, 393
	cause of 353
	danger signs of 361
	development of 184, 353
	early 352
	elimination of 355
	high risk of developing 161
	incidence of 183
	late 353
	lower levels of 247
	management of 361, 362
	mild 352
	moderate 352
	pathophysiology of 353*f*
	prevention 314, 355, 356, 358*t*, 360
		and cure 352
		measures for 354
	risk of 141, 159, 161, 163, 215, 245,
		257, 264, 266
	severe 268, 352, 352*t*
Ovarian induction 25
Ovarian rejuvenation 305
Ovarian reserve 25, 38, 43, 44, 212, 276
	assessment of 42, 289
	concept of 25
	diminished 25, 43, 213, 223*f*, 278
	estimate, tool for 40
	factors affecting 213, 213*f*
	markers of 23, 38
	screening tests 30*t*
	test 26, 290, 302
		abnormal 275
		types of 26*fc*
Ovarian response 212
	prediction 32*f*, 34*t*, 222
		index 31, 222
	predictor nomograms 224

	spectrum of 163
	unexpected 292
Ovarian sensitivity
	index 259
	to gonadotropins 258
Ovarian stimulation 85, 96, 99, 107, 181,
		184, 194, 195, 231, 249, 270,
		278, 284, 369, 370, 372, 375,
		391, 394
	advantages of mild 372
	agents, development of 232
	complications of 343
	cost of 395
	cycles 288
		mild 374
	disadvantages mild 372
	for in vitro fertilization
		advantages of mild 270*t*
		disadvantages of mild 270*t*
		mild 372
	for intrauterine insemination 185, 186
	gonadotropin for 107
	method of 219
	mild 270, 329, 392
	modified natural cycle 372
	on corpus luteum, effects of
		drugs for 330
	period of 261
	planning 293
	process 247
	progestin-primed 43, 219
	protocol 294
		for hyper-responders 257
		for normoresponders 245
		for poor responders 275
		mild 376
Ovarian stroma 42
Ovarian stromal
	blood flow 42
	flow 54, 54*f*
		measurement of 53, 56
Ovarian suppression 279
Ovarian surgery 275
	history of 215, 292
Ovarian theca cells 199
Ovarian volume 29, 41, 53, 55
	calculated 52*f*

Ovary 49, 88, 373
 B mode ultrasound of 54*f*
 on B mode ultrasound, measurement of three orthogonal diameters of 50*f*
 poor reserve 56*f*
 produce inhibin and activin 115
 stromal vessels, color Doppler image of 50*f*
Ovulation 13
 inducing drugs, types of 232
 induction 85, 102, 242, 315, 359, 369
  agents 315
  improves 312
  treatment for 109
 predictor kit 95*f*
 rate 94
 trigger 148, 160, 161, 280, 331, 355
 types of 232
Ovulatory cycles, normal 329
Ovulatory dysfunction 100
 treatment of 87
Ovulatory function 321
Ovum pick-up 162, 375*f*
Oxidative stress 197, 303
Oxygen species, reactive 197

P

Pain 346
Palinopsia 93
Palpitation 103
Paracentesis 362
Paracervical block 348
Parasympathetic nervous system 319
Peak systolic velocity 55
Pedicle artery sign 70
Pelvic
 inflammatory disease, signs of 72
 organ injury 347
 structures 347
Pelvis 72
Peptide hormone 319
Perform additional tests 425
Perifollicular blood flow 62
Perifollicular vessel 59
Persistence, lack of 234
Phosphatase 305
Phosphatidylinositol-3 kinase 305

Photophobia 93
Physiology 147
Pigment epithelium derived factor 163
Pioglitazone 318
Pituitary downregulation 164, 263
Pituitary dysfunction 92
Pituitary gland 101
Pituitary suppression regimens 277
Pituitary tumor 92
Placenta 329
Placental cell apoptosis 401
Plasma 117
 progesterone 62
Platelet-rich plasma 305
 use of 305
Plausible panacea 140
Political commitment 419
Polycystic ovarian
 disease 215, 219
 morphology 311*f*
Polycystic ovarian syndrome 17, 41, 43, 93, 102, 104, 106, 109, 174, 215, 245, 259, 261, 289, 292, 310, 312, 317, 318
 management of 100
 patients 153
 women 321
  insulin resistance in 312*f*
Polycystic ovary 139, 310
 syndrome, metformin use in 317*fc*
Polyp 202
Polyunsaturated fatty acid 198
Poor cytotoxic ability 400
Poor oocyte 278
 quality 301, 306
Poor ovarian reserve 38, 302
 patients 380
Poor ovarian response 275, 276, 284, 290, 382*f*
 diagnosis of 276, 302
 episodes of 302
 management of 379
 risk stratification of 276*t*
Poor responders, protocol for 250*f*
Poseidon's stratification 35*f*
Postmenopausal women 88
Postovulatory phase 13
Potential challenges 385
Practice family planning 431

Preantral follicle 3, 258
Preeclampsia 317
Pregnancy 92, 184, 316
    loss, early 198
    normal 153
    ongoing 152, 182
    outcomes 341
    patient's fitness for 424
    probability of 181
    produce 60
    promote safe 431
    rate 80, 94, 150, 174, 216, 241
        higher 235
        increase 220
        lower 147
    women desiring 87
Pregnant mares' serum 127
Pre-in vitro fertilization hysteroscopy 201
Premature ovarian
    failure 4
    insufficiency 289
Preovulatory follicles 236
Preovulatory scan 57
Prestimulation risk factor assessment 259*t*
Prestimulation treatment 277
Preterm deliveries 317
Primary care
    providers, identify 422
    services 426
Primary healthcare clinics 422
Primordial follicles 4
Prince's kiss analogy 128*f*
Progestational action,
        moderate-to-strong 267
Progesterone 17, 62, 73, 75, 96, 97, 137,
        138, 148, 174, 181, 251-253,
        303, 329, 331, 400
    administration
        advantages of routes of 334*t*
        disadvantages of routes of 334*t*
    alone 196
    capsules 332
    doses of 332, 334*t*
    low concentrations of 329
    premature 181
    pretreatment 196
    production of 13, 15, 18, 329
    receptor 64, 216-218
    role of 17

    supplementation 151, 334
    support 335
    synthesis 161
    with estrogen 332
Progesterone-primed ovarian
        stimulation 267, 270
    advantages of 270*t*
    disadvantages of 270*t*
    protocol 267
Progestin-induced menses 98
Progestogen 103, 277
    pretreatment 196
Prothrombin 216, 217
Protocol
    variability 339
    individualization of 187*f*, 240
Pseudogout 407
Psychological factors 215
Psychological stress on life,
        impact of 216*f*
Pulsatility index 64
Pulse repetition frequency 50, 70

Q

Quality of life 216*f*, 418

R

Radiotherapy 215
Raloxifene 94, 98
Randomized controlled
        trials 104, 221, 383
Recombinant follicle-stimulating
        hormone 55, 117, 248*f*-250*f*,
        259, 332, 333, 355, 383*f*, 392
    long-acting 117
Recombinant human
    chorionic gonadotropin 131, 372
    luteinizing hormone 359
Recombinant luteinizing
        hormone 140, 383*f*
Recruited primordial follicles 370
Rectovaginal endometriosis 103, 108
Recurrent implantation failure 398, 399*f*
Reference tools™ 416
Regulate menstrual cycles ovulation 320
Renal failure 406
Renal function test 361

Index

Renal impairment 314
   severe 104
Renin angiotensin system 353*f*
Reproductive age 211
   women of 67
Reproductive context 306
Reproductive health
   and age, educate about 430
   conditions 422
Reproductive outcome 257
Reproductive system 17
Reproductive tissues 88
Rescues corpus luteum 129
Resistance index 55, 64
Resources, protection of 420
Responders, moderate 292
Retrieved oocyte percentage 349
Retroperitoneal hematoma 346
Rheumatoid arthritis,
       exacerbation of 407
Ribonucleic acid, long non-coding 43
Rosiglitazone 317, 318

S

Safe abortion 431
Safety profile 104
   high 235
Saline 68
Scanty pericorpus luteal flow on color
       Doppler 63*f*
Scotomata 93
Search strategy 159, 160*fc*
Selective estrogen receptor modulator
       87, 88, 90, 94, 103, 108, 232
   chemical structure of 91*f*
   classification of 88, 90*t*
   evolution of 89*f*
   uses of 88, 90*t*
Self and fertility services,
       assessment of 429
Semen parameters 198, 199
Septicemia 404
Septum 202
Serum
   androgens, decreased 263
   C-reactive protein 381
   estradiol 290
   progesterone 341

   levels 181, 341
   threshold 340
   total 319
Sex and birth control, educate about 430
Sex hormone-binding globulin 310,
       311*f*, 312*f*
Sex steroid 329
Sexual intercourse 241
Sexually transmitted infection 419,
       419*f*, 431*f*
   prevent 431
Shanghai protocol 97, 98*f*
Sharply toothed 70
Short agonist stop protocol 176, 176*f*
Short protocol 175*f*
Sialic residues 115
Sickle cell anemia 288
Sildenafil 221, 282
Single dose
   fixed start 180*f*
   protocols 180*f*
Single embryo transfer 374
Single feeder vessel 70
Single recruitment episode theory 380
Single-nucleotide
       polymorphism 216, 218
Singleton pregnancy, triple of 391
Skin
   dry 403
   reaction 103
   thinning 403
Small growing follicles 27
Sodium bicarbonate 393
Solute carrier gene 218
Sonography-based automated
       volume count 252*f*
Sonohysterogram 68
Sonohysterography 72
Sperm membrane 198
Spiral arteries 63
Splenic enlargement 407
Splenomegaly 407
Stair step protocol 95, 233
Statins 312, 321
Step-down protocol 240
Step-up protocol 240
Stereochemical isomers 98
Stereoisomers 319

Steroid
  compounds 90
  levels of 376
  pathway 16f
Steroidogenesis 153
Stimulate follicular growth 101
Stimulate gonadotropin secretion 140
Stimulated cycles 7
Stimulates endothelial cell
          proliferation 353
Stimulates pituitary gonadotropin 232
Stimulation
  duration of 195, 303, 375
  mild 250, 279, 369, 373, 395
  response to 216
Stimulation cycle 373
  mild 373
  steps to perform dual 381
Stimulation drug and dose, type of 220
Stimulation protocols 291
  mild 250, 269, 279, 375f, 391
  type of 219, 248
Stomatitis 103
Strict fluid balance 357
Subcutaneous injection 174, 407
Subendometrial vascularization 78
Subendometrium 72
Support tool™ 416 425, 426f, 428, 429f,
          430f, 432f
Supraphysiologic estradiol level 330
Suprefact 174
Surge physiology 137
Surrogate luteinizing
          hormone surge 129
Synchronous growth 219
Synthetic progestogen 196
Systemic lupus erythematosus 288

T

Tacrolimus 407, 409
Tamoxifen 87, 90, 94, 98, 232, 234
Technology and services, identify
          available 421
Tensin homolog enzyme inhibitors 305
Testosterone 199, 200, 281, 302, 306
  gel 222
Tetrahedron-acetylenes 88
Tetraphenylethylene 88

Thalassemia 288
Theca interstitial stroma 42
Thiazolidinediones 312, 317
Third-generation aromatase inhibitor
          letrozole 100
Three-dimensional power Doppler 60f
  acquired volume of ovary 53f
  ultrasound 61f
Three-dimensional ultrasound acquired
          volume of ovary 52f
Thrombocytopenia 347, 407
Thrombophilia disorder 402
Thromboprophylaxis 361
Thyroid disease, uncontrolled 92
Toolbox, principles of 416
Tools pyramid 417f
Total body irradiation 293
Transabdominal sonography 67
Transient hypotension 407
Transvaginal oocyte
  pick-up 345
  retrieval 181f
Transvaginal sonography 67, 394
Transvaginal ultrasonography 290, 345
Transvaginal ultrasound 119, 233, 392
Treatment resources, identify 426
Trigger
  agents 142t
  choices 219
  timing of 11, 251
Triphenylethylene derivatives 90
Triptorelin 97, 161, 333
Trophoblast invasion 17
True love's kiss 127
Tubal factor 390
Tubal patency 391
Tuberculosis 404
Tumor necrosis factor 401f
  alpha 399, 404
Two-gonadotropin hypothesis 9f

U

Ultrasonography 26
Ultrasound and Doppler study for
          follicle, technique of 49
Upper vaginal fornix 347
Urinary abnormalities 407

Urinary follicle-stimulating hormone
    preparations 116
Urinary human chorionic
    gonadotropin 131
Uterine artery 63, 75, 78
    Doppler 79
    waveform, pulse Doppler
        analysis of 79
Uterine bleeding, abnormal 92
Uterine natural killer cells 400
Uterus 67, 88
    mid-positioned 67
    midsagittal section of 68*f*, 69*f*
    monitoring of 75

V

Vaginal bleeding 103
Vaginal cavity acts 393
Vaginal micronized progesterone 336
Vaginal progesterone 333
Validated immunological tests 398
Vascular endothelial growth factor 15,
    129, 135, 265, 341, 353, 353*f*,
    400
Vascularity index 51
Visual symptoms 234

Vitamin
    B 198
        complex group 319
    C 198
    D 43, 198
    E 198
Vocal calculated endometrium
        volume 80*f*
Vocal software 51
Vomiting 103, 234, 314

W

Walking egg
    nonprofit organization 393
    project 393
Weak acid 393
Weight change 103
Weight loss 314, 354
Woman's oocytes 301
Woman's ovary 26
Woman's pituitary gland 247

Z

Zuclomiphene 98, 232

EU GSPR Authorised Reprsentative
Logos Europe, 9 rue Nicolas Poussin
1700, La Rochelle, France
Phone: +33 (0) 6 67 93 73 78
E-mail: contact@logoseurope.eu